Biomarker Studies in Brain Aging

Biomarker Studies in Brain Aging

Editor: Maddy Evans

AMERICAN
MEDICAL PUBLISHERS
www.americanmedicalpublishers.com

AMERICAN
MEDICAL PUBLISHERS
www.americanmedicalpublishers.com

Cataloging-in-Publication Data

Biomarker studies in brain aging / edited by Maddy Evans.
p. cm.
Includes bibliographical references and index.
ISBN 978-1-63927-923-4
1. Brain--Diseases--Age factors. 2. Brain--Aging. 3. Biochemical markers.
4. Nervous system--Degeneration. 5. Older people--Diseases. 6. Geriatrics.
7. Aging. I. Evans, Maddy.
RC386.2 .B56 2023
616.8--dc23

American Medical Publishers,
41 Flatbush Avenue,
1st Floor, New York,
NY 11217, USA

ISBN 978-1-63927-923-4 (Hardback)

Contents

Preface

This book was inspired by the evolution of our times; to answer the curiosity of inquisitive minds. Many developments have occurred across the globe in the recent past which has transformed the progress in the field.

Biomarkers of aging refer to those biomarkers that can predict functional capacity at a later age more accurately than chronological age. Validated biomarkers of aging can enable interventions which can extend the lifespan, as any changes in the biomarkers can be observed during the life span of the organism. The levels of CD4 and CD8 memory T cells along with naive T cells are found to provide an estimate of lifespan. One of the significant biomarker of aging is the epigenetic clock, which has the capability to forecast human chronological age accurately. Some of the other prominent biomarkers of determining brain aging are proteomic clocks and neuroimaging age predictors. Furthermore, cell counts and blood chemistry can also be used for predicting chronological age accurately. This book is compiled in such a manner, that it will provide in-depth knowledge about the biomarker studies in brain aging. From theories to research to practical applications, case studies related to all contemporary topics of relevance to this area of study have been included herein. This book will provide comprehensive knowledge to the readers.

This book was developed from a mere concept to drafts to chapters and finally compiled together as a complete text to benefit the readers across all nations. To ensure the quality of the content we instilled two significant steps in our procedure. The first was to appoint an editorial team that would verify the data and statistics provided in the book and also select the most appropriate and valuable contributions from the plentiful contributions we received from authors worldwide. The next step was to appoint an expert of the topic as the Editor-in-Chief, who would head the project and finally make the necessary amendments and modifications to make the text reader-friendly. I was then commissioned to examine all the material to present the topics in the most comprehensible and productive format.

I would like to take this opportunity to thank all the contributing authors who were supportive enough to contribute their time and knowledge to this project. I also wish to convey my regards to my family who have been extremely supportive during the entire project.

Editor

1

Combined Assessment of Diffusion Parameters and Cerebral Blood Flow within Basal Ganglia in Early Parkinson's Disease

*Laura Pelizzari[1], Maria M. Laganà[1], Sonia Di Tella[1], Federica Rossetto[1], Niels Bergsland[1,2], Raffaello Nemni[1,3], Mario Clerici[1,3] and Francesca Baglio[1]**

[1] IRCCS, Fondazione Don Carlo Gnocchi, Milan, Italy, [2] Department of Neurology, Buffalo Neuroimaging Analysis Center, Jacobs School of Medicine and Biomedical Sciences, University at Buffalo, State University of New York, Buffalo, NY, United States, [3] Department of Pathophysiology and Transplantation, Università degli Studi di Milano, Milan, Italy

***Correspondence:**
Francesca Baglio
fbaglio@dongnocchi.it

Diffusion tensor imaging (DTI) is a sensitive tool for detecting brain tissue microstructural alterations in Parkinson's disease (PD). Abnormal cerebral perfusion patterns have also been reported in PD patients using arterial spin labeling (ASL) MRI. In this study we aimed to perform a combined DTI and ASL assessment in PD patients within the basal ganglia, in order to test the relationship between microstructural and perfusion alterations. Fifty-two subjects participated in this study. Specifically, 26 PD patients [mean age (SD) = 66.7 (8.9) years, 21 males, median (IQR) Modified Hoehn and Yahr = 1.5 (1–1.6)] and twenty-six healthy controls [HC, mean age (SD) = 65.2 (7.5), 15 males] were scanned with 1.5T MRI. Fractional anisotropy (FA), mean diffusivity (MD), axial diffusivity (AD), radial diffusivity (RD) maps were derived from diffusion-weighted images, while cerebral blood flow (CBF) maps were computed from ASL data. After registration to Montreal Neurological Institute standard space, FA, MD, AD, RD and CBF median values were extracted within specific regions of interest: substantia nigra, caudate, putamen, globus pallidus, thalamus, red nucleus and subthalamic nucleus. DTI measures and CBF were compared between the two groups. The relationship between diffusion parameters and CBF was tested with Spearman's correlations. False discovery rate (FDR)-corrected p-values lower than 0.05 were considered significant, while uncorrected p-values <0.05 were considered a trend. No significant FA, MD and RD differences were observed. AD was significantly increased in PD patients compared with HC in the putamen ($p = 0.005$, $p_{FDR} = 0.035$). No significant CBF differences were found between PD patients and HC. Diffusion parameters were not significantly correlated with CBF in the HC group, while a significant correlation emerged for PD patients in the caudate nucleus, for all DTI measures (with FA: $r = 0.543$, $p_{FDR} = 0.028$; with MD: $r = -0.661$, $p_{FDR} = 0.002$; with AD: $r = -0.628$, $p_{FDR} = 0.007$; with RD: $r = -0.635$, $p_{FDR} = 0.003$). This study showed that DTI is a more sensitive technique than ASL to detect alterations in the basal ganglia in the early phase of PD. Our results suggest that, although DTI and ASL convey different information, a relationship between microstructural integrity and perfusion changes in the caudate may be present.

Keywords: DTI, ASL, diffusion parameters, cerebral blood flow, Parkinson's disease

INTRODUCTION

Parkinson's disease (PD) is a progressive neurodegenerative disease that is characterized by early dopaminergic neuron loss in the substantia nigra pars compacta, leading to dopamine deficiency in the basal ganglia, and resulting in movement disorders (Kalia and Lang, 2015). Although non-motor symptoms such as sleep disorders, depression and cognitive impairment may be present, resting tremor, bradykinesia and rigidity are the hallmarks of the disease (Kalia and Lang, 2015; Obeso et al., 2017).

Parkinson's disease diagnosis still remains largely clinical, based on the three cardinal symptoms onset, (Postuma et al., 2015) while dopamine transporter (DaT) single photon emission computerized tomography is currently used to confirm the clinical diagnosis (Seifert and Wiener, 2013). Nevertheless, the search for biomarkers with magnetic resonance imaging (MRI) is an area of active research in the field of PD. A number of MRI-based methods have been proposed to provide sensitive and non-invasive quantitative biomarkers of neurodegeneration (Obeso et al., 2017). In this framework, diffusion tensor imaging (DTI) and arterial spin labeling (ASL) are advanced MRI techniques that specifically allow for tissue integrity assessment (Alexander et al., 2007) and cerebral blood flow (CBF) quantification, respectively (van Osch et al., 2018).

Parameters derived from DTI, such as fractional anisotropy (FA) and mean diffusivity (MD), are suitable for investigating microstructural changes in the brain. MD provides a measure of overall diffusivity, while FA quantifies the extent to which diffusion is characterized by a preferential orientation. In addition to FA and MD, axial diffusivity (AD) and radial diffusivity (RD) can also be computed from DTI data. AD represents the primary eigenvalue describing water diffusivity while RD is determined by the average of the two smaller eigenvalues. Alterations of FA, MD, AD, and RD in white matter (WM), cortical and subcortical gray matter (GM) have been previously reported in PD patients, mirroring neurodegeneration and possible brain reorganization due to the disease (Atkinson-Clement et al., 2017). Furthermore, DTI measures in the subcortical areas were shown to be sensitive makers of disease progression in PD, (Cochrane and Ebmeier, 2013; Scherfler et al., 2013; Wei et al., 2016; Atkinson-Clement et al., 2017) even at the early stages of the disease (Taylor et al., 2018). DTI changes in the substantia nigra of PD patients were observed to be associated with increasing dopaminergic deficits, reduced α-synuclein and total tau protein concentrations in cerebrospinal fluid, while diffusivity alterations in the thalamus were correlated with cognitive decline in PD (Zhang et al., 2016).

Together with neuronal degeneration, metabolic and perfusion parameters may also be altered in PD due to either neurovascular unit function changes or increased cerebrovascular disease burden associated with aging (Al-Bachari et al., 2014). Given the value of CBF as a biomarker in PD, ASL MRI is a promising technique for PD assessment since it allows absolute CBF assessment without using an exogenous contrast agent (Pyatigorskaya et al., 2014). Indeed, abnormal cerebral perfusion patterns in PD have been revealed using ASL (Melzer et al., 2011). In addition, this technique proved to be effective in detecting CBF alterations in non-demented PD patients (Syrimi et al., 2017) and arterial transit time changes in idiopathic PD (Al-Bachari et al., 2014).

The combined assessment of FA and CBF has recently been proposed as an effective method for investigating pathological changes in the early stages of PD (Wei et al., 2016). Decreased FA in the substantia nigra and reduced CBF in the basal ganglia were reported in the same group of patients, hinting that different neuro-pathological processes may underlie the degeneration in the subcortical regions primarily involved in the disease (Wei et al., 2016).

To the best of our knowledge, MD, AD, and RD have not been assessed together with CBF as of yet. Furthermore, a correlation analysis between DTI and ASL-derived parameters is still missing in PD. Therefore, in this study we aimed to perform a combined DTI and ASL assessment in early PD patients to investigate FA, MD, AD, RD, and CBF alterations in the basal ganglia regions with respect to healthy controls (HC). In addition, we aimed to evaluate the correlation between microstructural and perfusion parameters. Due to the neurovascular coupling, a potential link between them was expected.

MATERIALS AND METHODS

Subjects

Fifty-two subjects (26 PD patients and 26 HC) were included in this study. PD patients were consecutively recruited from the Neurorehabilitation Unit of the IRCCS Fondazione Don Gnocchi in Milan, while HC were enrolled between hospital personnel and volunteers. Only probable PD patients diagnosed according to the Movement Disorder Society Clinical Diagnostic Criteria for PD (Postuma et al., 2015) and with positive DaT scan were included in the study. Other inclusion criteria for PD group were: mild to moderate stages of the disease (Modified Hoehn and Yahr – H&Y<3), (Postuma et al., 2015) stable drug therapy with either L-Dopa or dopamine agonists, freezing assessed with Movement Disorder Society-sponsored revision of the Unified Parkinson's Disease Rating Scale (MDS-UPDRS) part II lower than 2, time spent with dyskinesias assessed with MDS-UPDRS part IV lower than 2. Left-handed subjects, people with history of psychiatric disorders, neurological diseases other than PD, cardiovascular and/or metabolic diseases were excluded from the study. All the enrolled PD patients were clinically evaluated by an experienced neurologist within 2 weeks of the MRI scan. Specifically, the H&Y Scale and the MDS-UPDRS were used to assess the severity of PD symptoms (Goetz et al., 2004). Levodopa equivalent daily dose (LEDD) was also calculated for each PD patient (Tomlinson et al., 2010). Montreal Cognitive Assessment (MoCA) was used to evaluate the cognitive status of all recruited subjects to exclude frank dementia. For PD patients, additional cognitive assessments included the Trail Making Test (TMT), phonemic fluency and semantic fluency.

The study was approved by the IRCCS Fondazione Don Carlo Gnocchi Ethics Committee and performed in accordance with the principles of the Helsinki Declaration. Written and informed consent was obtained from all the participants.

MRI Acquisition

All the enrolled subjects were scanned on a 1.5T Siemens Magnetom Avanto scanner, equipped with a 12-channel head coil. The MRI protocol included:

- Structural sequences:
  - A dual-echo turbo spin echo proton density PD/T2-weighted image [repetition time (TR) = 5550 ms, echo time (TE) = 23/103 ms, matrix size = 320 × 320 × 45, resolution 0.8 × 0.8 × 3 mm^3] to exclude the presence of WM hyperintensities beyond those expected as a part of normal aging;
  - A 3D high-resolution T1-weighted image obtained with a magnetization-prepared rapid acquisition with gradient echo (MPRAGE) sequence (TR = 1900 ms, TE = 3.37 ms, TI = 1100 ms, matrix size = 192 × 256 × 176, resolution 1 × 1 × 1 mm^3) as anatomical reference, and to evaluate GM volume differences between groups;
  - A 2D T1-weighted anatomical image with 5 mm-thick axial slices (TR/TE = 393/12 ms, matrix size = 128 × 128 × 26, resolution = 1.7 × 1.7 × 5 mm^3) as anatomical reference for CBF map registration;
- Diffusion-weighted echo planar images (EPI) along 64 directions (*b*-value = 1500 s/mm^2) and 3 b0 images (2 with A-P, 1 with P-A phase encoding) with the same parameters (TR/TE = 7800/109 ms, matrix size = 102 × 102 × 46, resolution = 2.5 × 2.5 × 2.5 mm^3);
- Multi-delay pseudo-continuous ASL (pCASL) sequence with background suppressed 3D gradient and spin echo (GRASE) readout (TR/TE = 3500/22.58 ms, labeling duration = 1500 ms, 5 post-labeling delays (PLD) = [700, 1200, 1700, 2200, 2700] ms, 12 pairs of tag/control images for each delay, matrix size = 64 × 64 × 32, resolution = 3.5 × 3.5 × 5 mm^3, distance between the center of imaging slices and labeling plane of 90 mm; 3 M0 images acquired with TR = 5000 ms) (Wang et al., 2013).

MRI Processing

A visual quality check was performed for all the acquired MRI data prior to any analysis. MRI data processing was performed with FMRIB's Software Library (FSL[1]) unless otherwise specified.

To avoid voxel misclassification during GM, WM and cerebrospinal fluid (CSF) automated segmentation, age-associated WM hyperintensities were identified (if any) on PD/T2-weighted images by an experienced neuroradiologist. Hyperintensities were segmented with Jim software, version 6.0[2], and the obtained masks were registered to corresponding MPRAGE images with Advanced Normalization Tools (ANTs[3]) in order to perform lesion filling. Non-brain tissue was removed from lesion-filled MPRAGE image, then brain tissue classification was performed with SIENAX (Smith et al., 2002).

For processing of the diffusion-weighted images, the susceptibility-induced off-resonance field was estimated with the topup tool (Andersson et al., 2003). The eddy tool was then used to simultaneously correct images for eddy currents and subject movement as well as susceptibility-induced geometric distortions (Andersson and Sotiropoulos, 2016). Diffusion tensor estimation for each voxel was performed with dtifit (Behrens et al., 2003) and FA maps were derived. Each FA map was registered to the Montreal Neurological Institute (MNI) FA template with non-linear transformation, and the tensor was warped accordingly. Then, MD, AD, and RD maps were derived.

ASL raw data were corrected for movement with ANTs, then tag images were subtracted from control ones. CBF maps were calculated with the oxford_asl tool (Chappell et al., 2009) (tissue T1 = 1.2 s, T1 of blood = 1.36 s, tagging efficiency = 0.8) (Wang et al., 2013; Laganà et al., 2018) and calibrated with the asl_calib tool (Chappell et al., 2009) by adjusting for CSF magnetization extracted from M0 images. Partial volume effect (PVE) correction was performed based on the assumption that CBF in the GM is 2.5 times greater than in the WM (Marshall et al., 2016). Finally, GM CBF maps were registered to MNI standard space. To do this, PVE-corrected CBF maps were first linearly registered to the respective 2D T1-weighted images, characterized by the same slice thickness of ASL data, using ANTs. Then, non-linear registration to MNI standard space was performed via the MPRAGE with ANTs.

For each subject, median values of CBF, FA, MD, AD, and RD were extracted within specific regions of interest (ROIs). Specifically, median CBF, FA, MD, AD, and RD values were computed across the voxels in each ROI, namely caudate, putamen, globus pallidus, thalamus, substantia nigra, red nucleus and subthalamic nucleus. The Harvard-Oxford atlas was used to generate caudate, putamen, globus pallidus, and thalamus masks. Substantia nigra, red nucleus and subthalamic nuclei were defined from the Multi-contrast PD25 atlas (Xiao et al., 2015) and registered to MNI standard space. All the ROIs were eroded with a gaussian kernel (sigma = 2 mm) before performing the extraction of the median values of the parameters of interest.

To check for potential GM volume differences between PD patients and HC within the basal ganglia, voxel-based morphometry (VBM) was performed. This analysis was used to exclude that potential differences in diffusion parameters could be due to GM atrophy. Specifically, each subject's GM map was non-linearly registered to MNI standard space, modulated with the Jacobian of the warp field and smoothed with a Gaussian kernel (sigma = 3 mm). GM volume voxel-wise comparison between the two groups was performed with the randomize tool, (Winkler et al., 2014) correcting for age and sex (ANCOVA), and using threshold-free cluster enhancement for cluster detection with 5000 permutations. The analysis was restricted to the basal ganglia regions of interest (i.e.,

[1] http://www.fmrib.ox.ac.uk/fsl

[2] http://www.xinapse.com/

[3] http://stnava.github.io/ANTs

substantia nigra, caudate, globus pallidus, putamen, thalamus, red nucleus and subthalamic nucleus). VBM results were family wise error (FWE) corrected at $p < 0.05$ to account for multiple comparisons.

Statistical Analysis

Normality of data distributions was tested with the Shapiro-Wilk test and parametric or non-parametric statistics were used accordingly.

Age and sex differences between PD and HC group were tested with an independent samples *t*-test and Chi-squared test, as appropriate.

Since L-Dopa or dopamine agonists may have an impact on CBF, (Chen et al., 2015; Lin et al., 2016) LEDD and CBF were non-parametrically correlated (Spearman's) with one another for all ROIs. In case of significant bivariate correlation, LEDD was included as a covariate.

The Mann-Whitney *U*-test was used to compare FA, MD, AD, RD and CBF measures between PD patients and HC. The relationship between each diffusion parameter and CBF was tested with Spearman's correlations, in PD and HC group separately. The Benjamini-Hochberg procedure was performed to control for the false discovery rate (FDR). FDR-corrected *p*-values lower that 0.05 were considered significant. Uncorrected *p*-values lower than 0.05 were considered as trends. Eta squared was computed to estimate the effect size and subsequently transformed to Cohen's d values. Effect size was classified as very small for $d < 0.2$, small for $0.2 \leq d < 0.5$, moderate for $0.5 \leq d < 0.8$ and large for $d \geq 0.8$.

Additional analyses to assess the relationship between diffusion and perfusion alterations and disease duration were performed and are described in **Supplementary Material** (see **Supplementary Table 1**). In addition, correlation analysis between FA, MD, AD, RD, and CBF and the neuropsychological test scores were performed and are shown in **Supplementary Material** (see **Supplementary Table 2**).

RESULTS

Demographics

PD and HC groups were age- and sex-matched ($p = 0.527$ and $p = 0.071$, respectively). PD patients and HC had a mean (standard deviation-SD) age of 66.7 (8.9) and 65.2 (7.5) years old, respectively. The PD group was characterized by a median (interquartile range-IQR) H&Y of 1.5 (1–1.6), and by a mean (SD) MDS-UPDRS III of 19.2 (11.2). The median adjusted MoCA (Santangelo et al., 2015) of the PD group and HC group was 24.3 and 25.6, respectively. Demographic and clinical characteristics of the two groups are reported in **Table 1**.

MRI Parameters Group Comparison

All the MRI images were classified as good quality scans and included in the analysis.

No significant correlation was found between CBF and LEDD in any ROI (results not shown). For this reason, LEDD was not considered as covariate in the following analysis.

TABLE 1 | Demographic and clinical characteristics of the participants of the study.

	HC (*n* = 26)	PD (*n* = 26)	*p*-value
Males, n (%)	15 (57.7)	21 (80.8)	0.071[a]
Age in yrs, mean (SD)	65.2 (7.5)	66.7 (8.9)	0.527[b]
H&Y median (IQR)	na	1.5 (1 – 1.6)	–
MDS-UPDRS III score during on periods, mean (SD)	na	19.2 (11.2)	–
Disease duration in yrs, median (IQR)	–	3 (2 – 4)	–
Onset laterality, left n (%)	–	10 (38.5)	–
Antiparkinsonian medications			
Levodopa-containing drugs, n (%)	–	11 (42.3)	–
Dopamine agonists, n (%)		11 (42.3)	
MAO-B inhibitors, n (%)		17 (65.4)	
LEDD, mean (SD)	–	214.2 (121.5)	–
Education level in yrs, median (IQR)	16 (13-18)	13 (8 – 17.3)	0.060[c]
MoCA, median (IQR)	25.6 (24.2-27.7)	24.3 (21.6 – 26.3)	**0.042**[c]
TMT, Part A, median (IQR)	na	41.5 (30.3 – 63.5)	–
TMT, Part B, median (IQR)	na	73.5 (58.3 – 110.5)	–
TMT, B-A, median (IQR)	na	40.0 (25.0 – 63.8)	–
Phonemic fluency, mean (SD)	na	32.7 (9.6)	–
Semantic fluency, mean (SD)	na	39.7 (10.4)	–

HC, healthy controls; IQR, interquartile range; LEDD, Levodopa daily dose equivalent; MAO-B, monoamine oxidase-B; Movement Disorder Society-sponsored revision of the Unified Parkinson's Disease Rating Scale (MDS-UPDRS), MoCA, Montreal Cognitive Assessment, n, number, na, not available, PD, Parkinson's disease, SD, standard deviation, TMT, Trail Making Test, yrs, years. MoCA scores were adjusted according to Santangelo et al. (2015), TMT according to Giovagnoli et al. (1996), phonemic fluency according to Carlesimo et al. (1996) and semantic fluency according to Novelli et al. (1986). Chi-squared test (a), independent samples Student's t-test (b), and Mann-Whitney test (c) were used to evaluate differences between PD and HC groups, as appropriate. P-values lower than 0.05 were considered significant (in bold).

No significant FA differences were observed. MD was significantly higher in PD patients with respect to HC in the substantia nigra ($p = 0.030$, $d = 0.631$), putamen ($p = 0.012$, $d = 0.742$) and red nucleus ($p = 0.036$, $d = 0.607$) but none of the results survived FDR correction. AD was found to be significantly higher in PD compared to HC in the putamen ($p = 0.005$, $d = 0.836$), even when correcting for multiple comparisons ($p_{FDR} = 0.035$). Increased RD was observed in PD for the putamen ($p = 0.039$, $d = 0.596$) and red nucleus ($p = 0.034$, $d = 0.616$), while higher CBF was found in the subthalamic nucleus ($p = 0.022$, $d = 0.669$) although significance was lost after FDR correction. Median FA, MD, AD, RD, and CBF values, and their IQR are reported in **Table 2**.

The VBM analysis did not show any significant GM volume differences between PD and HC groups within the basal ganglia regions.

Correlations Between DTI Parameters and CBF

No significant correlation was found between any of the diffusion parameters and CBF in HC group (**Supplementary Table 3**).

TABLE 2 | Median (IQR) values of FA, MD, AD, RD, and CBF for HC and PD groups within the ROIs.

Parameter	ROI	HC (n = 26)	PD (n = 26)	PD vs. HC		
				p	p_{FDR}	d
FA	Substantia Nigra	0.436 (0.411–0.463)	0.443 (0.422–0.457)	0.570	0.884	0.158
	Caudate	0.122 (0.114–0.136)	0.120 (0.109–0.141)	0.714	0.884	0.102
	Pallidum	0.241 (0.229–0.247)	0.237 (0.225–0.247)	0.884	0.884	0.041
	Putamen	0.140 (0.131–0.149)	0.139 (0.131–0.147)	0.840	0.884	0.056
	Thalamus	0.260 (0.250–0.271)	0.253 (0.244–0.261)	0.055	0.385	0.553
	Red Nucleus	0.372 (0.333–0.392)	0.355 (0.326–0.374)	0.305	0.712	0.287
	Subthalamic nucleus	0.437 (0.422–0.461)	0.434 (0.406–0.449)	0.257	0.712	0.319
MD [10^{-3} mm^2/sec]	Substantia Nigra	0.725 (0.698–0.759)	0.750 (0.731–0.775)	**0.030**	0.084	0.631
	Caudate	0.726 (0.706–0.850)	0.766 (0.715–1.004)	0.227	0.281	0.340
	Pallidum	0.736 (0.707–0.759)	0.743 (0.717–0.780)	0.464	0.464	0.204
	Putamen	0.685 (0.675–0.704)	0.704 (0.694–0.718)	**0.012**	0.084	0.742
	Thalamus	0.733 (0.725–0.763)	0.754 (0.739–0.770)	0.073	0.128	0.514
	Red nucleus	0.620 (0.595–0.647)	0.646 (0.621–0.658)	**0.036**	0.084	0.607
	Subthalamic nucleus	0.666 (0.651–0.690)	0.677 (0.660–0.701)	0.241	0.281	0.329
AD [10^{-3} mm^2/sec]	Substantia Nigra	1.117 (1.064–1.172)	1.147 (1.088–1.195)	0.188	0.373	0.372
	Caudate	0.836 (0.810–0.957)	0.874 (0.831–1.105)	0.162	0.373	0.396
	Pallidum	0.919 (0.891–0.977)	0.921 (0.890–0.994)	0.721	0.721	0.099
	Putamen	0.783 (0.769–0.802)	0.807 (0.792–0.825)	**0.005**	**0.035**	0.836
	Thalamus	0.947 (0.935–0.996)	0.968 (0.949–0.995)	0.213	0.373	0.350
	Red Nucleus	0.868 (0.830–0.914)	0.807 (0.792–0.825)	0.375	0.525	0.248
	Subthalamic Nucleus	0.995 (0.973–1.022)	0.987 (0.951–1.021)	0.674	0.721	0.117
RD [10^{-3} mm^2/sec]	Substantia Nigra	0.543 (0.498–0.563)	0.559 (0.538–0.579)	0.082	0.134	0.497
	Caudate	0.682 (0.656–0.801)	0.719 (0.662–0.957)	0.241	0.281	0.329
	Pallidum	0.650 (0.623–0.670)	0.663 (0.631–0.691)	0.365	0.365	0.253
	Putamen	0.637 (0.627–0.655)	0.653 (0.635–0.667)	**0.039**	0.124	0.596
	Thalamus	0.633 (0.625–0.660)	0.657 (0.639–0.674)	0.053	0.124	0.556
	Red nucleus	0.481 (0.470–0.527)	0.519 (0.500–0.530)	**0.034**	0.124	0.616
	Subthalamic nucleus	0.507 (0.488–0.537)	0.529 (0.495–0.547)	0.096	0.134	0.475
CBF [ml/min/100 g]	Substantia Nigra	26.86 (22.98–30.80)	24.86 (20.58–31.60)	0.634	0.840	0.132
	Caudate	21.63 (18.21–24.41)	20.75 (16.72–24.07)	0.608	0.840	0.142
	Pallidum	19.99 (18.21–24.43)	21.83 (19.65–24.84)	0.241	0.840	0.329
	Putamen	25.14 (21.54–29.18)	24.02 (21.50–28.47)	0.840	0.840	0.056
	Thalamus	25.92 (19.59–30.45)	23.44 (21.29–27.97)	0.687	0.840	0.112
	Red Nucleus	27.94 (23.39–33.87)	27.58 (23.47–32.28)	0.728	0.840	0.097
	Subthalamic Nucleus	22.65 (20.83–27.23)	28.56 (23.20–31.07)	**0.022**	0.154	0.669

AD, axial diffusivity; CBF, cerebral blood flow; FA, fractional anisotropy; d, Cohen's d; FDR, false discovery rate; HC, healthy controls; IQR, interquartile range; MD, mean diffusivity; n, number; PD, Parkinson's disease; RD, radial diffusivity; ROI, region of interest. The group differences were tested with Mann-Whitney test. Original p-values, FDR-corrected p-values and Cohen's d are reported. P-values lower than 0.05 were considered significant (in bold). Effect sizes were originally calculated as eta squared and subsequently transformed into Cohen's d values. Effect size was considered very small for $d < 0.2$, small for $0.2 \leq d < 0.5$, moderate for $0.5 \leq d < 0.8$, and large for $d \geq 0.8$. Note that obtained p-values lower than 0.05 are associated with moderate to large effect size.

Conversely, for the PD group, significant FDR-corrected correlations were found between CBF and all the diffusion parameters in the caudate nucleus (with FA: r = 0.543, p_{FDR} = 0.028; with MD: r = −0.661, p_{FDR} = 0.002; with AD: r = −0.628, p_{FDR} = 0.007; with RD: r = −0.635, p_{FDR} = 0.003; see **Table 3**). The scatterplots representing diffusion-vs.-perfusion measures in the caudate in the PD group are reported in **Figure 1**.

DISCUSSION

In the current study a combined assessment of DTI parameters and CBF within the basal ganglia was performed in a group of idiopathic PD patients to investigate the relationship between microstructural integrity and perfusion alterations. Three main findings were obtained. First, microstructural alteration was shown in the putamen, a region that is primarily involved in PD. In addition, no significant perfusion differences were observed between PD and HC in any of the considered ROIs. Finally, a significant correlation between DTI parameters and CBF emerged for PD patients in the caudate.

The presence of DTI alterations in PD has been extensively discussed over the last decade but without drawing final conclusions, as conflicting results have been reported (Cochrane and Ebmeier, 2013; Schwarz et al., 2013; Atkinson-Clement et al., 2017). Since the loss of dopaminergic neurons leads to the disruption of diffusion barriers, decreased FA and increased MD,

TABLE 3 | Spearman's correlation between local CBF and diffusion parameters in PD group (n = 26) within all the ROIs.

ROI	FA		MD		AD		RD	
	r	p_{FDR}	r	p_{FDR}	r	p_{FDR}	r	p_{FDR}
Substantia Nigra	+0.058	0.777	+0.015	0.941	−0.016	0.939	+0.201	0.692
Caudate	+0.543	**0.028**	−0.661	**0.002**	−0.628	**0.007**	−0.635	**0.003**
Pallidum	+0.382	0.126	−0.112	0.682	−0.032	0.939	−0.110	0.692
Putamen	−0.096	0.747	+0.320	0.391	+0.345	0.294	+0.0211	0.692
Thalamus	+0.128	0.747	−0.156	0.666	−0.175	0.688	−0.164	0.692
Red nucleus	−0.431	0.098	−0.236	0.572	−0.275	0.406	+0.024	0.906
Subthalamic Nucleus	+0.239	0.420	−0.284	0.666	−0.201	0.706	+0.123	0.692

AD, axial diffusivity; CBF, cerebral blood flow; FA, fractional anisotropy; FDR, false discovery rate; MD, mean diffusivity; PD, Parkinson's disease; RD, radial diffusivity; ROI, region of interest. P-values lower than 0.05 were considered significant (in bold).

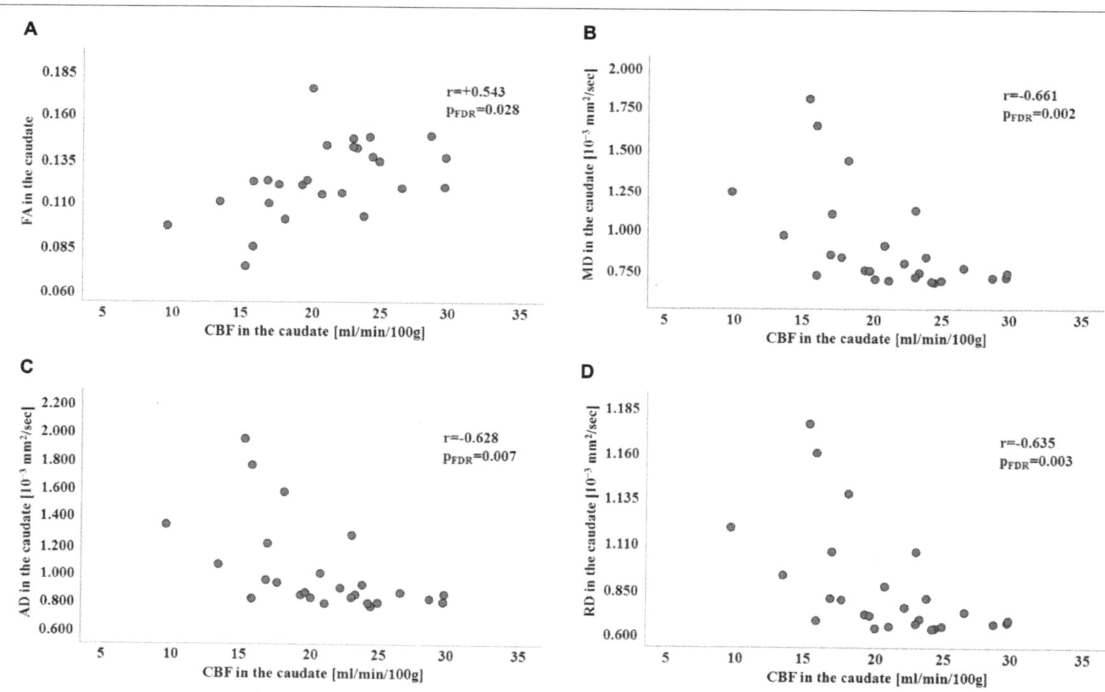

FIGURE 1 | Scatterplots showing FA, MD, AD, and RD in the caudate in relation to CBF in the PD group (panel **A–D**, respectively). Spearman's correlation coefficients and associated FDR-corrected p-values are shown (significant for p_{FDR} < 0.05). CBF, cerebral blood flow; FA, fractional anisotropy; FDR, false discovery rate; HC, healthy control; MD, mean diffusivity; AD, axial diffusivity; PD, Parkinson's disease; r-Spearman's correlation coefficient; RD, radial diffusivity.

AD and RD are expected in PD (Atkinson-Clement et al., 2017; Winklewski et al., 2018). Nevertheless, some recent studies also showed increased FA and decreased diffusivities in PD (Lenfeldt et al., 2015; Mole et al., 2016; Wen et al., 2016; Chen et al., 2018) In addition, varied multifocal patterns of abnormal DTI changes were reported, (Karagulle Kendi et al., 2008; Zhan et al., 2012) probably due to the multisystem involvement and the non-motor syndromes that characterize the disease (Hall et al., 2016). In the present study, significantly increased AD and a trend for higher MD and RD were found for PD patients in the putamen. The putamen is a key region for motor symptoms in PD, (Manza et al., 2016) since it is densely connected with the motor cortex. Therefore, its structural alterations are strongly associated with PD motor deficits (Nemmi et al., 2015) which are the cardinal symptoms of the disease. Notably, our PD group showed a trend for altered diffusivity also in the substantia nigra. Specifically, a trend for increased MD was observed, in line with several previous studies that reported altered nigral MD in PD (Scherfler et al., 2013; Schwarz et al., 2013; Du et al., 2014; Kamagata et al., 2016; Loane et al., 2016). Furthermore, a significant correlation between RD in the substantia nigra and TMT, part A score (**Supplementary Table 2**) was found. Conversely, no significant FA alterations were detected within the substantia nigra of PD patients in this study. Although this result is in contrast with several previous studies that reported reduced FA in PD, (Yoshikawa et al., 2004; Chan et al., 2007; Vaillancourt et al., 2009; Wei et al., 2016) heterogeneous FA alterations have been reported, so that FA in the substantia nigra has been considered insufficiently sensitive and specific to diagnose PD (Schuff et al., 2015; Hirata et al., 2017). The relatively limited sample size probably prevented us from consistently showing significant alterations of all the DTI parameters in the putamen and in the substantia nigra of our PD patients. However, the significantly altered AD in the putamen and the observed trends, associated with moderate to large effect sizes, suggest that DTI changes are present in the putamen and in the substantia nigra in early PD. The absence of group differences in terms of GM volumes within the regions showing DTI alterations highlighted that the loss of micro-structural integrity was without gross tissue loss (i.e., atrophy). Thus, the deafferentation of the nigrostriatal pathway likely induces a complex microstructural reorganization in the putamen and substantia nigra (Peran et al., 2010).

Besides DTI measures, ASL-derived CBF values were also tested in this study. No significant CBF differences between PD patients and HC were found within any of the ROIs. However, a trend for increased perfusion (significant before FDR-correction) was observed within the subthalamic nucleus. Hypermetabolism of the subthalamic nucleus, reflected by greater CBF, is in concordance with increased neuronal activity and an irregular firing pattern, as previously reported in PD (Hutchison et al., 1998; Blandini et al., 2000; Rodriguez-Oroz et al., 2001). The important role of the subthalamic nucleus in PD symptomatology and in direct-indirect pathway imbalance is supported by the dramatic clinical benefits experienced by PD patients after neurosurgery (both ablation and deep brain stimulation) targeting this structure (Obeso et al., 2017). Unlike in the DTI analysis, we did not detect any differences in putaminal perfusion in our PD patients. Our result of preserved CBF in the putamen is in line with some previous studies (Melzer et al., 2011; Al-Bachari et al., 2014; Pelizzari et al., 2019) but in contrast with a recent one that showed putaminal hypoperfusion in PD patients, both at early and middle stage of the disease (Wei et al., 2016). The considerable clinical heterogeneity that characterizes PD could have prevented us from identifying common patterns of CBF alterations in the basal ganglia in early PD patients. Investigating CBF in a wider cohort of PD patients at the early stage and accounting for motor symptom laterality onset is warranted to clarify the role of CBF changes in PD.

Interestingly, strongly significant correlations between all the DTI parameters and CBF were observed in the caudate nucleus of our PD patients, even though neither diffusion nor perfusion indices were altered. The caudate nucleus is known to be relatively spared at the early stage of the disease. A slower rate of dopaminergic decline in the caudate nucleus with respect to the putamen was reported by a previous study, with no significant changes in the caudate during the first years of the disease (Bruck et al., 2009). The dorsal caudate nucleus is connected with the dorsolateral prefrontal cortex, and it is part of the cognitive loop, which was proposed to be affected immediately after the motor one in PD (de la Fuente-Fernandez, 2012). Therefore, the absence of diffusion and perfusion changes in the caudate might be associated with the early disease stage. However, a correlation between DTI parameters and CBF was observed in this study. Specifically, PD patients who presented microstructural alterations in the caudate, showed also hypoperfusion. Both microstructural damage and perfusion alterations might be associated with disease duration (**Supplementary Table 1**), thus longitudinal studies are warranted to confirm their potential link with disease progression.

This study is not without limitations. The sample size was relatively small and the results remain to be confirmed in a larger number of patients. In addition, the relatively low resolution of ASL MRI, together with the small size of the ROIs, may have prevented us from showing the expected perfusion alterations. Another limitation that has to be mentioned is that the study was performed with a 1.5T MRI scanner. Although 3T scanners are characterized by a higher signal-to-noise ratio, the investigation of non-invasive markers to evaluate PD patients even with lower-field scanners, which are still prevalent in the clinical practice, is important in a translational perspective for diagnosis, treatment efficacy assessment and in terms of PD monitoring. The lack of a fine-grained neuropsychological assessment and the heterogeneity of our PD group in terms of laterality onset have also to be mentioned as limitations. This probably prevented us from showing consistent correlations between neuropsychological scores and MRI parameters (**Supplementary Table 2**). Finally, although we expected to find an association between perfusion changes and alterations of diffusion indices, only longitudinal studies may confirm the association with disease progression and allow for more firm conclusions to be drawn.

CONCLUSION

In conclusion, DTI appears to be a more sensitive technique than ASL to detect changes in basal ganglia regions of early PD patients when using 1.5T clinical scanners. However, since CBF in the caudate correlates with respective DTI parameters, both microstructural alterations and hypoperfusion may potentially be involved in caudate neurodegeneration and in the development of further symptoms in later stages of the disease.

AUTHOR CONTRIBUTIONS

LP, ML, NB, MC, and FB contributed conception and design of the study. RN recruited PD patients. FB performed the clinical evaluation of PD patients. SDT and FR performed the neuropsychological evaluation of PD patients. LP performed the image processing and the statistical analysis and wrote the first draft of the manuscript. All authors contributed to manuscript revision, read and approved the submitted version.

FUNDING

This study was in part funded by a grant awarded by the Annette Funicello Research Fund for Neurological Diseases and by the Italian Ministry of Health (Ricerca Corrente 2016–2018).

ACKNOWLEDGMENTS

Prof. Danny J. J. Wang (University of Southern California, CA, United States) and SIEMENS Healthineers provided us with the pCASL sequence. SDT received a scholarship from Crespi Spano Foundation.

REFERENCES

Al-Bachari, S., Parkes, L. M., Vidyasagar, R., Hanby, M. F., Tharaken, V., Leroi, I., et al. (2014). Arterial spin labelling reveals prolonged arterial arrival time in idiopathic Parkinson's disease. *Neuroimage Clin.* 6, 1–8. doi: 10.1016/j.nicl.2014.07.014

Alexander, A. L., Lee, J. E., Lazar, M., and Field, A. S. (2007). Diffusion tensor imaging of the brain. *Neurotherapeutics* 4, 316–329. doi: 10.1016/j.nurt.2007.05.011

Andersson, J. L., Skare, S., and Ashburner, J. (2003). How to correct susceptibility distortions in spin-echo echo-planar images: application to diffusion tensor imaging. *Neuroimage* 20, 870–888. doi: 10.1016/S1053-8119(03)00336-7

Andersson, J. L. R., and Sotiropoulos, S. N. (2016). An integrated approach to correction for off-resonance effects and subject movement in diffusion MR imaging. *Neuroimage* 125, 1063–1078. doi: 10.1016/j.neuroimage.2015.10.019

Atkinson-Clement, C., Pinto, S., Eusebio, A., and Coulon, O. (2017). Diffusion tensor imaging in Parkinson's disease: review and meta-analysis. *Neuroimage Clin.* 16, 98–110. doi: 10.1016/j.nicl.2017.07.011

Behrens, T. E., Woolrich, M. W., Jenkinson, M., Johansen-Berg, H., Nunes, R. G., Clare, S., et al. (2003). Characterization and propagation of uncertainty in diffusion-weighted MR imaging. *Magn. Reson. Med.* 50, 1077–1088. doi: 10.1002/mrm.10609

Blandini, F., Nappi, G., Tassorelli, C., and Martignoni, E. (2000). Functional changes of the basal ganglia circuitry in Parkinson's disease. *Prog. Neurobiol.* 62, 63–88. doi: 10.1016/s0301-0082(99)00067-2

Bruck, A., Aalto, S., Rauhala, E., Bergman, J., Marttila, R., and Rinne, J. O. (2009). A follow-up study on 6-[18F]fluoro-L-dopa uptake in early Parkinson's disease shows nonlinear progression in the putamen. *Mov. Disord.* 24, 1009–1015. doi: 10.1002/mds.22484

Carlesimo, G. A., Caltagirone, C., and Gainotti, G. (1996). The mental deterioration battery: normative data, diagnostic reliability and qualitative analyses of cognitive impairment. The group for the standardization of the mental deterioration battery. *Eur. Neurol.* 36, 378–384. doi: 10.1159/000117297

Chan, L. L., Rumpel, H., Yap, K., Lee, E., Loo, H. V., Ho, G. L., et al. (2007). Case control study of diffusion tensor imaging in Parkinson's disease. *J. Neurol. Neurosurg. Psychiatry* 78, 1383–1386. doi: 10.1136/jnnp.2007.121525

Chappell, M. A., Groves, A. R., Whitcher, B., and Woolrich, M. W. (2009). Variational bayesian inference for a nonlinear forward model. *IEEE J. MagazineIEEE Trans. Signal Processing* 57, 223–236. doi: 10.1109/tsp.2008.2005752

Chen, N. K., Chou, Y. H., Sundman, M., Hickey, P., Kasoff, W. S., Bernstein, A., et al. (2018). Alteration of diffusion-tensor magnetic resonance imaging measures in brain regions involved in early stages of Parkinson's Disease. *Brain Connect* 8, 343–349. doi: 10.1089/brain.2017.0558

Chen, Y., Pressman, P., Simuni, T., Parrish, T. B., and Gitelman, D. R. (2015). Effects of acute levodopa challenge on resting cerebral blood flow in Parkinson's Disease patients assessed using pseudo-continuous arterial spin labeling. *PeerJ* 3:e1381. doi: 10.7717/peerj.1381

Cochrane, C. J., and Ebmeier, K. P. (2013). Diffusion tensor imaging in parkinsonian syndromes: a systematic review and meta-analysis. *Neurology* 80, 857–864. doi: 10.1212/WNL.0b013e318284070c

de la Fuente-Fernandez, R. (2012). Frontostriatal cognitive staging in Parkinson's disease. *Parkinsons Dis.* 2012:561046. doi: 10.1155/2012/561046

Du, G., Lewis, M. M., Sterling, N. W., Kong, L., Chen, H., Mailman, R. B., et al. (2014). Microstructural changes in the substantia nigra of asymptomatic agricultural workers. *Neurotoxicol. Teratol.* 41, 60–64. doi: 10.1016/j.ntt.2013.12.001

Giovagnoli, A. R., Del Pesce, M., Mascheroni, S., Simoncelli, M., Laiacona, M., and Capitani, E. (1996). Trail making test: normative values from 287 normal adult controls. *Ital. J. Neurol. Sci.* 17, 305–309. doi: 10.1007/bf01997792

Goetz, C. G., Poewe, W., Rascol, O., Sampaio, C., Stebbins, G. T., Counsell, C., et al. (2004). Movement disorder society task force report on the hoehn and yahr staging scale: status and recommendations. *Mov. Disord.* 19, 1020–1028. doi: 10.1002/mds.20213

Hall, J. M., Ehgoetz Martens, K. A., Walton, C. C., O'Callaghan, C., Keller, P. E., Lewis, S. J., et al. (2016). Diffusion alterations associated with Parkinson's disease symptomatology: a review of the literature. *Parkinsonism Relat. Disord.* 33, 12–26. doi: 10.1016/j.parkreldis.2016.09.026

Hirata, F. C. C., Sato, J. R., Vieira, G., Lucato, L. T., Leite, C. C., Bor-Seng-Shu, E., et al. (2017). Substantia nigra fractional anisotropy is not a diagnostic biomarker of Parkinson's disease: a diagnostic performance study and meta-analysis. *Eur. Radiol.* 27, 2640–2648. doi: 10.1007/s00330-016-4611-0

Hutchison, W. D., Allan, R. J., Opitz, H., Levy, R., Dostrovsky, J. O., Lang, A. E., et al. (1998). Neurophysiological identification of the subthalamic nucleus in surgery for Parkinson's disease. *Ann. Neurol.* 44, 622–628. doi: 10.1002/ana.410440407

Kalia, L. V., and Lang, A. E. (2015). Parkinson's disease. *Lancet* 386, 896–912. doi: 10.1016/S0140-6736(14)61393-3

Kamagata, K., Hatano, T., Okuzumi, A., Motoi, Y., Abe, O., Shimoji, K., et al. (2016). Neurite orientation dispersion and density imaging in the substantia nigra in idiopathic Parkinson disease. *Eur. Radiol.* 26, 2567–2577. doi: 10.1007/s00330-015-4066-8

Karagulle Kendi, A. T., Lehericy, S., Luciana, M., Ugurbil, K., and Tuite, P. (2008). Altered diffusion in the frontal lobe in Parkinson disease. *AJNR Am. J. Neuroradiol.* 29, 501–505. doi: 10.3174/ajnr.A0850

Laganà, M. M., Mendozzi, L., Pelizzari, L., Bergsland, N. P., Pugnetti, L., Cecconi, P., et al. (2018). Are cerebral perfusion and atrophy linked in multiple sclerosis? Evidence for a multifactorial approach to assess neurodegeneration. *Curr. Neurovasc. Res.* 15, 282–291. doi: 10.2174/1567202616666181123164235

Lenfeldt, N., Larsson, A., Nyberg, L., Birgander, R., and Forsgren, L. (2015). Fractional anisotropy in the substantia nigra in Parkinson's disease: a complex picture. *Eur. J. Neurol.* 22, 1408–1414. doi: 10.1111/ene.12760

Lin, W. C., Chen, P. C., Huang, Y. C., Tsai, N. W., Chen, H. L., Wang, H. C., et al. (2016). Dopaminergic therapy modulates cortical perfusion in parkinson disease with and without dementia according to arterial spin labeled perfusion magnetic resonance imaging. *Medicine* 95:e2206. doi: 10.1097/MD.0000000000002206

Loane, C., Politis, M., Kefalopoulou, Z., Valle-Guzman, N., Paul, G., Widner, H., et al. (2016). Aberrant nigral diffusion in Parkinson's disease: a longitudinal diffusion tensor imaging study. *Mov. Disord.* 31, 1020–1026. doi: 10.1002/mds.26606

Manza, P., Zhang, S., Li, C. S., and Leung, H. C. (2016). Resting-state functional connectivity of the striatum in early-stage Parkinson's disease: cognitive decline and motor symptomatology. *Hum. Brain Mapp.* 37, 648–662. doi: 10.1002/hbm.23056

Marshall, O., Chawla, S., Lu, H., Pape, L., and Ge, Y. (2016). Cerebral blood flow modulation insufficiency in brain networks in multiple sclerosis: a hypercapnia MRI study. *J. Cereb. Blood Flow Metab.* 36, 2087–2095. doi: 10.1177/0271678X16654922

Melzer, T. R., Watts, R., MacAskill, M. R., Pearson, J. F., Rueger, S., Pitcher, T. L., et al. (2011). Arterial spin labelling reveals an abnormal cerebral perfusion pattern in Parkinson's disease. *Brain* 134(Pt 3), 845–855. doi: 10.1093/brain/awq377

Mole, J. P., Subramanian, L., Bracht, T., Morris, H., Metzler-Baddeley, C., and Linden, D. E. (2016). Increased fractional anisotropy in the motor tracts of Parkinson's disease suggests compensatory neuroplasticity or selective neurodegeneration. *Eur. Radiol.* 26, 3327–3335. doi: 10.1007/s00330-015-4178-1

Nemmi, F., Sabatini, U., Rascol, O., and Peran, P. (2015). Parkinson's disease and local atrophy in subcortical nuclei: insight from shape analysis. *Neurobiol. Aging* 36, 424–433. doi: 10.1016/j.neurobiolaging.2014.07.010

Novelli, G., Papagno, C., Capitani, E., Laiacona, M., Vallar, G., and Cappa, S. F. (1986). Tre test clinici di ricerca e produzione lessicale. Taratura su soggetti normali. *Arch. Psicol. Neurol. Psichiatr.* 4, 477–506.

Obeso, J. A., Stamelou, M., Goetz, C. G., Poewe, W., Lang, A. E., Weintraub, D., et al. (2017). Past, present, and future of Parkinson's disease: a special essay on the 200th Anniversary of the shaking palsy. *Mov. Disord.* 32, 1264–1310. doi: 10.1002/mds.27115

Pelizzari, L., Laganà, M. M., Rossetto, F., Bergsland, N., Galli, M., Baselli, G., et al. (2019). Cerebral blood flow and cerebrovascular reactivity correlate with severity of motor symptoms in Parkinson's disease. *Ther. Adv. Neurol. Disord.* 12:1756286419838354.

Peran, P., Cherubini, A., Assogna, F., Piras, F., Quattrocchi, C., Peppe, A., et al. (2010). Magnetic resonance imaging markers of Parkinson's disease nigrostriatal signature. *Brain* 133, 3423–3433. doi: 10.1093/brain/awq212

Postuma, R. B., Berg, D., Stern, M., Poewe, W., Olanow, C. W., Oertel, W., et al. (2015). MDS clinical diagnostic criteria for Parkinson's disease. *Mov. Disord.* 30, 1591–1601. doi: 10.1002/mds.26424

Pyatigorskaya, N., Gallea, C., Garcia-Lorenzo, D., Vidailhet, M., and Lehericy, S. (2014). A review of the use of magnetic resonance imaging in Parkinson's disease. *Ther. Adv. Neurol. Disord.* 7, 206–220. doi: 10.1177/1756285613511507

Rodriguez-Oroz, M. C., Rodriguez, M., Guridi, J., Mewes, K., Chockkman, V., Vitek, J., et al. (2001). The subthalamic nucleus in Parkinson's disease: somatotopic organization and physiological characteristics. *Brain* 124(Pt 9), 1777–1790. doi: 10.1093/brain/124.9.1777

Santangelo, G., Siciliano, M., Pedone, R., Vitale, C., Falco, F., Bisogno, R., et al. (2015). Normative data for the montreal cognitive assessment in an italian population sample. *Neurol. Sci.* 36, 585–591. doi: 10.1007/s10072-014-1995-y

Scherfler, C., Esterhammer, R., Nocker, M., Mahlknecht, P., Stockner, H., Warwitz, B., et al. (2013). Correlation of dopaminergic terminal dysfunction and microstructural abnormalities of the basal ganglia and the olfactory tract in Parkinson's disease. *Brain* 136(Pt 10), 3028–3037. doi: 10.1093/brain/awt234

Schuff, N., Wu, I. W., Buckley, S., Foster, E. D., Coffey, C. S., Gitelman, D. R., et al. (2015). Diffusion imaging of nigral alterations in early Parkinson's disease with dopaminergic deficits. *Mov. Disord.* 30, 1885–1892. doi: 10.1002/mds.26325

Schwarz, S. T., Abaei, M., Gontu, V., Morgan, P. S., Bajaj, N., and Auer, D. P. (2013). Diffusion tensor imaging of nigral degeneration in Parkinson's disease: a region-of-interest and voxel-based study at 3 T and systematic review with meta-analysis. *Neuroimage Clin.* 3, 481–488. doi: 10.1016/j.nicl.2013.10.006

Seifert, K. D., and Wiener, J. I. (2013). The impact of DaTscan on the diagnosis and management of movement disorders: a retrospective study. *Am. J. Neurodegener. Dis.* 2, 29–34.

Smith, S. M., Zhang, Y., Jenkinson, M., Chen, J., Matthews, P. M., Federico, A., et al. (2002). Accurate, robust, and automated longitudinal and cross-sectional brain change analysis. *Neuroimage* 17, 479–489. doi: 10.1006/nimg.2002.1040

Syrimi, Z. J., Vojtisek, L., Eliasova, I., Viskova, J., Svatkova, A., Vanicek, J., et al. (2017). Arterial spin labelling detects posterior cortical hypoperfusion in non-demented patients with Parkinson's disease. *J. Neural Transm.* 124, 551–557. doi: 10.1007/s00702-017-1703-1

Taylor, K. I., Sambataro, F., Boess, F., Bertolino, A., and Dukart, J. (2018). Progressive decline in gray and white matter integrity in de novo Parkinson's disease: an analysis of longitudinal parkinson progression markers initiative diffusion tensor imaging data. *Front. Aging Neurosci.* 10:318. doi: 10.3389/fnagi.2018.00318

Tomlinson, C. L., Stowe, R., Patel, S., Rick, C., Gray, R., and Clarke, C. E. (2010). Systematic review of levodopa dose equivalency reporting in Parkinson's disease. *Mov. Disord.* 25, 2649–2653. doi: 10.1002/mds.23429

Vaillancourt, D. E., Spraker, M. B., Prodoehl, J., Abraham, I., Corcos, D. M., Zhou, X. J., et al. (2009). High-resolution diffusion tensor imaging in the substantia nigra of de novo Parkinson disease. *Neurology* 72, 1378–1384. doi: 10.1212/01.wnl.0000340982.01727.6e

van Osch, M. J., Teeuwisse, W. M., Chen, Z., Suzuki, Y., Helle, M., and Schmid, S. (2018). Advances in arterial spin labelling MRI methods for measuring perfusion and collateral flow. *J. Cereb. Blood Flow Metab.* 38, 1461–1480. doi: 10.1177/0271678X17713434

Wang, D. J., Alger, J. R., Qiao, J. X., Gunther, M., Pope, W. B., Saver, J. L., et al. (2013). Multi-delay multi-parametric arterial spin-labeled perfusion MRI in acute ischemic stroke - Comparison with dynamic susceptibility contrast enhanced perfusion imaging. *Neuroimage Clin.* 3, 1–7. doi: 10.1016/j.nicl.2013.06.017

Wei, X., Yan, R., Chen, Z., Weng, R., Liu, X., Gao, H., et al. (2016). Combined diffusion tensor imaging and arterial spin labeling as markers of early Parkinson's disease. *Sci. Rep.* 6:33762. doi: 10.1038/srep33762

Wen, M. C., Heng, H. S., Ng, S. Y., Tan, L. C., Chan, L. L., and Tan, E. K. (2016). White matter microstructural characteristics in newly diagnosed Parkinson's disease: an unbiased whole-brain study. *Sci. Rep.* 6:35601. doi: 10.1038/srep35601

Winkler, A. M., Ridgway, G. R., Webster, M. A., Smith, S. M., and Nichols, T. E. (2014). Permutation inference for the general linear model. *Neuroimage* 92, 381–397. doi: 10.1016/j.neuroimage.2014.01.060

Winklewski, P. J., Sabisz, A., Naumczyk, P., Jodzio, K., Szurowska, E., and Szarmach, A. (2018). Understanding the physiopathology behind axial and radial diffusivity changes-what do we know? *Front. Neurol.* 9:92. doi: 10.3389/fneur.2018.00092

Xiao, Y., Fonov, V., Beriault, S., Al Subaie, F., Chakravarty, M. M., Sadikot, A. F., et al. (2015). Multi-contrast unbiased MRI atlas of a Parkinson's disease population. *Int. J. Comput. Assist. Radiol. Surg.* 10, 329–341. doi: 10.1007/s11548-014-1068-y

Yoshikawa, K., Nakata, Y., Yamada, K., and Nakagawa, M. (2004). Early pathological changes in the parkinsonian brain demonstrated by diffusion tensor MRI. *J. Neurol. Neurosurg. Psychiatry* 75, 481–484. doi: 10.1136/jnnp.2003.021873

Zhan, W., Kang, G. A., Glass, G. A., Zhang, Y., Shirley, C., Millin, R., et al. (2012). Regional alterations of brain microstructure in Parkinson's disease using diffusion tensor imaging. *Mov. Disord.* 27, 90–97. doi: 10.1002/mds.23917

Zhang, Y., Wu, I. W., Tosun, D., Foster, E., Schuff, N., and Parkinson's Progression Markers, I. (2016). Progression of regional microstructural degeneration in Parkinson's disease: a multicenter diffusion tensor imaging study. *PLoS One* 11:e0165540. doi: 10.1371/journal.pone.0165540

2

The Combination of DAT-SPECT, Structural and Diffusion MRI Predicts Clinical Progression in Parkinson's Disease

Sara Lorio[1,2,3], Fabio Sambataro[2,4], Alessandro Bertolino[2,5], Bogdan Draganski[3,6] and Juergen Dukart[2,7,8]*

[1] Developmental Neurosciences, UCL Great Ormond Street Institute of Child Health, University College London, London, United Kingdom, [2] Roche Pharma and Early Development, Neuroscience, Ophthalmology and Rare Diseases, F. Hoffmann-La Roche Ltd., Basel, Switzerland, [3] Laboratory for Research in Neuroimaging, Department of Clinical Neurosciences, Lausanne University Hospital, University of Lausanne, Lausanne, Switzerland, [4] Department of Experimental and Clinical Medical Sciences, University of Udine, Udine, Italy, [5] Department of Basic Medical Science, Neuroscience and Sense Organs, University of Bari, Bari, Italy, [6] Max Planck Institute for Human Cognitive and Brain Sciences, Leipzig, Germany, [7] Institute of Neuroscience and Medicine, Brain and Behaviour (INM-7), Research Centre Jülich, Jülich, Germany, [8] Institute of Systems Neuroscience, Medical Faculty, Heinrich Heine University Düsseldorf, Düsseldorf, Germany

***Correspondence:**
Sara Lorio
s.lorio@ucl.ac.uk

There is an increasing interest in identifying non-invasive biomarkers of disease severity and prognosis in idiopathic Parkinson's disease (PD). Dopamine-transporter SPECT (DAT-SPECT), diffusion tensor imaging (DTI), and structural magnetic resonance imaging (sMRI) provide unique information about the brain's neurotransmitter and microstructural properties. In this study, we evaluate the relative and combined capability of these imaging modalities to predict symptom severity and clinical progression in *de novo* PD patients. To this end, we used MRI, SPECT, and clinical data of *de novo* drug-naïve PD patients (n = 205, mean age 61 ± 10) and age-, sex-matched healthy controls (n = 105, mean age 58 ± 12) acquired at baseline. Moreover, we employed clinical data acquired at 1 year follow-up for PD patients with or without L-Dopa treatment in order to predict the progression symptoms severity. Voxel-based group comparisons and covariance analyses were applied to characterize baseline disease-related alterations for DAT-SPECT, DTI, and sMRI. Cortical and subcortical alterations in *de novo* PD patients were found in all evaluated imaging modalities, in line with previously reported midbrain-striato-cortical network alterations. The combination of these imaging alterations was reliably linked to clinical severity and disease progression at 1 year follow-up in this patient population, providing evidence for the potential use of these modalities as imaging biomarkers for disease severity and prognosis that can be integrated into clinical trials.

Keywords: Parkinson's disease, voxel-based morphometry, voxel-based quantification, covariance analysis, symptoms severity

INTRODUCTION

Parkinson's disease (PD) is primarily characterized by progressive accumulation of aggregated α-synuclein in the brainstem, leading to a degeneration of dopaminergic neurons in substantia nigra (Lang and Lozano, 1998; Xu et al., 2002; Braak et al., 2003; Kraemmer et al., 2014). This presumably toxic accumulation induces a progressive loss of dopaminergic input to the striatum and further degeneration of striato-cortical pathways, resulting in the occurrence of different motor and non-motor symptoms (Houk and Wise, 1995; Lang and Lozano, 1998; Kraemmer et al., 2014). Current PD drugs focus on the symptoms treatment, however, the main goal of pharmaceutical research is to develop drugs able to slow or even stop the clinical progression.

To improve the monitoring of disease progression and the evaluation of drug effectiveness, it is essential to identify biomarkers able to detect the neurodegenerative alterations at all circuitry levels. Such biomarkers should demonstrate a strong and reproducible correlation with pathological changes and symptoms severity in multicenter studies (McGhee et al., 2013).

Several imaging modalities have been suggested for that purpose in the literature. Dopamine transporter single photon emission tomography (DAT-SPECT) provides a semi-quantitative assessment of striatal dopaminergic deafferentation. It is a well-established diagnostic biomarker of PD, owing to the strong correlation between the amount of dopamine transporters in the striatum and the number of dopaminergic neurons in substantia nigra (Kraemmer et al., 2014). However, DAT-SPECT does not provide information on non-dopaminergic disease aspects, and its link to disease progression in *de novo* PD patients remains unclear (Kägi et al., 2010). Structural MRI (sMRI) and diffusion tensor imaging (DTI) are powerful tools to assess whole brain atrophy patterns and microstructural tissue integrity (Le Bihan et al., 2001; Ashburner et al., 2003; Burton et al., 2004). Several sMRI studies reported volumetric changes in PD using voxel-based morphometry (VBM) analysis (Burton et al., 2004; Nagano-Saito et al., 2005; Wattendorf et al., 2009). However, only few studies reported the association between volumetric changes or cortical thinning and PD symptoms severity, measured by neuropsychological scores for testing attention and memory, and olfactory alterations (Junqué et al., 2005; Camicioli et al., 2011; Melzer et al., 2012; Segura et al., 2014; Campabadal et al., 2017). Also microstructural brain changes assessed through DTI using mean diffusivity (MD) and fractional anisotropy (FA) maps were found in PD throughout different brain regions (Gattellaro et al., 2009; Peran et al., 2010; Wang et al., 2011; Zhang et al., 2011, 2015; Du et al., 2012; Zhan et al., 2012; Kim et al., 2013; Schwarz et al., 2013; Tan et al., 2015; Lim et al., 2016; Loane et al., 2016; Nagae et al., 2016). However, most of these studies measured structural changes in small, heterogeneous PD patient cohorts (e.g., highly varying disease duration), resulting in variable magnitude and directionality of the respective findings (McGhee et al., 2013; Meijer et al., 2013; Weingarten et al., 2015). Moreover single DTI measures failed to accurately assess disease severity and prognosis, hampering their application in standard clinical practice or as biomarkers in clinical trials (McGhee et al., 2013; Pyatigorskaya et al., 2014; Atkinson-Clement et al., 2017). In contrast, in a small proof-of-concept study in PD patients, multimodal MRI measures based on DTI and R2* maps have been shown to provide complementary information allowing for a better differentiation of patients and controls (Peran et al., 2010). However, the relative and combined value of MRI measures and DAT-SPECT as biomarkers of disease severity and prognosis remains unknown.

Despite imaging changes in individual brain regions can be used as diagnostic biomarker, theories on neuro-degenerative disease increasingly focus on the role of brain network alterations as potential predictors of early disease severity and prognosis (Helmich et al., 2010; Woo et al., 2017). In fact previous studies showed that PD targets regions that, in healthy individuals have a well-defined correlation patterns (Helmich et al., 2010; Woo et al., 2017). However, the interaction between changes in the striatal dopamine and the morphological and microstructural alterations in the striato-cortical circuits remains unclear. This interaction can be evaluated using structural covariance analysis, which examines whether an imaging measure in one region correlates with the variation of the same, or other modalities measures in other brain regions (Mechelli et al., 2005; Schmitt et al., 2009; Alexander-Bloch et al., 2013a). Complementary to functional MRI (fMRI) and DTI-based connectomics, population covariance in brain anatomy represents another source of information about inter-regional anatomical associations (Alexander-Bloch et al., 2013b). A crucial difference between fMRI, diffusion MRI networks, and structural covariance is that the latter estimates inter-regional correlations based on group of images, while the first two networks can be constructed from connectivity measures computed for an individual image (Alexander-Bloch et al., 2013a,b). Another challenge of the structural covariance networks might be the biological interpretation of the results (Alexander-Bloch et al., 2013a). However, recent studies showed that the structural covariance pattern are influenced by synaptic connectivity between brain regions, genetic and developmental relationships, and different degenerative processes (Gong et al., 2012; Chou et al., 2015; Chang et al., 2017; de Schipper et al., 2017; Oosterwijk et al., 2018; Yee et al., 2018). Therefore, we applied this method to investigate structural network alterations using MRI-based measurements and striatal dopamine transporter uptake derived from DAT-SPECT.

Here, we evaluated DAT-SPECT, DTI and sMRI as biomarkers of disease severity and progression in *de novo* PD patients. Disease severity was assessed longitudinally through the modified version of the unified Parkinson's disease rating scale (MDS-UPDRS) evaluated at baseline (same time point at which the imaging data was acquired) and at 1 year follow-up. We used well-established VBM, voxel-based quantification (VBQ) (Draganski et al., 2011) and structural covariance analyses to identify disease-related alterations in a large cohort of *de novo* PD patients. We then tested whether combinations of imaging alterations identified in drug-naïve *de novo* PD were associated with current clinical severity measured by baseline MDS-UPDRS scores. Moreover, we employed those imaging measure to predict the future disease progression quantified by the MDS-UPDRS variations between the two time points.

As the dopaminergic treatments taken by some patients after the baseline evaluation have substantial effects on the clinical symptoms measured with MDS-UPDRS, we accounted for those effects by applying the prediction models separately to the group of patients receiving medication and to the one without treatment employing off medication clinical assessment (Mueller et al., 2018; van Ruitenbeek et al., 2018).

MATERIALS AND METHODS

Subjects

Data of *de novo* PD patients (N = 205) and healthy controls (HC) (N = 105) included in this study were obtained from the Parkinson's Progression Markers Initiative (PPMI) database[1]. PPMI is a large multicenter study and each site independently received ethics approval of the protocol. This study was carried out in accordance with Good Clinical Practice (GCP) regulations and International Conference on Harmonization (ICH) guidelines. Written informed consent was obtained from all participants in accordance with the Declaration of Helsinki.

All subjects underwent sMRI, DTI, and DAT-SPECT at baseline, and had MDS-UPDRS 1, 2, 3, and total, acquired at baseline (BL) and after 1 year (TP1). *De novo* PD patients included in the PPMI database had a diagnosis confirmed by DAT-SPECT scans and Hoehn and Yahr stage I or II. The exclusion criteria were diagnosis of dementia, psychiatric disorders or other neurological disease detectable with MRI at baseline. At BL all patients were drug-naïve, while at TP1 some patients started drug treatment with L-Dopa, dopamine agonist, and other unspecified medications. Only categorical (yes/no) information was recorded on the respective treatment categories (L-Dopa, dopamine agonists or other PD medication) without information about the dosage. In the current study, we included patients remaining without drug treatment at TP1 (called as PD no med) and patients taking only L-Dopa treatment at TP1 (called as PD on med). The PD on med group was composed of patients having the MDS-UPDRS3 evaluation performed off medication (patients were asked not to take L-Dopa for 24 h before the evaluation). From the 205 patients, we identified 56 subjects for the PD no med group, and 44 subjects for the PD on med group.

Image Acquisition and Processing

Whole-brain MRI was performed using standardized protocols on different 3T scanners. All acquisition protocols included a standard T1-weighted MPRAGE sequence (TI/TR = 900/2,300 ms, TE = 2.98 ms, 1 mm isotropic resolution), and a 2D single-shot echo-planar DTI sequence for diffusion weighted images (TR/TE = 900/88 ms, 2 mm isotropic resolution, diffusion weighting along 64 gradient directions, b-value = 1000 s/mm^2).

DAT-SPECT images were obtained using different camera systems. Details about SPECT image reconstruction are available on the PPMI website (see footnote 1) (reconstructed image matrix 91 × 109 × 91, 2 mm isotropic resolution).

VBM analysis was performed on the T1-weighted images using automated tissue classification and enhanced subcortical tissue probability maps embedded into the unified segmentation framework of SPM12 (Ashburner and Friston, 2005; Lorio et al., 2016). Image registration to the MNI space was performed for each subject applying subject-specific diffeomorphic estimates obtained using DARTEL (Ashburner, 2007) with default settings on the gray and white matter tissue maps (respectively, GM and WM). The warped GM maps were scaled by the Jacobian determinants of the deformation fields to account for local compression and expansion due to linear and non-linear transformation (Ashburner and Friston, 2000), resulting in GM volume maps. The GM volume maps were then smoothed using an isotropic Gaussian kernel of 6 mm full width at half maximum (FWHM).

The DTI maps were calculated from the diffusion weighted data using a group of libraries called TEEM[2]. The pre-processing steps for the estimation of FA and MD maps included correction for distortions due to eddy currents and head motion (Rohde et al., 2004; Tao et al., 2009), and affine registration of the corrected diffusion weighted data to the T1-weighted images using FLIRT from FSL5.0[3] (Greve and Fischl, 2009).

For VBQ analysis, FA and MD maps were warped into MNI space using a non-linear registration approach based on the subject-specific diffeomorphic estimates (Ashburner, 2007), derived for the GM and WM maps without scaling by the Jacobian determinants. In order to enhance the specificity of the warped FA and MD values for brain tissue classes, we used the combination of weighting procedure with the GM and WM probability maps derived from the T1-weighted data, and Gaussian smoothing with a 6 mm FWHM isotropic smoothing kernel as described by Draganski et al. (2011). Separate FA and MD maps were generated for GM and WM sub-spaces.

DAT-SPECT data pre-processing was performed within SPM12 and included normalization to an average size DAT-SPECT template with subsequent normalization into the MNI space performed using the "normalization" function. Then the images were non-linearly warped from the MNI to the native space of the T1-weighted data using the spatial transformation parameters estimated for the GM and WM probability maps. This allowed the correction for partial volume effects using the modified Müller-Gartner method (Müller-Gärtner et al., 1992; Rousset et al., 1998) based on the convolution of the DAT-SPECT data with the tissue classification maps estimated from T1-weighted images. The GM SPECT images were then normalized to MNI space using parameters derived from T1-weighted data and scaled to the global mean GM signal for each subject. Finally, the SPECT images were smoothed with an isotropic Gaussian kernel of 6 mm FWHM.

Statistical Analysis and Voxel-Based Group Comparison

We used odds ratios and t-test, as implemented in Matlab 2012b, to assess gender and age differences between PD patients and

[1] www.ppmi-info.org

[2] http://teem.sourceforge.net/index.html

[3] www.fmrib.ox.ac.uk/fsl

HC, and between PD on med and PD no med groups (**Table 1**). We compared the values of MDS-UPDRS scales (1, 2, 3, and total) measured at BL, TP1 and the differences between the two time points, using two-sample *t*-tests between the respective groups (see **Table 1**). Only MDS-UPDRS 3 values measured off medication were compared at TP1. Fisher's exact test was used to compare the disease dominant side between PD on med and PD no med subgroups (see **Table 1**).

To test for local differences in GM volume maps, FA and MD between PD patients and HC, we used SPM12 to perform a voxel-wise t-statistic separately for every map and tissue class (GM and WM), using a flexible factorial design, controlling for sex, age, total intracranial volume (TIV) and image acquisition site. These tests were carried out using explicit masks defining GM and WM voxels. The masks were generated as follows: smoothed (FWHM of 5 mm isotropic), Jacobian-modulated tissue probability maps in MNI space were averaged across all subjects for each tissue class (GM and WM). Then binary masks were generated by applying a threshold of 20%, voxels for which neither the GM nor the WM probability exceeded that value were excluded from the analysis. This approach was used to ensure that each voxel was analyzed in only one subspace and that non-brain tissue was excluded.

Similarly, differences in DAT-SPECT were evaluated using voxel-based comparisons, restricting analyses to GM voxels and controlling for age and sex. We applied to all voxel-wise statistical analyses a family-wise error (FWE) corrected cluster threshold of $p < 0.05$ combined with a voxel-wise $p < 0.001$. We further estimated the effect size (Cohen's *d*) of the observed differences.

To test for differential interaction between striatal dopamine transporter uptake derived from DAT-SPECT and MRI-based measurements, we performed voxel-wise covariance analyses (Mechelli et al., 2005) between DAT-SPECT values in the putamen (region showing strongest differences between PD patients and HC) and GM volume, FA and MD maps. The putamen was delineated according to the basal ganglia human area template (Prodoehl et al., 2008). We computed separate covariance analyses for each MRI-based measure (GM volume, FA, MD) and each tissue type (gray and white matter for FA and MD), controlling for age, sex, TIV, disease dominant side and image acquisition site. The covariance analyses were carried out using GM and WM masks obtained as previously described.

An FWE-corrected cluster threshold of $p < 0.05$ combined with a voxel-wise $p < 0.001$ was applied for all analyses. To quantify the differential inter-modality correlations identified in the covariance analyses, we computed Spearman correlation coefficients between the putamen DAT-SPECT signal and the average value of the age and sex adjusted MRI-based measures showing significant between-group differences in the covariance analysis.

Prediction Models: Symptoms Severity and Disease Progression

To evaluate the combined value of imaging measures as biomarkers of symptoms severity we used multiple linear regression models to predict each MDS-UPDRS subscale. The MDS-UPDRS 1, 2, 3, and total were the dependent variables, while the models regressors were the mean imaging measures extracted from regions showing significant differences between PD patients and HC (group differences: FA in pons nuclei, prefrontal MD, DAT signal in putamen; covariance differences: prefrontal GM volume, brainstem MD). For regions identified in covariance analyses we included in the model an interaction

TABLE 1 | Demographic and clinical data of subjects included in the study.

Demographic		HC	PD	PD no med	PD on med	PD versus HC *p*-value	PD on med versus PD no med *p*-value
		Mean ± SD					
Number of subjects (m/f)		105 (74/31)	205 (143/62)	56 (34/22)	44 (28/16)	0.999	0.837
Age		58 ± 12	61 ± 10	59 ± 10.2	62.6 ± 10.1	0.207	0.084
MDS-UPDRS1	Baseline	2 ± 1	6 ± 4	5 ± 3	6 ± 4	**$<10^{-6}$***	**0.022***
	Follow-up	–	–	6 ± 4	7 ± 4	–	**0.030***
	Change	–	–	1 ± 2	2 ± 3	–	**0.041***
MDS-UPDRS2	Baseline	0.1 ± 0.03	6 ± 4	6 ± 3	7 ± 4	**$<10^{-6}$***	**0.012***
	Follow-up	–	–	7 ± 4	8 ± 4	–	**0.021***
	Change	–	–	2 ± 2	3 ± 2	–	**0.031***
MDS-UPDRS3	Baseline	0.6 ± 0.3	21 ± 9	19 ± 10	22 ± 9	**$<10^{-6}$***	0.121
	Follow-up	–	–	21 ± 11	24 ± 10	–	0.067
	Change	–	–	4 ± 9	5 ± 10	–	0.067
MDS-UPDRS total	Baseline	3 ± 1.8	33 ± 13	29 ± 10	34 ± 15	**$<10^{-6}$***	**0.031***
	Follow-up	–	–	32 ± 15	37 ± 16	–	0.069
	Change	–	–	7 ± 10	8 ± 9	–	0.100
Dominant side (left/right/equilateral)		–	78/117/10	20/35/1	20/22/2	–	0.309

HC, healthy controls; PD, Parkinson's disease patients, PD no med, patients without medications 1 year after baseline; PD on med, patients on L-Dopa treatment 1 year after the baseline. Bold characters and "" indicate a significant group difference (p < 0.05).*

term between the MRI measure and DAT-SPECT. All analyses were controlled for age, sex, and symptoms dominant side. The goodness of fit for each model was assessed using the determination coefficient (R^2), while the model overfit was evaluated by means of the leave-one-out adjusted R^2 coefficient. Additionally, we estimated the Pearson correlation coefficient between each of the above-mentioned imaging measures and the MDS-UPDRS 1, 2, 3, and total separately.

To test if the BL imaging measures were prognostic biomarkers of disease progression, we used multiple linear regression models for predicting the changes in MDS-UPDRS scores (ΔMDS-UPDRS) between TP1 and BL. The ΔMDS-UPDRS 1, 2, 3, and total were the dependent variables, while the model regressors were the FA values in pons nuclei, prefrontal MD, DAT signal in putamen, and the interaction between putamen DAT signal and prefrontal GM volume, brainstem MD, respectively. The longitudinal prediction models were computed using data of both PD no med and on med groups. Patients receiving dopamine agonists at TP1 were not included in this analysis due to the longer wash out time of those treatments and their potential effect on the off medication assessment of symptoms severity.

To account for the effect of L-Dopa treatment on the prediction models, we performed separate regression analyses for the PD on med and no med groups. Demographic and clinical details of the two subgroups are provided in **Table 1**. Moreover we computed the Pearson correlation coefficient between each of the imaging measures and the ΔMDS-UPDRS 1, 2, 3, and total separately for the PD on med and no med groups.

The multiple regression models for each MDS-UPDRS and ΔMDS-UPDRS subscales were considered as significant at $p < 0.05$. In case of a significant multiple regression model, single regressors were considered as significant at $p < 0.01$. The Pearson correlation coefficients were corrected for multiple comparison using the false discovery rate (FDR) at $q < 0.05$.

RESULTS

Demographic and Clinical Variables

Patients and HC were matched for gender and age, as shown in **Table 1**. The groups PD on med and PD no med did not differ with respect to sex, age, and disease dominant side (see **Table 1**). All clinical scores were significantly higher for patients as compared to HC (**Table 1**). The group PD on med showed significantly higher MDS-UPDRS 1, 2, and total scores at BL and TP1, as well as higher ΔMDS-UPDRS1 and ΔMDS-UPDRS2 in comparison to the PD no med group (**Table 1**). No significant differences were found for the MDS-UPDRS3 at BL, TP1, and ΔMDS-UPDRS3 between PD on med and no med groups.

Voxel-Based Group Comparison

In PD patients significantly higher FA values were found in the brainstem WM corresponding to the pontine tegmentum (**Table 2** and **Figure 1a**). Increased MD values were found in patients with respect to HC in the operculum (**Table 2** and **Figure 1b**). No significant differences between patients and HC were observed for GM volume.

In the structural covariance analyses, we found significant differences in the correlation between DAT-SPECT in the putamen and MD values in the pons nuclei across patients and HC. The Spearman correlation coefficients showed a significant positive correlation in PD patients ($\rho = 0.25$; $p < 0.001$), and a significant negative one in HC ($\rho = -0.52$; $p < 0.001$) (**Figures 2a,b**).

Furthermore, we found significant differences between patients and HC in the covariance analysis evaluating the association between DAT-SPECT signal in the putamen and GM volume in the left prefrontal, premotor cortex and in the insula. We observed a significant positive correlation ($\rho = 0.22$; $p < 0.001$) for patients, and a significant negative correlation for controls ($\rho = -0.44$; $p < 0.001$) (**Figures 2c,d**). No significant differences were found for structural covariance between DAT-SPECT and FA values across groups.

Prediction Models: Symptoms Severity and Disease Progression

The linear combinations of DAT-SPECT values in the putamen, and MRI differences found in the group comparison, significantly predicted the BL MDS-UPDRS2 and MDS-UPDRS total but not the other subscales (see **Tables 3, 4**). The MD values in the operculum, the DAT-SPECT signal in the putamen and age were the most significant predictors for the MDS-UPDRS2, as summarized in **Tables 3, 4**. The significant predictors for

TABLE 2 | Main differences for group comparisons and covariance analyses done at baseline between healthy controls (HC) and Parkinson's disease patients (PD).

Analysis	Region	Coordinates (mm)			*T*-value	Cluster size
		x	*y*	*z*		
FA maps: PD > HC	Left pontine tegmentum	−8	−21	−21	4.7	163
	Right pontine tegmentum	9	−22	−22	4.5	167
MD maps: PD > HC	Right operculum	58	9	−2	5	1571
Covariance DAT-MD: PD > HC	Pons nuclei	4	−26	−28	4	884
Covariance DAT-GM volume: PD > HC	Left prefrontal cortex	−44	20	34	4.6	681
	Left premotor cortex	−8	6	39	4.5	607
	Left insula	−54	−14	16	4	625
	Right insula	58	−12	14	4	686

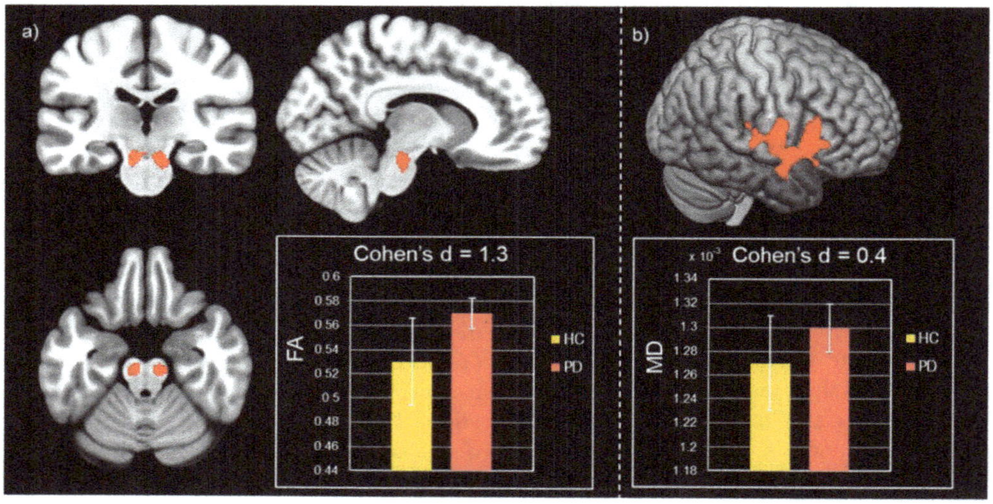

FIGURE 1 | Results of group comparisons for diffusion MRI measures. **(a)** Increased FA values in Parkinson's disease patients compared to healthy controls at pFWE < 0.05. **(b)** Higher MD values for Parkinson's disease patients with respect to healthy controls at pFWE < 0.05.

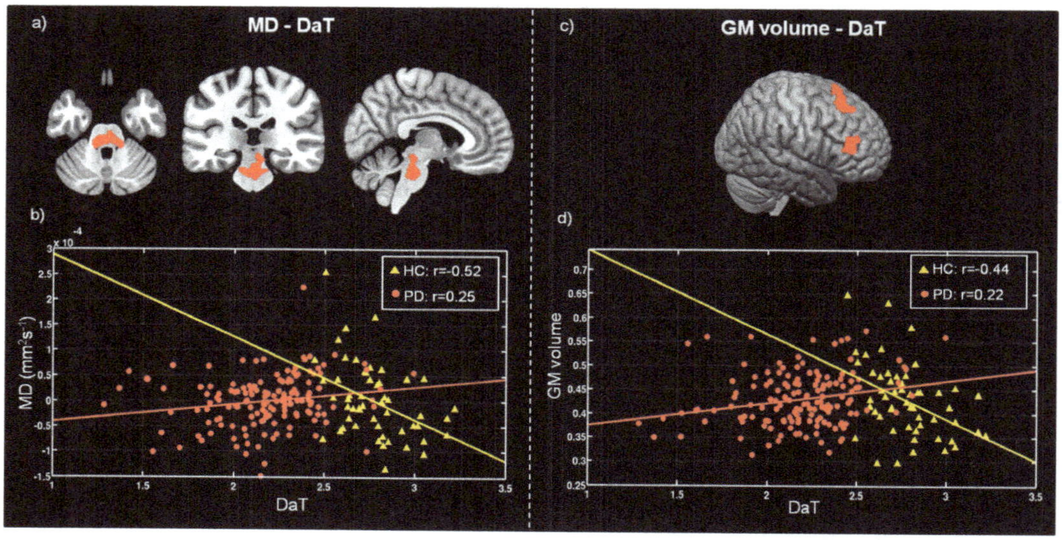

FIGURE 2 | Differences between healthy controls (HC) and Parkinson's disease patients (PD) in voxel-wise correlation of MD maps with DAT-SPECT measured in putamen **(a)**, and GM volume with mean DAT-SPECT in putamen **(c)**. **(b)** Scatter plot showing the correlation between the DAT-SPECT measured in the putamen and the mean MD values computed within the region highlighted in red on panel **(a)**, for HC (yellow triangles) and PD (red circles). **(d)** Scatter plot showing the correlation between the DAT-SPECT measured in the putamen and the mean GM volume estimated within the region highlighted in red on panel **(c)**, for HC (yellow triangles) and PD (red circles). Plot legend reports Spearman's correlation coefficients.

the MDS-UPDRS total were the MD values in the operculum, the putamen DAT-SPECT values, and the interaction between putamen DAT-SPECT – GM volume in premotor, prefrontal cortex and insula (see **Tables 3, 4**).

We did not find any significant correlation between the single imaging measures and the BS MDS-UPDRS scores.

For the longitudinal prediction models we found that the combination of BL DAT-SPECT and MRI measures was not able to significantly predict the ΔMDS-UPDRS scores for the group of patients with and without medication (see **Tables 3, 4**).

However the linear combination of BL imaging measures significantly predicted ΔMDS-UPDRS2 for the PD no med group, and ΔMDS-UPDRS1 and 2 for the PD on med (**Tables 3, 4**). The significant regressors for the prediction of ΔMDS-UPDRS2 in the PD no med group were GM volume in the premotor and prefrontal cortex, putamen DAT-SPECT, FA in the pontine tegmentum and the interaction between DAT signal in the putamen – GM volume in premotor, prefrontal cortex and insula (**Tables 3, 4**). For the PD on med, the significant predictors of ΔMDS-UPDRS1 were the MD in the pons nuclei,

TABLE 3 | Summary of the linear models explaining the MDS-UPDRS components at baseline (BL) and the MDS-UPDRS variation (ΔMDS-UPDRS) 1 year after the baseline.

Time point	Dependent variable	Model predictors: *p*-value										R^2	Adj R^2	*F*-, *p*-value
		GM vol in PFC and PMC	MD in OP	MD in PN	FA in PT	DAT in Put	Interaction DAT in Put – MD PN	Interaction DAT in Put – GM vol in PFC and PMC and IN	Age	Gender	Dominant side			
BL	MDS-UPDRS1	0.37	0.11	0.75	0.81	0.35	0.05	0.01	0.37	0.9	0.83	0.12	0.09	0.82, 0.57
	MDS-UPDRS2	**0.30**	**0.01***	**0.08**	**0.17**	**-2×10^{-4} ***	**0.39**	**0.10**	**0.01***	**0.87**	**0.12**	**0.38**	**0.29**	**4, 2×10^{-4}***
	MDS-UPDRS3	0.88	0.09	0.40	0.85	0.50	0.06	0.11	0.02	0.13	0.22	0.21	0.09	2, 0.08
	MDS-UPDRS tot	**0.9**	**0.002***	**0.23**	**0.50**	**0.006***	**0.03**	**0.002***	**0.01**	**0.31**	**0.70**	**0.31**	**0.21**	**4.85, 0.003***
Δ	MDS-UPDRS1 PD on med+no med	0.78	0.29	0.25	0.44	0.37	0.74	0.58	0.13	0.35	0.34	0.15	0.03	1.02, 0.43
	MDS-UPDRS1 PD on med	**0.87**	**0.70**	**0.003***	**0.47**	**0.01***	**0.002***	**0.32**	**0.008***	**0.96**	**0.87**	**0.47**	**0.27**	**5.7, 0.004***
	MDS-UPDRS1 PD no med	0.28	0.11	0.44	0.38	0.5	0.9	0.21	0.44	0.09	0.06	0.19	0.01	1, 0.41
	MDS-UPDRS2 PD on med+no med	0.02	0.30	0.36	0.03	0.03	0.03	0.80	0.01	0.12	0.18	0.22	0.09	1.71, 0.09
	MDS-UPDRS2 PD on med	**0.006***	**0.009***	**0.17**	**0.01***	**0.004***	**0.25**	**0.004***	**0.66**	**0.05**	**0.27**	**0.37**	**0.15**	**4.68, 0.01***
	MDS-UPDRS2 PD no med	**0.003***	**0.02**	**0.09**	**0.01***	**0.01***	**0.23**	**0.01***	**0.55**	**0.6**	**0.11**	**0.37**	**0.21**	**4.75, 0.01***
	MDS-UPDRS3 PD on med+no med	0.02	0.96	0.94	0.01	0.03	0.41	0.20	0.41	0.22	0.25	0.15	0.05	1.1, 0.38
	MDS-UPDRS3 PD on med	0.76	0.74	0.47	0.34	0.95	0.74	0.48	0.77	0.99	0.44	0.27	0.13	0.59, 0.83
	MDS-UPDRS3 PD no med	0.61	0.19	0.9	0.5	0.6	0.02	0.09	0.87	0.28	0.7	0.20	0.03	1.14, 0.35
	MDS-UPDRS tot PD on med+no med	0.02	0.98	0.92	0.01	0.01	0.03	0.71	0.08	0.98	0.38	0.17	0.03	1.3, 0.31
	MDS-UPDRS tot PD on med	0.82	0.58	0.69	0.58	0.5	0.06	0.61	0.79	0.58	0.38	0.21	0.05	0.89, 0.54
	MDS-UPDRS tot PD no med	0.14	0.24	0.03	0.34	0.04	0.73	0.37	0.86	0.16	0.22	0.27	0.11	1.69, 0.11

Models for the ΔMDS-UPDRS were estimated separately for the patients without medication 1 year after baseline (no med), for the patients on L-Dopa 1 year after baseline (on med) and for the patients of both groups together (on med + no med). The model predictors were the mean imaging values extracted from the following regions: IN, insula; OP, operculum; PFC, prefrontal cortex; PMC, premotor cortex; PN, pons nuclei; Put, putamen; PT, pontine tegmentum. We report the p-value for every regressor, and the determination coefficient (R^2), adjusted R^2, f-value, and p-value for every model. Bold characters and "" indicate a significant ($p < 0.05$) model – ($p < 0.01$) regressors.*

TABLE 4 | Summary of the slopes (β) of the linear regressions explaining the MDS-UPDRS components at baseline (BL) and the MDS-UPDRS variation (ΔMDS-UPDRS) 1 year after the baseline.

Time point	Dependent variable	Model predictors: β slope									
		GM vol in PFC and PMC	MD in OP	MD in PN	FA in PT	DAT in Put	Interaction DAT in Put – MD PN	Interaction DAT in Put – GM vol in PFC and PMC and IN	Age	Gender	Dominant side
BL	MDS-UPDRS1	2.8	−3.7	104.7	−1.8	8.6×10^4	-3.1×10^3	−9.4	10^4	0.1	−0.1
	MDS-UPDRS2	**−0.54**	**−19.8**	**50.2**	**−6.5**	$\mathbf{3.4 \times 10^4}$	$\mathbf{-1.5 \times 10^4}$	**9.8**	$\mathbf{1.1 \times 10^4}$	**−0.1**	**−0.7**
	MDS-UPDRS3	0.8	−6.7	149	−2.9	1.9×10^5	-1.9×10^4	3.7	2.6×10^4	0.23	3.3
	MDS-UPDRS tot	**3**	**−30.3**	**303**	**−11.2**	$\mathbf{3.1 \times 10^5}$	$\mathbf{3.8 \times 10^4}$	**4**	$\mathbf{4.8 \times 10^4}$	**0.36**	**3.1**
Δ	MDS-UPDRS1 PD on med+no med	−2	−9.1	19.2	−0.4	-3.2×10^4	-8.5×10^3	3.5	5.1×10^3	0.1	−1.1
	MDS-UPDRS1 PD on med	**−3.4**	**23.2**	**81.4**	**−1.9**	$\mathbf{-2.3 \times 10^5}$	$\mathbf{-2.6 \times 10^4}$	**−8.3**	$\mathbf{-3.1 \times 10^3}$	**0.1**	**−1.4**
	MDS-UPDRS1 PD no med	1.2	−14.5	−63.4	−1.3	5.6×10^3	-7.2×10^3	11.5	1.1×10^4	0.04	−1.7
	MDS-UPDRS2 PD on med+no med	2.3	−1	−29.7	−0.6	-7.5×10^4	6.4×10^3	7.6	1.7×10^4	−0.01	0.5
	MDS-UPDRS2 PD on med	**−9.4**	**−20.1**	**235**	**9.3**	$\mathbf{3.3 \times 10^4}$	$\mathbf{3.2 \times 10^4}$	**−24.1**	$\mathbf{1.5 \times 10^4}$	**0.07**	**2.9**
	MDS-UPDRS2 PD no med	**5.5**	**−26.8**	**−116.8**	**−2.8**	$\mathbf{-5.9 \times 10^4}$	**−865.3**	**9.5**	$\mathbf{2.3 \times 10^4}$	**−0.03**	**−0.5**
	MDS-UPDRS3 PD on med+no med	9.5	29.6	14.1	−1.3	-2.2×10^5	1.1×10^4	7.2	2.1×10^4	−0.1	−1
	MDS-UPDRS3 PD on med	−5	−42.8	447.3	13.6	3.3×10^5	1.1×10^5	−139.7	1.2×10^4	−0.03	2.7
	MDS-UPDRS3 PD no med	9.8	−31	−240.1	−2.9	-3.1×10^5	-4.2×10^3	15.2	2.5×10^4	0.02	−3
	MDS-UPDRS tot PD on med+no med	9.8	19.5	3.7	−2.3	-3.3×10^5	9.1×10^3	18.3	4.3×10^4	−0.01	−1.6
	MDS-UPDRS tot PD on med	−17.7	−40	763.8	21.1	1.3×10^5	1.1×10^5	−172.1	2.4×10^4	0.1	4.1
	MDS-UPDRS tot PD no med	16.5	−72.3	−420.3	−7.1	-3.6×10^5	-1.2×10^4	36.1	5.9×10^4	0.03	−5.3

Models for the ΔMDS-UPDRS were estimated separately for the patients without medication 1 year after baseline (no med), for the patients on L-Dopa 1 year after baseline (on med) and for the patients of both groups together (on med + no med). The model predictors were the mean imaging values extracted from the following regions: IN, insula; OP, operculum; PFC, prefrontal cortex; PMC, premotor cortex; PN, pons nuclei; Put, putamen; PT, pontine tegmentum. Bold characters indicate a significant ($p < 0.05$) model – ($p < 0.01$) regressors.

the DAT-SPECT in the putamen, interaction DAT – MD in the pons nuclei and age. The premotor and prefrontal GM volume, putamen DAT binding, MD in the pons nuclei and the interaction DAT in putamen – MD in pons nuclei significantly predicted ΔMDS-UPDRS2 for the PD on med group.

We did not find any significant correlation between the single imaging measures and the ΔMDS-UPDRS scores for both the PD no med and on med groups.

DISCUSSION

Here, we evaluated the relative and combined value of MRI and DAT-SPECT measures as biomarkers of disease severity and clinical progression in *de novo* PD patients. Consistent with prior literature, we identified DAT-SPECT and MRI abnormalities in patients compared to the HC (Brooks, 1998; Lee et al., 2000; Isaias et al., 2007; Gattellaro et al., 2009; Wang et al., 2011). Most importantly, we found that in combination, these imaging abnormalities could reliably predict both current clinical symptoms and their progression over time, suggesting that they could be used as prognostic biomarkers.

Clinical Variables

Prior to perform the image comparison and the prediction analysis of the clinical scores, we statistically compared the MDS-UPDRS across groups. As expected, we found significantly higher clinical scores for the PD patients with respect to the HC. Moreover, we observed significantly higher increase of the MDS-UPDRS 1, 2, and total scores at BL and TP1, as well as ΔMDS-UPDRS1 and ΔMDS-UPDRS2 for the PD group on med with respect to the PD no med group. Those results are in agreement with the fact that patients on medication exhibit more advanced disease stages. The lack of significant difference in MDS-UPDRS3 between the PD on med and PD no med groups might be explained by the fact that the motor assessment is a highly variable measure, involving both patient- and rater-dependent variability (Mentzel et al., 2016; Rahmim et al., 2017). The use of a longitudinal clinical assessment over 1 year might have increased this variability, confounding potential differences between the groups.

Regional Findings

Earlier studies have reported altered diffusion MRI measures across different brain areas in PD and associated animal models (Peran et al., 2010; Wang et al., 2011; Zhang et al., 2011, 2015; Du et al., 2012; Schwarz et al., 2013; Tan et al., 2015; Lim et al., 2016; Loane et al., 2016; Nagae et al., 2016). Consistent with those findings, we showed distinct patterns of MD alterations in the prefrontal cortex, suggesting underlying microstructure degradation that might be due to the loss of dopaminergic input into the striatum (Hornykiewicz, 1998; Mattay et al., 2002; Gattellaro et al., 2009; Zhan et al., 2012; Kim et al., 2013).

Furthermore, we found increased FA values in PD patients in midbrain regions corresponding to the location of pontine tegmentum. This region is affected by the alpha synuclein pathology at early disease stages (Braak et al., 2003; Mori et al., 2008; Venda et al., 2010), and it is associated with the patho-physiology of sleep behavior disorder frequently observed at prodromal disease stage (Iranzo et al., 2006; Burke and O'Malley, 2013). There is substantial controversy in the literature about the magnitude, directionality and neurobiological interpretation of FA changes in this region. While Wang et al. (2011) also found increased FA values in the substantia nigra, other studies reported lowered FA in PD patients in this region (Peran et al., 2010; Rolheiser et al., 2011; Du et al., 2012; Prakash et al., 2012; Zhang et al., 2016). The reason for this divergence remains unclear but might be related to the inclusion of more advanced PD patients in those studies.

Structural Network Findings

In agreement with previous research showing 40–60% loss of striatal dopaminergic innervations from substantia nigra in *de novo* PD patients, we found a significantly reduced DAT-SPECT signal in the striatum (Brooks, 1998; Lee et al., 2000; Isaias et al., 2007). Our findings on significant interactions between putamen DAT uptake and MD values in the pons nuclei are in line with the known disruption of brainstem projections to the striatum. More specifically, we found that a lower striatal DAT uptake was linked to lower MD values in PD patients, which was the opposite of what we observed in HC. This finding supports the idea that structural covariance might be more sensitive to axonal and neuronal damage in the ponto-mesencephalic tegmentum, which did not show significant MD changes in direct group comparisons. The pons nuclei represent the anatomical origin of projections modulating the dopaminergic action of the substantia nigra and they are under dopaminergic inhibitory control from the ventral tegmental area, which is known to degenerate in PD (Guiard et al., 2008). According to the physiological functions attributed to the noradrenergic system, impaired functioning of pons nuclei in PD results primarily in affective disorders (Remy et al., 2005), cognitive disturbances (Javoy-Agid and Agid, 1980), sleep disorders (Boeve et al., 2007), sensory impairment (Braak et al., 2003) and autonomic dysfunction (Orskov et al., 1987).

Furthermore, in PD patients we found a decrease in putamen DAT being linked to lower GM volume values in the premotor-prefrontal cortex, while in HC a reduction in putamen DAT was associated to a bigger GM volume. While, we did not detect any significant atrophy in those cortical regions using group comparisons, these findings suggested that progressive loss of striatal DAT uptake translates into GM volume loss in premotor-prefrontal regions. This result is in line with studies showing that significant GM volume loss is predominantly observed in more advanced PD patients exhibiting cognitive deficits (Beyer et al., 2007; Melzer et al., 2012). The clinical stage arises when the disease spreads from brainstem to basal ganglia nuclei and then to cortical regions in an ascending course (Lang and Lozano, 1998; Braak et al., 2003).

Prediction of Symptom Severity and Disease Progression

After identifying these alterations in patients compared to HC, we then evaluated their link to current disease severity and their prognostic value for future symptoms progression measured by the MDS-UPDRS subscales. We showed that the combination of the imaging measures was significantly related to the current clinical severity measured by MDS-UPDRS2 and MDS-UPDRS total. The imaging measures that better predicted the BL MDS-UPDRS2 were the MD values in the operculum and the DAT-SPECT signal in the putamen, while the MDS-UPDRS total was better predicted by the MD values in the operculum, the putamen DAT-SPECT values, and the interaction between putamen DAT-SPECT – GM volume in premotor, prefrontal cortex and insula. The absence of significant correlation between each of those imaging measures and the MDS-UPDRS2 and MDS-UPDRS total is in agreement with results previously reported literature (McGhee et al., 2013). Moreover this result highlights the fact that the combination of those imaging measures, rather than each single one, could be used as biomarker for predicting symptoms measured by MDS-UPDRS2.

The MDS-UPDRS2 is a subscale evaluating the subject's impairment in daily life activities (Goetz et al., 2008), and it is often used to evaluate symptoms severity perceived by the patient. Consequently MDS-UPDRS2 can be used to assess improvements related to pharmacological treatments or surgical therapies such as deep brain stimulation (Rodriguez-Oroz et al., 2005).

One key objective of the study was to evaluate the association between the imaging biomarkers and disease progression. As dopaminergic treatments have substantial effects on the clinical symptoms measured with MDS-UPDRS, those treatments represent a potential confound that needs to be controlled for. Due to this reason we first performed the predictive analysis of symptoms progression using the entire PD cohort and then we employed separate models for the PD no med and on med groups. For the patients on medications we employed the MDS-UPDRS scores assessed off medication. The off medication clinical assessments performed for the PPMI study were acquired asking the patients not to take PD medication the day before. While, the half-life of L-Dopa is short enough to achieve a sufficient wash out in 24 h, the half-life of dopamine agonists or other medications could be longer and therefore be not sufficient to estimate a proper off medication symptom severity (Brooks, 2008; Onofrj et al., 2009; Reichmann, 2009). For this reason, we restricted our analyses of the patients treated only with L-Dopa.

We found that GM volume extracted from the premotor cortex, putamen DAT, the interaction between both, and brainstem FA values were significant predictors for ΔMDS-UPDRS2 in the untreated patients. The ΔMDS-UPDRS2 in the group on medication was significantly predicted by the same measures with the addition of MD assessed in the pons nuclei. Though the separation of PD patients in no med and on med groups was performed to exclude confounds of treatment onto the MDS-UPDRS scales, the separate analyses could be also considered as independent replication samples of the prognostic link of MRI and DAT measures onto clinical symptoms measures. This consistency of the significant association between the identified structural measures and ΔMDS-UPDRS2 across both groups strengthens the confidence in these findings.

Finally, we found that the MD in the pons nuclei, putamen DAT-SPECT, interaction DAT – MD in the pons nuclei were significant predictors of ΔMDS-UPDRS1, which is associated to non-motor and cognitive deficits. However, the significant prediction of the ΔMDS-UPDRS1 was only observed in the on med group. Beside the possibility of being a false positive finding, this difference could also reflect the more severe phenotype in the on med group or the more complex effects of treatment onto clinical severity captured by MDS-UPDRS1. In fact the L-Dopa treatment of the on med group is likely to interfere with the clinical measures of symptoms severity as no off medication assessment was performed for the MDS-UPDRS1. Therefore it is important to replicate this association in an independent cohort in order to evaluate the prognostic ability of those imaging measures for the ΔMDS-UPDRS1.

The linear combination of DAT-SPECT and MRI measures was not able to significantly predict the symptoms progression at TP1 using the data of both PD no med and on med groups. This results might be indicative of the fact that using heterogeneous groups of patients could confound the reliability of predictive analysis (Miller and O'Callaghan, 2015; Tuite, 2016).

The lack of significant correlation between each of the imaging measures used in this study and the ΔMDS-UPDRS scores confirms previous literature results (McGhee et al., 2013). The crucial finding of this analysis was that the combination of DAT-SPECT imaging, structural and diffusion MRI achieved reliable prediction of some symptom severity scores and disease progression in 1 year in homogeneous cohort of patients, as reported by a previous study (Rahmim et al., 2017), while the single imaging measures failed to provide significant correlation with those scores. Many studies in literature assessed the correlations between disease severity-progression and brain changes in PD patients using uni-modal approaches (Burton et al., 2004; Nagano-Saito et al., 2005; Benninger et al., 2009; Wattendorf et al., 2009; Schwarz et al., 2013). The results cover different regions with a wide variety of repeatability and low correlations with clinical scores.

The findings obtained in the current study can be indicative of the presence of microstructural tissue changes induced by the disease in the early stages. In light of the correlation with the clinical progression, the combination of the imaging measures affected by those tissue changes could be employed as disease progression biomarker.

Cross-sectional and longitudinal studies in PD patients will be crucial to confirm our results and establish the value of the identified imaging alterations in more advanced and prodromal PD populations.

Limitations and Outlook

Here, we investigate the association between different imaging and clinical measures in a large cohort of *de novo* untreated PD patients. The acquisition of all those imaging modalities might be time-consuming and expensive, limiting their use in clinical protocols. However, recent advances in MRI hardware, such as improved scanner gradient performance, and software, such as parallel imaging and multi-band imaging sequences (Griswold et al., 2002; Setsompop et al., 2012; Uecker et al., 2014), can substantially reduce the time required for acquiring MRI data.

Despite the good correlation between brain changes and clinical scores, the study provides a reliable prediction only for some symptom subtypes. This might be due to the fact that the disease progression differentially affects the various cortical-subcortical circuits (Kish et al., 1988).

We find several potential structural and molecular imaging biomarkers altered in *de novo* PD patients. We further show the potential of these alterations as biomarkers of current symptom severity and their prognostic value with respect to evolution of specific PD symptom domains.

AUTHOR CONTRIBUTIONS

JD, FS, AB, and BD conceptualized the research project. JD organized the research project. SL executed the research project and statistical analysis, and wrote the first draft of manuscript. SL and JD designed the statistical analysis. JD critically reviewed the statistical analysis. SL, JD, FS, AB, and BD critically reviewed the manuscript.

FUNDING

Data used in the preparation of this article were obtained from the PPMI database (www.ppmi-info.org/data). For up-to-date information on the study, visit www.ppmi-info.org. PPMI – a public-private partnership – is funded by the Michael J. Fox Foundation for Parkinson's Research and funding partners, including Abbvie, Avid Radiopharmaceuticals, Biogen Idec, Briston-Myers Squibb, Covance, GE Healthcare, Genentech, GlaxoSmithKline, Lilly, Lundbeck, Merck, Meso Scale Discovery, Pfizer, Piramal, Roche, and UCB. SL was supported by the National Institute for Health Research Biomedical Research Centre at Great Ormond Street Hospital for Children NHS Foundation Trust, The Henry Smith Charity, and Action Medical Research (GN2214). BD was supported by the Swiss National Science Foundation (project grant no. 32003B_159780 and SPUM 33CM30_140332/1), Foundation Parkinson Switzerland, Foundation Synapsis. LREN is grateful to the Roger de Spoelberch and the Partridge Foundations for their generous support.

ACKNOWLEDGMENTS

We would like to thank David W. Carmichael for providing useful feedback on the manuscript.

REFERENCES

Alexander-Bloch, A., Giedd, J. N., and Bullmore, E. (2013a). Imaging structural co-variance between human brain regions. *Nat. Rev. Neurosci.* 14, 322–336. doi: 10.1038/nrn3465

Alexander-Bloch, A., Raznahan, A., Bullmore, E., and Giedd, J. (2013b). The convergence of maturational change and structural covariance in human cortical networks. *J. Neurosci.* 33, 2889–2899. doi: 10.1523/JNEUROSCI.3554-12.2013

Ashburner, J. (2007). A fast diffeomorphic image registration algorithm. *Neuroimage* 38, 95–113. doi: 10.1016/j.neuroimage.2007.07.007

Ashburner, J., Csernansky, J. G., Davatzikos, C., Fox, N. C., Frisoni, G. B., and Thompson, P. M. (2003). Computer-assisted imaging to assess brain structure in healthy and diseased brains. *Lancet Neurol.* 2, 79–88. doi: 10.1016/S1474-4422(03)00304-1

Ashburner, J., and Friston, K. J. (2000). Voxel-based morphometry–the methods. *Neuroimage* 11, 805–821. doi: 10.1006/nimg.2000.0582

Ashburner, J., and Friston, K. J. (2005). Unified segmentation. *Neuroimage* 26, 839–851. doi: 10.1016/j.neuroimage.2005.02.018

Atkinson-Clement, C., Pinto, S., Eusebio, A., and Coulon, O. (2017). Diffusion tensor imaging in Parkinson's disease: review and meta-analysis. *Neuroimage Clin.* 16, 98–110. doi: 10.1016/j.nicl.2017.07.011

Benninger, D. H., Thees, S., Kollias, S. S., Bassetti, C. L., and Waldvogel, D. (2009). Morphological differences in Parkinson's disease with and without rest tremor. *J. Neurol.* 256, 256–263. doi: 10.1007/s00415-009-0092-2

Beyer, M. K., Janvin, C. C., Larsen, J. P., and Aarsland, D. (2007). A magnetic resonance imaging study of patients with Parkinson's disease with mild cognitive impairment and dementia using voxel-based morphometry. *J. Neurol. Neurosurg. Psychiatry* 78, 254–259. doi: 10.1136/jnnp.2006.093849

Boeve, B. F., Silber, M. H., Saper, C. B., Ferman, T. J., Dickson, D. W., Parisi, J. E., et al. (2007). Pathophysiology of REM sleep behaviour disorder and relevance to neurodegenerative disease. *Brain J. Neurol.* 130, 2770–2788. doi: 10.1093/brain/awm056

Braak, H., Tredici, K. D., Rüb, U., de Vos, R. A. I., Jansen Steur, E. N. H., and Braak, E. (2003). Staging of brain pathology related to sporadic Parkinson's disease. *Neurobiol. Aging* 24, 197–211. doi: 10.1016/S0197-4580(02)00065-9

Brooks, D. J. (1998). The early diagnosis of Parkinson's disease. *Ann. Neurol.* 44, S10–S18. doi: 10.1002/ana.410440704

Brooks, D. J. (2008). Optimizing levodopa therapy for Parkinson's disease with levodopa/carbidopa/entacapone: implications from a clinical and patient perspective. *Neuropsychiatr. Dis. Treat.* 4, 39–47. doi: 10.2147/NDT.S1660

Burke, R. E., and O'Malley, K. (2013). Axon degeneration in Parkinson's disease. *Exp. Neurol.* 246, 72–83. doi: 10.1016/j.expneurol.2012.01.011

Burton, E. J., McKeith, I. G., Burn, D. J., Williams, E. D., and O'Brien, J. T. (2004). Cerebral atrophy in Parkinson's disease with and without dementia: a comparison with Alzheimer's disease, dementia with Lewy bodies and controls. *Brain* 127, 791–800. doi: 10.1093/brain/awh088

Camicioli, R., Sabino, J., Gee, M., Bouchard, T., Fisher, N., Hanstock, C., et al. (2011). Ventricular dilatation and brain atrophy in patients with Parkinson's disease with incipient dementia. *Mov. Disord.* 26, 1443–1450. doi: 10.1002/mds.23700

Campabadal, A., Uribe, C., Segura, B., Baggio, H. C., Abos, A., Garcia-Diaz, A. I., et al. (2017). Brain correlates of progressive olfactory loss in Parkinson's disease. *Parkinsonism Relat. Disord.* 41, 44–50. doi: 10.1016/j.parkreldis.2017.05.005

Chang, Y.-T., Hsu, S.-W., Tsai, S.-J., Chang, Y.-T., Huang, C.-W., Liu, M.-E., et al. (2017). Genetic effect of MTHFR C677T polymorphism on the structural covariance network and white-matter integrity in Alzheimer's disease. *Hum. Brain Mapp.* 38, 3039–3051. doi: 10.1002/hbm.23572

Chou, K.-H., Lin, W.-C., Lee, P.-L., Tsai, N.-W., Huang, Y.-C., Chen, H.-L., et al. (2015). Structural covariance networks of striatum subdivision in patients with Parkinson's disease. *Hum. Brain Mapp.* 36, 1567–1584. doi: 10.1002/hbm.22724

de Schipper, L. J., van der Grond, J., Marinus, J., Henselmans, J. M. L., and van Hilten, J. J. (2017). Loss of integrity and atrophy in cingulate structural covariance networks in Parkinson's disease. *Neuroimage Clin.* 15, 587–593. doi: 10.1016/j.nicl.2017.05.012

Draganski, B., Ashburner, J., Hutton, C., Kherif, F., Frackowiak, R. S. J., Helms, G., et al. (2011). Regional specificity of MRI contrast parameter changes in normal ageing revealed by voxel-based quantification (VBQ). *Neuroimage* 55, 1423–1434. doi: 10.1016/j.neuroimage.2011.01.052

Du, G., Lewis, M. M., Sen, S., Wang, J., Shaffer, M. L., Styner, M., et al. (2012). Imaging nigral pathology and clinical progression in Parkinson's disease. *Mov. Disord.* 27, 1636–1643. doi: 10.1002/mds.25182

Gattellaro, G., Minati, L., Grisoli, M., Mariani, C., Carella, F., Osio, M., et al. (2009). White matter involvement in idiopathic Parkinson disease: a diffusion tensor imaging study. *Am. J. Neuroradiol.* 30, 1222–1226. doi: 10.3174/ajnr.A1556

Goetz, C. G., Tilley, B. C., Shaftman, S. R., Stebbins, G. T., Fahn, S., Martinez-Martin, P., et al. (2008). Movement Disorder Society-sponsored revision of the Unified Parkinson's Disease Rating Scale (MDS-UPDRS): scale presentation and clinimetric testing results. *Mov. Disord.* 23, 2129–2170. doi: 10.1002/mds.22340

Gong, G., He, Y., Chen, Z. J., and Evans, A. C. (2012). Convergence and divergence of thickness correlations with diffusion connections across the human cerebral cortex. *Neuroimage* 59, 1239–1248. doi: 10.1016/j.neuroimage.2011.08.017

Greve, D. N., and Fischl, B. (2009). Accurate and robust brain image alignment using boundary-based registration. *Neuroimage* 48, 63–72. doi: 10.1016/j.neuroimage.2009.06.060

Griswold, M. A., Jakob, P. M., Heidemann, R. M., Nittka, M., Jellus, V., Wang, J., et al. (2002). Generalized autocalibrating partially parallel acquisitions (GRAPPA). *Magn. Reson. Med.* 47, 1202–1210. doi: 10.1002/mrm.10171

Guiard, B. P., El Mansari, M., and Blier, P. (2008). Cross-talk between dopaminergic and noradrenergic systems in the rat ventral tegmental area, locus ceruleus, and dorsal hippocampus. *Mol. Pharmacol.* 74, 1463–1475. doi: 10.1124/mol.108.048033

Helmich, R. C., Derikx, L. C., Bakker, M., Scheeringa, R., Bloem, B. R., and Toni, I. (2010). Spatial remapping of cortico-striatal connectivity in Parkinson's disease. *Cereb. Cortex* 20, 1175–1186. doi: 10.1093/cercor/bhp178

Hornykiewicz, O. (1998). Biochemical aspects of Parkinson's disease. *Neurology* 51, S2–S9. doi: 10.1212/WNL.51.2_Suppl_2.S2

Houk, J. C., and Wise, S. P. (1995). Feature article: distributed modular architectures linking basal ganglia, cerebellum, and cerebral cortex: their role in planning and controlling action. *Cereb. Cortex* 5, 95–110. doi: 10.1093/cercor/5.2.95

Iranzo, A., Molinuevo, J. L., Santamaría, J., Serradell, M., Martí, M. J., Valldeoriola, F., et al. (2006). Rapid-eye-movement sleep behaviour disorder as an early marker for a neurodegenerative disorder: a descriptive study. *Lancet Neurol.* 5, 572–577. doi: 10.1016/S1474-4422(06)70476-8

Isaias, I. U., Benti, R., Cilia, R., Canesi, M., Marotta, G., Gerundini, P., et al. (2007). [123I]FP-CIT striatal binding in early Parkinson's disease patients with tremor vs. akinetic-rigid onset. *Neuroreport* 18, 1499–1502. doi: 10.1097/WNR.0b013e3282ef69f9

Javoy-Agid, F., and Agid, Y. (1980). Is the mesocortical dopaminergic system involved in Parkinson disease? *Neurology* 30, 1326–1330.

Junqué, C., Ramírez-Ruiz, B., Tolosa, E., Summerfield, C., Martí, M.-J., Pastor, P., et al. (2005). Amygdalar and hippocampal MRI volumetric reductions in Parkinson's disease with dementia. *Mov. Disord.* 20, 540–544. doi: 10.1002/mds.20371

Kägi, G., Bhatia, K. P., and Tolosa, E. (2010). The role of DAT-SPECT in movement disorders. *J. Neurol. Neurosurg. Psychiatry* 81, 5–12. doi: 10.1136/jnnp.2008.157370

Kim, H. J., Kim, S. J., Kim, H. S., Choi, C. G., Kim, N., Han, S., et al. (2013). Alterations of mean diffusivity in brain white matter and deep gray matter in Parkinson's disease. *Neurosci. Lett.* 550, 64–68. doi: 10.1016/j.neulet.2013.06.050

Kish, S. J., Shannak, K., and Hornykiewicz, O. (1988). Uneven pattern of dopamine loss in the striatum of patients with idiopathic Parkinson's disease. Pathophysiologic and clinical implications. *N. Engl. J. Med.* 318, 876–880. doi: 10.1056/NEJM198804073181402

Kraemmer, J., Kovacs, G. G., Perju-Dumbrava, L., Pirker, S., Traub-Weidinger, T., and Pirker, W. (2014). Correlation of striatal dopamine transporter imaging with post mortem *Substantia nigra* cell counts. *Mov. Disord.* 29, 1767–1773. doi: 10.1002/mds.25975

Lang, A. E., and Lozano, A. M. (1998). Parkinson's disease. *N. Engl. J. Med.* 339, 1044–1053. doi: 10.1056/NEJM199810083391506

Le Bihan, D., Mangin, J.-F., Poupon, C., Clark, C. A., Pappata, S., Molko, N., et al. (2001). Diffusion tensor imaging: concepts and applications. *J. Magn. Reson. Imaging* 13, 534–546. doi: 10.1002/jmri.1076

Lee, C. S., Samii, A., Sossi, V., Ruth, T. J., Schulzer, M., Holden, J. E., et al. (2000). In vivo positron emission tomographic evidence for compensatory changes in presynaptic dopaminergic nerve terminals in Parkinson's disease. *Ann. Neurol.* 47, 493–503. doi: 10.1002/1531-8249(200004)47:4<493::AID-ANA13>3.0.CO;2-4

Lim, J.-S., Shin, S. A., Lee, J.-Y., Nam, H., Lee, J.-Y., and Kim, Y. K. (2016). Neural substrates of rapid eye movement sleep behavior disorder in Parkinson's disease. *Parkinsonism Relat. Disord.* 23, 31–36. doi: 10.1016/j.parkreldis.2015.11.027

Loane, C., Politis, M., Kefalopoulou, Z., Valle-Guzman, N., Paul, G., Widner, H., et al. (2016). Aberrant nigral diffusion in Parkinson's disease: a longitudinal diffusion tensor imaging study. *Mov. Disord.* 31, 1020–1026. doi: 10.1002/mds.26606

Lorio, S., Fresard, S., Adaszewski, S., Kherif, F., Chowdhury, R., Frackowiak, R. S., et al. (2016). New tissue priors for improved automated classification of subcortical brain structures on MRI. *Neuroimage* 130, 157–166. doi: 10.1016/j.neuroimage.2016.01.062

Mattay, V. S., Tessitore, A., Callicott, J. H., Bertolino, A., Goldberg, T. E., Chase, T. N., et al. (2002). Dopaminergic modulation of cortical function in patients with Parkinson's disease. *Ann. Neurol.* 51, 156–164. doi: 10.1002/ana.10078

McGhee, D. J., Royle, P. L., Thompson, P. A., Wright, D. E., Zajicek, J. P., and Counsell, C. E. (2013). A systematic review of biomarkers for disease progression in Parkinson's disease. *BMC Neurol.* 13:35. doi: 10.1186/1471-2377-13-35

Mechelli, A., Friston, K. J., Frackowiak, R. S., and Price, C. J. (2005). Structural covariance in the human cortex. *J. Neurosci.* 25, 8303–8310. doi: 10.1523/JNEUROSCI.0357-05.2005

Meijer, F. J. A., Bloem, B. R., Mahlknecht, P., Seppi, K., and Goraj, B. (2013). Update on diffusion MRI in Parkinson's disease and atypical parkinsonism. *J. Neurol. Sci.* 332, 21–29. doi: 10.1016/j.jns.2013.06.032

Melzer, T. R., Watts, R., MacAskill, M. R., Pitcher, T. L., Livingston, L., Keenan, R. J., et al. (2012). Grey matter atrophy in cognitively impaired Parkinson's disease. *J. Neurol. Neurosurg. Psychiatry* 83, 188–194. doi: 10.1136/jnnp-2011-300828

Mentzel, T. Q., Lieverse, R., Levens, A., Mentzel, C. L., Tenback, D. E., Bakker, P. R., et al. (2016). Reliability and validity of an instrument for the assessment of bradykinesia. *Psychiatry Res.* 238, 189–195. doi: 10.1016/j.psychres.2016.02.011

Miller, D. B., and O'Callaghan, J. P. (2015). Biomarkers of Parkinson's disease: present and future. *Metabolism* 64, S40–S46. doi: 10.1016/j.metabol.2014.10.030

Mori, F., Tanji, K., Zhang, H.-X., Nishihira, Y., Tan, C.-F., Takahashi, H., et al. (2008). Maturation process of TDP-43-positive neuronal cytoplasmic inclusions in amyotrophic lateral sclerosis with and without dementia. *Acta Neuropathol.* 116, 193–203. doi: 10.1007/s00401-008-0396-9

Mueller, K., Jech, R., Ballarini, T., Holiga, Š., Růžička, F., Piecha, F. A., et al. (2018). Modulatory effects of levodopa on cerebellar connectivity in Parkinson's disease. *Cerebellum* doi: 10.1007/s12311-018-0981-y [Epub ahead of print].

Müller-Gärtner, H. W., Links, J. M., Prince, J. L., Bryan, R. N., McVeigh, E., Leal, J. P., et al. (1992). Measurement of radiotracer concentration in brain gray matter using positron emission tomography: MRI-based correction for partial volume effects. *J. Cereb. Blood Flow Metab.* 12, 571–583. doi: 10.1038/jcbfm.1992.81

Nagae, L. M., Honce, J. M., Tanabe, J., Shelton, E., Sillau, S. H., and Berman, B. D. (2016). Microstructural changes within the basal ganglia differ between Parkinson disease subtypes. *Front. Neuroanat.* 10:17. doi: 10.3389/fnana.2016.00017

Nagano-Saito, A., Washimi, Y., Arahata, Y., Kachi, T., Lerch, J. P., Evans, A. C., et al. (2005). Cerebral atrophy and its relation to cognitive impairment in Parkinson disease. *Neurology* 64, 224–229. doi: 10.1212/01.WNL.0000149510.41793.50

Onofrj, M., Bonanni, L., De Angelis, M. V., Anzellotti, F., Ciccocioppo, F., and Thomas, A. (2009). Long half-life and prolonged-release dopamine receptor agonists: a review of ropinirole prolonged-release studies. *Parkinsonism Relat. Disord.* 15(Suppl. 4), S85–S92. doi: 10.1016/S1353-8020(09)70842-9

Oosterwijk, C. S., Vriend, C., Berendse, H. W., van der Werf, Y. D., and van den Heuvel, O. A. (2018). Anxiety in Parkinson's disease is associated with reduced structural covariance of the striatum. *J. Affect. Disord.* 240, 113–120. doi: 10.1016/j.jad.2018.07.053

Orskov, L., Jakobsen, J., Dupont, E., de Fine Olivarius, B., and Christensen, N. J. (1987). Autonomic function in Parkinsonian patients relates to duration of disease. *Neurology* 37, 1173–1178. doi: 10.1212/WNL.37.7.1173

Peran, P., Cherubini, A., Assogna, F., Piras, F., Quattrocchi, C., Peppe, A., et al. (2010). Magnetic resonance imaging markers of Parkinson's disease nigrostriatal signature. *Brain* 133, 3423–3433. doi: 10.1093/brain/awq212

Prakash, B. D., Sitoh, Y.-Y., Tan, L. C. S., and Au, W. L. (2012). Asymmetrical diffusion tensor imaging indices of the rostral *Substantia nigra* in Parkinson's disease. *Parkinsonism Relat. Disord.* 18, 1029–1033. doi: 10.1016/j.parkreldis.2012.05.021

Prodoehl, J., Yu, H., Little, D. M., Abraham, I., and Vaillancourt, D. E. (2008). Region of interest template for the human basal ganglia: comparing EPI and standardized space approaches. *Neuroimage* 39, 956–965. doi: 10.1016/j.neuroimage.2007.09.027

Pyatigorskaya, N., Gallea, C., Garcia-Lorenzo, D., Vidailhet, M., and Lehericy, S. (2014). A review of the use of magnetic resonance imaging in Parkinson's disease. *Ther. Adv. Neurol. Disord.* 7, 206–220. doi: 10.1177/1756285613511507

Rahmim, A., Huang, P., Shenkov, N., Fotouhi, S., Davoodi-Bojd, E., Lu, L., et al. (2017). Improved prediction of outcome in Parkinson's disease using radiomics analysis of longitudinal DAT SPECT images. *Neuroimage Clin.* 16, 539–544. doi: 10.1016/j.nicl.2017.08.021

Reichmann, H. (2009). Dopamine agonist therapy in advanced Parkinson's disease. *J. Mov. Disord.* 2, 10–13. doi: 10.14802/jmd.09003

Remy, P., Doder, M., Lees, A., Turjanski, N., and Brooks, D. (2005). Depression in Parkinson's disease: loss of dopamine and noradrenaline innervation in the limbic system. *Brain J. Neurol.* 128, 1314–1322. doi: 10.1093/brain/awh445

Rodriguez-Oroz, M. C., Obeso, J. A., Lang, A. E., Houeto, J.-L., Pollak, P., Rehncrona, S., et al. (2005). Bilateral deep brain stimulation in Parkinson's disease: a multicentre study with 4 years follow-up. *Brain* 128, 2240–2249. doi: 10.1093/brain/awh571

Rohde, G. K., Barnett, A. S., Basser, P. J., Marenco, S., and Pierpaoli, C. (2004). Comprehensive approach for correction of motion and distortion in diffusion-weighted MRI. *Magn. Reson. Med.* 51, 103–114. doi: 10.1002/mrm.10677

Rolheiser, T. M., Fulton, H. G., Good, K. P., Fisk, J. D., McKelvey, J. R., Scherfler, C., et al. (2011). Diffusion tensor imaging and olfactory identification testing in early-stage Parkinson's disease. *J. Neurol.* 258, 1254–1260. doi: 10.1007/s00415-011-5915-2

Rousset, O. G., Ma, Y., and Evans, A. C. (1998). Correction for partial volume effects in PET: principle and validation. *J. Nucl. Med.* 39, 904–911.

Schmitt, J. E., Lenroot, R. K., Ordaz, S. E., Wallace, G. L., Lerch, J. P., Evans, A. C., et al. (2009). Variance decomposition of MRI-based covariance maps using genetically informative samples and structural equation modeling. *Neuroimage* 47, 56–64. doi: 10.1016/j.neuroimage.2008.06.039

Schwarz, S. T., Abaei, M., Gontu, V., Morgan, P. S., Bajaj, N., and Auer, D. P. (2013). Diffusion tensor imaging of nigral degeneration in Parkinson's disease: a region-of-interest and voxel-based study at 3 T and systematic review with meta-analysis. *Neuroimage Clin.* 3, 481–488. doi: 10.1016/j.nicl.2013.10.006

Segura, B., Baggio, H. C., Marti, M. J., Valldeoriola, F., Compta, Y., Garcia-Diaz, A. I., et al. (2014). Cortical thinning associated with mild cognitive impairment in Parkinson's disease. *Mov. Disord.* 29, 1495–1503. doi: 10.1002/mds.25982

Setsompop, K., Cohen-Adad, J., Gagoski, B. A., Raij, T., Yendiki, A., Keil, B., et al. (2012). Improving diffusion MRI using simultaneous multi-slice echo planar imaging. *Neuroimage* 63, 569–580. doi: 10.1016/j.neuroimage.2012.06.033

Tan, W.-Q., Yeoh, C.-S., Rumpel, H., Nadkarni, N., Lye, W.-K., Tan, E.-K., et al. (2015). Deterministic tractography of the nigrostriatal-nigropallidal pathway in Parkinson's disease. *Sci. Rep.* 5:17283. doi: 10.1038/srep17283

Tao, R., Fletcher, P. T., Gerber, S., and Whitaker, R. T. (2009). A variational image-based approach to the correction of susceptibility artifacts in the alignment of diffusion weighted and structural MRI. *Inf. Process. Med. Imaging* 21, 664–675. doi: 10.1007/978-3-642-02498-6_55

Tuite, P. (2016). Magnetic resonance imaging as a potential biomarker for Parkinson's disease. *Transl. Res.* 175, 4–16. doi: 10.1016/j.trsl.2015.12.006

Uecker, M., Lai, P., Murphy, M. J., Virtue, P., Elad, M., Pauly, J. M., et al. (2014). ESPIRiT — an eigenvalue approach to autocalibrating parallel MRI: where SENSE meets GRAPPA. *Magn. Reson. Med.* 71, 990–1001. doi: 10.1002/mrm.24751

van Ruitenbeek, P., Hernaus, D., and Mehta, M. A. (2018). A proof-of-principle study of the effect of combined haloperidol and levodopa administration on working memory-related brain activation in humans. *Hum. Psychopharmacol.* 33:e2675. doi: 10.1002/hup.2675

Venda, L. L., Cragg, S. J., Buchman, V. L., and Wade-Martins, R. (2010). α-Synuclein and dopamine at the crossroads of Parkinson's disease. *Trends Neurosci.* 33, 559–568. doi: 10.1016/j.tins.2010.09.004

Wang, J.-J., Lin, W.-Y., Lu, C.-S., Weng, Y.-H., Ng, S.-H., Wang, C.-H., et al. (2011). Parkinson disease: diagnostic utility of diffusion kurtosis imaging. *Radiology* 261, 210–217. doi: 10.1148/radiol.11102277

Wattendorf, E., Welge-Lussen, A., Fiedler, K., Bilecen, D., Wolfensberger, M., Fuhr, P., et al. (2009). Olfactory impairment predicts brain atrophy in Parkinson's disease. *J. Neurosci.* 29, 15410–15413. doi: 10.1523/JNEUROSCI.1909-09.2009

Weingarten, C. P., Sundman, M. H., Hickey, P., and Chen, N. (2015). Neuroimaging of Parkinson's disease: expanding views. *Neurosci. Biobehav. Rev.* 59, 16–52. doi: 10.1016/j.neubiorev.2015.09.007

Woo, C.-W., Chang, L. J., Lindquist, M. A., and Wager, T. D. (2017). Building better biomarkers: brain models in translational neuroimaging. *Nat. Neurosci.* 20, 365–377. doi: 10.1038/nn.4478

Xu, J., Kao, S.-Y., Lee, F. J. S., Song, W., Jin, L.-W., and Yankner, B. A. (2002). Dopamine-dependent neurotoxicity of alpha-synuclein: a mechanism for selective neurodegeneration in Parkinson disease. *Nat. Med.* 8, 600–606. doi: 10.1038/nm0602-600

Yee, Y., Fernandes, D. J., French, L., Ellegood, J., Cahill, L. S., Vousden, D. A., et al. (2018). Structural covariance of brain region volumes is associated with both structural connectivity and transcriptomic similarity. *Neuroimage* 179, 357–372. doi: 10.1016/j.neuroimage.2018.05.028

Zhan, W., Kang, G. A., Glass, G. A., Zhang, Y., Shirley, C., Millin, R., et al. (2012). Regional alterations of brain microstructure in Parkinson's disease using diffusion tensor imaging. *Mov. Disord.* 27, 90–97. doi: 10.1002/mds.23917

Zhang, K., Yu, C., Zhang, Y., Wu, X., Zhu, C., Chan, P., et al. (2011). Voxel-based analysis of diffusion tensor indices in the brain in patients with Parkinson's disease. *Eur. J. Radiol.* 77, 269–273. doi: 10.1016/j.ejrad.2009.07.032

Zhang, Y., Wu, I.-W., Buckley, S., Coffey, C. S., Foster, E., Mendick, S., et al. (2015). Diffusion tensor imaging of the nigrostriatal fibers in Parkinson's disease. *Mov. Disord.* 30, 1229–1236. doi: 10.1002/mds.26251

Zhang, Y., Wu, I.-W., Tosun, D., Foster, E., Schuff, N., and Parkinson's Progression Markers Initiative (2016). Progression of regional microstructural degeneration in Parkinson's disease: a multicenter diffusion tensor imaging study. *PLoS One* 11:e0165540. doi: 10.1371/journal.pone.0165540

3

Distinct Brain Regions in Physiological and Pathological Brain Aging

*Jin San Lee[1,2,3], Yu Hyun Park[1,2], Seongbeom Park[1,2], Uicheul Yoon[4], Yeongsim Choe[1,2], Bo Kyoung Cheon[1,2], Alice Hahn[1,2], Soo Hyun Cho[5], Seung Joo Kim[6], Jun Pyo Kim[1,2], Young Hee Jung[1,2], Key-Chung Park[3], Hee Jin Kim[1,2], Hyemin Jang[1,2], Duk L. Na[1,2] and Sang Won Seo[1,2,7,8]**

[1] Department of Neurology, Samsung Medical Center, Sungkyunkwan University School of Medicine, Seoul, South Korea, [2] Neuroscience Center, Samsung Medical Center, Seoul, South Korea, [3] Department of Neurology, Kyung Hee University Hospital, Seoul, South Korea, [4] Department of Biomedical Engineering, Daegu Catholic University, Gyeongsan, South Korea, [5] Department of Neurology, Chonnam National University Medical School, Gwangju, South Korea, [6] Department of Neurology, Gyeongsang National University School of Medicine and Gyeongsang National University Changwon Hospital, Changwon, South Korea, [7] Samsung Alzheimer Research Center, Center for Clinical Epidemiology, Samsung Medical Center, Seoul, South Korea, [8] Department of Health Sciences and Technology, Clinical Research Design and Evaluation, SAIHST, Sungkyunkwan University, Seoul, South Korea

Correspondence:
Sang Won Seo
sangwonseo@empal.com;
sangwonseo@empas.com

Background: Studying structural brain aging is important to understand age-related pathologies, as well as to identify the early manifestations of the Alzheimer's disease (AD) continuum. In this study, we investigated the long-term trajectory of physiological and pathological brain aging in a large number of participants ranging from the 50s to over 80 years of age.

Objective: To explore the distinct brain regions that distinguish pathological brain aging from physiological brain aging using sophisticated measurements of cortical thickness.

Methods: A total of 2,823 cognitively normal (CN) individuals and 2,675 patients with AD continuum [874 with subjective memory impairment (SMI), 954 with amnestic mild cognitive impairment (aMCI), and 847 with AD dementia] who underwent a high-resolution 3.0-tesla MRI were included in this study. To investigate pathological brain aging, we further classified patients with aMCI and AD according to the severity of cognitive impairment. Cortical thickness was measured using a surface-based method. Multiple linear regression analyses were performed to evaluate age, diagnostic groups, and cortical thickness.

Results: Aging extensively affected cortical thickness not only in CN individuals but also in AD continuum patients; however, the precuneus and inferior temporal regions were relatively preserved against age-related cortical thinning. Compared to CN individuals, AD continuum patients including those with SMI showed a decreased cortical thickness in the perisylvian region. However, widespread cortical thinning including the precuneus and inferior temporal regions were found from the late-stage aMCI to the moderate to severe AD. Unlike the other age groups, AD continuum patients aged over 80 years showed prominent cortical thinning in the medial temporal region with relative sparing of the precuneus.

Conclusion: Our findings suggested that the precuneus and inferior temporal regions are the key regions in distinguishing between physiological and pathological brain aging. Attempts to differentiate age-related pathology from physiological brain aging at a very early stage would be important in terms of establishing new strategies for preventing accelerated pathological brain aging.

Keywords: physiological brain aging, pathological brain aging, cortical thickness, Alzheimer's disease, precuneus, inferior temporal region

INTRODUCTION

Aging is a physiological process that affects all tissues and organs including the human brain. The functional capabilities of the brain show a gradually progressive decline during aging, as with other organs. Specifically, declines in memory, conceptual reasoning, and processing speed are commonly observed in the elderly (Blazer et al., 2015). To date, the underlying cellular and molecular mechanisms of brain aging have been established in the context of mitochondrial dysfunction, impaired molecular waste disposal, aberrant neuronal network activity, oxidative damage, dysregulation of neuronal calcium homeostasis, and inflammation (Mattson and Arumugam, 2018).

Alzheimer's disease (AD) is a slowly progressing, irreversible neurodegenerative disease with a long preclinical phase (Masters et al., 2015). Regarded as a pre-dementia phase of AD, amnestic mild cognitive impairment (aMCI) is characterized by the development of noticeable memory problems, which do not affect the independence of functional abilities (Albert et al., 2011). Based on the concept of the paradigm shift in focus from AD dementia to preclinical AD in clinical trials, early-stage aMCI with milder cognitive impairments has emerged as a new classification rather than late-stage aMCI (Aisen et al., 2010). Furthermore, subjective memory impairment (SMI), a self-experienced persistent memory decline without objective cognitive deterioration, may represent the first symptomatic manifestation of AD (Jessen et al., 2014; Rabin et al., 2017). Therefore, both the clinical symptomatology and the underlying process of AD pathology have been conceptualized as part of the AD continuum which includes: SMI, aMCI, and AD dementia (Sperling et al., 2011).

Studying structural brain aging is of interest for the understanding of age-related pathology, as well as for the identification of the early manifestations of the AD continuum. Indeed, a previous study from our group showed that physiological brain aging occurs from the age of 40 years and continues past the age of 80 years (Lee et al., 2018). Cortical thickness in the dorsolateral prefrontal cortex and inferior parietal lobule was affected by aging earlier in life, but cortical thickness was relatively preserved in the precuneus, inferior temporal, and lateral occipital cortices until later in life. However, neuroimaging studies of AD have shown greater cortical atrophy in the medial temporal, posterior parietotemporal, posterior cingulate, and precuneus in early stage of disease (Jack, et al., 1997; Scahill et al., 2002; Damoiseaux et al., 2012). Also, there have been reports showing that cortical atrophy precedes cognitive decline and can be used to detect early changes in AD (Hampel et al., 2008; Jack et al., 2009). Additionally, patients with aMCI exhibit significant atrophy in the hippocampus, parahippocampal gyrus, and entorhinal cortex compared to cognitively normal (CN) individuals (Killiany et al., 2000; Wolf et al., 2001). Even in SMI stage, significant cortical atrophy in the entorhinal cortex, posterior cingulate gyrus, and inferior parietal cortex is observed (Peter et al., 2014; Meiberth et al., 2015; Schultz et al., 2015). To our knowledge, however, there have been no studies comparing cortical atrophy according to the age group in AD continuum patients, which can be regarded as pathological aging, with physiological brain aging. Considering that aging is a strong risk factor for AD (Scheltens et al., 2016), attempts to differentiate age-related pathology from physiological brain aging at a very early stage are important for establishing new strategies to prevent accelerated pathological brain aging.

In this study, we therefore investigated the long-term trajectory of physiological and pathological brain aging in a large cohort comprising individuals ranging from the 50s to over 80 years of age. Our main objective was to explore specific brain regions in order to distinguish pathological brain aging from physiological brain aging using sophisticated measurements of cortical thickness. We hypothesized that there would be distinct brain regions between physiological and pathological brain aging. To address different stages of the AD continuum, we studied seven groups of participants according to the severity of cognitive impairment: CN; SMI; early-stage aMCI; late-stage aMCI; very mild AD; mild AD; and moderate to severe AD.

MATERIALS AND METHODS

Study Participants

Cognitively normal individuals were recruited from the Health Promotion Center of the Samsung Medical Center (Seoul, South Korea). The study population comprised men and women aged 50 years or older who underwent a comprehensive health screening exam from January 1, 2009 to December 31, 2014. There were 3,290 eligible participants who attended a preventative medical check-up, which included an assessment of cognitive function and dementia status. All study participants underwent a high-resolution 3.0-Tesla brain MRI, including three-dimensional (3D) volume images, as a part of their dementia assessment. The assessment procedure used for the participants has been described in detail elsewhere (Lee et al., 2016). We excluded participants who had any of the following conditions: 202 participants with missing data on education years or Mini-Mental State Examination (MMSE) score; 178 participants with significant cognitive impairments defined as an MMSE scores below the 16th percentile in age-, sex-, and education-matched norms or through an interview conducted by a qualified neurologist; and 136 participants with unreliable analyses of cortical thickness due to head motion, blurring of the MRI, inadequate registration to a standardized stereotaxic space, misclassification of the tissue type, or inexact surface extraction. Therefore, the final sample size was 2,823 participants (1,427 men and 1,396 women).

In addition, a total of 3,619 AD continuum patients were recruited from the Memory Disorders Clinic of Samsung Medical Center from March 1, 2007 to December 31, 2013. Our recruitment from the memory clinic was focused on enriching the number of patients with clinical AD, subcortical vascular dementia, MCI, or SMI. However, only a small minority of the recruited group had frontotemporal lobar dementia, dementia with Lewy bodies, or other degenerative dementias. We selected 2,770 patients at the age of 50 or older who were clinically diagnosed with SMI, aMCI, or AD dementia. The clinical diagnosis was established at a multi-disciplinary conference applying standard research criteria for SMI, aMCI, and dementia syndromes. In detail, all of the SMI patients met the following criteria (Rabin et al., 2015): (1) subjective memory complaints by patients or caregivers; (2) no objective cognitive dysfunction as evidenced by scores from evaluations on any cognitive domains; and (3) not suffering dementia. Patients were diagnosed with aMCI using the Petersen criteria (Petersen, 2004) with the following modifications, which have been previously described in detail (Seo et al., 2009): (1) a subjective cognitive complaint by the patient or his/her caregiver; (2) normal Activities of Daily Living (ADL) score determined clinically and with the instrumental ADL scale; (3) an objective cognitive decline below the 16th percentile [−1.0 standard deviation (SD)] of age- and education-matched norms in at least one of four cognitive domains (language, visuospatial, memory, or frontal-executive function) on neuropsychological tests; and (4) absence of dementia. Patients with AD dementia fit the NINCDS-ADRDA criteria for probable AD (McKhann et al., 2011). In this study, we excluded patients who met the Diagnostic and Statistical Manual of Mental Disorders (Fourth Edition) criteria for psychotic or mood disorder, such as schizophrenia or major depressive disorder. All patients underwent a standardized diagnostic assessment protocol including a high-resolution 3.0-Tesla MRI for neurodegenerative and cerebrovascular diseases and detailed neuropsychological tests. We excluded 95 patients with an unreliable analysis of the cortical thickness due to head motion, blurring of the MRI, inadequate registration to a standardized stereotaxic space, misclassification of tissue type, or inexact surface extraction. Therefore, the final sample size of the AD continuum patients was 2,675 (874 with SMI, 954 with aMCI, and 847 with AD).

Laboratory tests were conducted in all patients to rule out other causes of cognitive impairment. These tests included complete blood count, vitamin B12, folate, metabolite profile, thyroid function tests, and syphilis serology. Apolipoprotein E (*APOE*) genotyping was performed in 658 (23.3%) of the 2,823 CN individuals, 700 (80.1%) of the 874 patients with SMI, 803 (84.2%) of the 954 patients with aMCI, and 639 (75.4%) of the 847 patients with AD dementia, respectively. All study participants were excluded if they had a cerebral, cerebellar, or brainstem infarction; hemorrhage; brain tumor; hydrocephalus; severe cerebral white matter hyperintensities (deep white matter ≥ 2.5 cm and caps or band ≥ 1.0 cm); or severe head trauma by personal history.

Standard Protocol Approvals, Registrations, and Patient Consent

This study was approved by the Institutional Review Board at the Samsung Medical Center. In addition, all methods were carried out in accordance with the approved guidelines. A written informed consent was obtained from all participants prior to the study.

Neuropsychological Assessments

All AD continuum patients underwent neuropsychological tests using a standardized neuropsychological battery (Ahn et al., 2010). This included tests for attention, language, praxis, elements of Gerstmann syndrome, visuoconstructive function, verbal and visual memory, and frontal/executive function. The series also included digit span tests (forward and backward); the Korean version of the Boston Naming Test; the Rey-Osterrieth Complex Figure Test (RCFT), which involves copying, immediate and 20-min delayed recall, and recognition; the Seoul Verbal Learning Test (SVLT), which includes three learning-free recall trials of 12 words, a 20-min delayed recall trial for these 12 items, and a recognition test; a phonemic and semantic Controlled Oral Word Association Test; and a Stroop Test, which involves word and color reading of 112 items during a 2-min period. Each score was converted into a standardized score (Z score) based on age-, sex, and education-adjusted norms (Ahn et al., 2010). Scores lower than −1.0 SD from the age-, sex-, and education-adjusted norms were considered abnormal. The results of neuropsychological tests in AD continuum patients are presented in **Supplementary Table 1**.

Classification of aMCI and AD

To investigate pathological brain aging, we further classified patients with aMCI or AD according to the severity of cognitive impairment. In aMCI patients, memory function was considered abnormal when delayed recall scores on either the SVLT or RCFT were lower than −1.0 SD from the baseline memory test results (Ye et al., 2013). Patients with performances between −1.0 and −1.5 SD of the age-, sex-, and education-adjusted norms were diagnosed with early-stage aMCI (305 patients), while those with performances lower than −1.5 SD were classified as late-stage aMCI (649 patients). In AD patients, dementia severity was classified based on the clinical dementia rating (CDR) score (Morris et al., 2001): very mild AD (CDR 0.5, 282 patients), mild AD (CDR 1, 411 patients), and moderate to severe AD (CDR 2 and 3, 154 patients).

Brain MRI Scans

All study participants underwent a 3D volumetric brain MRI scan. An Achieva 3.0-Tesla MRI scanner (Philips, Best,

Netherlands) was used to acquire a 3D T1 Turbo Field Echo (TFE) MRI data using the following imaging parameters: sagittal slice thickness, 1.0 mm with 50% overlap; no gap; repetition time of 9.9 ms; echo time of 4.6 ms; flip angle of 8°; and matrix size of 240 × 240 pixels reconstructed to 480 × 480 over a field view of 240 mm.

Cortical Thickness Measurements

T1-weighted MR images were automatically processed using the standard Montreal Neurological Institute image processing software (CIVET) to measure cortical thickness. This software has been well-validated and extensively described elsewhere including in aging/atrophied brain studies (Lerch and Evans, 2005; Singh et al., 2006). In summary, native MR images were first registered into a standardized stereotaxic space using an affine transformation (Collins et al., 1994). Non-uniformity artifacts were corrected using the N3 algorithm, and the registered and corrected volumes were classified as GM, white matter (WM), cerebrospinal fluid (CSF), and background using an artificial neural net classifier (Sled et al., 1998). The surfaces of the inner and outer cortices were automatically extracted by deforming a spherical mesh onto the gray/white boundary of each hemisphere using the Constrained Laplacian-Based Automated Segmentation with Proximities algorithm, which has also been well-validated and extensively described elsewhere (Kim J.S. et al., 2005).

Cortical thickness was calculated as the Euclidean distance between the linked vertices of the inner and outer surfaces after application of an inverse transformation matrix to the cortical surfaces and reconstructing them in the native space (Kim J.S. et al., 2005; Im et al., 2006). To control for brain size, we computed the intracranial volume (ICV) using classified tissue information and a skull mask acquired from the T1-weighted image (Smith, 2002). ICV was defined as the total volume of GM, WM, and CSF, with consideration of the voxel dimension. Classified GM, WM, CSF, and background within the mask were transformed back into the individual native space.

To compare the thicknesses of corresponding regions among the participants, the thicknesses were spatially registered on an unbiased iterative group template by matching the sulcal folding pattern using surface-based registration involving sphere-to-sphere warping (Lyttelton et al., 2007). For global and lobar regional analyses, we used the lobe-parcellated group template that had been previously divided into frontal, temporal, parietal, and occipital lobes using SUMA[1] (Im et al., 2006). Average thickness values of the whole vertex in each hemisphere and lobar region were used for global analysis.

Statistical Analysis

The Student's *t*-test, Chi-square test, and analysis of variance with Bonferroni *post hoc* tests were used as appropriate to compare the demographic and clinical characteristics of the groups (diagnostic or age groups). To evaluate the relationship between age (continuous) and cortical thickness, we used multiple linear regression analysis after controlling for sex, education years (continuous), ICV, vascular risk factors (hypertension, diabetes mellitus, and hyperlipidemia), and history of ischemic heart disease or stroke.

For cortical thickness analyses of MRI data from CN individuals and AD continuum patients, we used a MATLAB-based toolbox (available free online at the University of Chicago website[2]). Diffusion smoothing with a full-width half-maximum of 20 mm was used to blur each cortical thickness map, leading to an increased signal-to-noise ratio and statistical power (Lerch and Evans, 2005). We entered age (continuous or categorical) as a predictor and vertex-by-vertex cortical thickness as an outcome to analyze the relationship between cortical thickness and age in the surface model. A linear regression analysis was then performed after controlling for sex, education years (continuous), ICV, vascular risk factors (hypertension, diabetes mellitus, and hyperlipidemia), and history of ischemic heart disease or stroke. The cortical surface model contained 81,924 vertices; thus, correction for multiple comparisons was performed using a random field theory correction at a probability value of 0.05. Statistical analyses were performed using SPSS version 20.0 (SPSS, Inc., Chicago, IL, United States).

RESULTS

Characteristics of the Study Participants

Table 1 shows the demographic and clinical characteristics of the study participants. The mean (SD) ages of the CN, SMI, aMCI, and AD dementia group were 64.1 (6.9), 65.9 (8.5), 71.1 (8.4), and 73.0 (9.2) years, respectively. Significant differences in the mean age among the four groups were noted. The proportion of female was highest in the SMI group (72.2%), while it was lowest in the CN group (49.5%). The AD dementia group had the lowest education years and ICV, but the proportion of *APOE* ε4 carriers was highest among the four groups. The number of study participants in each group is presented in **Supplementary Table 2**. In the CN, aMCI, and AD dementia groups, we combined the age groups of the 90 and 100s into the over-80 groups due to the small number of participants in these age groups.

Mean Cortical Thickness of Each Age Group According to the Diagnostic Groups

The mean and SD of the cortical thickness for each age group according to the diagnostic groups is presented in **Table 2**. In the CN, SMI, and aMCI (early- and late-stages) groups, the mean cortical thickness in the global, frontal, temporal, parietal, and occipital regions decreased as the age increased. However, among patients with very mild and mild AD, the 50s group had a lower mean cortical thickness in the parietal and occipital regions than the 60 and 70s groups. Among patients with moderate to severe AD, the 50s group exhibited

[1]http://afni.nimh.nih.gov

[2]http://galton.uchicago.edu/faculty/InMemoriam/worsley/research/surfstat/

TABLE 1 | Demographic and clinical characteristics of the study participants (N = 5,498).

	Total	CN	SMI	aMCI			AD dementia			
				Total	Early-stage	Late-stage	Total	Very mild	Mild	Moderate to severe
N	5,498	2,823	874	954	305	649	847	282	411	154
Age, years	67.0 (8.6)	64.1 (6.9)^{a,b,c}	65.9 (8.5)^{a,d,e}	71.1 (8.4)^{b,d,f}	70.3 (8.2)	71.5 (8.5)	73.0 (9.2)^{c,e,f}	72.5 (9.3)	73.0 (8.7)	73.9 (10.3)
Age range, years	50–101	50–91	50–89	50–99	50–88	50–99	50–101	50–101	51–91	50–91
Female	3,160 (57.5)	1,396 (49.5)^{a,b,c}	631 (72.2)^{a,d,e}	575 (60.3)^{b,d,f}	200 (65.6)	375 (57.8)	558 (65.9)^{c,e,f}	179 (63.5)	263 (64.0)	116 (75.3)
Education, years	11.6 (4.9)	12.7 (4.3)^{a,b,c}	11.1 (5.0)^{a,e}	10.5 (5.1)^{b,f}	9.3 (5.8)	11.1 (4.6)	9.6 (5.5)^{c,e,f}	9.6 (5.6)	9.8 (5.6)	9.3 (5.1)
APOE ε4 present*	890 (31.8)	124 (18.8)^{b,c}	149 (21.3)^{d,e}	290 (36.1)^{b,d,f}	71 (28.3)	219 (39.7)	327 (51.2)^{c,e,f}	125 (53.9)	152 (50.0)	50 (48.5)
MMSE, score	26.2 (4.5)	28.1 (1.7)^{b,c}	28.3 (2.1)^{d,e}	25.7 (3.4)^{b,d,f}	26.0 (3.5)	25.5 (3.3)	18.4 (5.3)^{c,e,f}	21.3 (3.9)	18.6 (4.2)	12.6 (5.5)
CDR, score	0.7 (0.5)	–	0.0 (0.0)	0.5 (0.1)^{f}	0.5 (0.1)	0.5 (0.1)	1.0 (0.6)^{f}	0.5 (0.0)	1.0 (0.0)	2.1 (0.3)
Hypertension	2,395 (43.6)	1,303 (46.2)^{a,}	294 (33.6)^{a,d,e}	425 (44.5)^{d}	130 (42.6)	295 (45.5)	373 (44.0)^{e}	130 (46.1)	175 (42.6)	68 (44.2)
DM	1,173 (21.3)	476 (16.9)^{a,b,c}	183 (20.9)^{a,d,e}	271 (28.4)^{b,d}	78 (25.6)	193 (29.7)	243 (28.7)^{c,e}	83 (29.4)	117 (28.5)	43 (27.9)
Hyperlipidemia	1,660 (30.2)	935 (33.1)^{b,c}	273 (31.2)^{e}	259 (27.1)^{b,f}	78 (25.6)	181 (27.9)	193 (22.8)^{c,e,f}	69 (24.5)	94 (22.9)	30 (19.5)
History of IHD	490 (8.9)	158 (5.6)^{a,b,c}	119 (13.6)^{a,e}	130 (13.6)^{b,f}	45 (14.8)	85 (13.1)	83 (9.8)^{c,e,f}	30 (10.6)	39 (9.5)	14 (9.1)
History of stroke	196 (3.6)	80 (2.8)^{b,c}	23 (2.6)^{d,e}	49 (5.1)^{b,d}	16 (5.2)	33 (5.1)	44 (5.2)^{c,e}	20 (7.1)	19 (4.6)	5 (3.2)
ICV (cm^3)	1,332.9 (126.4)	1,358.4 (122.4)^{a,b,c}	1,313.7 (121.9)^{a,e}	1,311.5 (123.8)^{b,f}	1,314.5 (126.0)	1,310.1 (122.7)	1,291.9 (128.5)^{c,e,f}	1,295.4 (121.6)	1,293.2 (129.4)	1,282.0 (138.6)

*Values are mean (SD) or N (%). *APOE genotyping was performed in 658 (23.3%) of the 2,823 CN individuals, 700 (80.1%) of the 874 patients with SMI, 803 (84.2%) of the 954 patients with aMCI, and 639 (75.4%) of the 847 patients with AD dementia, respectively.* ^{a,b,c,d,e,f}*Scores in each row are significantly different in the analysis of variance with Bonferroni's corrections, Chi-square or Fisher's exact tests:* ^{a}*CN vs. SMI;* ^{b}*CN vs. aMCI;* ^{c}*CN vs. AD dementia;* ^{d}*SMI vs. aMCI;* ^{e}*SMI vs. AD dementia;* ^{f}*aMCI vs. AD dementia. N, number; SD, standard deviation; CN, cognitively normal; SMI, subjective memory impairment; aMCI, amnestic mild cognitive impairment; AD, Alzheimer's disease; APOE, apolipoprotein E; MMSE, Mini-Mental State Examination; CDR, clinical dementia rating; DM, diabetes mellitus; IHD, ischemic heart disease; ICV, intracranial volume.*

TABLE 2 | Mean and SD of the cortical thickness for each age group according to the diagnostic groups.

Age group	*N*	Global	Frontal	Temporal	Parietal	Occipital
CN						
50s	694	3.08 (0.10)	3.13 (0.10)	3.23 (0.15)	2.95 (0.14)	2.72 (0.12)
60s	1,509	3.05 (0.10)	3.10 (0.11)	3.22 (0.15)	2.92 (0.13)	2.70 (0.12)
70s	572	2.99 (0.12)	3.04 (0.13)	3.16 (0.17)	2.85 (0.14)	2.63 (0.13)
Over-80	48	2.98 (0.16)	3.03 (0.16)	3.14 (0.19)	2.83 (0.17)	2.63 (0.16)
SMI						
50s	224	3.09 (0.09)	3.16 (0.10)	3.28 (0.10)	2.93 (0.10)	2.70 (0.11)
60s	348	3.04 (0.10)	3.11 (0.11)	3.24 (0.11)	2.89 (0.11)	2.65 (0.11)
70s	247	2.96 (0.12)	3.02 (0.13)	3.14 (0.15)	2.80 (0.13)	2.58 (0.13)
Over-80	55	2.91 (0.13)	2.98 (0.14)	3.06 (0.14)	2.77 (0.15)	2.54 (0.12)
Early-stage aMCI						
50s	35	3.11 (0.09)	3.18 (0.10)	3.30 (0.10)	2.96 (0.08)	2.73 (0.10)
60s	96	3.03 (0.10)	3.10 (0.11)	3.23 (0.11)	2.88 (0.11)	2.65 (0.12)
70s	137	2.92 (0.12)	2.98 (0.14)	3.08 (0.14)	2.78 (0.13)	2.56 (0.12)
Over-80	37	2.85 (0.14)	2.92 (0.15)	3.01 (0.16)	2.71 (0.15)	2.49 (0.14)
Late-stage aMCI						
50s	62	3.03 (0.13)	3.11 (0.14)	3.21 (0.16)	2.87 (0.13)	2.66 (0.12)
60s	193	2.98 (0.12)	3.05 (0.12)	3.15 (0.15)	2.82 (0.13)	2.61 (0.12)
70s	288	2.89 (0.13)	2.96 (0.14)	3.04 (0.16)	2.74 (0.13)	2.54 (0.13)
Over-80	106	2.82 (0.13)	2.89 (0.14)	2.95 (0.16)	2.68 (0.13)	2.49 (0.14)
Very mild AD						
50s	35	2.88 (0.15)	3.00 (0.13)	3.05 (0.18)	2.65 (0.19)	2.49 (0.20)
60s	56	2.90 (0.16)	2.99 (0.14)	3.04 (0.20)	2.74 (0.19)	2.53 (0.19)
70s	125	2.84 (0.14)	2.92 (0.15)	2.97 (0.17)	2.70 (0.15)	2.50 (0.14)
Over-80	66	2.77 (0.15)	2.85 (0.15)	2.89 (0.19)	2.65 (0.17)	2.45 (0.16)
Mild AD						
50s	43	2.78 (0.10)	2.91 (0.12)	2.91 (0.15)	2.55 (0.12)	2.41 (0.15)
60s	82	2.81 (0.14)	2.91 (0.13)	2.93 (0.18)	2.65 (0.15)	2.47 (0.17)
70s	198	2.81 (0.15)	2.90 (0.15)	2.91 (0.19)	2.69 (0.17)	2.50 (0.15)
Over-80	88	2.78 (0.13)	2.85 (0.13)	2.87 (0.17)	2.67 (0.15)	2.47 (0.15)
Moderate to severe AD						
50s	20	2.64 (0.16)	2.73 (0.20)	2.79 (0.22)	2.44 (0.13)	2.34 (0.18)
60s	29	2.62 (0.17)	2.74 (0.18)	2.69 (0.21)	2.48 (0.20)	2.32 (0.22)
70s	54	2.66 (0.17)	2.76 (0.17)	2.69 (0.22)	2.55 (0.17)	2.37 (0.18)
Over-80	51	2.71 (0.18)	2.79 (0.18)	2.76 (0.23)	2.62 (0.19)	2.41 (0.19)

Values are N or mean cortical thickness (SD). N, number; SD, standard deviation; CN, cognitively normal; SMI, subjective memory impairment; aMCI, amnestic mild cognitive impairment; AD, Alzheimer's disease.

the lowest mean cortical thickness in the frontal, parietal, and occipital regions.

Relationship Between Age and Cortical Thickness According to the Diagnostic Groups

Table 3 shows the relationships between age and cortical thickness according to the diagnostic groups. Multiple linear regression analyses showed that age was negatively correlated with cortical thickness in the global, frontal, temporal, parietal, and occipital regions in the CN, SMI, and aMCI (early- and late-stages) groups (all $P < 0.001$). In the very mild AD groups, age was negatively correlated with cortical thickness in the global ($P < 0.001$), frontal ($P < 0.001$), and temporal regions ($P < 0.001$), but not in the parietal ($P = 0.079$) and occipital ($P = 0.061$) regions. Age was positively correlated with cortical thickness in the parietal region in the mild AD ($P = 0.001$) and moderate to severe AD ($P < 0.001$) groups. The 3D reconstruction for the correlation between age and cortical

TABLE 3 | Relationship between age and cortical thickness according to the diagnostic groups.

	Global			Frontal			Temporal			Parietal			Occipital		
	B	**SE**	**P**	**B**	**SE**	**P**	**B**	**SE**	**P**	**B**	**SE**	**P**	**B**	**SE**	**P**
CN															
Age	−0.004	< 0.001	< 0.001	−0.004	< 0.001	< 0.001	−0.004	< 0.001	< 0.001	−0.005	< 0.001	< 0.001	−0.005	< 0.001	< 0.001
SMI															
Age	−0.006	< 0.001	< 0.001	−0.006	< 0.001	< 0.001	−0.007	0.001	< 0.001	−0.005	< 0.001	< 0.001	−0.006	< 0.001	< 0.001
Early-stage aMCI															
Age	−0.009	0.001	< 0.001	−0.009	0.001	< 0.001	−0.012	0.001	< 0.001	−0.009	0.001	< 0.001	−0.008	0.001	< 0.001
Late-stage aMCI															
Age	−0.008	0.001	< 0.001	−0.008	0.001	< 0.001	−0.010	0.001	< 0.001	−0.007	0.001	< 0.001	−0.006	0.001	< 0.001
Very mild AD															
Age	−0.005	0.001	< 0.001	−0.006	0.001	< 0.001	−0.007	0.001	< 0.001	−0.002	0.001	0.079	−0.002	0.001	0.061
Mild AD															
Age	−0.001	0.001	0.416	−0.002	0.001	0.009	−0.003	0.001	0.012	0.003	0.001	0.001	0.002	0.001	0.095
Moderate to severe AD															
Age	0.002	0.001	0.179	0.001	0.001	0.436	< 0.001	0.002	0.827	0.006	0.001	< 0.001	0.002	0.002	0.193

B (SE): β value (standard error of the mean). Multiple linear regression analysis was performed after controlling for sex, education years (continuous), ICV, vascular risk factors (hypertension, diabetes mellitus, and hyperlipidemia), and history of ischemic heart disease or stroke. CN, cognitively normal; SMI, subjective memory impairment; aMCI, amnestic mild cognitive impairment; AD, Alzheimer's disease.

thickness of the diagnostic groups is presented in **Figure 1**. The topography of age-related cortical thinning was widespread and severe in the CN, SMI, and aMCI groups. However, the precuneus and inferior temporal regions were relatively preserved against the effects of age (**Figures 1A–C**). In the AD group, increasing age was associated with cortical thinning in the medial and ventrolateral prefrontal, medial and lateral temporal, medial occipital, precentral, and post-central regions (**Figure 1D**).

Topographical Differences in Cortical Thickness of Each Age Group Based on the Diagnostic Groups Compared to Age Group-Matched CN Individuals

Figure 2 shows the topographical differences in cortical thickness of each age group based on the diagnostic groups compared to the age-matched CN group. From the SMI to moderate to severe AD stages, cortical thinning occurred in the perisylvian region and spread widely in the 60 and 70s groups. Notably, the precuneus and inferior temporal regions, which were relatively preserved against age-related cortical thinning, were especially affected at the late-stage aMCI stage and cortical thinning occurred across most of the cortices in the moderate to severe AD stage. However, cortical thinning of the paracentral lobule and anterior cingulate regions were relatively less affected until later in life, even at the stage of moderate to severe AD. Compared to the over-80 CN group, the over-80 late-stage aMCI group showed cortical thinning in the dorsolateral prefrontal, perisylvian, and medial temporal regions. However, the precuneus, paracentral lobule, anterior cingulate, medial occipital regions were relatively preserved until the moderate to severe AD stage.

DISCUSSION

In this study, we investigated the trajectory of physiological and pathological brain aging in a large population of 5,498 participants using sophisticated measurements of cortical thickness. The major findings of the study were as follows. First, aging extensively affected cortical thinning not only in CN individuals but also in AD continuum patients; however, the precuneus and inferior temporal regions were relatively preserved against age-related cortical thinning. Second, compared to CN individuals, AD continuum patients showed a decreased cortical thickness in the perisylvian region even in the SMI stage. However, widespread cortical thinning including the precuneus and inferior temporal regions were found in late-stage aMCI and moderate to severe AD. Third, unlike the other age groups, the over-80 AD continuum patients showed prominent cortical thinning in the medial temporal region with relative sparing of the precuneus. Taken together, our findings provide some important insights into the difference between physiological and pathological brain aging.

Age-related cortical thinning was widespread and severe in the CN, SMI, and aMCI groups, whereas in the AD group, increasing age was not associated with cortical thinning in the dorsolateral prefrontal, parietal, and lateral occipital regions. Besides, age

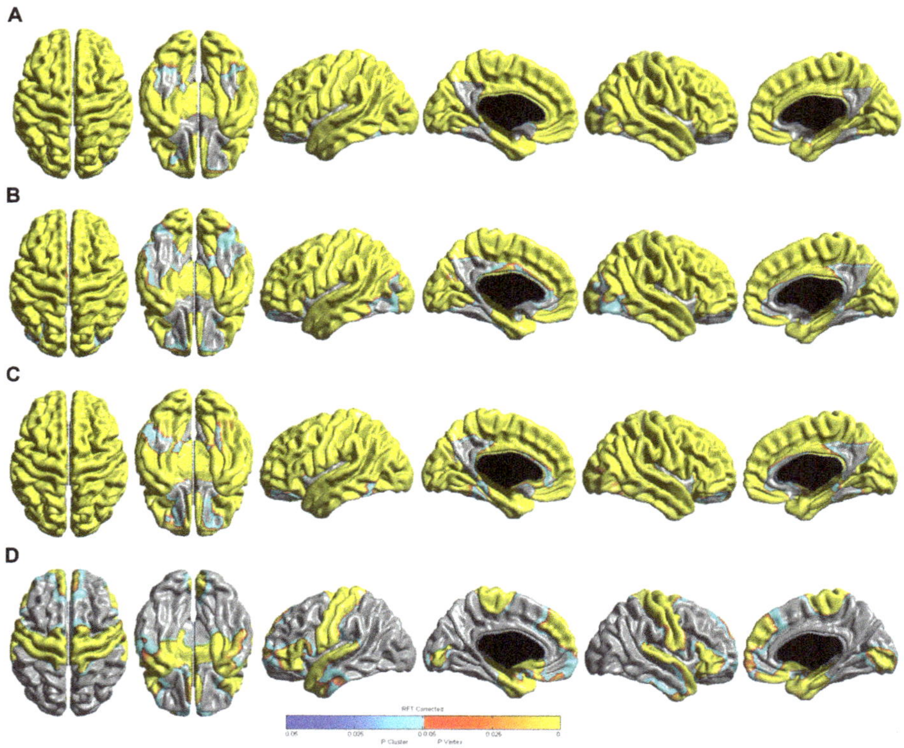

FIGURE 1 | Three-dimensional reconstruction of the correlation between age (continuous) and cortical thickness in the **(A)** CN, **(B)** SMI, **(C)** aMCI, and **(D)** AD groups. RFT-corrected (*P*-value < 0.05) results were adjusted for sex, education years, ICV, vascular risk factors (hypertension, diabetes mellitus, and hyperlipidemia), and history of ischemic heart disease or stroke. The color scale from blue to yellow indicates statistically significant age-related cortical thinning. CN, cognitively normal; SMI, subjective memory impairment; aMCI, amnestic mild cognitive impairment; AD, Alzheimer's disease; RFT, random field theory; ICV, intracranial volume.

was positively correlated with mean cortical thickness in the parietal region in the mild AD and moderate to severe AD groups. In AD patients, the age of symptom onset is known to determine distinctive radiologic features (Kim E.J. et al., 2005; Cho et al., 2013); specifically, patients with early-onset AD have greater cortical atrophy in the lateral parietal region and precuneus than those with late-onset AD (Frisoni et al., 2007; Ossenkoppele et al., 2015a). This could be explained by the brain reserve hypothesis (Stern, 2002), which postulates that early-onset AD have a greater brain reserve than late-onset AD and therefore more severe imaging abnormalities despite having similar cognitive performance. We therefore suggest that early-onset AD is more severely affected by pathological brain aging than physiological brain aging.

To evaluate pathological brain aging more specifically, we classified the AD continuum patients into six groups according to the severity of cognitive worsening. Through comparisons with CN individuals in each age group, we minimalized the effects of physiological aging and evaluated the distinct brain regions associated with physiological and pathological brain aging. Cortical thinning in the perisylvian region was found from the SMI group and spread widely as pathological brain aging progressed. Previous studies have shown that SMI patients, compared to CN individuals, had AD-like cortical atrophy patterns (Peter et al., 2014; Meiberth et al., 2015; Schultz et al., 2015). However, some studies did not find significant differences between SMI patients and CN individuals (Selnes et al., 2012; Jung et al., 2016). This disparity is probably due to the fact that SMI is a heterogeneous group that includes preclinical AD or various conditions that can affect cognition, such as anxiety and depression (Jessen et al., 2014). Nonetheless, we found that there was a distinctive cortical thinning region – the perisylvian area – between the SMI and CN groups with a large sample size. The perisylvian area has been linked to the lateral cholinergic pathway (Selden et al., 1998). Considering that the cholinergic system plays an important role in learning and memory (Hasselmo, 2006), our findings may provide clues for future research on SMI, as a part of AD continuum.

Another noteworthy finding was that widespread cortical thinning including the precuneus and inferior temporal regions were found from the late-stage aMCI to the moderate to severe AD. As mentioned above, the precuneus and inferior temporal regions were relatively preserved against the effects of aging in the CN, SMI, and aMCI groups; however, these regions exhibited cortical thinning that clearly distinguished between the early- and late-stage aMCI. The precuneus has been reported to have a central role in highly integrated tasks, including episodic memory retrieval, visuospatial processing, and self-consciousness (Cavanna and Trimble, 2006). The current literature suggests that

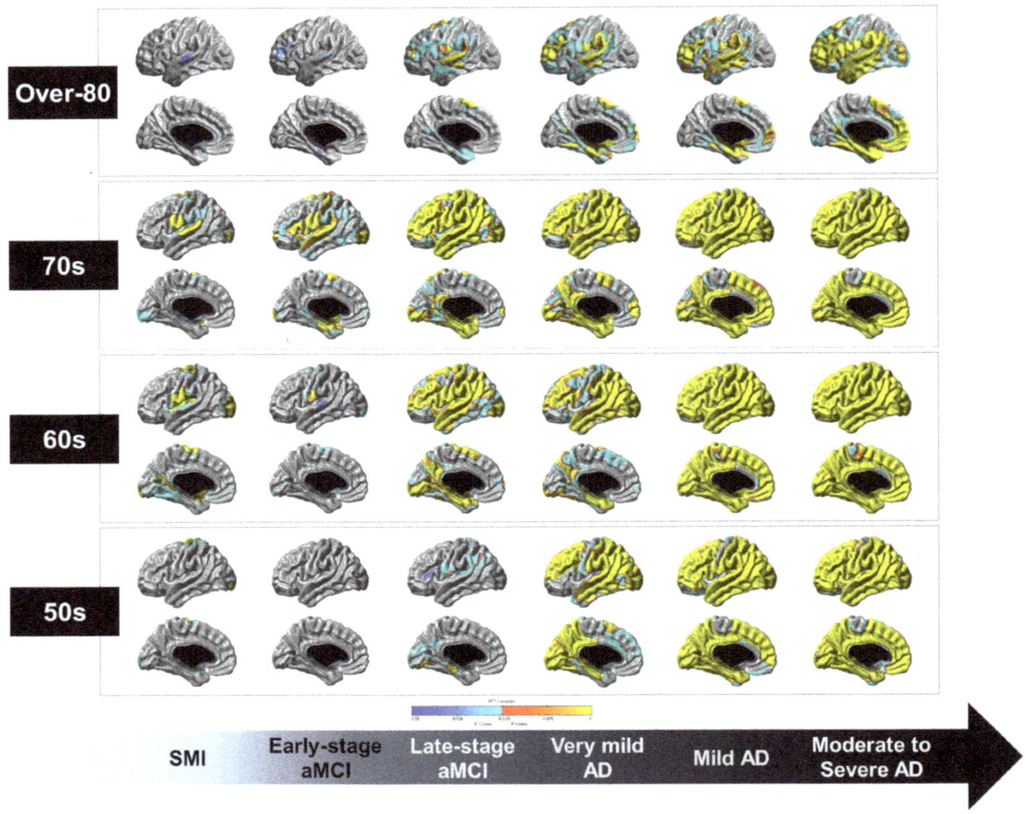

FIGURE 2 | Topographical differences in the cortical thickness of each age group based on the diagnostic groups compared to age group-matched CN individuals. RFT-corrected (*P*-value < 0.05) results were adjusted for sex, education years, ICV, vascular risk factors (hypertension, diabetes mellitus, and hyperlipidemia), and history of ischemic heart disease or stroke. The color scale from blue to yellow indicates statistically significant topographical differences in cortical thinning of each age group. CN, cognitively normal; SMI, subjective memory impairment; aMCI, amnestic mild cognitive impairment; AD, Alzheimer's disease; RFT, random field theory; ICV, intracranial volume.

the precuneus is particularly vulnerable to the early deposition of β-amyloid (Sperling et al., 2009) and seems to be affected even in the early-stages of AD (Greicius et al., 2004; Klunk et al., 2004; Minners et al., 2016). In addition, the inferior temporal region is considered particularly important for the ventral stream and has been implicated in object recognition and semantic processing (Grill-Spector et al., 2000; Kellenbach et al., 2005). Previous studies also demonstrated that the inferior temporal region is affected during the prodromal stage of AD and may underlie some of the early AD-related clinical dysfunctions (Convit et al., 2000; Scheff et al., 2011). We therefore suggest that the precuneus and inferior temporal regions are key regions in distinguishing between physiological and pathological brain aging, although cortical thinning is initiated in the perisylvian region, even at the SMI stage.

Interestingly, unlike the other age groups, the over-80 AD continuum patients showed minimal cortical thinning in the perisylvian region from SMI; however, prominent cortical thinning was found in the medial temporal region with relative sparing of the precuneus. This might be due to the specific pattern of cortical thinning that occurs in late-onset AD. In fact, previous studies from our group showed that patients with late-onset AD presented cortical thinning mostly in the medial temporal region, while early-onset AD patients had prominent cortical thinning in the precuneus (Seo et al., 2011; Cho et al., 2013). Alternatively, considering 25–50% of the oldest-old have "low" or "none" neuritic amyloid plaque density (Neltner et al., 2016), this may be partly explained by suspected non-Alzheimer pathology or primary age-related tauopathy (PART). As aging progresses, burdens of neurodegenerative and cerebrovascular diseases increase (Braak et al., 2011; Thal et al., 2012). Moreover, a meta-analysis showed that the frequency of amyloid positivity actually decreased with aging in patients with clinical AD dementia (Ossenkoppele et al., 2015b). Recent studies demonstrated that the oldest-old patients with PART showed significantly less extensive tau lesions beyond the medial temporal lobe differing from those in AD (Jellinger, 2018; Bell et al., 2019). As a result, the oldest-old patients may be clinically misdiagnosed with AD. Further studies are needed to determine the underlying pathology in the oldest-old patients with clinical AD dementia.

The strengths of the study include the large number of participants (N = 5,498) and the sophisticated measurements of cortical thickness using the same type of scanner with the same scan parameters across different waves of data collection.

However, several limitations should be acknowledged when interpreting the results. First, our study was designed to be cross-sectional, precluding claims of causality. The cross-sectional design did not take into account individual differences in the process of aging. Second, in the present study, CN individuals were recruited from individuals seeking a comprehensive preventive health exam not covered by national medical insurance, which might not be completely representative of the general population. Third, we did not have additional biomarkers indicating AD pathology, such as CSF biomarkers, molecular imaging or neuropathological data from the participants. Finally, despite the large sample size, some subgroups such as the 50s and over-80 groups in early-stage aMCI or the 50s group in very mild AD, were relatively small.

Nevertheless, our findings provide an important clue to understanding the mechanism of brain aging. Early identification of age-related pathology in physiological brain aging may be important to establish new strategies for preventing accelerated pathological brain aging, in keeping with the paradigm shift in focus from AD dementia to preclinical AD in the development of therapeutic interventions.

AUTHOR CONTRIBUTIONS

JL and SS conceived and designed the study, and drafted and revised the manuscript. JL, SC, SK, JK, YJ, HK, HJ, DN, and SS acquired the data. JL, YP, SP, UY, YC, BC, AH, SC, SK, JK, YJ, K-CP, HK, HJ, DN, and SS analyzed and interpreted the data. SS approved the final manuscript.

FUNDING

This research was supported by the Brain Research Program through the National Research Foundation of Korea (NRF) funded by the Ministry of Science, ICT & Future Planning (2016M3C7A1913844), by the NRF grant funded by the Korea Government (2017R1A2B2005081), by a grant of the Korea Health Technology R&D Project through the Korea Health Industry Development Institute, funded by the Ministry of Health & Welfare, South Korea (HI17C1915), and by a fund (2018-ER6203-00) by Research of Korea Centers for Disease Control and Prevention.

REFERENCES

Ahn, H. J., Chin, J., Park, A., Lee, B. H., Suh, M. K., Seo, S. W., et al. (2010). Seoul neuropsychological screening battery-dementia version (SNSB-D): a useful tool for assessing and monitoring cognitive impairments in dementia patients. *J. Korean Med. Sci.* 25, 1071–1076. doi: 10.3346/jkms.2010.25.7.1071

Aisen, P. S., Petersen, R. C., Donohue, M. C., Gamst, A., Raman, R., Thomas, R. G., et al. (2010). Clinical core of the Alzheimer's disease neuroimaging initiative: progress and plans. *Alzheimers Dement* 6, 239–246. doi: 10.1016/j.jalz.2010.03.006

Albert, M. S., DeKosky, S. T., Dickson, D., Dubois, B., Feldman, H. H., Fox, N. C., et al. (2011). The diagnosis of mild cognitive impairment due to Alzheimer's disease: recommendations from the national institute on aging-Alzheimer's association workgroups on diagnostic guidelines for Alzheimer's disease. *Alzheimers Dement* 7, 270–279. doi: 10.1016/j.jalz.2011.03.008

Bell, W. R., An, Y., Kageyama, Y., English, C., Rudow, G. L., Pletnikova, O., et al. (2019). Neuropathologic, genetic, and longitudinal cognitive profiles in primary age-related tauopathy (PART) and Alzheimer's disease. *Alzheimers Dement* 15, 8–16. doi: 10.1016/j.jalz.2018.07.215

Blazer, D. G., Yaffe, K., and Liverman, C. T. (eds) (2015). *Cognitive Aging: Progress in Understanding and Opportunities for Action.* Washington DC: National Academies Press.

Braak, H., Thal, D. R., Ghebremedhin, E., and Del Tredici, K. (2011). Stages of the pathologic process in Alzheimer disease: age categories from 1 to 100 years. *J. Neuropathol. Exp. Neurol.* 70, 960–969. doi: 10.1097/NEN.0b013e318232a379

Cavanna, A. E., and Trimble, M. R. (2006). The precuneus: a review of its functional anatomy and behavioural correlates. *Brain* 129(Pt 3), 564–583. doi: 10.1093/brain/awl004

Cho, H., Jeon, S., Kang, S. J., Lee, J. M., Lee, J. H., Kim, G. H., et al. (2013). Longitudinal changes of cortical thickness in early- versus late-onset Alzheimer's disease. *Neurobiol. Aging* 34, 1921.e9–1921.e15. doi: 10.1016/j.neurobiolaging.2013.01.004

Collins, D. L., Neelin, P., Peters, T. M., and Evans, A. C. (1994). Automatic 3D intersubject registration of MR volumetric data in standardized Talairach space. *J. Comput. Assist. Tomogr.* 18, 192–205. doi: 10.1097/00004728-199403000-00005

Convit, A., de Asis, J., de Leon, M. J., Tarshish, C. Y., De Santi, S., and Rusinek, H. (2000). Atrophy of the medial occipitotemporal, inferior, and middle temporal gyri in non-demented elderly predict decline to Alzheimer's disease. *Neurobiol. Aging* 21, 19–26. doi: 10.1016/s0197-4580(99)00107-4

Damoiseaux, J. S., Prater, K. E., Miller, B. L., and Greicius, M. D. (2012). Functional connectivity tracks clinical deterioration in Alzheimer's disease. *Neurobiol. Aging* 33, 828.e19–828.e30. doi: 10.1016/j.neurobiolaging.2011.06.024

Frisoni, G. B., Pievani, M., Testa, C., Sabattoli, F., Bresciani, L., Bonetti, M., et al. (2007). The topography of grey matter involvement in early and late onset Alzheimer's disease. *Brain* 130(Pt 3), 720–730. doi: 10.1093/brain/awl377

Greicius, M. D., Srivastava, G., Reiss, A. L., and Menon, V. (2004). Default-mode network activity distinguishes Alzheimer's disease from healthy aging: evidence from functional MRI. *Proc. Natl. Acad. Sci. U.S.A.* 101, 4637–4642. doi: 10.1073/pnas.0308627101

Grill-Spector, K., Kushnir, T., Hendler, T., and Malach, R. (2000). The dynamics of object-selective activation correlate with recognition performance in humans. *Nat. Neurosci.* 3, 837–843. doi: 10.1038/77754

Hampel, H., Burger, K., Teipel, S. J., Bokde, A. L., Zetterberg, H., and Blennow, K. (2008). Core candidate neurochemical and imaging biomarkers of Alzheimer's disease. *Alzheimers Dement* 4, 38–48. doi: 10.1016/j.jalz.2007.08.006

Hasselmo, M. E. (2006). The role of acetylcholine in learning and memory. *Curr. Opin. Neurobiol* 16, 710–715. doi: 10.1016/j.conb.2006.09.002

Im, K., Lee, J. M., Lee, J., Shin, Y. W., Kim, I. Y., Kwon, J. S., et al. (2006). Gender difference analysis of cortical thickness in healthy young adults with surface-based methods. *Neuroimage* 31, 31–38. doi: 10.1016/j.neuroimage.2005.11.042

Jack, C. R. Jr., Lowe, V. J., Weigand, S. D., Wiste, H. J., Senjem, M. L., Knopman, D. S., et al. (2009). Serial PIB and MRI in normal, mild cognitive impairment and Alzheimer's disease: implications for sequence of pathological events in Alzheimer's disease. *Brain* 132(Pt 5), 1355–1365. doi: 10.1093/brain/awp062

Jack, C. R., Petersen, R. C., Xu, Y. C., Waring, S. C., O'Brien, P. C., Tangalos, E. G., et al. (1997). Medial temporal atrophy on MRI in normal aging and very mild Alzheimer's disease. *Neurology* 49, 786–794. doi: 10.1212/wnl.49.3.786

Jellinger, K. A. (2018). Different patterns of hippocampal tau pathology in Alzheimer's disease and PART. *Acta Neuropathol.* 136, 811–813. doi: 10.1007/s00401-018-1894-z

Jessen, F., Amariglio, R. E., van Boxtel, M., Breteler, M., Ceccaldi, M., Chetelat, G., et al. (2014). A conceptual framework for research on subjective cognitive decline in preclinical Alzheimer's disease. *Alzheimers Dement* 10, 844–852. doi: 10.1016/j.jalz.2014.01.001

Jung, N. Y., Seo, S. W., Yoo, H., Yang, J. J., Park, S., Kim, Y. J., et al. (2016). Classifying anatomical subtypes of subjective memory impairment. *Neurobiol. Aging* 48, 53–60. doi: 10.1016/j.neurobiolaging.2016.08.010

Kellenbach, M. L., Hovius, M., and Patterson, K. (2005). A pet study of visual and semantic knowledge about objects. *Cortex* 41, 121–132. doi: 10.1016/s0010-9452(08)70887-6

Killiany, R. J., Gomez-Isla, T., Moss, M., Kikinis, R., Sandor, T., Jolesz, F., et al. (2000). Use of structural magnetic resonance imaging to predict who will get Alzheimer's disease. *Ann. Neurol.* 47, 430–439. doi: 10.1002/1531-8249(200004)47:4<430::aid-ana5>3.3.co;2-9

Kim, E. J., Cho, S. S., Jeong, Y., Park, K. C., Kang, S. J., Kang, E., et al. (2005). Glucose metabolism in early onset versus late onset Alzheimer's disease: an SPM analysis of 120 patients. *Brain* 128(Pt 8), 1790–1801. doi: 10.1093/brain/awh539

Kim, J. S., Singh, V., Lee, J. K., Lerch, J., Ad-Dab'bagh, Y., MacDonald, D., et al. (2005). Automated 3-D extraction and evaluation of the inner and outer cortical surfaces using a laplacian map and partial volume effect classification. *Neuroimage* 27, 210–221. doi: 10.1016/j.neuroimage.2005.03.036

Klunk, W. E., Engler, H., Nordberg, A., Wang, Y., Blomqvist, G., Holt, D. P., et al. (2004). Imaging brain amyloid in Alzheimer's disease with Pittsburgh Compound-B. *Ann. Neurol.* 55, 306–319. doi: 10.1002/ana.20009

Lee, J. S., Kim, S., Yoo, H., Park, S., Jang, Y. K., Kim, H. J., et al. (2018). Trajectories of physiological brain aging and related factors in people aged from 20 to over-80. *J. Alzheimers. Dis.* 65, 1237–1246. doi: 10.3233/jad-170537

Lee, J. S., Shin, H. Y., Kim, H. J., Jang, Y. K., Jung, N. Y., Lee, J., et al. (2016). Combined effects of physical exercise and education on age-related cortical thinning in cognitively normal individuals. *Sci. Rep.* 6:24284. doi: 10.1038/srep24284

Lerch, J. P., and Evans, A. C. (2005). Cortical thickness analysis examined through power analysis and a population simulation. *Neuroimage* 24, 163–173. doi: 10.1016/j.neuroimage.2004.07.045

Lyttelton, O., Boucher, M., Robbins, S., and Evans, A. (2007). An unbiased iterative group registration template for cortical surface analysis. *Neuroimage* 34, 1535–1544. doi: 10.1016/j.neuroimage.2006.10.041

Masters, C. L., Bateman, R., Blennow, K., Rowe, C. C., Sperling, R. A., and Cummings, J. L. (2015). Alzheimer's disease. *Nat. Rev. Dis. Primers* 1:15056. doi: 10.1038/nrdp.2015.56

Mattson, M. P., and Arumugam, T. V. (2018). Hallmarks of brain aging: adaptive and pathological modification by metabolic states. *Cell Metab.* 27, 1176–1199. doi: 10.1016/j.cmet.2018.05.011

McKhann, G. M., Knopman, D. S., Chertkow, H., Hyman, B. T., Jack, C. R. Jr., Kawas, C. H., et al. (2011). The diagnosis of dementia due to Alzheimer's disease: recommendations from the national institute on aging-Alzheimer's association workgroups on diagnostic guidelines for Alzheimer's disease. *Alzheimers Dement* 7, 263–269. doi: 10.1016/j.jalz.2011.03.005

Meiberth, D., Scheef, L., Wolfsgruber, S., Boecker, H., Block, W., Traber, F., et al. (2015). Cortical thinning in individuals with subjective memory impairment. *J. Alzheimers Dis.* 45, 139–146. doi: 10.3233/jad-142322

Miners, J. S., Palmer, J. C., and Love, S. (2016). Pathophysiology of hypoperfusion of the precuneus in early Alzheimer's disease. *Brain Pathol.* 26, 533–541. doi: 10.1111/bpa.12331

Morris, J. C., Storandt, M., Miller, J. P., McKeel, D. W., Price, J. L., Rubin, E. H., et al. (2001). Mild cognitive impairment represents early-stage Alzheimer disease. *Arch. Neurol.* 58, 397–405.

Neltner, J. H., Abner, E. L., Jicha, G. A., Schmitt, F. A., Patel, E., Poon, L. W., et al. (2016). Brain pathologies in extreme old age. *Neurobiol. Aging* 37, 1–11. doi: 10.1016/j.neurobiolaging.2015.10.009

Ossenkoppele, R., Cohn-Sheehy, B. I., La Joie, R., Vogel, J. W., Moller, C., Lehmann, M., et al. (2015a). Atrophy patterns in early clinical stages across distinct phenotypes of Alzheimer's disease. *Hum. Brain Mapp.* 36, 4421–4437. doi: 10.1002/hbm.22927

Ossenkoppele, R., Jansen, W. J., Rabinovici, G. D., Knol, D. L., van der Flier, W. M., van Berckel, B. N., et al. (2015b). Prevalence of amyloid PET positivity in dementia syndromes: a meta-analysis. *JAMA* 313, 1939–1949. doi: 10.1001/jama.2015.4669

Peter, J., Scheef, L., Abdulkadir, A., Boecker, H., Heneka, M., Wagner, M., et al. (2014). Gray matter atrophy pattern in elderly with subjective memory impairment. *Alzheimers Dement* 10, 99–108. doi: 10.1016/j.jalz.2013.05.1764

Petersen, R. C. (2004). Mild cognitive impairment as a diagnostic entity. *J. Intern. Med.* 256, 183–194. doi: 10.1111/j.1365-2796.2004.01388.x

Rabin, L. A., Smart, C. M., and Amariglio, R. E. (2017). Subjective cognitive decline in preclinical Alzheimer's disease. *Annu. Rev. Clin. Psychol.* 13, 369–396. doi: 10.1146/annurev-clinpsy-032816-045136

Rabin, L. A., Smart, C. M., Crane, P. K., Amariglio, R. E., Berman, L. M., Boada, M., et al. (2015). Subjective cognitive decline in older adults: an overview of self-report measures used across 19 international research Studies. *J. Alzheimers Dis.* 48(Suppl. 1), S63–S86. doi: 10.3233/jad-150154

Scahill, R. I., Schott, J. M., Stevens, J. M., Rossor, M. N., and Fox, N. C. (2002). Mapping the evolution of regional atrophy in Alzheimer's disease: unbiased analysis of fluid-registered serial MRI. *Proc. Natl. Acad. Sci. U.S.A.* 99, 4703–4707. doi: 10.1073/pnas.052587399

Scheff, S. W., Price, D. A., Schmitt, F. A., Scheff, M. A., and Mufson, E. J. (2011). Synaptic loss in the inferior temporal gyrus in mild cognitive impairment and Alzheimer's disease. *J. Alzheimers Dis.* 24, 547–557. doi: 10.3233/jad-2011-101782

Scheltens, P., Blennow, K., Breteler, M. M., de Strooper, B., Frisoni, G. B., Salloway, S., et al. (2016). Alzheimer's disease. *Lancet* 388, 505–517. doi: 10.1016/s0140-6736(15)01124-1

Schultz, S. A., Oh, J. M., Koscik, R. L., Dowling, N. M., Gallagher, C. L., Carlsson, C. M., et al. (2015). Subjective memory complaints, cortical thinning, and cognitive dysfunction in middle-aged adults at risk for AD. *Alzheimers Dement* 1, 33–40. doi: 10.1016/j.dadm.2014.11.010

Selden, N. R., Gitelman, D. R., Salamon-Murayama, N., Parrish, T. B., and Mesulam, M. M. (1998). Trajectories of cholinergic pathways within the cerebral hemispheres of the human brain. *Brain* 121(Pt 12), 2249–2257. doi: 10.1093/brain/121.12.2249

Selnes, P., Fjell, A. M., Gjerstad, L., Bjornerud, A., Wallin, A., Due-Tonnessen, P., et al. (2012). White matter imaging changes in subjective and mild cognitive impairment. *Alzheimers Dement* 8(5 Suppl.), S112–S121. doi: 10.1016/j.jalz.2011.07.001

Seo, S. W., Cho, S. S., Park, A., Chin, J., and Na, D. L. (2009). Subcortical vascular versus amnestic mild cognitive impairment: comparison of cerebral glucose metabolism. *J. Neuroimaging* 19, 213–219. doi: 10.1111/j.1552-6569.2008.00292.x

Seo, S. W., Im, K., Lee, J. M., Kim, S. T., Ahn, H. J., Go, S. M., et al. (2011). Effects of demographic factors on cortical thickness in Alzheimer's disease. *Neurobiol. Aging* 32, 200–209. doi: 10.1016/j.neurobiolaging.2009.02.004

Singh, V., Chertkow, H., Lerch, J. P., Evans, A. C., Dorr, A. E., and Kabani, N. J. (2006). Spatial patterns of cortical thinning in mild cognitive impairment and Alzheimer's disease. *Brain* 129(Pt 11), 2885–2893. doi: 10.1093/brain/awl256

Sled, J. G., Zijdenbos, A. P., and Evans, A. C. (1998). A nonparametric method for automatic correction of intensity nonuniformity in MRI data. *IEEE Trans. Med. Imaging* 17, 87–97. doi: 10.1109/42.668698

Smith, S. M. (2002). Fast robust automated brain extraction. *Hum. Brain Mapp.* 17, 143–155. doi: 10.1002/hbm.10062

Sperling, R. A., Aisen, P. S., Beckett, L. A., Bennett, D. A., Craft, S., Fagan, A. M., et al. (2011). Toward defining the preclinical stages of Alzheimer's disease: recommendations from the national institute on aging-Alzheimer's association workgroups on diagnostic guidelines for Alzheimer's disease. *Alzheimers Dement* 7, 280–292. doi: 10.1016/j.jalz.2011.03.003

Sperling, R. A., Laviolette, P. S., O'Keefe, K., O'Brien, J., Rentz, D. M., Pihlajamaki, M., et al. (2009). Amyloid deposition is associated with impaired default network function in older persons without dementia. *Neuron* 63, 178–188. doi: 10.1016/j.neuron.2009.07.003

Stern, Y. (2002). What is cognitive reserve? Theory and research application of the reserve concept. *J. Int. Neuropsychol. Soc.* 8, 448–460. doi: 10.1017/s1355617702813248

Thal, D. R., Grinberg, L. T., and Attems, J. (2012). Vascular dementia: different forms of vessel disorders contribute to the development of dementia in the elderly brain. *Exp. Gerontol.* 47, 816–824. doi: 10.1016/j.exger.2012.05.023

4

Effects of Brain Parcellation on the Characterization of Topological Deterioration in Alzheimer's Disease

Zhanxiong Wu[1,2]*, Dong Xu*[1,3]*, Thomas Potter*[2]*, Yingchun Zhang*[2*] *and the Alzheimer's Disease Neuroimaging Initiative*[†]

[1] *School of Electronic Information, Hangzhou Dianzi University, Hangzhou, China,* [2] *Department of Biomedical Engineering, University of Houston, Houston, TX, United States,* [3] *Zhejiang Key Laboratory of Equipment Electronics, Hangzhou, China*

Correspondence:
Yingchun Zhang
yzhang94@uh.edu

[†] *Data used in preparation of this article were obtained from the Alzheimer's Disease Neuroimaging Initiative (ADNI) database (adni.loni.usc.edu). As such, the investigators within the ADNI contributed to the design and implementation of ADNI and/or provided data but did not participate in analysis or writing of this report. A complete listing of ADNI investigators can be found at: http://adni.loni.usc.edu/wp-content/uploads/how_to_apply/ADNI_Acknowledgement_List.pdf*

Alzheimer's disease (AD) causes the progressive deterioration of neural connections, disrupting structural connectivity (SC) networks within the brain. Graph-based analyses of SC networks have shown that topological properties can reveal the course of AD propagation. Different whole-brain parcellation schemes have been developed to define the nodes of these SC networks, although it remains unclear which scheme can best describe the AD-related deterioration of SC networks. In this study, four whole-brain parcellation schemes with different numbers of parcels were used to define SC network nodes. SC networks were constructed based on high angular resolution diffusion imaging (HARDI) tractography for a mixed cohort that includes 20 normal controls (NC), 20 early mild cognitive impairment (EMCI), 20 late mild cognitive impairment (LMCI), and 20 AD patients, from the Alzheimer's Disease Neuroimaging Initiative. Parcellation schemes investigated in this study include the OASIS-TRT-20 (62 regions), AAL (116 regions), HCP-MMP (180 regions), and Gordon-rsfMRI (333 regions), which have all been widely used for the construction of brain structural or functional connectivity networks. Topological characteristics of the SC networks, including the network strength, global efficiency, clustering coefficient, rich-club, characteristic path length, k-core, rich-club coefficient, and modularity, were fully investigated at the network level. Statistical analyses were performed on these metrics using Kruskal-Wallis tests to examine the group differences that were apparent at different stages of AD progression. Results suggest that the HCP-MMP scheme is the most robust and sensitive to AD progression, while the OASIS-TRT-20 scheme is sensitive to group differences in network strength, global efficiency, k-core, and rich-club coefficient at *k*-levels from 18 and 39. With the exception of the rich-club and modularity coefficients, AAL could not significantly identify group differences on other topological metrics. Further, the Gordon-rsfMRI atlas only significantly differentiates the groups on network strength, characteristic path length, k-core, and rich-club coefficient. Results show that the topological examination of SC networks with different parcellation schemes can provide important complementary AD-related information and thus contribute to a more accurate and earlier diagnosis of AD.

Keywords: Alzheimer's disease, mild cognitive impairment, high angular resolution diffusion imaging, structural connectivity network, fiber tracking

INTRODUCTION

As the leading cause of dementia in elderly adults, Alzheimer's disease (AD) is a progressive neurodegenerative disorder characterized by increasing cognitive and behavioral deficits (Mueller et al., 2005). Preceding AD, the mild cognitive impairment (MCI) phase presents with significant cognitive or behavioral deficits and an increased risk of developing dementia (Winblad et al., 2004; Jessen et al., 2014; Daianu et al., 2015; Mckenna et al., 2016). Understanding the physiological deterioration caused by MCI and AD provides an opportunity to develop future treatments and predict AD onset. Many post-mortem histological and *in-vivo* imaging studies have demonstrated widespread white matter (WM) alterations in MCI and AD patients (Brun and Englund, 1986; Rose et al., 2000; Bozzali et al., 2002; Nir et al., 2015). The WM degeneration and neuronal death linked to AD progression then creates abnormal connectivity patterns between anatomically related brain regions (Lo et al., 2010). Specifically, demyelination and axonal degeneration cause drastic reductions in WM volume, which may contribute to alterations in structural connectivity (SC) network efficacy. Therefore, AD-related cognitive and behavioral deficits may be directly linked the disconnection of brain regions (Delbeuck et al., 2003; Sorg et al., 2009; Lo et al., 2010), such that altered SC topological patterns reflect the propagation stage of AD.

High angular resolution diffusion imaging (HARDI) has provided an ability to extensively study brain networks in clinical neuroscience (Nguyen et al., 2018). The recent development of accurate and sophisticated HARDI-based tractography methods has encouraged the exploration of regional connectivity and topological network measures, which can quantify MCI and AD-linked brain changes. Graph theory has been frequently employed to detect SC network differences across normal control (NC), MCI, and AD groups, and a variety of topological measures sensitive to SC network disruption can be computed to reveal how AD affects the human connectome. Particular measures of interest include *k*-core, rich-club efficiency, nodal degree, characteristic path length, clustering coefficient, and global efficiency. To perform statistical analysis on SC networks, Kim et al. presented a multi-resolution analysis framework (Kim et al., 2015), in which a Wavelet representation of each anatomical connection was derived at multiple resolutions to analyze AD-related alterations. In Daianu et al. (2015), rich-club properties at a range of degree thresholds were calculated, and their findings indicated that brain network disruptions occurred predominately in the low-degree (<16) regions of the connectome in AD. In Daianu et al. (2013b), *k*-core was computed to understand the brain network breakdown caused by AD. In Lo et al. (2010), the alterations of various network properties were examined, indicating that AD patients exhibit shorter path lengths, decreased global efficiency, and reduced nodal efficiency. Yao et al. (2010) explored the characteristics of SC networks in MCI and AD, finding that the MCI groups showed a loss of hub regions in the temporal lobe and altered inter-regional correlations, and that the topological measures of the MCI SC networks exhibited intermediate values. Most of these findings suggest that AD is related to the disruption of structural connectivity, which is characterized by the loss of rich-club organization and network efficiency. Together, the findings suggest that AD is associated with a disrupted topological organization of SC networks, thus providing structural evidence for abnormalities in the SC network integrity of AD patients.

Graph-based analysis of brain structural networks provides a chance to understand how AD-linked structural connectivity abnormalities underlie the cognitive and behavioral deficits of patients. Specifically, the definition of network nodes is one of the most critical steps in network topological analysis, as it assigns the network structure and density for subsequent assessment. Different whole-brain parcellation schemes have been developed to define network nodes, although the effect that these schemes have on the detection of AD propagation stages remains unknown. Accurate brain parcellation provides a foundation for understanding the functional and structural organization of the human brain. During graph-based analysis of the SC networks derived from HARDI, brain parcellation is a key step for the construction of brain anatomical brain network architecture. This step is not trivial, however; the division of the cortex into different numbers of regions affects the structure of the SC network, such that the resulting topological properties of the generated SC network can be significantly changed by the scale of the chosen parcellation atlas (Proix et al., 2016). Considering that brain parcellation schemes are fundamental to the isolation and selection of brain regions, their application plays an important role in revealing the abnormal topological organization of SC networks in MCI and AD.

Cognitive studies have demonstrated that the cerebral cortex is comprised of distinct cortical areas that are interconnected through WM fibers (Sporns et al., 2004; delEtoile and Adeli, 2017). Network analysis represents cortical regions and their connections as a series of nodes and edges, respectively (Lo et al., 2010). Previous investigation have typically relied on a single type of whole-brain parcellation scheme to construct SC networks, such as the 96-region Harvard-Oxford atlas used in Shao et al. (2012), 113-region Harvard-Oxford atlas used in Zhan et al. (2015a), 162-region IIT3 atlas used in Kim et al. (2015), and 68-region Desikan-Killiany atlas used in Daianu et al. (2013b) and Daianu et al. (2015). Each of these schemes presents a different number of parcels, and the effect this has on AD-related SC topological changes has not comprehensively characterized. In this study, SC networks are constructed for NC, early mild cognitive impairment (EMCI), late mild cognitive impairment (LMCI), and AD subjects based on HARDI tractography to fully characterize the manner in which patterns of SC network topological metrics change based on parcellation schemes. Four different whole-brain parcellation schemes over a range of parcellation scales (62, 116, 180, and 333 regions) were used to define SC network nodes: the OASIS-TRT-20 (62 regions) (Klein and Tourville, 2012), AAL (116 regions) (Tzourio-Mazoyer et al., 2002), HCP-MMP (180 regions) (Glasser et al., 2016), and Gordon-rsfMRI (333 regions) (Gordon et al., 2014). Edges were then estimated through deterministic fiber tracking based on orientation distribution function (ODF) fields, which was derived from HARDI images (Iturria-Medina et al., 2008; Descoteaux

TABLE 1 | Demographics information for ANDI participants, arranged into NC, EMCI, LMCI, and AD groups.

	NC	EMCI	LMCI	AD
N	20	20	20	20
Gender	8M/12F	13M/7F	11M/9F	10M/10F
Age range (years)	66–87	62–88	61–85	61–90
Mean age (*SD*)	76.85 (6.67)	77.90 (7.26)	75.60 (5.65)	74.15 (7.94)

et al., 2009; Côté et al., 2013; Yeh et al., 2013; Christiaens et al., 2015). To determine if SC topological characteristics changed with different cortical parcellation schemes as AD progressed, SC network topological assessments were performed on a mixed ADNI cohort of 20 NC, 20 early MCI (EMCI), 20 late MCI (LMCI), and 20 AD subjects. Finally, to explore the influence that different cortical parcellation schemes exert on the graph-based analysis of brain SC networks in AD propagation, Kruskal-Wallis tests were employed to identify group differences in network strength, global efficiency, characterized path length, cluster coefficient, *k*-core, and modularity coefficient. Additionally, linear regression analysis was used to examine the changing trajectories of rich-club coefficients for NC, EMCI, LMCI, and AD groups.

MATERIALS AND METHODS

Data

Data used in the preparation of this article were obtained from the Alzheimer's Disease Neuroimaging Initiative (ADNI) database (adni.loni.usc.edu). The ADNI was launched in 2003 as a public-private partnership, led by Principal Investigator Michael W. Weiner, MD. The primary goal of the ADNI has been to test whether serial magnetic resonance imaging (MRI), positron emission tomography (PET), other biological markers, and clinical and neuropsychological assessment can be combined to measure the progression of mild cognitive impairment (MCI) and early AD (Jack et al., 2008; Risacher et al., 2009; Petersen et al., 2010). In this study, 80 subjects were selected from the ADNI database and arranged into NC, EMCI, LMCI, and AD groups according to their ADNI classification. **Table 1** shows the demographics of the participants, including age and gender. All 80 participants underwent whole-brain MRI scanning using 3T GE Medical Systems scanners. The acquisition protocol included a T1-weighted image (acquisition matrix = 256 × 256 × 196, voxel size = 1.05 × 1.05 × 1.2 mm^3, TR = 6.96 ms, TE = 2.83 ms). Furthermore, the participants were scanned with DWI echo planar imaging (EPI) protocol. Specifically, five images with no diffusion sensitization (b0 images) and 41 images along 41 diffusion directions were acquired (b = 1,000 s/mm^2) with the following parameters: acquisition matrix = 128 × 128 × 55, voxel size = 2.7 × 2.7 × 2.7 mm^3, TR=7,200.0 ms, TE = 56.0 ms.

SC Network Construction

We evaluated the influence of cortex parcellation schemes on the topological characterization of AD propagation by systematically varying the number of brain parcellated regions. The cerebral cortex of each subject was parcellated into 62, 116, 180, or 333 regions, according to the parcellation templates of OASIS-TRT-20 (Klein and Tourville, 2012), AAL (Tzourio-Mazoyer et al., 2002), HCP-MMP (Glasser et al., 2016), and Gordon-rsfMRI (Gordon et al., 2014), respectively. These four parcellation templates were all spatially normalized into Montreal Neurological Institute (MNI) space (Fonov et al., 2011), and are visualized from different views in **Figure S1**. Before tracking, the parcellation labels of these templates were used to segment whole brain into clusters of cortical regions. The parcellation templates were co-registered from MNI space (1 mm^3) to DWI space via T1-weighted images using a 12-degree-of-freedom transformation matrix, using Freesurfer 6.0.0 and DSI Studio.

The construction of subject-specific SC networks requires a number of complex steps, including cortical parcellation, fiber tractography, and connection strength estimation, as shown in **Figure 1**. To determine the structural connectivity between each pair of cortical regions, deterministic ODF-based tractography was used. First, the eddy current effects and motion artifacts in the DWI images were corrected using the DiffusionKit toolbox (Xie et al., 2016). DWI images were then denoised using singular value decomposition and non-local means methods, as described in Wu et al. (2018a). Second, a model-free general q-ball imaging (GQI) reconstruction method was employed to estimate ODFs from the HARDI images, with high sensitivity and specificity to WM characteristics and pathology (Yeh and Tseng, 2011). The whole-brain fiber tracking was performed using DSI Studio software (Yeh et al., 2013), with a fractional anisotropy (FA) threshold of 0.2 and a track-turning angular threshold of 60° between each two connections. Cortical connections were established between any set of cortical regions that a fiber bundle passed through or ended in. ODF-based tracking was chosen for this application, as it can resolve multiple fiber populations, including crossing, branching, and merging fibers, and thereby produces more accurate results than DT-based tracking methods (Barnett, 2009; Zhan et al., 2015b; Wu et al., 2018b). The number of reconstructed fibers between different regions were then used to define SC network edges (Hagmann et al., 2007; Houenou et al., 2007; Li et al., 2009), while each parcellated region was regarded as a network node.

Network Topological Metrics

Graph theory provides a set of measures to concisely quantify the topological properties of brain networks and describe interrelationships between brain regions of interest (ROIs) (represented by nodes in SC networks). Graph-based analysis of brain SC topological patterns allows for the quantification of a broad range of network characteristics. The most common measures used to describe the integrity of healthy or diseased brain networks include network strength, characteristic path length, efficiency, clustering coefficient, *k*-core, rich-club coefficient, and modularity (Sporns, 2010). Topological characterization was performed using the GRETNA (http://www.nitrc.org/projects/gretna/) (Wang et al., 2015) and Brain Connectivity Toolbox (BCT) toolboxes (https://sites.google.com/site/bctnet/) (Rubinov and Sporns, 2010). The utilized network

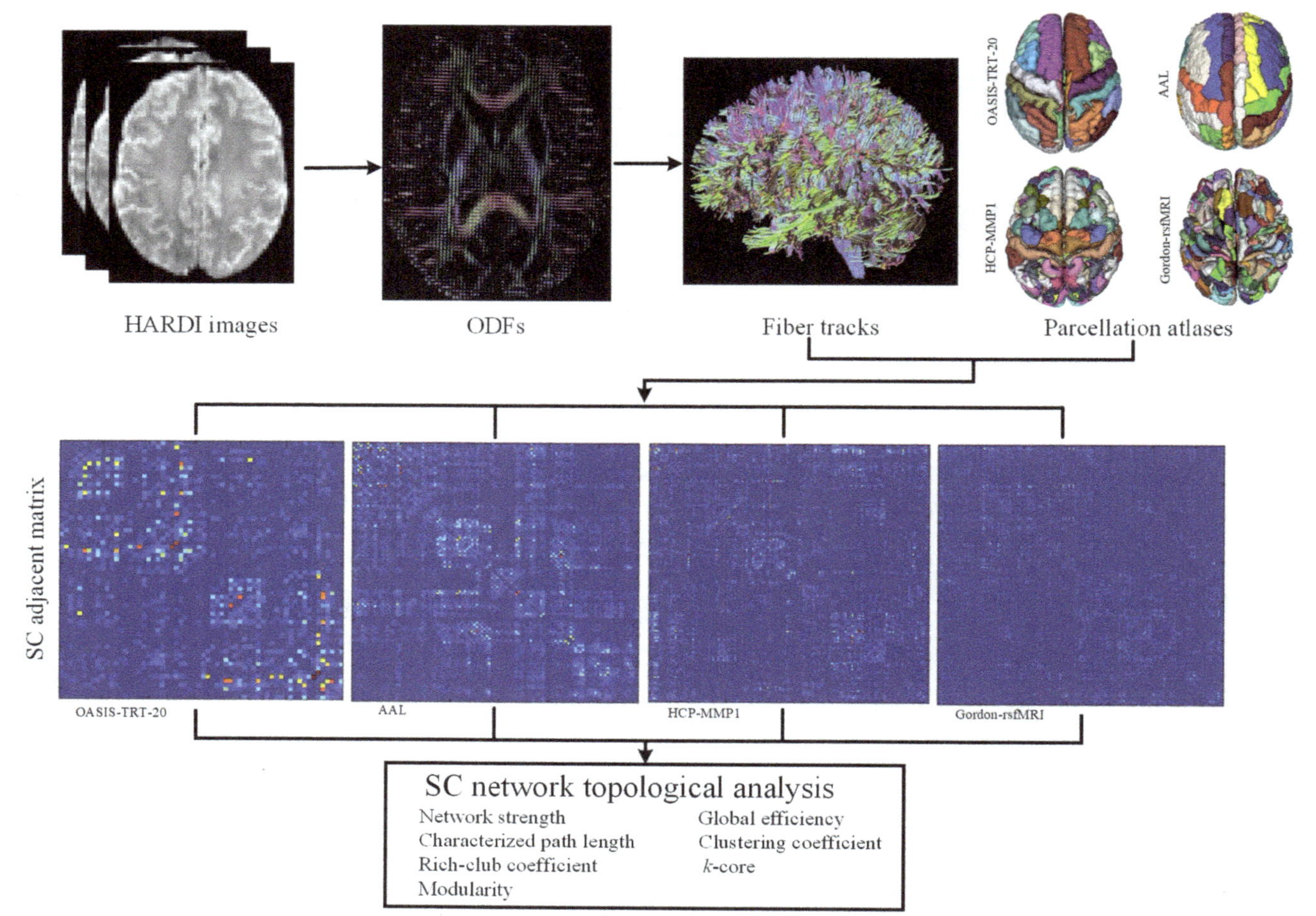

FIGURE 1 | Flowchart of SC network topological analysis. Four parcellation atlases were employed to define the nodes of the SC networks, including OASIS-TRT-20 (62 regions) (Klein and Tourville, 2012), AAL (116 regions) (Tzourio-Mazoyer et al., 2002), HCP-MMP (180 regions) (Glasser et al., 2016), and Gordon-rsfMRI (333 regions) (Gordon et al., 2014). ODFs were computed from HARDI images with a general q-ball imaging (GQI) computational model. Whole-brain tractography was performed using the DSI-Studio tool, and edges were determined by the number of neural connections between each pair of parcellated regions.

metrics are briefly described below (Cao et al., 2013; Daianu et al., 2013a, 2015).

Network Strength

For a SC network G with N nodes and K edges, we calculated the strength of G as Cao et al. (2013):

$$S_p(G) = \frac{1}{N} \sum_{i \in G} S(i) \tag{1}$$

where $S(i)$ is the sum of the edge weights linking to node i. The strength of a network is the average of the connection strengths across all of the nodes in the network. This metric reflects the extent to which network nodes are connected.

Clustering Coefficient

The clustering coefficient C_p of a network is the average of the clustering coefficient over all nodes, which indicates the extent of local interconnectivity or cliquishness in a network (Watts and Strogatz, 1998).

$$C(i) = \frac{2}{k_i(k_i - 1)} \sum_{j,k} (w_{ij} w_{jk} w_{ki})^{1/3} \tag{2}$$

Where k_i is the degree of node i, and w is connection weight. The clustering coefficient will be zero if all nodes are isolated or have just one connection (Watts and Strogatz, 1998).

$$C_p = \frac{1}{N} \sum_{i \in G} C(i) \tag{3}$$

Characteristic Path Length

The path length between any pair of nodes is defined as the sum of the edge lengths along this path. In this study, the length of each edge was assigned by computing the reciprocal of the edge weight, $\frac{1}{w_{ij}}$. The characteristic path length of G was then computed as Cao et al. (2013):

$$L_c(G) = \frac{1}{N(N-1)} \sum\nolimits_{i \neq j \in G} L_{ij} \tag{4}$$

where L_{ij} defined as the shortest path between node i and node j. This metric quantifies the ability for information to be propagated in parallel.

Network Efficiency

The global efficiency of G measures the efficiency of parallel information transfer throughout the network, which can be computed as follows (Cao et al., 2013):

$$E_{glob}(G) = \frac{1}{N(N-1)} \sum\nolimits_{i \neq j \in G} \frac{1}{L_{ij}} \tag{5}$$

where L_{ij} is the shortest path length between nodes i and j in G.

k-Core Decomposition

To model the basic architecture of SC networks, a k-core decomposition algorithm that disentangles the hierarchical structure of the networks was proposed in Daianu et al. (2013b). This k-core decomposition outputs a network core that consists of highly and mutually interconnected nodes. This is accomplished by recursively removing nodes with degrees lower than k, such that k serves as a degree threshold for nodes, ultimately identifying dense subsets of the graph.

Rich-Club Coefficient

"Rich-club" is a network property that describes how high-degree network nodes are more interconnected than would be expected by chance. The rich-club coefficient is the ratio of the number of connections among nodes of degree k (or higher) to the total possible number of connections for those nodes (Daianu et al., 2015). In this study, Rich-club coefficients were calculated at a range of degree thresholds. The rich-club coefficient can be determined as:

$$R(k) = \frac{E_{>k}}{N_{>k}(N_{>k} - 1)} \tag{6}$$

where R is rich-club coefficient, $E_{>k}$ is the number of connections among nodes of degree k or higher, and $N_{>k}(N_{>k} - 1)$ is the total possible number of connections if those nodes were fully connected.

Modularity

Modularity or community structure is a property that is common to brain SC networks, which divides SC network nodes into groups such that structural connections within each group are dense while connections between the groups are sparse. The study of modularity structures in SC networks can provide invaluable help in understanding and visualizing the structure of SC networks. Modularization is an optimization process in which the maximal value of Q—the quantity known as modularity—is obtained over all possible divisions of a network (Newman,

TABLE 2 | The topological metrics (mean ± std) of SC networks in each group, including network strength S_P, global efficiency E_{glob}, characterized path length L_C, and cluster coefficient C_P.

	CN				EMCI				LMCI				AD			
	OASIS	AAL	HCP	Gordon	OASIS	AAL	HCP	Gordon	OASIS	AAL	HCP	Gordon	OASIS	AAL	HCP	Gordon
S_P	3.06 ± 1.14	4.59 ± 0.87	3.80 ± 1.60	1.92 ± 0.55	2.40 ± 0.82	4.31 ± 1.16	2.81 ± 1.36	1.65 ± 0.58	2.39 ± 1.14	4.18 ± 0.91	2.81 ± 1.10	1.50 ± 0.52	1.89 ± 0.81	3.86 ± 0.88	1.95 ± 0.97	1.36 ± 0.45
E_{glob}	0.12 ± 0.03	0.11 ± 0.02	0.08 ± 0.02	0.05 ± 0.01	0.10 ± 0.02	0.10 ± 0.01	0.07 ± 0.02	0.05 ± 0.01	0.10 ± 0.03	0.10 ± 0.02	0.07 ± 0.02	0.05 ± 0.01	0.09 ± 0.03	0.10 ± 0.02	0.05 ± 0.02	0.05 ± 0.01
L_C	12.73 ± 2.97	12.75 ± 2.68	17.78 ± 4.96	21.79 ± 1.26	14.44 ± 4.26	13.15 ± 2.33	19.87 ± 4.50	31.89 ± 1.49	14.18 ± 3.85	13.26 ± 2.51	21.01 ± 6.08	21.91 ± 1.67	15.85 ± 4.01	13.92 ± 2.45	24.98 ± 7.41	23.30 ± 2.03
C_P	0.06 ± 0.01	0.05 ± 0.01	0.04 ± 0.01	0.03 ± 0.01	0.05 ± 0.01	0.05 ± 0.01	0.04 ± 0.01	0.03 ± 0.01	0.05 ± 0.01	0.05 ± 0.01	0.04 ± 0.01	0.03 ± 0.01	0.05 ± 0.01	0.05 ± 0.01	0.03 ± 0.01	0.03 ± 0.01

OASIS, AAL, HCP, and Gordon represent OASIS-TRT-20 (62 regions), AAL (116 regions), HCP-MMP (180 regions), and Gordon-rsfMRI (333 regions), respectively.

2006). Larger Q values are indicative of a highly modular network organization, while lower Q values indicate a more uniform network structure (Newman and Girvan, 2004). In this study, the *community_louvain* function of the BCT was used to calculate the modularity for the identified SC networks. The employed Louvain optimization is a simple, efficient, and easy-to-implement method for identifying modules in large networks. The optimization comprises two steps. First, the method searches for small modules by optimizing modularity locally. Second, it aggregates the nodes that belong to the same module and builds a new network wherein each node represents a module identified in the first step. These steps are iterated until a maximum of modularity value is attained and a hierarchy of modules is generated (Blondel et al., 2008; Lancichinetti and Fortunato, 2009). Modularity (Q) is defined as:

$$Q = \frac{1}{2m}\sum_{i,j}\left[w_{ij} - \frac{k_i k_j}{2m}\right]\delta(c_i, c_j) \quad (7)$$

where w_{ij} denotes the linking weight between node i and node j; k_i, and k_j are the sums of the weights of the edges attached to nodes i and j, respectively; m is the total link weight in the network overall; and $\delta(c_i, c_j)$ is 1 when nodes i and j are assigned to the same module and 0 otherwise.

Topological Metric Estimation

After SC network nodes were determined using four different parcellation schemes, ODF-based tractography was employed to calculate the structural connectivity for each subject. Connection

TABLE 3 | *P*-values of Kruskal-Wallis testing for S_p, E_{glob}, L_C, and C_p differences among the NC, EMCI, LMCI, and AD groups.

	OASIS	AAL	HCP	Gordon
S_p	**0.0017**	0.0782	**0.0007**	**0.0032**
E_{glob}	**0.0080**	0.8482	**0.0015**	0.9816
L_C	0.0637	0.3627	**0.0019**	**0.0003**
C_p	0.0514	0.9988	**0.0207**	0.9538

The significant p-values are shown in bold. OASIS, AAL, HCP, and Gordon represent OASIS-TRT-20 (62 regions), AAL (116 regions), HCP-MMP (180 regions), and Gordon-rsfMRI (333 regions), respectively. S_p denotes network strength. E_{glob} is global network efficiency. L_C is characterized path length. C_p is clustering coefficient.

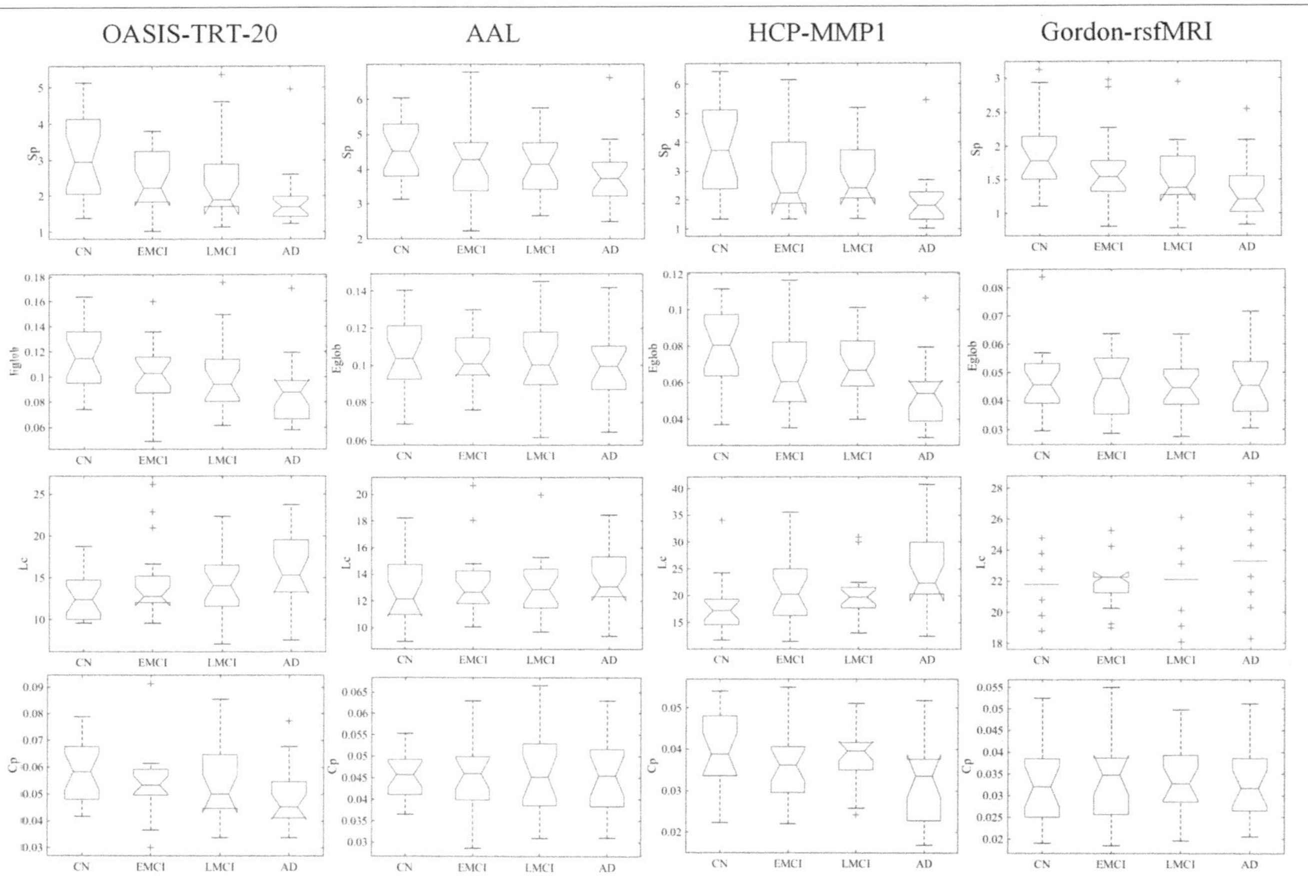

FIGURE 2 | Group median and interquartile ranges of the SC topological metrics for each group, including network strength S_p, global efficiency E_{glob}, characterized path length L_C, and cluster coefficient C_p. *P*-values derived from Kruskal-Wallis tests assessing SC topological differences among NC, EMCI, LMCI, and AD for each parcellation scheme are reported in **Table 3**.

strength values were normalized from [0, 1] and self-connections were excluded. Group average SC matrices were computed for each parcellation scheme. Afterwards, topological measures were estimated using the codes provided in the BCT and GRETNA, including network strength, global efficiency, characterized path length, cluster coefficient, k-core, rich-club coefficient, and modularity. Separate from other measures, k-core measurement directly reflects how the SC network breaks down as cognitive impairment increases, quantifying how AD affects the human connectome (Daianu et al., 2013b). k acts as a degree threshold for network nodes by which k-core decomposition creates a subnetwork that consists of highly and mutually interconnected nodes by recursively removing the nodes with degrees lower than k. In this study, we used k-core analysis to access AD-related anatomical network changes under different whole-brain parcellation schemes including OASIS-TRT-20, AAL, HCP-MMP, and Gordon-rsfMRI. When using a k threshold <17, AD subjects cannot be discriminated from NC and MCI subjects (Daianu et al., 2015). Thus, thresholds of $k = 20$ and $k = 30$ are typically chosen for comparative computations. The rich-club coefficient is the ratio of the number of connections among nodes of degree k or higher to the total possible number of connections if those nodes were fully connected (Daianu et al., 2015). This coefficient was computed at a range of k-value thresholds from 17 to 39. When the threshold is <17, the coefficient is close to 1 (Daianu et al., 2015). Modularity optimization is a complete subdivision of the network into non-overlapping modules (Fortunato, 2010), which maximizes the number of within-module edges and minimizes the number of between-module edges. In this study, we used a Louvain community detection algorithm provided in BCT to achieve sub-module decomposition.

Statistical Analysis

To evaluate discriminating power for AD progressing phases of the network metrices corresponding to different parcellation schemes, statistical analyses were separately performed on each of them using Kruskal-Wallis tests. Additionally, a linear regression model was fitted to rich-club coefficient over a range of k-levels from 17 to 39 (Daianu et al., 2015), which was calculated using different whole-brain parcellation schemes. The intercepts and slopes of these regression models generally reflect the associations between rich-club coefficient and progressive AD phases. P-values lower than 0.05 were considered statistically significant.

RESULTS

The group-averaged SC matrices of NC, EMCI, LMCI, and AD groups are depicted in **Figure S2**. The calculated network metrics (mean $\pm$ std) for each parcellation method are listed in **Table 2**, including network strength S_p, global efficiency E_{glob}, characterized path length L_c, and cluster coefficient C_p. The mean and standard deviation of group network metrics computed for each parcellation scheme are reported in **Table 2**, with median values and interquartile differences represented in **Figure 2**. P-values derived from Kruskal-Wallis tests assessing the SC differences among NC, EMCI, LMCI, and AD groups for each parcellation scheme are reported in **Table 3** (significant values are shown in bold). Significant group differences in S_p, E_{glob}, L_c, and C_p values were observed when HCP-MMP

TABLE 4 | P-values of Kruskal-Wallis testing for k-core differences among the NC, EMCI, LMCI, and AD groups.

	OASIS	AAL	HCP	Gordon
$k = 20$	**0.0038**	0.2345	**0.0105**	**0.0014**
$k = 30$	**0.0040**	0.1696	**0.0024**	**0.0023**

The significant p-values are shown in bold. OASIS, AAL, HCP, and Gordon represent OASIS-TRT-20 (62 regions), AAL (116 regions), HCP-MMP (180 regions), and Gordon-rsfMRI (333 regions), respectively.

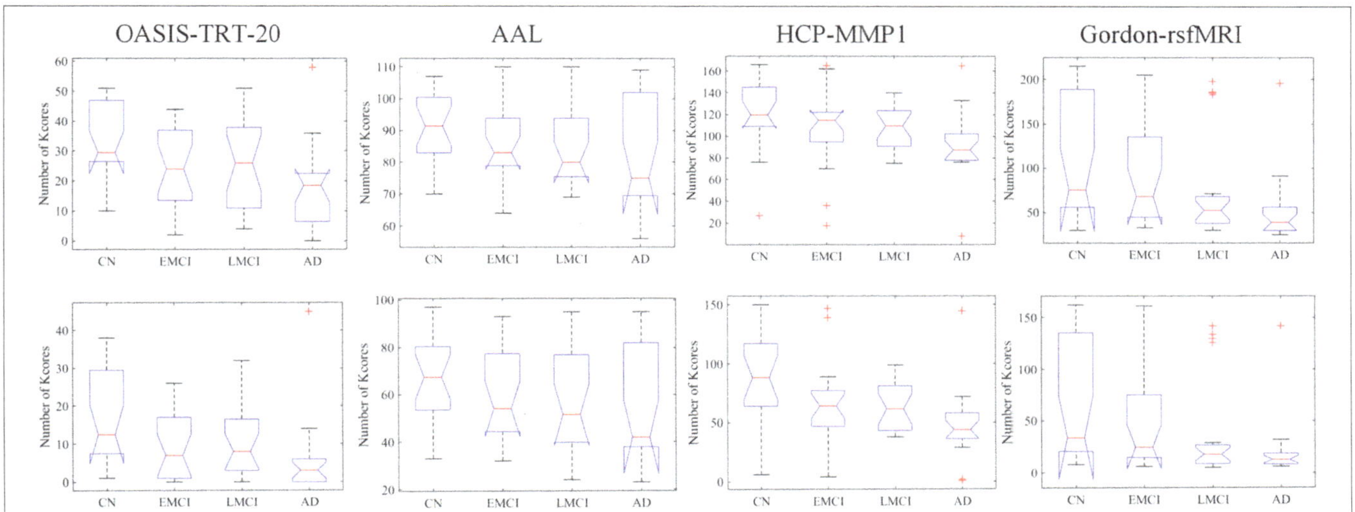

FIGURE 3 | Group median and interquartile ranges of k-core network nodes for each group, typically at the thresholds of $k = 20$ and $k = 30$. P-values derived from Kruskal-Wallis tests assessing SC topological differences among NC, EMCI, LMCI, and AD for each parcellation scheme are reported in **Table 4**.

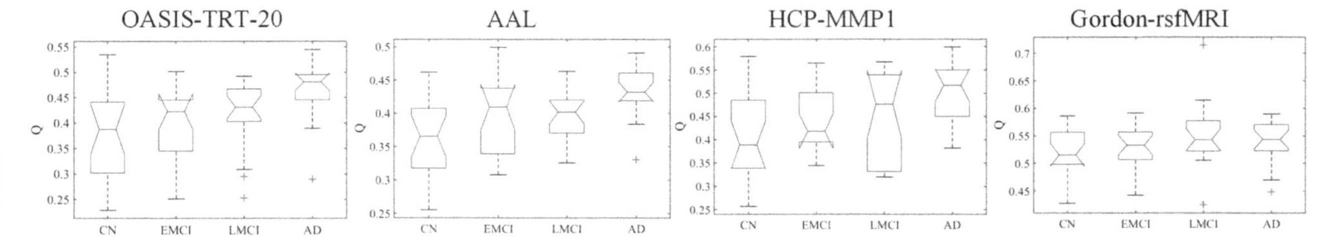

FIGURE 4 | Group median and interquartile ranges of Q coefficient of modularity structure for each group. *P*-values derived from Kruskal-Wallis tests assessing SC topological differences among NC, EMCI, LMCI, and AD for each parcellation scheme are reported in **Table 5**.

TABLE 5 | *P*-values of Kruskal-Wallis testing for modularity differences among the NC, EMCI, LMCI, and AD groups.

	OASIS	AAL	HCP	Gordon
Q of modularity	**0.0004**	**0.0008**	**0.0148**	0.1540

The significant p-values are shown in bold. OASIS, AAL, HCP, and Gordon represent OASIS-TRT-20 (62 regions), AAL (116 regions), HCP-MMP (180 regions), and Gordon-rsfMRI (333 regions), respectively.

was used as parcellation scheme ($p = 0.0007$, $p = 0.0015$, $p = 0.0019$, and $p = 0.0207$, respectively). No group differences were found for any AAL-based SC indexes. Significant group differences were found in S_p and L_c ($p = 0.0032$ and $p = 0.0003$, respectively) but not in f E_{glob} and C_p for SC matrices constructed with Gordon-rsfMRI nodes. For OASIS-TRT-20 parcellation, significant differences in S_p and E_{glob} were found among the NC, EMCI, LMCI and AD ($p = 0.0017$ and $p = 0.0080$, respectively). No significant group differences in L_c and C_p values were observed for OASIS parcellation.

At the typical thresholds of $k = 20$ and $k = 30$, Kruskal-Wallis tests were performed on the number of k-core network nodes of NC, EMCI, LMCI, and AD groups. **Figure 3** shows group median and interquartile ranges, and the corresponding p-values are provided in **Table 4**. The results indicate that significant group differences in terms of k-core were detected when OASIS-TRT-20, HCP-MMP, and Gordon-rsfMRI were used as parcellation schemes ($p = 0.0038/0.0040$, $p = 0.0105/0.0024$, and $p = 0.0014/0.0023$, respectively). For AAL parcellation, no significant group differences in k-core number were observed ($p = 0.2345/0.1696$).

The topological metric of Q quantifies the extent to which SC networks may be subdivided into clearly delineated groups. **Figure 4** shows group median and interquartile ranges of modularity statistic Q across different parcellation schemes, and **Table 5** shows the p-values with significant values in bold. Results indicate that significant group differences were detected when OASIS-TRT-20, AAL, and HCP-MMP parcellation schemes were used to define network nodes ($p = 0.0004$, $p = 0.0008$, and $p = 0.0148$, respectively). For Gordon-rsfMRI parcellation, no significant group differences in Q were observed ($p = 0.1540$).

To evaluate discriminatory efficacy of different parcellation schemes on rich-club coefficient, Kruskal-Wallis tests on the rich-club coefficient $R(k)$ at each of the k-levels from 17 to 39

TABLE 6 | *P*-values of Kruskal-Wallis testing for rich-club coefficient differences among the NC, EMCI, LMCI, and AD groups.

k-level	OASIS	AAL	HCP	Gordon
17	0.0965	**0.0002**	**0.0013**	**<0.0001**
18	**0.0045**	**0.0002**	**0.0007**	**<0.0001**
19	**<0.0001**	**0.0002**	**0.0008**	**<0.0001**
20	**<0.0001**	**<0.0001**	**0.0006**	**<0.0001**
21	**<0.0001**	**0.0002**	**0.0004**	**<0.0001**
22	**<0.0001**	**0.0004**	**0.0005**	**<0.0001**
23	**<0.0001**	**0.0015**	**0.0007**	**<0.0001**
24	**0.0002**	**0.0005**	**0.0004**	**<0.0001**
25	**<0.0001**	**0.0005**	**0.0005**	**<0.0001**
26	**0.0004**	**0.0005**	**0.0003**	**<0.0001**
27	**0.0002**	**0.0002**	**0.0003**	**<0.0001**
28	**0.0001**	**0.0002**	**0.0002**	**<0.0001**
29	**<0.0001**	**0.0001**	**0.0006**	**<0.0001**
30	**<0.0001**	**0.0003**	**0.0009**	**<0.0001**
31	**<0.0001**	**0.0005**	**0.0006**	**<0.0001**
32	**<0.0001**	**0.0005**	**0.0006**	**<0.0001**
33	**<0.0001**	**0.0006**	**0.0007**	**<0.0001**
34	**<0.0001**	**0.0006**	**0.0005**	**0.0002**
35	**<0.0001**	**0.0010**	**0.0006**	**0.0003**
36	**<0.0001**	**0.0007**	**0.0009**	**0.0005**
37	**0.0001**	**0.0008**	**<0.0001**	**0.0008**
38	**<0.0001**	**0.0006**	**0.0008**	**0.0012**
39	**0.0003**	**0.0007**	**0.0012**	**0.0032**

The significant p-values are shown in bold. OASIS, AAL, HCP, and Gordon represent OASIS-TRT-20 (62 regions), AAL (116 regions), HCP-MMP (180 regions), and Gordon-rsfMRI (333 regions), respectively.

(Daianu et al., 2015) were performed (p-values at each k-level are shown in **Table 6**), a linear regression model was fit to $R(k)$ as it was calculated over the k-levels from 17 to 39. The results in **Table 6** indicate that the rich-club coefficients computed based on AAL, HCP-MMP, and Gordon-rsfMRI over the k-levels from 17 to 39 are significantly sensitive to the group differences across NC, EMCI, LMCI, and AD (the corresponding p-values are <0.05). Except for the rich-club coefficients computed based on the OASIS_TRT_20 atlas at k-level $= 17$ ($p = 0.0965$), the coefficients at k-level between 18 and 39 are able to significantly differentiate the groups (the corresponding p-values are <0.05).

Figure 5 shows the linear regression fitted results which reflects the changing trend of rich-club coefficient over the k-levels from 17 to 39.

DISCUSSION

To this point, evaluating the effects of brain parcellation on the topological characterization of SC networks has been a challenging task, largely due to the lack of universally-accepted parcellation templates that can be used as a reference (Arslan et al., 2017). To provide an effective comparison, this study applied different parcellation schemes and ODF-based tractography to build SC networks for NC, EMCI, LMCI, and AD subjects. Four whole-brain parcellation techniques were used to define the nodes of these SC networks with different number of parcels, and connections were estimated by measuring the pairwise number of neural fiber bundles. To assess the impact of parcellation scheme on the ability to identify differences among NC, EMCI, LMCI, and AD, we explored the topological organization of SC networks. Our findings provide evidence that parcellation schemes have significant impact on topological characterization of brain structural connectivity networks in AD propagation.

After the topological measures were derived from subject-specific adjacency matrices, Kruskal-Wallis tests were employed to investigate their sensitivity to the NC, EMCI, LMCI, and AD groups under each parcellation scheme. Tested measures included network strength, global efficiency, clustering coefficient, characteristic path length, k-core, rich-club coefficient, and modularity. We found that these measures were generally sensitive to the selection of parcellation scheme. When interpreting the SC-related results of AD-related studies, the parcellation effect on the calculated measures is a factor that needs to be taken into consideration.

Overall, characteristic path length increased with AD progression in all tested parcellation schemes while network strength, global efficiency, and clustering coefficient decreased, as shown in **Table 2** and **Figure 2**. This is consistent with the results in Lo et al. (2010), Yao et al. (2010), and Daianu et al. (2013a). When the HCP-MMP (180 nodes) parcellation was used to define network nodes, the metrics, including S_p, E_{glob}, L_c, and C_p, displayed significant differences between the NC, EMCI, LMCI, and AD groups. In contrary, AAL atlas cannot discriminate group differences in terms of S_p, E_{glob}, C_p, L_c. The OASIS-TRT-20 scheme was unable to differentiate group differences in terms of C_p and L_c, while Gordon_rsfMRI scheme cannot recognize group differences in terms of E_{glob} and C_p. From the results, we could conclude that network strength $S_p$was most robust and sensitive to the characterization of topological deterioration in MCI and AD, while clustering coefficient C_p lacked robustness to whole-brain parcellation atlases. These findings align with a previous study which investigated structural connectivity and the sensitivity of network measures to the parcel number of the parcellation scheme (Zalesky et al., 2010).

k-core patterns in the SC networks were then explored, from which the most highly interconnected subnetworks were determined. Kruskal-Wallis test was then performed to determine if k-core regions remained intact or were altered by AD progression by eliminating the least reliable anatomical connections (Daianu et al., 2013b). In this study, we analyzed the k-core feature at $k = 20$ and $k = 30$, as $k = 16$ has been reported as the minimum value at which the majority of nodes in networks would remain connected. As Daianu et al. (2013b) explored, some k-core nodes are lost with AD progression (**Figure 3**). We used the number of k-core nodes as a measure to investigate AD-related network disruption. Significant group differences in the k-core patterns of the NC, EMCI, LMCI, and AD groups were found under the OASIS-TRT-20, HCP-MMP, and Gordon_rsfMRI parcellation schemes. Regardless of k-level, group difference could not be detected when using AAL atlas.

Modularity was then used to measure the extent to which a network is optimally partitioned into functional subgroups (Rubinov and Sporns, 2011). Due to the breakdown of anatomical connections, the modularity structures of the SC networks exhibited apparent alterations (**Figure 4**). The breakdown of global informative connections involving the medial prefrontal, posterior parietal, and insular cortices were already apparent in MCI, suggesting that progressive damage to fiber connections begins during the predementia stages of AD (Acosta-Cabronero et al., 2009; Sorg et al., 2009; Sperling et al., 2010; Shao et al., 2012). AD patients then show reduced associative white matter fiber density in the cingulum, the splenium of the corpus callosum, and the superior longitudinal fasciculus (Rose et al., 2000). Coherence studies have further identified disturbed interhemispheric functional connectivity in AD (Brun and Englund, 1986; Wada et al., 1998; Delbeuck et al., 2003). According to Kruskal-Wallis testing, the NC, EMCI, LMCI, and AD groups showed significantly different Q values under most parcellation schemes, with the lone exception of the Gordon_rsfMRI333 parcellation. Further, our results indicate that a loss of k-core nodes should increase modularity (**Figure 4**). This supports the concept that, in addition to mediating internetwork interactions, k-core nodes are involved in maintaining the modular structure of functional networks through decreasing network connectivity (Hwang et al., 2017). In accordance with (Daianu et al., 2015), findings here indicate that the breakdown of anatomical connections affected by MCI and AD could increase the modularity coefficient.

Highly connected k-core nodes serve as communication hubs, facilitating integrative information processing. These hubs have high nodal degrees and tend to form a rich club—a set of nodes that are densely interconnected. The rich-club coefficient is a related but separate concept from k-core, as it evaluates a range of k-core thresholds from 17 to 39. The rich-club coefficient is defined as the ratio of the number of connections among nodes of degree k or higher to the total possible number of connections if those nodes were fully connected (Daianu et al., 2015). Significant group differences in rich-club coefficient were detected when AAL, HCP-MMP, and Gordon_rsfMRI333 parcellation schemes were used to define SC network nodes. Under the OASIS scheme, no significant group differences were detected at k-level $= 17$. Although some conditional differences were limited, these results help better understand nodal degree alterations in AD. Finally,

A

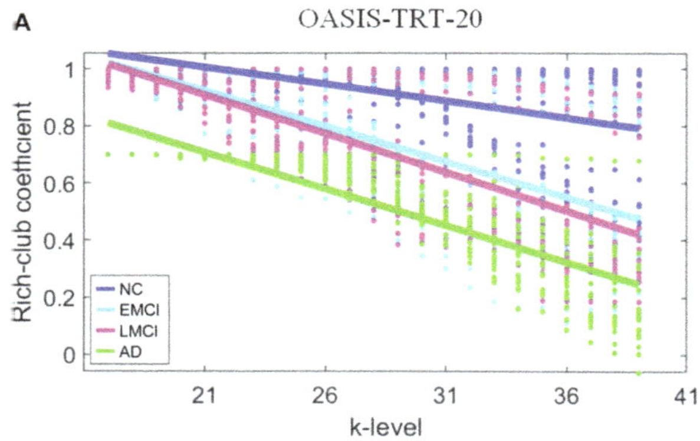

	NC	EMCI	LMCI	AD
r^2	0.8639	0.9919	0.9913	0.9004
p-value	1.4847e-10	1.8939e-23	4.2060e-23	5.4745e-12

B

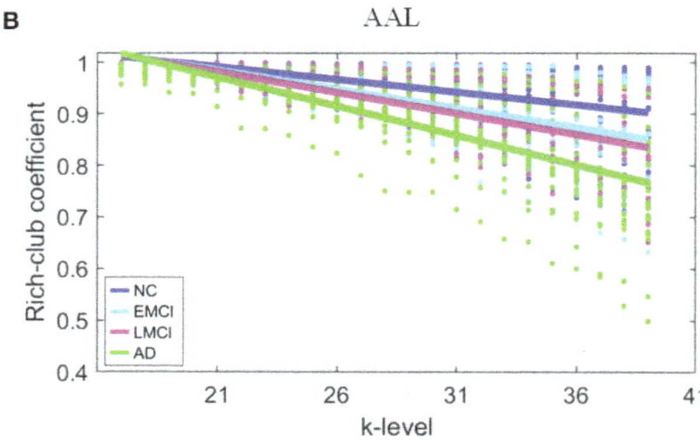

	NC	EMCI	LMCI	AD
r^2	0.9206	0.9438	0.9443	0.9556
p-value	5.0111e-13	1.3075e-14	1.1995e-14	1.1109e-15

C

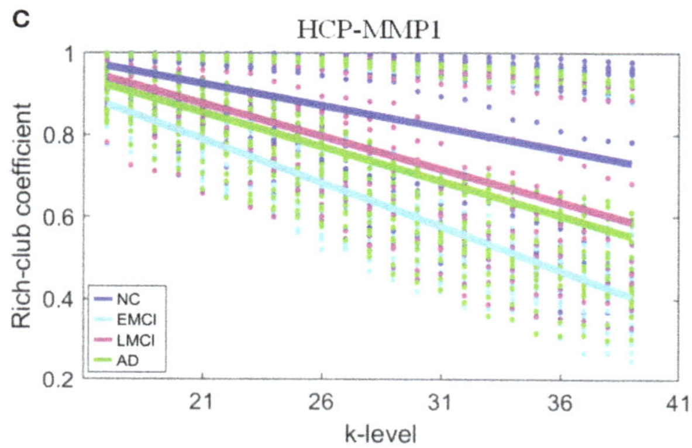

	NC	EMCI	LMCI	AD
r^2	0.9982	0.9897	0.9965	0.9901
p-value	2.6758e-30	2.4486e-22	2.9584e-27	1.6197e-22

D

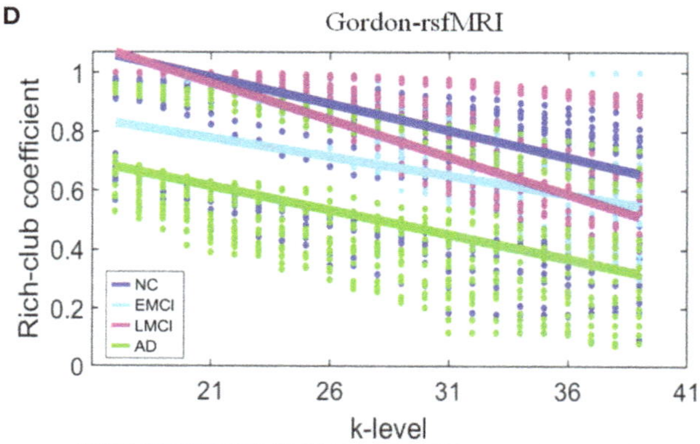

	NC	EMCI	LMCI	AD
r^2	0.9956	0.9605	0.9904	0.9668
p-value	3.4757e-26	3.1986e-16	1.2321e-19	5.1955e-17

FIGURE 5 | Linear regression of rich-club coefficient over a range of *k*-level from 17 to 39. NC, EMCI, LMCI, and AD groups are represented by blue, cyan, magenta, and green colors, respectively. **(A)** OASIS-TRT-20, **(B)** AAL, **(C)** HCP-MMP, and **(D)** Gordon-rsfMRI.

the changing trends of rich-club coefficients over *k*-level was investigated using linear regression by fitting models with the metrics as predictors for AD propagation. The results indicate that the trends in this metric were different depending on the parcellation scheme used during SC network construction (**Figure 5**). Overall, rich-club coefficient changes in EMCI, LMCI, and AD accompany a decrease in *k*-core nodes.

From these results, it can be concluded that whole-brain parcellations exert significant influence on the topological characterization of brain structural connectivity networks in AD propagation. Future AD-related structural network studies should attempt to use metrics that are largely robust to the underlying parcellation scheme when attempting to predict AD progression. While it was not possible in this study due to limited available information, the incorporation of clinical and neuropsychological information (such as the Clinical Dementia Rating or Mini-Mental State Examination) should also be considered during analysis. Further, the effect of applied parcellation schemes should be considered during the interpretation of results, as even the most robust measures exhibit some degree of scheme-based variability. As tractography methods could greatly influence the construction of SC networks, a more sophisticated HARDI-based tractography approach may improve the credibility of SC matrices in future.

CONCLUSION

Brain parcellation influences the construction of SC network and their topological properties. This work aims to comprehensively explore effect of brain parcellation atlases on characterization of topological deterioration in MCI and AD. There is increasing evidence that widespread network disruptions exist in MCI and AD, and that topological characterization can provide useful biomarkers for the detection of AD progression. In this study

ODF-based tractography was employed to construct SC networks from a mixed cohort of 20 NC, 20 EMCI, 20 LMCI, and 20 AD from ADNI under different whole-brain parcellation schemes across multiple spatial scales. The influence of parcellation scheme on the differentiation of the NC, EMCI, LEMCI, and AD groups was then demonstrated. Results suggest differences in the parcellation schemes used to generate SC networks affect the ability for network measures to distinguish structural differences between the NC, EMCI, LMCI, and AD groups. While this study has underlined the importance of the brain parcellation schemes in the SC network analysis of AD progression, further research is required to fully understand the relationship between SC networks and the underlying neural substrates of EMCI, LMCI, and AD at the network level.

AUTHOR CONTRIBUTIONS

ZW and YZ: study design. ZW: data acquisition. ZW, DX, TP, and YZ: analysis and interpretation, manuscript drafting, and final approval.

FUNDING

The research is supported in part by Natural Science Foundation of Zhejiang Province (LY17E070007), National Natural Science Foundation of China (51207038), China Scholarship Council, and the University of Houston. Data collection and sharing for this project was funded by the Alzheimer's Disease Neuroimaging Initiative (ADNI) (National Institutes of Health Grant U01 AG024904) and DOD ADNI (Department of Defense award number W81XWH-12-2-0012). ADNI is funded by the National Institute on Aging, the National Institute of Biomedical Imaging and Bioengineering, and through generous contributions from the following: AbbVie, Alzheimer's Association; Alzheimer's Drug Discovery Foundation; Araclon Biotech; BioClinica, Inc.; Biogen; Bristol-Myers Squibb Company; CereSpir, Inc.; Cogstate; Eisai Inc.; Elan Pharmaceuticals, Inc.; Eli Lilly and Company; EuroImmun; F. Hoffmann-La Roche Ltd and its affiliated company Genentech, Inc.; Fujirebio; GE Healthcare; IXICO Ltd.; Janssen Alzheimer Immunotherapy Research & Development, LLC.; Johnson & Johnson Pharmaceutical Research & Development LLC.; Lumosity; Lundbeck; Merck & Co., Inc.; Meso Scale Diagnostics, LLC.; NeuroRx Research; Neurotrack Technologies; Novartis Pharmaceuticals Corporation; Pfizer Inc.; Piramal Imaging; Servier; Takeda Pharmaceutical Company; and Transition Therapeutics. The Canadian Institutes of Health Research is providing funds to support ADNI clinical sites in Canada. Private sector contributions are facilitated by the Foundation for the National Institutes of Health (www.fnih.org). The grantee organization is the Northern California Institute for Research and Education, and the study is coordinated by the Alzheimer's Therapeutic Research Institute at the University of Southern California. ADNI data are disseminated by the Laboratory for Neuro Imaging at the University of Southern California.

SUPPLEMENTARY MATERIAL

The four parcellation templates were all spatially normalized into Montreal Neurological Institute (MNI) space (Fonov et al., 2011), and are visualized from different views (left, right, top, and bottom views) in **Figure S1**.

Group-averaged SC matrices were obtained by averaging the matrices of all subjects within each group, as shown in **Figure S2**.

Figure S1 | Cerebral cortex parcellation schemes with different numbers of parcels, including OASIS-TRT-20 (62 regions), AAL (116 regions), HCP-MMP (180 regions), and Gordon-rsfMRI (333 regions). The character *M* represents the number of parcellated regions. These schemes are shown from left, right, bottom, and top brain views, respectively. Full index of the parcellated regions can be found in Tzourio-Mazoyer et al. (2002), Klein and Tourville (2012), Gordon et al. (2014), and Glasser et al. (2016).

Figure S2 | The group-averaged structural connectivity matrices of NC, EMCI, LMCI, and AD subjects. The strength values were normalized from [0, 1], and self-connections were excluded. From top to bottom, the dimensions of the adjacency matrices are 62 × 62, 116 × 116, 180 × 180, and 333 × 333, respectively.

REFERENCES

Acosta-Cabronero, J., Willianms, G. B., Pengas, G., and Nestor, P. J. (2009). Absolute diffusivities define the landscape of white matter degeneration in Alzheimer's disease. *Brain* 133, 529–539. doi: 10.1093/brain/awp257

Arslan, S., Ktena, S. I., Makropoulos, A., Robinson, E. C., Rueckert, D., and Parisot, S. (2017). Human brain mapping: a systematic comparison of parcellation methods for the human cerebral cortex. *NeuroImage* 170, 5–30. doi: 10.1016/j.neuroimage.2017.04.014

Barnett, A. (2009). Theory of Q-ball imaging redux: Implications for fiber tracking. *Magn. Reson. Med.* 62, 910–923. doi: 10.1002/mrm.22073

Blondel, V. D., Guillaume, J. L., Lambiotte, R., and Lefebvre, E. (2008). Fast unfolding of communities in large networks. *J. Stat. Mechan.* 10:P10008. doi: 10.1088/1742-5468/2008/10/P10008

Bozzali, M., Falini, A., Franceschi, M., Cercignani, M., Zuffi, M., Scotti, G., et al. (2002). White matter damage in Alzheimer's disease assessed *in vivo* using diffusion tensor magnetic resonance imaging. *J. Neurol. Neurosurg. Psychiatry* 72, 742–746. doi: 10.1136/jnnp.72.6.742

Brun, A., and Englund, E. (1986). A white matter disorder in dementia of the Alzheimer type: a pathoanatomical study. *Ann. Neurol.* 19, 253–262. doi: 10.1002/ana.410190306

Côté, M. A., Girard, G., Boré, A., Garyfallidis, E., Houde, J. C., and Descoteaux, M. (2013). Tractometer: towards validation of tractography pipelines. *Med. Image Anal.* 17, 844–857. doi: 10.1016/j.media.2013.03.009

Cao, Q., Shu, N., An, L., Wang, P., Sun, L., Xia, M. R., et al. (2013). Probabilistic diffusion tractography and graph theory analysis reveal abnormal white matter structural connectivity networks in drug-naive boys with attention deficit/hyperactivity disorder. *J. Neurosci.* 33, 10676–10687. doi: 10.1523/JNEUROSCI.4793-12.2013

Christiaens, D., Reisert, M., Dhollander, T., Sunaert, S., Suetens, P., and Maes, F. (2015). Global tractography of multi-shell diffusion-weighted imaging data using a multi-tissue model. *Neuroimage* 123, 89–101. doi: 10.1016/j.neuroimage.2015.08.008

Daianu, M., Dennis, E. L., Jahanshad, N., Nir, T. M., Toga, A. W., Jack, C. R. Jr., et al. (2013a). "Alzheimer's disease disrupts rich club organization in brain connectivity networks," in 2013 *IEEE 10th International Symposium on Biomedical Imaging (ISBI)* (San Francisco, CA), 266–269. doi: 10.1109/ISBI.2013.6556463

Daianu, M., Jahanshad, N., Nir, T. M., Jack C. R. Jr, Weiner, M. W., Bernstein, M. A., et al. (2015). Rich club analysis in the Alzheimer's disease connectome reveals a relatively undisturbed structural core network. *Hum. Brain Mapp.* 36, 3087–3103. doi: 10.1002/hbm.22830

Daianu, M., Jahanshad, N., Nir, T. M., Toga, A. W., Jack C. R. Jr, Weiner, M. W., et al. (2013b). Breakdown of brain connectivity between normal aging and Alzheimer's disease: a structural k-core network analysis. *Brain Connect.* 3, 407–422. doi: 10.1089/brain.2012.0137

Delbeuck, X., Van der Linden, M., and Collette, F. (2003). Alzheimer' disease as a disconnection syndrome? *Neuropsychol. Rev.* 13, 79–92. doi: 10.1023/A:1023832305702

deEtoile, J., and Adeli, H. (2017). Graph theory and brain connectivity in Alzheimer's disease. *Neuroscientist* 23, 616–626. doi: 10.1177/1073858417702621

Descoteaux, M., Deriche, R., Knosche, T. R., and Anwander, A. (2009). Deterministic and probabilistic tractography based on complex fibre orientation distributions. *IEEE Trans. Med. Imaging* 28, 269–286. doi: 10.1109/TMI.2008.2004424

Fonov, V., Evans, A. C., Botteron, K., Almli, C. R., McKinstry, R. C., and Collins, D. L. (2011). Unbiased average age-appropriate atlases for pediatric studies. *Neuroimage* 54, 313–327. doi: 10.1016/j.neuroimage.2010.07.033

Fortunato, S. (2010). Community detection in graphs. *Phys. Rep.* 486, 75–174. doi: 10.1016/j.physrep.2009.11.002

Glasser, M. F., Coalson, T. S., Robinson, E. C., Hacker, C. D., Harwell, J., and Yacoub, E. (2016). A multi-modal parcellation of human cerebral cortex. *Nature* 536, 171–178. doi: 10.1038/nature18933

Gordon, E. M., Laumann, T. O., Adeyemo, B., Huckins, J. F., Kelley, W. M., and Petersen, S. E. (2014). Generation and evaluation of a cortical area parcellation from resting-state correlations. *Cereb. Cortex* 26, 288–303. doi: 10.1093/cercor/bhu239

Hagmann, P., Kurant, M., Gigandet, X., Thiran, P., Wedeen, V. J., Meuli, R., et al. (2007). Mapping human whole-brain structural networks with diffusion MRI. *PLoS ONE* 2:e597. doi: 10.1371/journal.pone.0000597

Houenou, J., Wessa, M., Douaud, G., Leboyer, M., Chanraud, S., Perrin, M., et al. (2007). Increased white matter connectivity in euthymic bipolar patients: diffusion tensor tractography between the subgenual cingulate and the amygdalo-hippocampal complex. *Mol. Psychiatry* 12, 1001–10. doi: 10.1038/sj.mp.4002010

Hwang, K., Bertolero, M., Liu, W., and D'Esposito, M. (2017). The human thalamus is an integrative hub for functional brain networks. *J. Neurosci.* 37, 5594–5607. doi: 10.1101/056630

Iturria-Medina, Y., Sotero, R. C., Canales-Rodríguez, E. J., Alemán-Gómez, Y., and Melie-García, L. (2008). Studying the human brain anatomical network via diffusion-weighted MRI and graph theory. *Neuroimage* 40, 1064–1076. doi: 10.1016/j.neuroimage.2007.10.060

Jack, C. R., Bernstein, M. A., Fox, N. C., Thompson, P., Alexander, G., and Harvey, D. (2008). The Alzheimer's disease neuroimaging initiative (ADNI): MRI methods. *J. Magn. Reson. Imaging* 27, 685–691. doi: 10.1002/jmri.21049

Jessen, F., Wolfsgruber, S., Wiese, B., Bickel, H., Mosch, E., Kaduszkiewic, H., et al. (2014). AD dementia risk in late MCI, in early MCI, and in subjective memory impairment. *Alzheimer's Dementia* 10, 76–83. doi: 10.1016/j.jalz.2012.09.017

Kim, W. H., Adluru, N., Chung, M. K., Okonkwo, O. C., Johnson, S. C., Bendlin, B. B., et al. (2015). Multi-resolution statistical analysis of brain connectivity graphs in preclinical Alzheimer's disease. *Neuroimage* 118, 103–117. doi: 10.1016/j.neuroimage.2015.05.050

Klein, A., and Tourville, J. (2012). 101 labeled brain images and a consistent human cortical labeling protocol. *Front. Neurosci.* 6:171. doi: 10.3389/fnins.2012.00171

Lancichinetti, A., and Fortunato, S. (2009). Community detection algorithms: a comparative analysis. *Phys. Rev. E* 80:056117. doi: 10.1103/PhysRevE.80.056117

Li, Y., Liu, Y., Li, J., Qin, W., Li, K., Yu, C., et al. (2009). Brain anatomical network and intelligence. *PLoS Comput. Biol.* 5:e1000395. doi: 10.1371/journal.pcbi.1000395

Lo, C. Y., Wang, P. N., Chou, K. H., Wang, J., He, Y., and Lin, C. P. (2010). Diffusion tensor tractography reveals abnormal topological organization in structural cortical networks in Alzheimer's disease. *J. Neurosci.* 30, 16876–16885. doi: 10.1523/JNEUROSCI.4136-10.2010

Mckenna, F., Koo, B. B., and Killiany, R. (2016). Comparison of ApoE-related brain connectivity differences in early MCI and normal aging populations: an fMRI study. *Brain Imaging Behav.* 10, 970–983. doi: 10.1007/s11682-015-9451-z

Mueller, S. G., Weiner, M. W., Thal, L. J., Petersen, R. C., Jack, C. R., Jagust, W., et al. (2005). Ways toward an early diagnosis in Alzheimer's disease: the Alzheimer's Disease Neuroimaging Initiative (ADNI). *Alzheimer's Dement.* 1, 55–66. doi: 10.1016/j.jalz.2005.06.003

Newman, M. E. (2006). Modularity and community structure in networks. *Proc. Natl. Acad. Sci. U.S.A.* 103, 8577–8582. doi: 10.1073/pnas.0601602103

Newman, M. E., and Girvan, M. (2004). Finding and evaluating community structure in networks. *Phys. Rev. E* 69:026113. doi: 10.1103/PhysRevE.69.026113

Nguyen, T., Potter, T., Grossman, R., and Zhang, Y. (2018). Characterization of dynamic changes of current source localization based on spatiotemporal fMRI constrained EEG source imaging. *J. Neural Eng.* 15:036017. doi: 10.1088/1741-2552/aa9fb2

Nir, T. M., Villalon-Reina, J. E., Prasad, G., Jahanshad, N., Joshi, S. H., and Toga, A. W. (2015). Diffusion weighted imaging-based maximum density path analysis and classification of Alzheimer's disease. *Neurobiol. Aging* 36, S132–S140. doi: 10.1016/j.neurobiolaging.2014.05.037

Petersen, R. C., Aisen, P. S., Beckett, L. A., Donohue, M. C., Gamst, A. C., and Harvey, D. J. (2010). Alzheimer's disease Neuroimaging Initiative (ADNI) clinical characterization. *Neurology* 74, 201–209. doi: 10.1212/WNL.0b013e3181cb3e25

Proix, T., Spiegler, A., Schirner, M., Rothmeier, S., Ritter, P., and Jirsa, V. K. (2016). How do parcellation size and short-range connectivity affect dynamics in large-scale brain network models? *NeuroImage* 142, 135–149. doi: 10.1016/j.neuroimage.2016.06.016

Risacher, S. L., Saykin, A. J., Wes, J. D., Shen, L., Firpi, H. A., and McDonald, B. C. (2009). Baseline MRI predictors of conversion from MCI to probable AD in the ADNI cohort. *Curr. Alzheimer Res.* 6, 347–361. doi: 10.2174/156720509788929273

Rose, S. E., Chen, F., Chalk, J. B., Zelaya, F. O., Strugnell, W. E., and Benson, M. (2000). Loss of connectivity in Alzheimer's disease: an evaluation of white matter tract integrity with colour coded MR diffusion tensor imaging. *J. Neurol. Neurosurg. Psychiatry* 69, 528–530. doi: 10.1136/jnnp.69.4.528

Rubinov, M., and Sporns, O. (2010). Complex network measures of brain connectivity: uses and interpretations. *Neuroimage* 52, 1059–1069. doi: 10.1016/j.neuroimage.2009.10.003

Rubinov, M., and Sporns, O. (2011). Weight-conserving characterization of complex functional brain networks. *Neuroimage* 56, 2068–2079. doi: 10.1016/j.neuroimage.2011.03.069

Shao, J., Myers, N., Yang, Q., Feng, J., Plant, C., and Böhm, C. (2012). Prediction of Alzheimer's disease using individual structural connectivity networks. *Neurobiol. Aging* 33, 2756–2765. doi: 10.1016/j.neurobiolaging.2012.01.017

Sorg, C., Riedl, V., Perneczky, R., Kurz, A., and Wohlschlager, A. M. (2009). Impact of Alzheimer's disease on the functional connectivity of spontaneous brain activity. *Curr. Alzheimer Res.* 6, 541–553. doi: 10.2174/156720509790147106

Sperling, R. A., Dickerson, B. C., Pihlajamaki, M., Vannini, P., LaViolette, P. S., and Vitolo, O. V. (2010). Functional alterations in memory networks in early Alzheimer's disease. *Neuromol. Med.* 12, 27–43. doi: 10.1007/s12017-009-8109-7

Sporns, O. (2010). *Networks of the Brain.* Cambridge, MA: MIT press. doi: 10.7551/mitpress/8476.001.0001

Sporns, O., Chialvo, D. R., Kaiser, M., and Hilgetag, C. C. (2004). Organization, development and function of complex brain networks. *Trends Cogn. Sci.* 8, 418–425. doi: 10.1016/j.tics.2004.07.008

Tzourio-Mazoyer, N., Landeau, B., Papathanassiou, D., Crivello, F., Etard, O., and Delcroix, N. (2002). Automated anatomical labeling of activations in SPM using a macroscopic anatomical parcellation of the MNI MRI single-subject brain.

Neuroimage 15, 273–289. doi: 10.1006/nimg.2001.0978

Wada, Y., Nanbu, Y., Koshino, Y., Yamaguchi, N., and Hashimoto, T. (1998). Reduced interhemispheric EEG coherence in Alzheimer disease: analysis during rest and photic stimulation. *Alzheimer Dis. Assoc. Disord.* 12, 175–81. doi: 10.1097/00002093-199809000-00009

Wang, J., Wang, X., Xia, M., Liao, X., Evans, A., and He, Y. (2015). GRETNA: a graph theoretical network analysis toolbox for imaging connectomics. *Front. Hum. Neurosci.* 9:386. doi: 10.3389/fnhum.2015.00386

Watts, D. J., and Strogatz, S. H. (1998). Collective dynamics of 'small-world' networks. *Nature* 393, 440–442. doi: 10.1038/30918

Winblad, B., Palmer, K., Kivipelto, M., Jelic, V., Fratiglioni, L., and Wahlund, L. O. (2004). Mild cognitive impairment–beyond controversies, towards a consensus: report of the International Working Group on Mild Cognitive Impairment. *J. Internal Med.* 256, 240–246. doi: 10.1111/j.1365-2796.2004.01380.x

Wu, Z., Potter, T., Wu, D., and Zhang, Y. (2018a). Denoising high angular resolution diffusion imaging data by combining singular value decomposition and non-local means filter. *J. Neurosci. Methods* 312, 105–113. doi: 10.1016/j.jneumeth.2018.11.020

Wu, Z., Yu, X., Liu, Y., and Hong, M. (2018b). A PSO-Powell Hybrid Method to Extract Fiber Orientations from ODF. *Comput. Math. Methods Med.* 2018:7680164. doi: 10.1155/2018/7680164

Xie, S., Chen, L., Zuo, N., and Jiang, T. (2016). DiffusionKit: a light one-stop solution for diffusion MRI data analysis. *J. Neurosci. Methods* 273, 107–119. doi: 10.1016/j.jneumeth.2016.08.011

Yao, Z., Zhang, Y., Lin, L., Zhou, Y., Xu, C., and Jiang, T. (2010). Abnormal cortical networks in mild cognitive impairment and Alzheimer's Disease. *PLoS Comput. Biol.* 6:e1001006. doi: 10.1371/journal.pcbi.1001006

Yeh, F. C., and Tseng, W. Y. I. (2011). NTU-90: a high angular resolution brain atlas constructed by q-space diffeomorphic reconstruction. *Neuroimage* 58, 91–99. doi: 10.1016/j.neuroimage.2011.06.021

Yeh, F. C., Verstynen, T. D., Wang, Y., Fernández-Miranda, J. C., and Tseng, W. Y. I. (2013). Deterministic diffusion fiber tracking improved by quantitative anisotropy. *PLoS ONE* 8:e80713. doi: 10.1371/journal.pone.0080713

Zalesky, A., Fornito, A., Harding, I. H., Cocchi, L., Yücel, M., Pantelis, C., et al. (2010). Whole-brain anatomical networks: does the choice of nodes matter? *Neuroimage* 50, 970–983. doi: 10.1016/j.neuroimage.2009.12.027

Zhan, L., Liu, Y., Wang, Y., Zhou, J., Jahanshad, N., Ye, J., et al. (2015a). Boosting brain connectome classification accuracy in Alzheimer's disease using higher-order singular value decomposition. *Front. Neurosci.* 9:257. doi: 10.3389/fnins.2015.00257

Zhan, L., Zhou, J., Wang, Y., Jin, Y., Jahanshad, N., and Prasad, G. (2015b). Comparison of nine tractography algorithms for detecting abnormal structural brain networks in Alzheimer's disease. *Front. Aging Neurosci.* 7;48. doi: 10.3389/fnagi.2015.00048

5

Amyloid-β Load is Related to Worries, but not to Severity of Cognitive Complaints in Individuals with Subjective Cognitive Decline: The SCIENCe Project

Sander C. J. Verfaillie[1,2,3], Tessa Timmers[1,2,3], Rosalinde E. R. Slot[1,3], Chris W. J. van der Weijden[2,3], Linda M. P. Wesselman[1,3], Niels D. Prins[1,3], Sietske A. M. Sikkes[1,3,4], Maqsood Yaqub[2,3], Annemiek Dols[1,3,5], Adriaan A. Lammertsma[2,3], Philip Scheltens[1,3], Rik Ossenkoppele[1,3,6], Bart N. M. van Berckel[2,3] and Wiesje M. van der Flier[1,3,4]*

[1] Department of Neurology and Alzheimer Center, Amsterdam University Medical Center, Vrije Universiteit Amsterdam, Amsterdam, Netherlands, [2] Department of Radiology and Nuclear Medicine, Amsterdam Neuroscience, Amsterdam University Medical Center, Vrije Universiteit Amsterdam, Amsterdam, Netherlands, [3] Amsterdam Neuroscience, Amsterdam, Netherlands, [4] Department of Epidemiology and Biostatistics, Amsterdam Neuroscience, Amsterdam University Medical Center, Vrije Universiteit Amsterdam, Amsterdam, Netherlands, [5] Department of Old Age Psychiatry, Amsterdam Neuroscience, GGZ inGeest, Amsterdam University Medical Center, Vrije Universiteit Amsterdam, Amsterdam, Netherlands, [6] Clinical Memory Research Unit, Lund University, Malmö, Sweden

Correspondence:
Sander C. J. Verfaillie
s.verfaillie@vumc.nl

Objective: Subjective cognitive decline (SCD) is associated with an increased risk of Alzheimer's Disease (AD). Early disease processes, such as amyloid-β aggregation measured with quantitative PET, may help to explain the phenotype of SCD. The aim of this study was to investigate whether quantitative amyloid-β load is associated with both self- and informant-reported cognitive complaints and memory deficit awareness in individuals with SCD.

Methods: We included 106 SCD patients (mean ± SD age: 64 ± 8, 45%F) with 90 min dynamic [^{18}F]florbetapir PET scans. We used the following questionnaires to assess SCD severity: cognitive change index (CCI, self and informant reports; 2 × 20 items), subjective cognitive functioning (SCF, four items), and five questions "Do you have complaints?" (yes/no) for memory, attention, organization and language), and "Does this worry you? (yes/no)." The Rivermead Behavioral Memory Test (RBMT)-Stories (immediate and delayed recall) was used to assess objective episodic memory. To investigate the level of self-awareness, we calculated a memory deficit awareness index (Z-transformed (inverted self-reported CCI minus episodic memory); higher index, heightened self-awareness) and a self-proxy index (Z-transformed self- minus informant-reported CCI). Mean cortical [^{18}F]florbetapir binding potential (BP_{ND}) was derived from the PET data. Logistic and linear regression analyses, adjusted for age, sex, education, and depressive symptoms, were used to investigate associations between BP_{ND} and measures of SCD.

Results: Higher mean cortical [^{18}F]florbetapir BP_{ND} was associated with SCD-related worries (odds ratio = 1.76 [95%CI = 1.07 ± 2.90]), but not with other SCD questionnaires (informant and self-report CCI or SCF, total scores or individual items, all $p > 0.05$). In addition, higher mean cortical [^{18}F]florbetapir BP_{ND} was associated with a higher memory deficit awareness index (Beta = 0.55), with an interaction between BP_{ND} and education ($p = 0.002$). There were no associations between [^{18}F]florbetapir BP_{ND} and self-proxy index (Beta = 0.11).

Conclusion: Amyloid-β deposition was associated with SCD-related worries and heightened memory deficit awareness (i.e., hypernosognosia), but not with severity of cognitive complaints. Our findings indicate that worries about self-perceived decline may reflect an early symptom of amyloid-β related pathology rather than subjective cognitive functioning.

Keywords: subjective cognitive decline (SCD), Alzheimer's diseaese, amyloid PET, self-awareness, early - biomarkers

INTRODUCTION

Amyloid-β plaques and neurofibrillary tangles are neuropathological hallmarks of Alzheimer's disease (AD), which start to appear 10–20 years before the onset of dementia (Jack et al., 2013). Self-perceived cognitive decline in cognitively normal individuals is associated with a three- to six fold increased risk of AD (Schmand et al., 1996; Geerlings et al., 1999; Jessen et al., 2010). As such, a proportion of individuals with subjective cognitive decline (SCD) may harbor the earliest pathological changes associated with AD (Verfaillie et al., 2016, 2018a,b), particularly amyloid-β accumulation (i.e., preclinical AD) (Buckley et al., 2016; Perrotin et al., 2016; Hu et al., 2018).

Only a minority of individuals with SCD will develop AD within a few years (Slot et al., 2018a), but it is conceivable that individuals with preclinical AD exhibit a specific phenotype of cognitive complaints compared with individuals without underlying AD. There are many questionnaires to investigate the nature and severity of SCD, but the appropriate items enabling prediction of conversion to mild cognitive impairment (MCI) and dementia have not yet been identified (Rabin et al., 2015, 2017). There are various methodological challenges associated with SCD assessment, one of which is that cognitive complaints tend to vary as a function of demographic characteristics, such as level of education and age (Rabin et al., 2015). In addition, these factors can also act in synergy; for example, it has been shown that cognitive complaints in highly educated individuals are associated with increased risk of progression to AD, while this is not found in individuals with lower education levels (Jonker et al., 2000; van Oijen et al., 2007). SCD *plus* criteria were proposed in an effort to increase the likelihood of identifying preclinical AD in individuals with SCD. One of these criteria suggests that especially individuals who worry about their self-perceived cognitive decline are more likely to have preclinical AD, but associations between worries and amyloid-β load have not been confirmed in prospective studies yet (Geerlings et al., 1999; Jessen et al., 2010, 2014). Furthermore, former studies investigating associations between amyloid-β load and various SCD questionnaires have generated highly inconsistent results in cognitively normal individuals (Rodda et al., 2010; Amariglio et al., 2012; Mielke et al., 2012; Perrotin et al., 2012, 2016; Buckley et al., 2013; Holland et al., 2015; Snitz et al., 2015). These discrepancies could be due to the less precise amyloid-β positron emission tomography (PET) semi-quantitative cut-off values in preclinical stages of AD (Villeneuve et al., 2015), and variability of implemented SCD questionnaires, including the lack of informant reports or objective memory tests relative to self-reports (Rabin et al., 2015, 2017).

Another approach is to explore whether preclinical AD is linked to the insight in cognitive deficits (i.e., self-awareness) rather than to the severity of SCD. The degree of memory deficit awareness takes into account the contribution of objective memory performance or informant reports relative to self-reports of cognitive decline (Barba et al., 1995; Perrotin et al., 2015). A lack of awareness of memory deficits, anosognosia, is a striking symptom in patients with AD dementia (Barba et al., 1995; Perrotin et al., 2015). On the contrary, it is has been suggested that the earliest changes in cognition during preclinical stages of the disease are best perceived by the individual including a heightened sense of self-awareness for early brain changes (i.e., hypernosognosia) (Caselli et al., 2014; Langer and Levine, 2014). In a recent study self-awareness was defined as a discrepancy score between subjective and objective episodic memory performance and they found that cognitively normal individuals harboring amyloid-β pathology had a heightened sense of self-awareness (Vannini et al., 2017). It has, however, not yet been investigated whether the earliest changes in cognition are best perceived by the individual rather than the observer or objective memory tests in a memory clinic setting.

We hypothesized that increased amyloid-β load is related to specific cognitive complaints and heightened level of self-awareness. Therefore, the purpose of the present study was to investigate whether amyloid-β load, as measured using quantitative PET, may help to explain the phenotype of SCD in cognitively normal individuals who initially have been referred to a memory clinic. A second aim was to investigate whether amyloid-β load is associated with altered levels of self-awareness and informant reports of cognitive change.

MATERIALS AND METHODS

We included 106 SCD memory-clinic patients with [^{18}F]florbetapir PET scans from the ongoing Subjective Cognitive ImpairmENt Cohort (SCIENCe) study (Slot et al., 2018b). Subjects were referred to our memory clinic by their general practitioner or medical specialist because of cognitive complaints. Prior to inclusion via the memory clinic, all patients underwent a standardized dementia screening according to the procedures of the Amsterdam Dementia Cohort (Van Der Flier et al., 2014). Screening included extensive neuropsychological assessment, physical and neurologic examination as well as laboratory serum tests (hemoglobin, thrombocytes, leucocytes, TSH, MCH, MCV, erycytes), and brain magnetic resonance imaging (MRI). A Dutch translation of the mini-mental state examination (MMSE) was used to screen for global cognition (Folstein et al., 1975). Clinical diagnosis was established by consensus in a multidisciplinary team. Individuals were labeled as having SCD when they presented with cognitive complaints, and results of clinical investigations were within normal range. Criteria for MCI, dementia, or any other neurological or psychiatric (e.g., major depression) disorders known to cause cognitive complaints were not met (Jessen et al., 2014; Molinuevo et al., 2017). In addition, we used the Hospital Anxiety and Depression Scale- Anxiety subscale (HADS-A) and Center for Epidemiological Studies Depression Scale (CES-D) scale to evaluate (subclinical) anxiety and depressive symptoms (cut-off $\geq$ 16), respectively (Radloff, 1977; Zigmond and Snaith, 1983). The study had been approved by the Medical Ethics Review Committee of the VU University Medical Center. All patients provided written informed consent.

Image Acquisition and Analyses

Ninety minutes dynamic [^{18}F]florbetapir PET scans were acquired on a PET/CT scanner (n = 59 on an Ingenuity TF and n = 47 on a Gemini TF, both from Philips Medical Systems, Best, Netherlands). PET images were corrected for attenuation, scatter, randoms, decay and dead time using standard software provided by Philips Healthcare. Three-dimensional T1-weighted MRI scans were co-registered to the PET scans, and regions of interest (Hammers template, n = 68 regions of interest [ROI]) were defined on the MRI scan (in native space) and superimposed onto the dynamic PET scan to obtain regional time activity curves using PVElab (Hammers et al., 2003; Rask et al., 2004). Receptor parametric mapping (RPM) with optimized settings (parameters settings 0.01–0.1, 50 basis functions) and cerebellar gray matter as reference region was used to generate images of binding potential (BP_{ND}) relative to the non-displaceable compartment (Lammertsma and Hume, 1996; Gunn et al., 1997; Golla et al., 2018). From the BP_{ND} images, gray matter volume-weighted mean cortical BP_{ND} values were obtained. To investigate potential regional specificity, volume-weighted bilateral frontal, temporal (medial and lateral), and parietal cortical BP_{ND} values were also extracted. In addition, standardized uptake value (SUV, 50–70 min post-injection) images were visually assessed by a trained and experienced reader (BvB), leading to "normal" or "abnormal" classification of amyloid accumulation (for more details regarding visual reading of [^{18}F]florbetapir PET images, please see https://www.accessdata.fda.gov/drugsatfda_docs/label/2012/202008s000lbl.pdf).

SCD Assessment

We used four questionnaires with the following characteristics: two self-, one informant-based questionnaires, and one which was composed of five cognitive questions to assess SCD. The maximal time window between these assessments and the PET scan was 1 year (median = 3 months). We used both self- and informant reports of the Dutch translation of the Cognitive Change Index (CCI self and informant versions; each 20 questions [range 0–4], total score: 20–100) to assess cognitive function compared to 5 years ago (Rattanabannakit et al., 2016). We used the Subjective Cognitive Functioning (SCF, self-report) questionnaire (4 questions, range: −12 to +12) to assess self-experienced cognitive decline over a one-year time period.(Van Der Flier et al., 2014) SCF scores were inverted in such a way that higher scores reflect more complaints, comparable to the CCI. Finally, we used a structured patient interview to assess SCD. We used the following question "What complaints do you report?". Based on the individuals' spontaneous response the following cognitive domains were scored "yes/no": memory, attention, organization, language, together with the follow-up question: "Does this worry you?" (Geerlings et al., 1999; Jessen et al., 2010). In addition, for descriptive purposes, the following question was used to inquire SCD onset "when was the first time that you talked with a physician about these problems?"

Memory Self-Awareness Indexes

To investigate the level of self-awareness, two index scores were calculated. First, the memory deficit awareness index, was defined for each participant by calculating the difference between subjective and objective episodic memory scores (Barba et al., 1995; Perrotin et al., 2015; Vannini et al., 2017). In concordance with previous studies we used episodic memory (%remembered = [immediate/delayed recall] * 100%) for the memory deficit awareness index, i.e., the Rivermead Behavioral Memory Test (RBMT)-Stories. To allow comparison between both measures, (1) the CCI-self was inverted in such a way that, similar to the objective memory score, a lower score indicated more severe subjective memory impairment; (2) both objective and the subjective memory scores were Z-transformed (Barba et al., 1995; Perrotin et al., 2015; Vannini et al., 2017). A positive index score reflects heightened self-awareness (hypernosognosia), whereas negative scores lowered self-awareness (anosognosia) (Barba et al., 1995; Perrotin et al., 2015; Vannini et al., 2017). To test the robustness of the memory deficit awareness index, we repeated the aforementioned procedures while using the Dutch version of the Rey auditory verbal learning test (RAVLT; immediate [5 trials summed] and delayed recall). Second, a self-proxy index (self-reported CCI minus informant-reported CCI) was calculated. A positive index score reflects more self-reported cognitive complaints than informant-reported complaints (hypernosognosia), whereas negative scores reflect more informant-based complaints than self-reported complaints (anosognosia).

Statistical Analyses

Statistical analyses were performed using Statistical Package for the Social Sciences (SPSS, IBM v22). We used linear regression (for continuous outcome measures) or binary logistic regression (for dichotomous outcome measures) analyses to investigate associations between mean cortical [^{18}F]florbetapir BP_{ND} (independent variable) and measures of SCD (i.e., CCI, SCF [total and single items scores], complaints questions). Analyses were adjusted for age, sex, education and depressive symptoms (CES-D). As cognitive complaints in highly educated individuals may be more predictive of dementia (Jonker et al., 2000; van Oijen et al., 2007), we also tested for an interaction education*[^{18}F]florbetapir BP_{ND}. We repeated analyses for cortical lobar [^{18}F]florbetapir BP_{ND}. Linear regression analyses, adjusted for age, sex, education and depressive symptoms, were used to investigate associations between [^{18}F]florbetapir BP_{ND} (independent variable) and memory self-awareness indexes (dependent variables; separate models). In addition, we also tested for an interaction education*[^{18}F]florbetapir BP_{ND}. Associations were considered significant if $p < 0.05$.

RESULTS

Demographic and clinical data are presented in **Table 1**. Individuals (43% females) were (mean ± SD) 64 ± 8 years old and had an MMSE of 29 ± 1. Twenty-four individuals (23%) showed abnormal amyloid-β accumulation. On average, subjects had a mean cortical BP_{ND} of 0.18 ± 0.15 (**Figure 1**; frontal cortex 0.18 ± 0.18, temporal cortex 0.13 ± 0.13, cingulate cortex 0.25 ± 0.19, parietal cortex 0.22 ± 0.17). On average, individuals reported lower subjective cognitive functioning than 1 year earlier (SCF = −1.54 ± 2.92), and slight to occasional problems (CCI self-report: 41.23 ± 15.05; CCI informant report: 37.17 ± 16.44) compared to 5 years ago. There were no differences between self- and informant-based reports regarding the degree of cognitive change over a 5 year period (i.e., both CCI versions). About 68% ($n = 73$), 34% ($n = 36$), 13% ($n = 14$) and 25% ($n = 27$) of the individuals reported complaints in the domains of memory, language, organization and attention, respectively, whilst 47% ($n = 50$) felt worried about their self-perceived decline.

Associations between mean cortical [^{18}F]florbetapir BP_{ND} and measures of SCD are presented in **Table 2**. Adjusted for age, sex, education and depressive symptoms (CES-D), higher mean cortical (**Figure 2**) [^{18}F]florbetapir BP_{ND} was associated with two-fold increased risk of SCD-related worries, but neither with any item nor total score of the SCF nor CCI (neither informant-based nor self-reported) nor dichotomous memory (**Figure 2**), attention, organization or language questions (all $p > 0.05$). There were no interaction effects between mean cortical [^{18}F]florbetapir BP_{ND} and education for any of the SCD questionnaire outcomes (all $p > 0.05$). If we repeated analyses with cortical lobar [^{18}F]florbetapir BP_{ND}, we found that frontal

TABLE 1 | Clinical and demographic data.

	Total group (*N* = 106)
Demographics	
Male/female (*n*, %)	46/60 (43%M)
Age (years)	63.83 (7.65)
Education (range: 1–7)	5.79 (1.07)
SCD onset (% within last 5 years)	83%
Depressive symptoms (CES-D)	8.5 (7.0)
Anxiety (HADS-A anxiety subscale)	3.8 (3.2)
Amyloid imaging	
Net injected dose (MBq)	312 (38)
Specific activity (MBq/μg)	2.72 (1.76)
Visual assessment of SUV_{50-70} images (n abnormal [%])	24 (23%)
Mean cortical amyloid load ([^{18}F]florbetapir BP_{ND})	0.18 (0.15)
Frontal cortex	0.18 (0.17)
Temporal cortex	0.13 (0.13)
Parietal cortex	0.22 (0.17)
Cingulate cortex	0.25 (0.19)
Episodic memory	
RBMT stories (version A+B) immediate recall	20.37 (5.94)
RBMT stories (version A+B) delayed recall	16.73 (6.20)
Rey auditory verbal learning test (RAVLT immediate recall (5 trials)	45.36 (8.97)
Rey auditory verbal learning test delayed recall	9.28 (3.18)
SCD questionnaires	
SCF	−1.54 (2.92)
CCI self-reported	41.23 (15.05)
CCI informant-based	37.17 (16.44)
Memory question *n* "yes" (%)	73 (68%)
Attention question *n* "yes" (%)	27 (25%)
Organization question *n* "yes" (%)	14 (13%)
Language question *n* "yes" (%)	36 (34%)
Worry question *n* "yes" (%)	50 (47%)

Data are presented as means (standard deviations) or percentages. Education level was assessed using the Verhage classification in accordance with the Dutch educational system. SCD onset was based upon individuals' self-reports. Depressive symptoms were assessed with the CES-D.

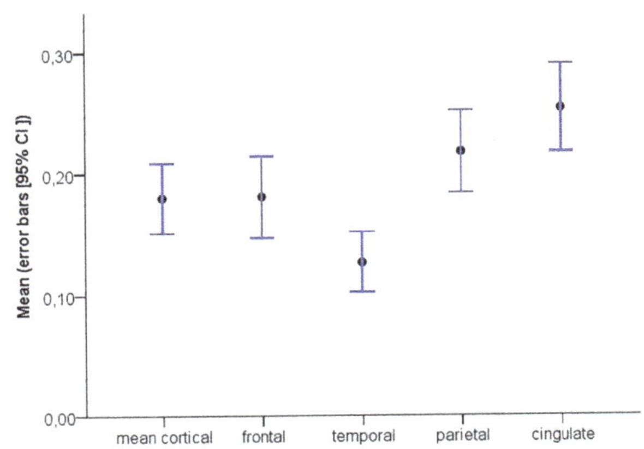

FIGURE 1 | Distribution of global and regional [^{18}F]florbetapir BP_{ND} with corresponding 95% confidence intervals.

TABLE 2 | Associations between mean cortical amyloid-β load and SCD.

		p-values
SCD questionnaires		
SCF	0.16 (−2.73 ± 1.92)	0.16
CCI self-reported	−0.10 (−10.01 ± 9.69)	0.30
CCI informant-based	0.01 (0.54 ± 10.38)	0.96
Memory question*	0.72 (0.46 ± 1.12)	0.14
Worry question*	1.76 (1.07 ± 2.90)	0.02
Episodic memory		
RBMT stories (% recall)	−0.16 (−1.09 ± 0.63)	0.09
RAVLT (% recall)	−0.09 (−0.62 ± 0.67)	0.35
Memory self-awareness indexes		
Self-awareness index (RMBT-based)	0.55 (4.82 ± 1.23)	< 0.001
Interaction Education*BPnd	−0.58 (−5.23 ± 1.61)	0.002
Self-awareness index (RAVLT-based)	0.38 (3.30 ± 1.27)	0.01
Interaction Education*BPnd	−0.42 (−3.69 ± 1.65)	0.03
Self-proxy index	0.11 (0.71 ± 0.69)	0.31

*Data are presented as standardized Beta (unstandardized beta +standard error) or *odd ratios (95% confidence intervals). Analyses were adjusted for age, sex, education and depressive symptoms. Analyses between amyloid-β load, self-proxy and self-awareness indexes were based on mean cortical amyloid-β load. Self-awareness indexes; positive associations (i.e., betas) reflect heightened self-awareness (hypernosognosia) in relation with higher amyloid-β load, whereas negative scores reflect lowered self-awareness (anosognosia).*

(Odds ratio (OR) [95% confidence interval] = 1.70 [1.05–2.76]), cingulate (OR = 1.70 [1.06–2.73]), parietal (OR = 1.72 [1.08–2.74]), and temporal (OR = 1.86 [1.10–3.14]) cortical regions were associated with SCD-related worries, but not with other SCD questionnaires (all $p > 0.05$). Results remained essentially comparable when we repeated analyses while additionally adjusting for PET/CT scanner systems (data not shown).

We furthermore investigated associations between mean cortical [^{18}F]florbetapir BP_{ND} and two self-awareness indexes. We found that higher mean cortical [^{18}F]florbetapir BP_{ND} was associated with a higher memory deficit awareness index (i.e., hypernosognosia) (**Table 2** and **Figure 2**), with an interaction between BP_{ND} and education implying that this effect was stronger for individuals with relatively lower education (please see the full statistical models in **Supplementary Table S1**). When we repeated analyses with the memory deficit awareness index based on the RAVLT we found comparable results (**Table 2** and **Figure 2E** right panel). There were no associations between mean cortical BP_{ND} and the self-proxy index, indicating that amyloid load was not related to discrepancy scores between self- and informant reports (based on the CCI).

DISCUSSION

The main finding of the present study is that amyloid-β load is associated with an approximately two-fold increased risk of SCD-related worries and a heightened memory-deficit self-awareness, but not with severity or specific cognitive complaints.

Amyloid-β load may insidiously affect cognition and self-perceived decline prior to symptom onset (Perrotin et al., 2012; Snitz et al., 2015; Baker et al., 2017), which could be amongst others a reason for individuals to visit a memory clinic. Some population-based and mixed population and memory clinic studies have shown that amyloid-β load is related to SCD (Amariglio et al., 2012; Mielke et al., 2012; Perrotin et al., 2012, 2016; Snitz et al., 2015), but other studies did not find this association with SCD (Buckley et al., 2013; Holland et al., 2015). To the best of our knowledge, associations between amyloid-β load and cognitive complaints have not been investigated in a pure memory clinic sample, and earlier findings could have been affected by the recruitment policy, particularly in the case of mixed recruitment studies (Jansen et al., 2015; Slot et al., 2018a). Therefore, it remains unclear to what extent amyloid-β is contributing to the phenotype of SCD in individuals who seek medical evaluation for their complaints (Jonker et al., 2000; Stewart, 2012). In the present study we investigated relatively young individuals with a recent SCD onset (<5 years), and compared to literature (Jansen et al., 2015; Ossenkoppele et al., 2015), a substantial fraction of almost one out of four showed abnormal amyloid-β accumulation. We furthermore used quantitative PET (i.e., BP_{ND}) because it can more accurately determine amyloid-β load than standardized uptake ratio values (SUVr), which is especially important to capture potentially early – subtle – disease processes, and SCD-related worries are related to a sixteen and six fold increased risk of clinical progression, respectively (Jessen et al., 2010; Van Harten et al., 2013; Buckley et al., 2016), and we now show that they associated with each other in cognitively normal individuals. The SCD *plus* criteria have suggested that the presence of SCD-related worries are associated with an increased risk of future cognitive decline (Jessen et al., 2014), and our results support this notion.

Apart from the relationship with SCD-related worries, no associations between amyloid-β load and any of the SCD questionnaires or single items that measure various aspects of cognitive change were observed, indicating that these questionnaires are not specific for amyloid-β accumulation in a memory clinic. There is much controversy about which questionnaire can be used to unveil cognitive normal individuals at increased risk for AD, but the present results indicate that it does not necessarily matters which questionnaire, but rather whether the SCD assessment includes a "worry" inquiry. Earlier studies have used SUVr to assess abnormal amyloid-β accumulation, which have generated inconsistent results (Mielke et al., 2012; Perrotin et al., 2012, 2016; Holland et al., 2015; Snitz et al., 2015). Compared with BP_{ND}, SUVr is liable to overestimation of amyloid-β load together with a higher variability (van Berckel et al., 2013), which could hamper a correct interpretation and reduce statistical power especially in early disease stages (Yaqub et al., 2008; van Berckel et al., 2013; Golla et al., 2018). Other possible explanations for our findings are recruitment criteria used and the operationalization of SCD (Perrotin et al., 2016; Molinuevo et al., 2017). A recent study has demonstrated elevated levels of amyloid-β load in memory clinic SCD patients compared with community-dwelling individuals without SCD, but not compared with community-recruited subjects with SCD (Perrotin et al., 2016). The present investigations were restricted to individuals with SCD, who had visited a memory clinic for their self-perceived

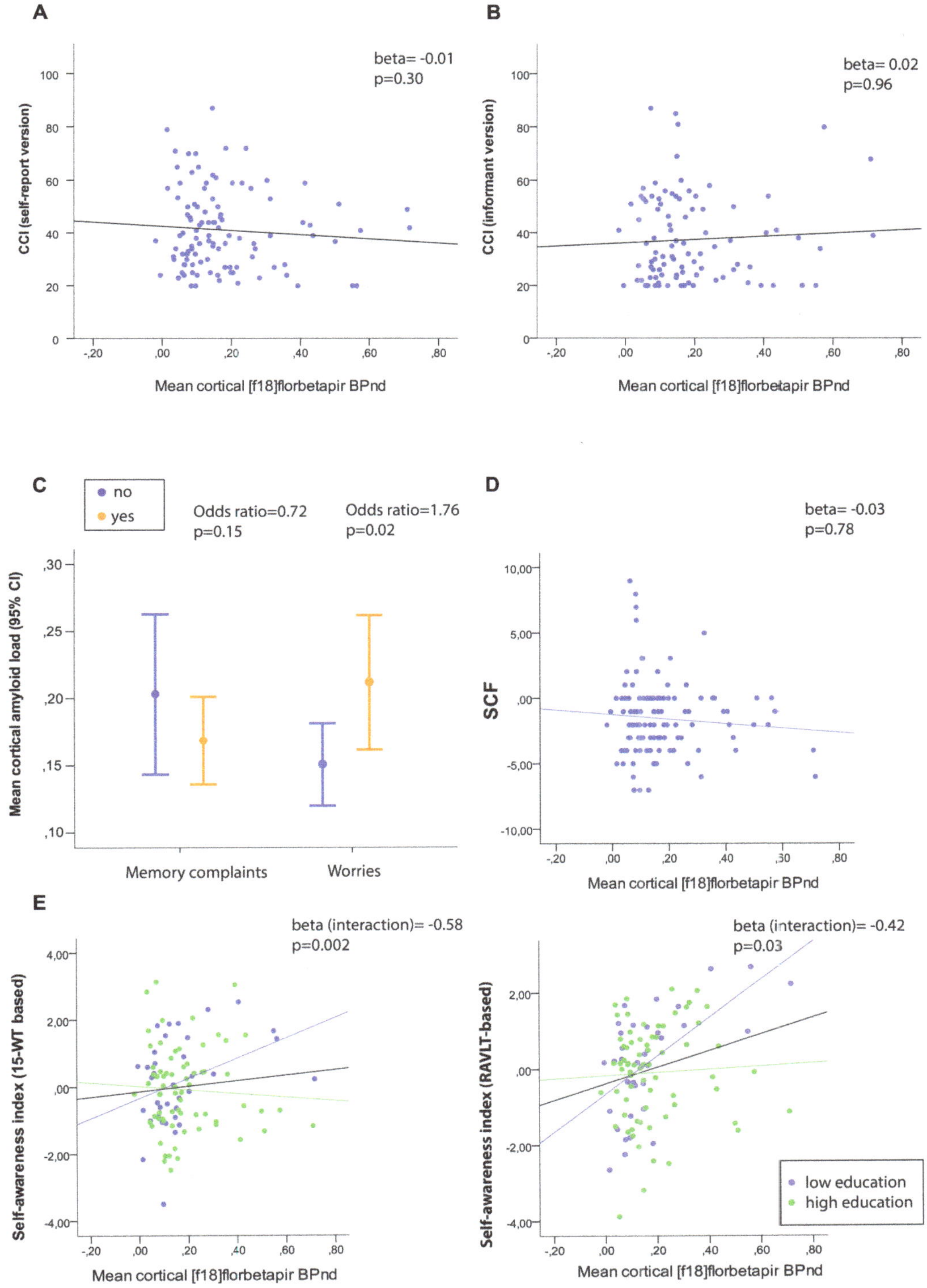

FIGURE 2 | (A) Mean cortical amyloid-beta load in relation to raw (untransformed) scores of the self-report cognitive change index (CCI) and **(B)** informant-based CCI, and **(D)** the subjective cognitive functioning (SCF) questionnaire. **(C)** Mean cortical amyloid-beta load stratified for memory complaints (yes/no) and worries (yes/no). **(E)** Associations between mean cortical amyloid load and self-awareness index based on the RBMT % delayed recall (left) and RAVLT % delayed recall (right) with stratification for low and high education level. Memory deficit awareness index: A positive index score reflects heightened self-awareness (hypernosognosia), whereas negative scores lowered self-awareness (anosognosia).

decline. By definition these individuals experience cognitive complaints, but these may be caused by various factors other than amyloid-β accumulation. For example, it has been shown that memory clinic SCD patients have higher (subclinical) depressive symptoms compared with community-dwelling individuals with SCD (Perrotin et al., 2016). In the present study, however, individuals with a current psychiatric diagnosis were excluded prior to enrolment. In addition, analyses were adjusted for depressive symptoms, which makes it unlikely that mental illness was responsible for the lack of associations. Nevertheless, irrespective of the nature of cognitive complaints, higher mean cortical amyloid-β load was associated with SCD related worries, and this appeared to be consistent for all cortical lobar regions.

It has been claimed that earliest changes in cognition are best perceived by the individual rather than by an observer (Caselli et al., 2014). In order to investigate the awareness of memory deficits, two discrepancy scores were calculated to adjust cognitive complaints for episodic memory performance (i.e., memory deficit awareness index) and informant reports (i.e., self-proxy index). Although SCD conceptually refers to the self-perception of cognitive decline and does not require confirmation by informants, we did not find different associations between amyloid-β and the self-proxy index. In line with a study on cognitively normal individuals from the community (Vannini et al., 2017), we found a positive relation between amyloid-β load and memory deficit awareness, which indicated that individuals with increased amyloid-β load showed heightened memory deficit awareness or hypernosognosia. We furthermore found that associations were dependent on the level of education. The previous indicates that when taking into account the degree of delayed memory recall with cognitive complaints this could result in a stronger relationship with amyloid-β load, particularly for individuals with relatively lower education levels. Earlier studies have used this index to investigate anosognosia, and showed that AD patients have an impaired memory deficit awareness, i.e., more severe episodic memory performance compared with self-rated cognitive performance (Barba et al., 1995; Perrotin et al., 2015). In the present study we found opposite patterns compared to patients with AD dementia (Perrotin et al., 2015). Although it needs to be interpreted with care, these positive associations could reflect a higher level of memory deficit self-awareness in individuals with elevated amyloid-beta accumulation (Vannini et al., 2017). The index scores seemed to be slightly driven by episodic memory performance, and our findings imply that higher amyloid-β load can be observed in cases when individuals' self-rated cognitive complaints are less severe than their episodic memory performance, which is in line with studies showing that episodic memory starts to deteriorate early in the disease course (Hanseeuw et al., 2017; Lim et al., 2018).

Although individuals with SCD who visit a memory clinic are a clinically relevant group since they seek help for their complaints and are at increased risk for clinical progression (Geerlings et al., 1999; Jonker et al., 2000; Jessen et al., 2010), some limitations need to be acknowledged. First, while we have incorporated every available SCD item from our cohort, there may be other questionnaires which are better able to isolate SCD due to preclinical AD. On the other hand, the use of other SCD questionnaires may not provide very different results, because questionnaires will likely show high correlations, and typically inquire about memory complaints (Rabin et al., 2015). In addition, questionnaires rely on self-perception of cognitive decline, which in the present study did not show any relation with amyloid-β load or could have been distorted by other non-AD or subthreshold psychiatry SCD phenotypes (Buckley et al., 2015; Slot et al., 2018b). Notwithstanding, our results indicate that not SCD severity, but rather worries about self-perceived decline can be relevant. Second, we have not included individuals without cognitive complaints, therefore we cannot extrapolate our findings to the general population. On the other hand, we do expect that individuals who feel worried about their cognitive decline will most likely visit a memory clinic. Third, our memory self-awareness index seemed driven by relatively lower, but non-significant, episodic memory performance in individuals with higher amyloid-β burden. Lastly, the present study had a cross-sectional design. Therefore, it is not possible to make inferences as to whether individuals with more severe amyloid-β accumulation and SCD related worries will show an increased risk of clinical progression to symptomatic stages of AD. Future longitudinal studies are necessary to fully elucidate these associations, while taking into account the effects of concomitant AD pathology such as tau burden (measured with PET, CSF or blood) and hippocampal atrophy.

In conclusion, amyloid-β load was associated with SCD related worries and higher memory deficit self-awareness (i.e., hypernosognosia), but not with severity or specific pattern of cognitive complaints. Our findings indicate that worries about self-perceived decline may therefore help to identify amyloid-β related SCD.

AUTHOR CONTRIBUTIONS

SV acquired, analyzed, and interpreted the data, drafted the manuscript, and approved the final content of the manuscript. TT, CvdW, LW, and RS acquired the data, critically revised the manuscript, and approved the final content of the manuscript. RO, SS, NP, AD, MY, BvB, and AL conceived and designed the study, analyzed and interpreted the data, drafted the manuscript and enhanced its intellectual content, and approved the final content of the manuscript. PS and WvdF conceived and designed the study, enhanced the intellectual content of the manuscript, and approved the final content of the manuscript.

FUNDING

WvdF is recipient of a research grant for the SCIENCe project from Gieske-Strijbis Fonds. SV and RS are supported by a research grant from Gieske-Strijbis Fonds. SS is supported by grants from JPND Euro-SCD and Zon-MW (Off-Road). The VUmc Alzheimer Center is supported by Alzheimer Nederland and Stichting VUmc Fonds. Research of the VUmc Alzheimer Center is part of the neurodegeneration research program of the Amsterdam Neuroscience. [^{18}F]Florbetapir PET scans were made possible by Avid Radiopharmeuticals Inc. SV, RS, TT, LW, CvdW, SS, NP, AD, RO, AL, MY, and BvB report no conflict of interest. SP received grant support (for the institution) from GE Healthcare, Danone Research, Piramal and MERCK. In the past 2 years he has received consultancy/speaker fees from Lilly, GE Healthcare, Novartis, Forum, Sanofi, Nutricia, Probiodrug and EIP Pharma. All funding is paid to the institution. WvdF received grant support from ZonMW, NWO, EU-FP7, Alzheimer Nederland, CardioVascular Onderzoek Nederland, Stichting Dioraphte, Gieskes-Strijbis Fonds, Boehringer Ingelheim, Piramal Neuroimaging, Roche BV, Janssen Stellar, Combinostics. All funding is paid to the institution.

ACKNOWLEDGMENTS

We would like to acknowledge the participants of the SCIENCe cohort for dedicating their time and energy to this study.

REFERENCES

Amariglio, R. E., Becker, J. A., Carmasin, J., Wadsworth, L. P., Lorius, N., Sullivan, C., et al. (2012). Subjective cognitive complaints and amyloid burden in cognitively normal older individuals. *Neuropsychologia* 50, 2880–2886. doi: 10.1016/j.neuropsychologia.2012.08.011

Baker, J. E., Lim, Y. Y., Pietrzak, R. H., Hassenstab, J., Snyder, P. J., Masters, C. L., et al. (2017). Cognitive impairment and decline in cognitively normal older adults with high amyloid-β: a meta-analysis. *Alzheimers Dement.* 6, 108–121. doi: 10.1016/j.dadm.2016.09.002

Barba, G. D., Parlato, V., Iavarone, A., and Boller, F. (1995). Anosognosia, intrusions and "frontal" functions in Alzheimer's disease and depression. *Neuropsychologia* 33, 247–259. doi: 10.1016/0028-3932(94)00091-3

Buckley, R., Saling, M. M., Ames, D., Rowe, C. C., Lautenschlager, N. T., MacAulay, S. L., et al. (2013). Factors affecting subjective memory complaints i. The AIBL aging study: biomarkers, memory, affect, and age. *Int. Psychogeriatr.* 25, 1307–1315. doi: 10.1017/S1041610213000665

Buckley, R. F., Maruff, P., Ames, D., Bourgeat, P., Martins, R. N., Masters, C. L., et al. (2016). Subjective memory decline predicts greater rates of clinical progression in preclinical Alzheimer's disease. *Alzheimers Dement.* 12, 796–804. doi: 10.1016/j.jalz.2015.12.013

Buckley, R. F., Saling, M. M., Frommann, I., Wolfsgruber, S., and Wagner, M. (2015). Subjective cognitive decline from a phenomenological perspective: a review of the qualitative literature. *J. Alzheimers Dis.* 48, S125–S140. doi: 10.3233/JAD-150095

Caselli, R. J., Chen, K., Locke, D. E. C., Lee, W., Roontiva, A., Bandy, D., et al. (2014). Subjective cognitive decline: self and informant comparisons. *Alzheimers Dement.* 10, 93–98. doi: 10.1016/j.jalz.2013.01.003

Folstein, M. F., Folstein, S. E., and McHugh, P. R. (1975). Mini-mental state". A practical method for grading the cognitive state of patients for the clinician. *J. Psychiatr. Res.* 12, 198–193. doi: 10.1016/0022-3956(75)90026-6

Geerlings, M. I., Jonker, C., Bouter, L. M., Adèr, H. J., and Schmand, B. (1999). Association between memory complaints and incident Alzheimer's disease in elderly people with normal baseline cognition. *Am. J. Psychiatry* 156, 531–537. doi: 10.1176/ajp.156.4.531

Golla, S. S. V., Verfaillie, S. C. J., Boellaard, R., Adriaanse, S. M., Zwan, M. D., Schuit, R. C., et al. (2018). Quantification of [18F]florbetapir: a test – retest tracer kinetic modelling study. *J. Cereb. Blood Flow Metab.* doi: 10.1177/0271678X18783628 [Epub ahead of print].

Gunn, R. N., Lammertsma, A. A., Hume, S. P., and Cunningham, V. J. (1997). Parametric imaging of ligand-receptor binding in PET using a simplified reference region model. *Neuroimage* 6, 279–287. doi: 10.1006/nimg.1997.0303

Hammers, A., Allom, R., Koepp, M. J., Free, S. L., Myers, R., Lemieux, L., et al. (2003). Three-dimensional maximum probability atlas of the human brain, with particular reference to the temporal lobe. *Hum. Brain Mapp.* 19, 224–247. doi: 10.1002/hbm.10123

Hanseeuw, B. J., Betensky, R. A., Schultz, A. P., Papp, K. V., Mormino, E. C., Sepulcre, J., et al. (2017). Fluorodeoxyglucose metabolism associated with tau-amyloid interaction predicts memory decline. *Ann. Neurol.* 81, 583–596. doi: 10.1002/ana.24910

Holland, D., Lim, Y. Y., Buckley, R. F., Pietrzak, R. H., Snyder, P. J., Ames, D., et al. (2015). Amyloid-β related memory decline is not associated with subjective or informant rated cognitive impairment in healthy adults. *J. Alzheimers Dis.* 43, 677–686. doi: 10.3233/JAD-140678

Hu, X., Teunissen, C. E., Spottke, A., Heneka, M. T., Düzel, E., Peters, O., et al. (2018). Smaller medial temporal lobe volumes in individuals with subjective cognitive decline and biomarker evidence of Alzheimer's disease—Data from three memory clinic studies. *Alzheimers Dement.* doi: 10.1016/j.jalz.2018.09.002 [Epub ahead of print].

Jack, C. R., Knopman, D. S., Jagust, W. J., Petersen, R. C., Weiner, M. W., Aisen, P. S., et al. (2013). Tracking pathophysiological processes in Alzheimer's disease: an updated hypothetical model of dynamic biomarkers. *Lancet Neurol.* 12, 207–216. doi: 10.1016/S1474-4422(12)70291-0

Jansen, W. J., Ossenkoppele, R., Knol, D. L., Tijms, B. M., Scheltens, P., Verhey, F. R. J., et al. (2015). Prevalence of cerebral amyloid pathology in persons without dementia. *JAMA* 313, 1924–1938. doi: 10.1001/jama.2015.4668

Jessen, F., Amariglio, R. E., van Boxtel, M., Breteler, M., Ceccaldi, M., Chételat, G., et al. (2014). A conceptual framework for research on subjective cognitive decline in preclinical Alzheimer's disease. *Alzheimers Dement.* 10, 844–852. doi: 10.1016/j.jalz.2014.01.001

Jessen, F., Wiese, B., Bachmann, C., Eifflaender-Gorfer, S., Haller, F., Kölsch, H., et al. (2010). Prediction of dementia by subjective memory impairment: effects of severity and temporal association with cognitive impairment. *Arch. Gen. Psychiatry* 67, 414–422. doi: 10.1001/archgenpsychiatry.2010.30

Jonker, C., Geerlings, M. I., and Schmand, B. (2000). Are memory complaints predictive for dementia? A review of clinical and population-based studies. *Int. J. Geriatr. Psychiatry* 15, 983–991. doi: 10.1002/1099-1166(200011)15:11<983::AID-GPS238>3.0.CO;2-5

Lammertsma, A. A., and Hume, S. P. (1996). Simplified reference tissue model for PET receptor studies. *Neuroimage* 4, 153–158. doi: 10.1006/nimg.1996.0066

Langer, K. G., and Levine, D. N. (2014). Babinski, J. (1914). Contribution to the study of the mental disorders in hemiplegia of organic cerebral origin (anosognosia). Translated by K.G. Langer & D.N. levine. Translated from the original Contribution à l'Étude des troubles mentaux dans l'hémiplé. *Cortex* 61, 5–8. doi: 10.1016/j.cortex.2014.04.019

Lim, Y., Kalinowski, P., Pietrzak, R. H., Laws, S. M., Burnham, S. C., Ames, D., et al. (2018). Association of β-Amyloid and apolipoprotein E ε4 with memory decline in preclinical alzheimer disease. *JAMA Neurol.* 75, 488–494. doi: 10.1001/jamaneurol.2017.4325

Mielke, M. M., Wiste, H. J., Weigand, S. D., Knopman, D. S., Lowe, V. J., Roberts, R. O., et al. (2012). Indicators of amyloid burden in a population-based study of cognitively normal elderly. *Neurology* 79, 1570–1577. doi: 10.1212/WNL.0b013e31826e2696

Molinuevo, J. L., Rabin, L. A., Amariglio, R., Buckley, R., Dubois, B., Ellis, K. A., et al. (2017). Implementation of subjective cognitive decline criteria in research studies. *Alzheimers Dement.* 13, 296–311. doi: 10.1016/j.jalz.2016.09.012

Ossenkoppele, R., Jansen, W. J., Rabinovici, G. D., Knol, D. L., Van Der Flier, W. M., Van Berckel, B. N. M., et al. (2015). Prevalence of amyloid PET positivity in dementia syndromes: a meta-analysis. *JAMA* 313, 1939–1949. doi: 10.1001/jama.2015.4669

Perrotin, A., Desgranges, B., Landeau, B., Mézenge, F., La Joie, R., Egret, S., et al. (2015). Anosognosia in Alzheimer disease: disconnection between memory and self-related brain networks. *Ann. Neurol.* 78, 477–486. doi: 10.1002/ana.24462

Perrotin, A., La Joie, R., de La Sayette, V., Barré, L., Mézenge, F., Mutlu, J., et al. (2016). Subjective cognitive decline in cognitively normal elders from the community or from a memory clinic: differential affective and imaging correlates. *Alzheimers Dement.* 13, 550–560. doi: 10.1016/j.jalz.2016.08.011

Perrotin, A., Mormino, E. C., Madison, C. M., Hayenga, A. O., and Jagust, W. J. (2012). Subjective cognition and amyloid deposition imaging: a Pittsburgh Compound B positron emission tomography study in normal elderly individuals. *Arch. Neurol.* 69, 223–229. doi: 10.1001/archneurol.2011.666

Rabin, L. A., Smart, C. M., and Amariglio, R. E. (2017). Subjective cognitive decline in preclinical Alzheimer's disease. *Annu. Rev. Clin. Psychol.* 13, 369–396. doi: 10.1146/annurev-clinpsy-032816-045136

Rabin, L. A., Smart, C. M., Crane, P. K., Amariglio, R. E., Berman, L. M., Boada, M., et al. (2015). Subjective cognitive decline in older adults: an overview of self-report measures used across 19 international research studies. *J. Alzheimers Dis.* 48(Suppl. 1), S63–S86. doi: 10.3233/JAD-150154

Radloff, L. S. (1977). The CES-D Scale: a self-report depression scale for research in the general population. *Appl. Psychol. Measure.* 1, 385–401. doi: 10.1177/014662167700100306

Rask, T., Svarer, C., Dyrby, T., Comerci, M., Berkouk, K., Baron, J. C., et al. (2004). "PVElab: software for correction of functional images for partial volume errors," in *Proceedings of the 10th Meeting of the Organisation for Human Brain Mapping*, Budapest.

Rattanabannakit, C., Risacher, S. L., Gao, S., Lane, K. A., Brown, S. A., McDonald, B. C., et al. (2016). The cognitive change index as a measure of self and informant perception of cognitive decline: relation to neuropsychological tests. *J. Alzheimers Dis.* 51, 1145–1155. doi: 10.3233/JAD-150729

Rodda, J., Okello, A., Edison, P., Dannhauser, T., Brooks, D. J., and Walker, Z. (2010). 11C-PIB PET in subjective cognitive impairment. *Eur. Psychiatry* 25, 123–125. doi: 10.1016/j.eurpsy.2009.07.011

Schmand, B., Jonker, C., Hooijer, C., and Lindeboom, J. (1996). Subjective memory complaints may announce dementia. *Neurology* 46, 121–125. doi: 10.1212/WNL.46.1.121

Slot, R. E. R., Sikkes, S. A., Berkhof, J., Brodaty, H., Buckley, R., Cavedo, E., et al. (2018a). Subjective cognitive decline and rates of incident Alzheimer's disease and non-Alzheimer's disease dementia. *Alzheimers Dement.* doi: 10.1016/j.jalz.2018.10.003 [Epub ahead of print].

Slot, R. E. R., Verfaillie, S. C. J., Overbeek, J. M., Timmers, T., Wesselman, L. M. P., Teunissen, C. E., et al. (2018b). Subjective cognitive impairment cohort (science): study design and first results. *Alzheimers Res. Ther.* 10:76. doi: 10.1186/s13195-018-0390-y

Snitz, B. E., Weissfeld, L. A., Cohen, A. D., Lopez, O. L., Nebes, R. D., Aizenstein, H. J., et al. (2015). Subjective cognitive complaints, personality and brain amyloid-beta in cognitively normal older adults. *Am. J. Geriatr. Psychiatry* 23, 985–993. doi: 10.1016/j.jagp.2015.01.008

Stewart, R. (2012). Subjective cognitive impairment. *Curr. Opin. Psychiatry* 25, 445–450. doi: 10.1097/YCO.0b013e3283586fd8

van Berckel, B. N. M., Ossenkoppele, R., Tolboom, N., Yaqub, M., Foster-Dingley, J. C., Windhorst, A. D., et al. (2013). Longitudinal amyloid imaging using 11C-PiB: methodologic considerations. *J. Nucl. Med.* 54, 1570–1576. doi: 10.2967/jnumed.112.113654

Van Der Flier, W. M., Pijnenburg, Y. A. L., Prins, N., Lemstra, A. W., Bouwman, F. H., Teunissen, C. E., et al. (2014). Optimizing patient care and research: the Amsterdam dementia cohort. *J. Alzheimers Dis.* 41, 313–327. doi: 10.3233/JAD-132306

Van Harten, A. C., Visser, P. J., Pijnenburg, Y. A. L., Teunissen, C. E., Blankenstein, M. A., Scheltens, P., et al. (2013). Cerebrospinal fluid Aβ42 is the best predictor of clinical progression in patients with subjective complaints. *Alzheimers Dement.* 9, 481–487. doi: 10.1016/j.jalz.2012.08.004

van Oijen, M., de Jong, F. J., Hofman, A., Koudstaal, P. J., and Breteler, M. M. B. (2007). Subjective memory complaints, education, and risk of Alzheimer's disease. *Alzheimers Dement.* 3, 92–97. doi: 10.1016/j.jalz.2007.01.011

Vannini, P., Amariglio, R., Hanseeuw, B., Johnson, K. A., McLaren, D. G., Chhatwal, J., et al. (2017). Memory self-awareness in the preclinical and prodromal stages of Alzheimer's disease. *Neuropsychologia* 99, 343–349. doi: 10.1016/j.neuropsychologia.2017.04.002

Verfaillie, S. C. J., Pichet Binette, A., Vachon-Presseau, E., Tabrizi, S., Savard, M., Bellec, P., et al. (2018a). Subjective cognitive decline is associated with altered default mode network connectivity in individuals with a family history of Alzheimer's disease. *Biol. Psychiatry Cogn. Neurosci. Neuroimaging* 3, 463–472. doi: 10.1016/j.bpsc.2017.11.012

Verfaillie, S. C. J., Slot, R. E. R., Dicks, E., Prins, N. D., Overbeek, J. M., Teunissen, C. E., et al. (2018b). A more randomly organized grey matter network is associated with deteriorating language and global cognition in individuals with subjective cognitive decline. *Hum. Brain Mapp.* 39, 3143–3151. doi: 10.1002/hbm.24065

Verfaillie, S. C. J., Tijms, B., Versteeg, A., Benedictus, M. R., Bouwman, F. H., Scheltens, P., et al. (2016). Thinner temporal and parietal cortex is related to incident clinical progression to dementia in patients with subjective cognitive decline. *Alzheimers Dement.* 5, 43–52. doi: 10.1016/j.dadm.2016.10.007

Villeneuve, S., Rabinovici, G. D., Cohn-Sheehy, B. I., Madison, C., Ayakta, N., Ghosh, P. M., et al. (2015). Existing Pittsburgh Compound-B positron emission tomography thresholds are too high: statistical and pathological evaluation. *Brain* 138, 2020–2033. doi: 10.1093/brain/awv112

Yaqub, M., Tolboom, N., Boellaard, R., van Berckel, B., van Tilburg, E., Luurtsema, G., et al. (2008). Simplified parametric methods for [11C]PIB studies. *Neuroimage* 42, 76–86. doi: 10.1016/J.NEUROIMAGE.2008.04.251

Zigmond, A. S., and Snaith, R. P. (1983). The hospital anxiety and depression scale. *Acta Psychiatr. Scand.* 67, 361–370. doi: 10.1111/j.1600-0447.1983.tb09716.x

6

Cognitive Profiles of Aging in Multiple Sclerosis

*Dejan Jakimovski[1,2], Bianca Weinstock-Guttman[1], Shumita Roy[1], Michael Jaworski III[1], Laura Hancock[3], Alissa Nizinski[1], Pavitra Srinivasan[1], Tom A. Fuchs[1,2], Kinga Szigeti[1], Robert Zivadinov[1,2,4] and Ralph H. B. Benedict[1]**

[1] Department of Neurology, Jacobs School of Medicine and Biomedical Sciences, University at Buffalo – The State University of New York, Buffalo, NY, United States, [2] Buffalo Neuroimaging Analysis Center, Department of Neurology, Jacobs School of Medicine and Biomedical Sciences, University at Buffalo – The State University of New York, Buffalo, NY, United States, [3] Department of Neurology, University of Wisconsin School of Medicine and Public Health, Madison, WI, United States, [4] Clinical Translational Science Institute, Center for Biomedical Imaging, University at Buffalo – The State University of New York, Buffalo, NY, United States

Correspondence:
Ralph H. B. Benedict
benedict@buffalo.edu

Background: Increasingly favorable mortality prognosis in multiple sclerosis (MS) raises questions regarding MS-specific cognitive aging and the presence of comorbidities such as Alzheimer's disease (AD).

Objective: To assess elderly with MS (EwMS) and age-matched healthy controls (HCs) using both MS- and AD-specific psychometrics.

Methods: EwMS (n = 104) and 56 HCs were assessed on a broad spectrum of language, visual-spatial processing, memory, processing speed, and executive function tests. Using logistic regression analysis, we examined cognitive performance differences between the EwMS and HC groups. Cognitive impairment (CI) was defined using a −1.5 SD threshold relative to age and education years-matched HCs, in two cognitive domains.

Results: CI was observed in 47.1% of EwMS with differences most often seen on tests emphasizing cognitive processing speed as measured by Symbol Digit Modalities Test (SDMT) ($d = 0.9$, $p < 0.001$) and verbal fluency (both category-based $d = 0.87$, $p < 0.001$; letter-based $d = 0.67$, $p < 0.001$). After adjusting for age, sex and years of education, MS/HC diagnosis was best predicted ($R^2 = 0.27$) by differences in category-based verbal fluency (Wald = 9.935, $p = 0.002$) and SDMT (Wald = 13.937, $p < 0.001$).

Conclusion: This study confirms the common hallmark of slowed cognitive processing speed in MS among elderly patients. Defective verbal fluency, less often observed in younger cohorts, may represent emerging cognitive pathology due to other etiologies.

Keywords: aging, MS, cognition, processing speed, verbal fluency

INTRODUCTION

Multiple sclerosis (MS) is a chronic demyelinating disease of the central nervous system (CNS) which presents with acute inflammatory episodes and co-occurring widespread neurodegeneration (Reich et al., 2018). These neuropathological processes are not only linked to physical disability progression, but also to cognitive impairment (Benedict et al., 2014). The increasingly favorable mortality prognosis with new disease modifying therapies raises new questions about quality of life, the influence of frailty, prevalence of comorbidities, and cognitive aging among the elderly with MS (EwMS) (Sanai et al., 2016; Koch-Henriksen et al., 2017).

Alzheimer's disease (AD) and its prodromal state, amnestic mild cognitive impairment (aMCI), are among the many comorbidities expected to increase within the aging population. Furthermore, the progressive MS phase is associated with neurodegenerative features resembling an AD-like phenotype. Although both diseases may lead to dementia, their cognitive hallmarks are thought to differ. MS patients commonly present with slowed cognitive processing speed (CPS) and deficient learning, a cognitive profile frequently associated with lesion disruption of neural networks and atrophy of major hubs that facilitate information exchange (e.g., thalamus) (Van Schependom et al., 2015; Bergsland et al., 2018). Contrarily, AD is characterized by progressive decline in episodic memory, rapid forgetting, and impairments in semantic language. These defects are associated with neurodegeneration starting within the hippocampus, and entorhinal cortex (Hyman et al., 1984; McKhann et al., 2011; Reitz et al., 2011). The prevalence of MS in the United States is now estimated at one million persons, and the average age of the population is increasing (Nelson et al., 2019). Therefore, the possibility that an EwMS patient may develop AD should be considered with new onset cognitive complaints (Luczynski et al., 2018). Nevertheless, only a few case reports of MS and AD dual diagnosis are found in the literature (Luczynski et al., 2018). Therefore, understanding the cognitive profiles EwMS is highly warranted.

In a preliminary cross-sectional investigation, we compared EwMS (an average of 60 years old) with age and education-matched aMCI and AD patients (Roy et al., 2018). On a test of semantic verbal fluency, we found no significant difference between cognitively impaired MS and aMCI patients (Roy et al., 2018). Therefore, one may propose that as the MS cognitive decline progresses, additional cognitive features apart from processing speed are likely to emerge. Herein we endeavored to comprehensively examine the cognitive profile of a larger group of EwMS and age-matched healthy controls (HCs) using MS and AD-specific psychometric tests. We hypothesized that if EwMS have a true impairment in the language aspects of verbal fluency, this deficit should remain significant after controlling for the influence of cognitive processing speed.

MATERIALS AND METHODS

Study Population

The study sample was composed of prospectively enrolled EwMS and HCs. The inclusion criteria for EwMS were (1) age $\geq$50 years old, (2) neuropsychological and clinical examination, and (3) MS diagnosis per 2010-revised McDonald criteria (Polman et al., 2011). The exclusion criteria for the EwMS consisted of (1) history of psychiatric and major depressive disorder prior to the onset of MS, (2) active relapse within 30 days of the examination, and (3) use of corticosteroids within 30 days of the study. Inclusion and exclusion criteria for HCs were (1) $\geq$50 years old, (2) neuropsychological examination, (3) self-reported intact cognition, (4) no history of neurological or medical illness that might impact cognitive function, and (5) no diagnosis of major depressive disorder. Furthermore, HCs with mini-mental state examination (MMSE) performance lower than 28 were excluded. Both the EwMS and HCs were additionally screened with the beck depression inventory-II fastscreen (BDI-FS).

Clinical examination was performed by a neurologist and physical disability was assessed using the expanded disability status scale (EDSS) (Kurtzke, 1983). The Timed 25-Foot Walk (T25FW) and 9-Hole Peg Test (9PHT) were additional measures of lower and upper extremity function, respectively. The EwMS were classified by disease course as relapsing-remitting MS (RRMS) and progressive MS (PMS). The study was approved by the Institutional Review Board (IRB) and all participants signed an informed consent form.

Neuropsychological Examination

The neuropsychological examination was performed by trained examiners under supervision of a board-certified neuropsychologist (RHBB) and included tests traditionally regarded as MS and AD-specific (Strauss et al., 2006). The cognitive domains, their participating tests, and corresponding references are shown in **Table 1**.

The exam included the Minimal Assessment of Cognitive Function in Multiple Sclerosis (MACFIMS) battery (Benedict et al., 2002) which evaluates several domains, including: processing speed/working memory [Paced Auditory Serial Addition Test (PASAT) (Gronwall, 1977) and Symbol Digit Modalities Test (SDMT) (Smith, 1982)], learning and memory [learning trials for California Verbal Learning Test–second edition (CVLT-II) (Delis et al., 2000) and Brief Visuospatial Memory Test-Revised (BVMT-R) (Benedict, 1997)], language [Controlled Oral Word Association Test (COWAT) (Ruff et al., 1996)] and executive function [number of correct sorts and description scores from the Sorting subtest of the Delis-Kaplan Executive Function System (D-KEFS) (Delis et al., 2001)].

Participants also completed neuropsychological measures that are traditionally utilized for detecting AD-specific cognitive impairments (Strauss et al., 2006). These tests included those measuring the domains of memory [Logical Memory from the Wechsler Memory Scale-Revised (WMS-R) (Wechsler, 1945)], language [Boston Naming Test (BNT) (Goodglass et al., 1983)], two categories of semantic fluency (total number of categorical items generated in one minute; animals and supermarket items), and visuospatial skill [Beery Visual-Motor Integration (VMI) (Beery, 2010) and clock drawing test (Agrell and Dehlin, 1998)]. The MMSE was also performed as an additional assessment of descriptive global cognitive functioning. For all performed psychometric tests, higher scores indicate better cognitive performance.

TABLE 1 | Cognitive domains and their respective tests.

Abbreviation	Name	References
Processing speed/working memory		
PASAT-3	Paced Auditory Serial Addition Test (3 second version)	Gronwall, 1977
SDMT	Symbol Digit Modalities Test	Smith, 1982
Learning and memory		
CVLT-II total learning trials	California Verbal Learning Test (total score)	Delis et al., 2000
CVLT-II short delay	California Verbal Learning Test (short delay score)	Delis et al., 2000
CVLT-II long delay	California Verbal Learning Test (long delay score)	Delis et al., 2000
CVLT-II recognition index	California Verbal Learning Test (recognition index)	Delis et al., 2000
BVMT-R total learning trials	Brief Visuospatial Memory Test – Revised (total immediate score)	Benedict, 1997
BVMT-R delay	Brief Visuospatial Memory Test – Revised (long delay score)	Benedict, 1997
BVMT-R recognition index	Brief Visuospatial Memory Test – Revised (recognition index)	Benedict, 1997
WMS-R Logical Memory IR	Wechsler Memory Scale – Revised (immediate recall score)	Wechsler, 1945
WMS-R Logical Memory DR	Wechsler Memory Scale – Revised (delayed recall score)	Wechsler, 1945
WMS-R Logical Memory MR	Wechsler Memory Scale – Revised (memory retention)	Wechsler, 1945
Spatial processing		
Beery VMI	Beery-Buktenica Visual-Motor Integration Test	Beery, 2010
Clock drawing test	N/A	Agrell and Dehlin, 1998
Executive function		
D-KEFS sorting CS	Delis-Kaplan Executive Function System (correct sorts score)	Delis et al., 2001
D-KEFS sorting DS	Delis-Kaplan Executive Function System (description score)	Delis et al., 2001
Language		
COWAT	Controlled Oral Word Association Test	Ruff et al., 1996
BNT	Boston Naming Test	Goodglass et al., 1983
Animal fluency	N/A	Ruff et al., 1996
Supermarket items fluency	N/A	Ruff et al., 1996
Total verbal fluency	N/A	Ruff et al., 1996

Statistical Analysis

All statistical tests were performed using SPSS version 25.0 (IBM, Armonk, NY, United States). The distribution of the variables was examined using both Kolmogorov-Smirnov and Shapiro-Wilk tests of normality. The differences in demographics and cognitive raw scores between EwMS and HCs were determined by χ^2–test for categorical variables, ANOVA or t-test for continuous, normally distributed variables, and Mann Whitney U-test for continuous, not normally distributed variables. To control for the multiple comparisons, Benjamini-Hochberg procedure was employed and adjusted $p < 0.05$ were considered statistically significant.

In order to delineate the degree of cognitive impairment across various cognitive domains while controlling for age, z-scores derived from the age-matched HCs were calculated. EwMS with z-score performance lower than -1.5 on at least two different cognitive domains were classified as cognitively impaired. The number of tests within each corresponding domain are shown in **Table 1**.

The impact of CPS on differences in cognitive performance between EwMS and HCs was additionally determined by analysis of covariance (ANCOVA) adjusted for SDMT scores.

Lastly, a multivariate logistic regression model determining the specific cognitive differences between the EwMS and the HCs was constructed. The model was composed of an initial force-entered block which corrected for differences in sex, age, and years of education. Furthermore, a second step-wise inclusion block determined the strength and order of cognitive variables which provided the greatest explanatory value in differentiating EwMS and HCs. For each derived step, the respective R^2, Wald coefficient, and p-values were reported.

RESULTS

Demographic and Clinical Characteristics

The EwMS ($n = 104$) and HCs ($n = 56$) were similar in age (62.1 vs. 62.3 years, $p = 0.919$), years of education (15.2 vs. 15.6 years, $p = 0.213$) and sex ratio (75.0% vs. 62.5% females, $p = 0.09$). The MS group had a mean disease duration of 20.5 years, median EDSS scores of 3.5 (IQR 3.0–6.0), and ratio of RRMS/PMS of 73/31. Regarding disease modifying therapy (DMT), most EwMS were prescribed interferon-β (32, 30.8%), followed by glatiramer acetate (28, 17.3%), oral DMT medications (15, 14.4%), natalizumab (6, 5.8%), off-label medication (1, 0.9%), and the rest of the EwMS were not on any DMT (32, 30.8%).

The EwMS were more disabled when compared to the HCs in both lower and upper extremity function (T25FW, 6.7s vs. 4.7s, $p < 0.001$; and 9PHT, 24.7s vs. 21.5s, $p < 0.001$). The MS

TABLE 2 | Demographic and clinical characteristics of the EwMS and HCs samples.

Demographic and clinical characteristics	EwMS (n = 104)	HCs (n = 56)	Cohen's d	p-value
Female, n (%)	78 (75.0)	35 (62.5)	–	0.09
Age mean (SD)	62.1 (6.3)	62.3 (8.1)	0.028	0.919
Years of education, mean (SD)	15.2 (2.3)	15.6 (2.3)	0.174	0.213
EDSS, median (IQR)	3.5 (3.0 – 6.0)	–	–	–
Disease duration, mean (SD)	20.5 (11.9)	–	–	–
RRMS/PMS	73/31	–	–	–
T25FW, median (IQR)	6.7 (5.1 – 9.1)	4.7 (4.1 – 5.1)	**0.514**	**<0.001**
9-PHT, median (IQR)	24.1 (22.1 – 29.5)	21.5 (20.4 – 23.5)	**0.532**	**<0.001**
BDI-II, median (IQR)	1.0 (0.0 – 2.75)	0.0 (0.0 – 2.0)	**0.374**	**0.027**
Disease modifying therapy, n (%)				
Interferon-β	32 (30.8)	–	–	–
Glatiramer acetate	18 (17.3)	–	–	–
Natalizumab	6 (5.8)	–	–	–
No DMT	32 (30.8)	–	–	–
Oral DMT*	15 (14.4)	–	–	–
Off-label medications	1 (0.9)	–	–	–

*EwMS, elderly persons with multiple sclerosis; HCs, healthy controls; SD, standard deviation; IQR, interquartile ratio; RRMS, relapsing-remitting multiple sclerosis; PMS, progressive multiple sclerosis; BDI-II, Beck Depression Inventory; T25FW, Timed 25-Foot Walk; 9PHT, 9 Peg Hole Test; DMT, disease modifying therapy. Mann Whitney U-test, χ^2, and Student's t-test were used accordingly. P-value lower than 0.05 was considered statistically significant. *Oral DMTs include teriflunamide (9), dimethyl fumarate (5), and fingolimod (1). Use of off-label medications included only one case with rituximab. P-values lower than 0.05 were considered statistically significant and shown in bold.*

group also had higher depression scores (BDI-FS of 1.0 vs. 0.0, p = 0.005). All demographic and clinical information are shown in **Table 2**.

Cognitive Performance, and *Z*-Score-Derived Domain-Specific Impairment Rates in the EwMS

The raw scores from the neuropsychological examination of the EwMS and HCs on both the MACFIMS and AD-specific batteries are shown in **Table 3**. EwMS had lower raw scores when compared to the age-matched controls on both total learned and short delay recall in CVLT-II (49.7 vs. 54.9, d = 0.45, p = 0.018 and 9.8 vs. 11.2, d = 0.38, p = 0.045, respectively), SDMT (46.3 vs. 55.4, d = 0.91, p < 0.001), letter verbal fluency (35.8 vs. 43.0, d = 0.67, p = 0.001) and category verbal fluency (17.3 vs. 20.3, d = 0.67, p = 0.001; 20.9 vs. 25.7, d = 0.84, p < 0.001; and 38.2 vs. 45.9, d = 0.87, p < 0.001, for animal category, supermarket category and total score, respectively). Furthermore, the EwMS had lower immediate recall and delayed recall scores on WMS-R logical memory performance (23.7 vs. 26.4, d = 0.39, p = 0.045 and 18.8 vs. 21.7, d = 0.38, p = 0.048). No other group differences were observed.

To investigate the influence of processing speed on our findings, we performed an analysis of covariance in which the COWAT differences (letter-based and category-based fluency) were adjusted by CPS performance (SDMT score as covariate). The performance on SDMT had a significant influence on letter-based verbal fluency performance ($F_{1,156}$ = 39.5 r = 0.49, p < 0.001). In the final model, EwMS and HCs were not significantly different in letter-based fluency scores when CPS was controlled ($F_{1,156}$ = 3.9, p = 0.057). Processing speed also influenced the performance on total categorical verbal fluency ($F_{1,156}$ = 34.2, r = 0.425, p < 0.001) and on both animal-specific ($F_{1,156}$ = 12.2, r = 0.242, p = 0.001), and supermarket items-specific category ($F_{1,156}$ = 39.7, r = 0.476, p < 0.001). Despite the large SDMT effect, categorical verbal fluency remained significantly different between the EwMS and HCs (adjusted p = 0.036, adjusted p < 0.001, and adjusted p = 0.001, for animals, supermarket items, and total categorical verbal fluency, respectively).

Based on the HC-derived z-scores, the differences in processing speed and verbal fluency represented the most commonly affected domains in the EwMS. More than a quarter (27.9%) of EwMS had categorical verbal fluency impairment relative to HCs (22.1 and 24.0% for individual animal and supermarket tests, respectively). 25.0% were impaired on the letter-based verbal fluency, and 25.9% as impaired on the SDMT. Overall, 47.1% of the EwMS were classified as cognitively impaired on at least two different domain-specific tests. **Table 4** portrays the impairment rate observed for each cognitive test.

Both the multivariate logistic regression model blocks and derived step-wise predictors are shown in **Table 5**. The diagnosis of MS was best predicted by differences in category-based verbal fluency (Wald = 9.935, p = 0.002) and SDMT (Wald = 13.937, p < 0.001). Together with the force-entered block containing age, sex and years of education, the final step-wise model was able to explain 27% of the diagnosis variance (Nagelkerke R^2 = 0.27). In terms of odds ratio (OR), for every point decrease in categorical verbal fluency, the chance of MS diagnosis increased for 8.1% [Exp(B) = 0.919]. Similarly, for every point decrease

TABLE 3 | Cognitive performance of the EwMS and HCs populations on the minimal assessment for cognitive function in multip e sclerosis (MACFIMS) battery.

Cognitive test	EwMS (n = 104)	HCs (n = 56)	Cohen's d	p-value	BH-adjusted p-value*
CVLT-II total learning trials	49.7 (12.5)	54.9 (10.4)	**0.452**	**0.005**	**0.018**
CVLT-II short delay	9.8 (4.1)	11.2 (3.3)	**0.376**	**0.02**	**0.045**
CVLT-II long delay	10.7 (3.9)	11.9 (3.3)	0.581	0.029	0.053
CVLT-II recognition index	2.9 (1.0)	3.3 (0.7)	0.463	0.111	0.167
BVMT-R total learning trials	19.9 (7.1)	22.5 (5.6)	0.407	0.018	0.05
BVMT-R delay	8.1 (2.7)	8.5 (2.7)	0.148	0.309	0.412
BVMT-R recognition index	5.5 (0.8)	5.5 (0.9)	0.0	0.634	0.667
SDMT	46.3 (10.8)	55.4 (9.2)	**0.907**	**<0.001**	**<0.001**
PASAT-3	41.5 (13.2)	45.8 (12.3)	0.337	0.05	0.077
D-KEFS sorting CS[a]	9.0 (2.8)	9.3 (2.2)	0.119	0.579	0.644
D-KEFS sorting DS[a]	33.6 (10.8)	34.9 (8.9)	0.131	0.448	0.559
BNT	56.1 (3.8)	56.9 (3.3)	0.225	0.179	0.256
Letter-based verbal fluency	35.8 (11.2)	43.0 (10.2)	**0.672**	**<0.001**	**<0.001**
Animal-based fluency	17.3 (4.7)	20.3 (4.3)	**0.666**	**<0.001**	**0.001**
Supermarket items-based fluency	20.9 (5.5)	25.7 (5.9)	**0.842**	**<0.001**	**<0.001**
Total categorical fluency	38.2 (8.8)	45.9 (8.9)	**0.870**	**<0.001**	**<0.001**
Beery VMI	23.2 (3.3)	24.2 (2.6)	0.337	0.03	0.05
Clock drawing test	8.9 (1.2)	9.1 (1.2)	0.167	0.505	0.594
WMS-R logical memory IR	23.7 (7.1)	26.4 (6.4)	**0.399**	**0.018**	**0.045**
WMS-R logical memory DR	18.8 (7.3)	21.7 (8.1)	**0.376**	**0.024**	**0.048**
WMS-R logical memory MR	78.1% (14.8%)	79.3% (18.3%)	0.072	0.641	0.641

*EwMS, elderly persons with multiple sclerosis; HC, healthy controls; MACFIMS, Minimal Assessment of Cognitive Function in Multiple Sclerosis; CVLT-II, California Verbal Learning Test; BVMT-R, Brief Visuospatial Memory Test – Revised; SDMT, Symbol Digit Modalities Test; PASAT-3, 3 second Paced Auditory Serial Addition Test; D-KEFS, Delis-Kaplan Executive Function System; CS, number of correct sorts; DS, description score; BNT, Boston Naming Test; VMI, Visual-Motor Integration; WMS-R, Wechsler Memory Scale – Revised; IR, immediate recall; DR, delayed recall; MR, memory retention. All variables are shown as the mean (SD) raw scores. For all tests, higher scores relate to better cognitive performance. Letter-based and categorical verbal fluency were examined by Controlled Oral Word Association Test (COWAT). Student's t-test was used *Benjamini-Hochberg adjusted p-value <0.05 was considered statistically significant and shown in bold. [a]77 out of 104 EwMS patients had available D-KEFS scores.*

TABLE 4 | The ratio and percentage of cognitive impairment in the EwMS patients.

Psychometric test	Impairment ratio	Psychometric test	Impairment ratio
CVLT-II total learning trials	23/104 (22.1%)	D-KEFS Sorting DS	14/77 (13.5%)
CVLT-II short delay	23/104 (22.1%)	BNT	10/104 (9.6%)
CVLT-II long delay	18/104 (17.3%)	Animal-based fluency	23/104 (22.1%)
CVLT-II recognition index	21/104 (20.2%)	Supermarket items-based fluency	25/104 (24.0%)
BVMT-R total learning trials	23/104 (22.1%)	Total categorical fluency	29/104 (27.9%)
BVMT-R delay	11/104 (10.6%)	Beery VMI	23/104 (22.1%)
BVMT-R recognition index	12/104 (11.5%)	Clock drawing test	14/104 (13.5%)
SDMT	27/104 (25.9%)	WMS-R logical memory IR	19/104 (18.3%)
PASAT-3	18/104 (17.3%)	WMS-R logical memory DR	11/104 (10.6%)
Letter-based verbal fluency	26/104 (25.0%)	WMS-R logical memory MR	6/104 (5.8%)
D-KEFS Sorting CS	17/77 (16.3%)		

CVLT-II, California Verbal Learning Test; SD, short delay; LD, long delay; BVMT-R, Brief Visuospatial Memory Test – Revised; SDMT, Symbol Digit Modalities Test; PASAT-3, 3 second Paced Auditory Serial Addition Test; COWAT, Controlled Oral Word Association Test; D-KEFS, Delis-Kaplan Executive Function System; CS, number of correct sorts; DS, description score; BNT, Boston Naming Test; VMI, Visual-Motor Integration; WMS-R, Wechsler Memory Scale – Revised; IR, immediate recall; DR, delayed recall; MR, memory retention. Cognitive impairment was defined as a score <−1.5 SD relative to mean HC performance on the respective test. Letter-based and categorical verbal fluency were examined by Controlled Oral Word Association Test (COWAT).

in SDMT, the change of MS diagnosis is increased for 9.3% [Exp(B) = 0.907].

Lastly, we investigated the associations between verbal fluency and cognitive processing speed with the overall disability scores as depicted by EDSS. Within the total sample of EwMS, EDSS scores were associated with both total verbal fluency (Spearman's ranked correlation, $r_s = -0.292$, $p = 0.003$) and SDMT performance ($r_s = -0.398$, $p < 0.001$). Due to the nature of EDSS scoring system, we further delineated the EwMS into groups within the lower range of the score (EDSS scores between 0 and 4.0 which depend and reflect the neurological examination) and within the higher range of the score (EDSS scores $\geq$4.0

TABLE 5 | Logistic regression model determining the cognitive differences between the EwMS and HCs.

	Nagelkerke R^2	Wald coefficient	Exp(B)	*p*-value
Block 1	0.04			
Sex		3.186	1.914	0.074
Age		0.022	0.996	0.883
Years of education		1.973	0.901	0.16
Block 2				
Step 1:	0.218			
SDMT		22.992	0.885	**<0.001**
Step 2:	0.27			
SDMT		13.937	0.907	**<0.001**
Supermarket items-based fluency		9.935	0.919	**0.002**

EwMS, elderly with multiple sclerosis; HCs, healthy controls; SDMT, Symbol Digit Modalities Test. Block 1 force-entered the demographic characteristics (sex, age and years of education) regardless if they were significantly associated with the diagnosis. A second step-wise block included only significant differentiators between the EwMS and HCs. P-values lower than 0.05 were considered statistically significant and shown in bold.

which solemnly depends on the walking ability) (van Munster and Uitdehaag, 2017; Jakimovski et al., 2018a). As expected, the associations between cognitive performance and EDSS scores were mainly present within the subset of EwMS with lower EDSS scores (total verbal fluency $r_s = -0.341$, $p = 0.001$ and SDMT $r_s = -0.398$, $p < 0.001$).

DISCUSSION

The main findings from this comprehensive neuropsychological evaluation of EwMS and age-matched HCs are grounded in two main themes. First, in addition to the previously established processing speed impairment, EwMS present with poorer verbal fluency (for both letter and category). Second, these findings were further extended by the logistic regression model which highlighted verbal fluency performance as second major differentiator between EwMS and HCs.

Currently there are few published analyses examining the question of comorbid aMCI/AD and cognitive aging in EwMS. Muller et al. (2013) used an AD-specific battery to examine 120 total age-, sex-, and education-matched SPMS, aMCI, and HCs and found word list recognition as the single metric distinguishing SPMS from aMCI – recognition memory was preserved in SPMS and defective in aMCI. Furthermore, they additionally showed that SPMS patients had similar performance on both letter-based and category-based verbal fluency when compared to the aMCI patients and significantly lower than HCs (Muller et al., 2013). In a similar study, EwMS were impaired on both processing speed and categorical fluency (Cohen's $d = 0.68$) when compared to HCs (Roth et al., 2018). Therefore, both studies are conforming to the present results showing a high rate of processing speed impairment and diminished verbal fluency performance in EwMS, but no differences in the recognition indices of both verbal memory and visuospatial processing (Roy et al., 2018). Although language impairment is classically associated with an AD cognitive profile, the deficits in processing speed and verbal fluency were not accompanied by deficits in naming and memory consolidation. Therefore, the verbal fluency deficits found here are likely attributable to MS rather than co-morbid aMCI/AD.

Verbal fluency tasks allow the participants only 1 min to produce as many words that start with a certain letter of the alphabet or are part of a specific category (e.g., animals or supermarket items). Given this predetermined time limitation, verbal fluency performance may potentially be moderated by processing speed, as we found in our adjusted model. Report by Roth et al. (2018) showed that the EwMS have poorer categorical fluency when compared to HCs; however, after adjusting for CPS performance, these differences became non-significant. The discrepancy between our results and theirs is, however, minuscule (d 0.87 vs. 0.68 in Roth et al., 2018) – the partial correlation survived in our study with $p = 0.036$ with more statistical power by virtue of a larger sample. Devising new language tests that are less dependent on CPS would be of value in this area of investigation. Finally, determining the nature of the language impairment and its association with specific structural MS changes will allow better understanding of this particular cognitive ability. For example, while examining neurodegenerative MS patterns, studies demonstrated accelerated atrophy of the entorhinal cortex and the bilateral temporal lobes in a population of older (on average of 57 years old) SPMS patients (Steenwijk et al., 2016). These neurodegenerative changes located within AD-associated areas may provide explanation for the emerging semantic and logical memory deficit seen in our EwMS.

One limitation of this study is its cross-sectional research design. In order to better evaluate cognitive aging trajectories, ideally, one would evaluate these same cognitive functions over a period of three or more years, and include not only EwMS, but also aMCI patients. MRI-derived neurodegenerative outcome measures, amyloid PET imaging, assessment of known AD risk factors and the effect of other age-related comorbidities may further determine the nature of the semantic fluency impairment seen in EwMS (Jakimovski et al., 2018b). Lastly, global disability scores which are currently used in the MS field are not suitable in depicting the increasingly prevalent cognitive impairment within the aging MS population.

CONCLUSION

In conclusion, roughly half of EwMS are impaired on tests of cognitive processing speed or verbal fluency. The deficit in verbal fluency is not a hallmark feature of MS associated cognitive disorder for the wider MS population, and may represent a unique quality in the EwMS neurocognitive profile. Further studies investigating the additional disease-related factors which influence cognitive aging in EwMS are warranted.

AUTHOR CONTRIBUTIONS

RB and DJ conceived and designed the study. All authors analyzed and interpreted the data and critically revised the manuscript for important intellectual content. RB, RZ, and BW-G supervised the study.

The protocol was approved by the University at Buffalo Institutional Review Board.

FUNDING

This study was supported in part by a grant from the Biogen IIS Aging, US-mSG-15-10855 grant to BW-G.

REFERENCES

Agrell, B., and Dehlin, O. (1998). The clock-drawing test. *Age Ageing* 27, 399–403.

Beery, K. (2010). *Beery VMI Administration, Scoring, and Teaching Manual.* Bloomington: Pearson.

Benedict, R. H. (1997). *Brief Visuospatial Memory Test–Revised: Professional Manual.* Lutz, FL: PAR.

Benedict, R. H., Fischer, J. S., Archibald, C. J., Arnett, P. A., Beatty, W. W., Bobholz, J., et al. (2002). Minimal neuropsychological assessment of MS patients: a consensus approach. *Clin. Neuropsychol.* 16, 381–397. doi: 10.1076/clin.16.3.381.13859

Benedict, R. H., Morrow, S., Rodgers, J., Hojnacki, D., Bucello, M. A., Zivadinov, R., et al. (2014). Characterizing cognitive function during relapse in multiple sclerosis. *Mult. Scler.* 20, 1745–1752. doi: 10.1177/1352458514533229

Bergsland, N., Schweser, F., Dwyer, M. G., Weinstock-Guttman, B., Benedict, R. H. B., and Zivadinov, R. (2018). Thalamic white matter in multiple sclerosis: a combined diffusion-tensor imaging and quantitative susceptibility mapping study. *Hum. Brain Mapp.* 39, 4007–4017. doi: 10.1002/hbm.24227

Delis, D. C., Kaplan, E., and Kramer, J. H. (2001). *Delis-Kaplan Executive Function System® (D-KEFS®): Examiner's Manual: Flexibility of Thinking, Concept Formation, Problem Solving, Planning, Creativity, Impluse Control, Inhibition.* Bloomington: Pearson.

Delis, D. C., Kramer, J., Kaplan, E., and Ober, B. A. (2000). *CVLT-II: California Verbal Learning Test: Adult Version.* New York, NY: The Psychological Corporation.

Goodglass, H., Kaplan, E., and Weintraub, S. (1983). *Boston Naming Test.* Philadelphia, PA: Lea & Febiger.

Gronwall, D. (1977). Paced auditory serial-addition task: a measure of recovery from concussion. *Percept. Motor Skills* 44, 367–373. doi: 10.2466/pms.1977.44.2.367

Hyman, B. T., Van Hoesen, G. W., Damasio, A. R., and Barnes, C. L. (1984). Alzheimer's disease: cell-specific pathology isolates the hippocampal formation. *Science* 225, 1168–1170. doi: 10.1126/science.6474172

Jakimovski, D., Benedict, R., Marr, K., Gandhi, S., Bergsland, N., Weinstock-Guttmam, B., et al. (2018a). Lower total cerebral arterial flow contributes to cognitive perofrmance in multiple sclerosis patients. *Mult. Scler.* doi: 10.1177/1352458518819608 [Epub ahead of print].

Jakimovski, D., Weinstock-Guttman, B., Hagemeier, J., Vaughn, C. B., Kavak, K. S., Gandhi, S., et al. (2018b). Walking disability measures in multiple sclerosis patients: correlations with MRI-derived global and microstructural damage. *J. Neurol. Sci.* 393, 128–134. doi: 10.1016/j.jns.2018.08.020

Koch-Henriksen, N., Laursen, B., Stenager, E., and Magyari, M. (2017). Excess mortality among patients with multiple sclerosis in Denmark has dropped significantly over the past six decades: a population based study. *J. Neurol. Neurosurg. Psychiatry* 88, 626–631. doi: 10.1136/jnnp-2017-315907

Kurtzke, J. F. (1983). Rating neurologic impairment in multiple sclerosis: an expanded disability status scale (EDSS). *Neurology* 33, 1444–1452.

Luczynski, P., Laule, C., Hsiung, G. R., Moore, G. R. W., and Tremlett, H. (2018). Coexistence of multiple sclerosis and Alzheimer's disease: a review. *Mult. Scler. Relat. Disord.* 27, 232–238. doi: 10.1016/j.msard.2018.10.109

McKhann, G. M., Knopman, D. S., Chertkow, H., Hyman, B. T., Jack, C. R. Jr., Kawas, C. H., et al. (2011). The diagnosis of dementia due to Alzheimer's disease: recommendations from the national institute on aging-Alzheimer's association workgroups on diagnostic guidelines for Alzheimer's disease. *Alzheimers Dement.* 7, 263–269. doi: 10.1016/j.jalz.2011.03.005

Muller, S., Saur, R., Greve, B., Melms, A., Hautzinger, M., Fallgatter, A. J., et al. (2013). Recognition performance differentiates between elderly patients in the long term course of secondary progressive multiple sclerosis and amnestic mild cognitive impairment. *Mult. Scler.* 19, 799–805. doi: 10.1177/1352458512461392

Nelson, L. M., Wallin, M. T., Marrie, R. A., Culpepper, W. J., Langer-Gould, A., Campbell, J., et al. (2019). A new way to estimate neurologic disease prevalence in the United States: Illustrated with MS. *Neurology* 92, 1–13. doi: 10.1212/WNL.0000000000007044

Polman, C. H., Reingold, S. C., Banwell, B., Clanet, M., Cohen, J. A., Filippi, M., et al. (2011). Diagnostic criteria for multiple sclerosis: 2010 revisions to the McDonald criteria. *Ann. Neurol.* 69, 292–302. doi: 10.1002/ana.22366

Reich, D. S., Lucchinetti, C. F., and Calabresi, P. A. (2018). Multiple sclerosis. *N. Engl. J. Med.* 378, 169–180.

Reitz, C., Brayne, C., and Mayeux, R. (2011). Epidemiology of Alzheimer disease. *Nat. Rev. Neurol.* 7, 137–152. doi: 10.1038/nrneurol.2011.2

Roth, A. K., Denney, D. R., Burns, J. M., and Lynch, S. G. (2018). Cognition in older patients with multiple sclerosis compared to patients with amnestic mild cognitive impairment and healthy older adults. *Neuropsychology* 32, 654–663. doi: 10.1037/neu0000453

Roy, S., Drake, A., Snyder, S., Cline, B., Khan, A., Fuchs, T., et al. (2018). Preliminary investigation of cognitive function in aged multiple sclerosis patients: challenges in detecting comorbid Alzheimer's disease. *Mult. Scler. Relat. Disord.* 22, 52–56. doi: 10.1016/j.msard.2018.03.008

Ruff, R., Light, R., Parker, S., and Levin, H. (1996). Benton controlled oral word association test: reliability and updated norms. *Arch. Clin. Neuropsychol.* 11, 329–338. doi: 10.1016/0887-6177(95)00033-x

Sanai, S. A., Saini, V., Benedict, R. H., Zivadinov, R., Teter, B. E., Ramanathan, M., et al. (2016). Aging and multiple sclerosis. *Mult. Scler.* 22, 717–725.

Smith, A. (1982). *Symbol Digit Modalities Test.* Los Angeles, CA: Western Psychological Services.

Steenwijk, M. D., Geurts, J. J., Daams, M., Tijms, B. M., Wink, A. M., Balk, L. J., et al. (2016). Cortical atrophy patterns in multiple sclerosis are non-random and clinically relevant. *Brain* 139, 115–126. doi: 10.1093/brain/awv337

Strauss, E., Sherman, E., and Spreen, O. (2006). *A Compendium of Neuropsychological Tests: Administration, Norms, and Commentary.* Oxford: Oxford University Press.

7

Assessment of Amyloid Deposition in Patients with Probable REM Sleep Behavior Disorder as a Prodromal Symptom of Dementia with Lewy Bodies Using PiB-PET

Ryota Kobayashi[1*], Hiroshi Hayashi[1], Shinobu Kawakatsu[2], Nobuyuki Okamura[3], Masanori Yoshioka[4] and Koichi Otani[1]

[1] Department of Psychiatry, Yamagata University School of Medicine, Yamagata, Japan, [2] Department of Neuropsychiatry, Aizu Medical Center, Fukushima Medical University, Aizuwakamatsu, Japan, [3] Department of Pharmacology, Faculty of Medicine, Tohoku Medical and Pharmaceutical University, Sendai, Japan, [4] Department of Radiology, Yamagata University Hospital, Yamagata, Japan

***Correspondence:**
Ryota Kobayashi
ryo.kobayashi@med.id.yamagata-u.ac.jp

Introduction: Dementia with Lewy bodies (DLB) often exhibits REM sleep behavior disorder (RBD) at its prodromal stage. Meanwhile, DLB is often comorbid with Alzheimer's disease (AD)-type pathology. In typical AD, amyloid-β deposition begins considerably before the onset of dementia and has already reached a plateau at the stage of mild cognitive impairment. However, it is not known when amyloid accumulation starts in DLB with AD-type pathology. In the present study, we examined amyloid deposition in patients with RBD as a prodromal symptom of DLB using [11C]-Pittsburgh compound B positron emission tomography (PiB-PET).

Methods: The subjects were 12 patients with probable RBD as diagnosed by the Japanese RBD screening questionnaire. They also showed abnormality in 123I-metaiodobenzylguanidine myocardial scintigraphy, a biomarker for DLB. For comparison, 11 patients with probable DLB were included. Applying PMOD software to the PiB-PET images, the global cortical distribution volume ratio was calculated and a ratio >1.3 was regarded as PiB-positive.

Results: Two of the RBD patients (16.7%) and eight of the DLB patients (72.7%) were PiB-positive. The amyloid-positive rate was significantly lower in the RBD group than in the DLB group ($P = 0.012$).

Conclusion: The prevalence of amyloid deposition in RBD as a prodromal symptom of DLB was significantly lower than that in DLB, suggesting that amyloid accumulation does not always begin at the early stage of DLB.

Keywords: Dementia with Lewy bodies, REM sleep behavior disorder, Alzheimer's disease, amyloid-β, prodromal stage, PiB-PET

INTRODUCTION

Dementia with Lewy bodies (DLB) is the second most common dementia after Alzheimer's disease (AD) (1). DLB reduces quality of life and lifespan to a greater extent than AD (2); therefore, early diagnosis of and intervention for DLB are important. Recently, prodromal symptoms of DLB have attracted attention, and REM sleep behavior disorder (RBD), dysautonomia, olfactory dysfunction, and psychiatric symptoms have been reported to precede the onset of DLB by several years (3). RBD is a parasomnia characterized by dream-enacting behaviors without muscle atonia during REM sleep (4). Idiopathic patients with RBD have a high affinity for DLB as reflected by abnormality in 123I-metaiodobenzylguanidine (MIBG) myocardial scintigraphy (5), a biomarker for DLB (1), and have a high possibility of developing Lewy body disease (LBD), which includes DLB. In observational studies, the median interval between the diagnosis of RBD and that of a defined neurodegenerative syndrome was 4 years (6).

Patients with DLB are often accompanied by AD-type pathology [e.g., (7, 8)], and this is comorbidity is associated with a worse prognosis [e.g., (8, 9)]. Therefore, early detection of and intervention for AD-type pathology may be beneficial (9). Since [11C]-Pittsburgh compound B positron emission tomography (PiB-PET) has emerged as a standard amyloid-β (Aβ) imaging method, many studies have demonstrated amyloid accumulation in DLB. According to a systematic review of PiB-PET studies, the positive rate of Aβ accumulation in patients with DLB is as high as 68% (10). This finding suggests a high rate of comorbid AD-type pathology in DLB.

In typical AD, deposition of Aβ starts ~15 years prior to the onset of symptoms, and amyloid PET shows positive findings in the mild cognitive impairment (MCI) phase or even in the preclinical phase of the disease (11). Furthermore, Aβ deposition has reached almost a plateau at the stage of MCI (11). On the other hand, the onset of Aβ accumulation in the course of DLB is not known. However, in light of the high rate of amyloid positivity in DLB mentioned above (10), it is not surprising that Aβ accumulation has already started in the prodromal stage of DLB.

The purpose of this study was to investigate amyloid deposition in RBD as a prodromal symptom of DLB using PiB-PET. We performed PiB-PET in patients with probable RBD as a prodromal symptom of DLB (MIBG myocardial scintigraphy confirmed), and in those with probable DLB (MIBG myocardial scintigraphy and/or dopamine transporter imaging confirmed), and compared the rates of amyloid positivity between these two groups.

METHODS

Subjects

The subjects were 12 patients with probable RBD who visited the Department of Psychiatry at Yamagata University Hospital between February 2014 and March 2019. The diagnosis of probable RBD was made using the Japanese RBD screening questionnaire (RBDSQ-J) (4), which has high sensitivity and specificity for idiopathic RBD. Furthermore, all patients showed abnormal findings in MIBG myocardial scintigraphy according to the criteria of Nakajima et al. (12). They also received general physical, psychiatric and neurological examinations, extensive laboratory tests, and magnetic resonance imaging. Patients with a history of cerebrovascular diseases, neurodegenerative diseases, diabetes mellitus, and psychiatric diseases were excluded. Absence of visual hallucination, cognitive fluctuation or Parkinson's symptoms was confirmed by detailed clinical examinations. For comparison, 11 patients with probable DLB from our hospital were included. These patients showed abnormal findings in MIBG myocardial scintigraphy and/ or dopamine transporter imaging, and fulfilled the criteria for probable DLB developed by McKeith et al. (1). The Ethics Committee of Yamagata University School of Medicine approved the present study, and written informed consent for participation was obtained from all patients.

PET Imaging

[11C]-PiB was synthesized at our institution's PET facility as described previously (11). PET scans were performed using a PET/Computed Tomography scanner (Biograph mCT, Siemens Healthineers, Tokyo, Japan) in three-dimensional scanning mode. [11C]-PiB was injected into an antecubital vein at a mean (SD) dose of 555 (185) MBq (10 MBq/kg body weight), followed immediately by a 70-min dynamic acquisition. The PET images were reconstructed into 25 time frames (6×10, 3×20, 2×60, 2×180, and 12×300 s) using the standard ordered subset expectation maximization algorithm (subset 21, iteration 4), point spread function and time of flight. These images were analyzed with PMOD software (version 3.409, PMOD Technologies Ltd., Zurich, Switzerland). Global cortical PiB retention was calculated using the Logan graphical analysis method, with the cerebellar cortex as the reference tissue input function, and expressed as the distribution volume ratio (DVR) (13). A global cortical DVR >1.3 was regarded as PiB-positive (13).

Apolipoprotein E (APOE) Genotyping

APOE genotypes were determined using restriction fragment length polymorphism analysis. One patient from each group refused a blood sampling for genotyping.

Statistical Analysis

Differences in demographic and clinical data of the subjects were tested using Student's t-test or Fisher's exact test, as appropriate. Fisher's exact test was used to compare the PiB-positive rate between the RBD group and the DLB group. Statistical analyses were performed using SPSS software (version 25, IBM, New York, USA) and a P-value <0.05 was considered statistically significant.

RESULTS

Demographic and clinical data of the subjects are shown in **Table 1**. There was no significant difference in age, duration of education or presence of the APOE ε4-allele between the RBD and DLB groups. Scores of the Mini Mental State Examination were significantly ($P < 0.001$) higher in the RBD group than in the DLB group. There was no significant difference in the frequency of the APOE ε4-allele, a known risk factor for AD pathology (9).

Based on the global cortical DVR, two of the RBD patients (16.7%) and eight of the DLB patients (72.7%) were classified as PiB-positive (**Figure 1**). The prevalence of amyloid deposition was significantly ($P = 0.012$) lower in the RBD group than in the DLB group. The detailed demographic, cognitive, genetic, and PiB-PET data of individual subjects are provided in **Table S1**.

TABLE 1 | Demographic and clinical data of subjects.

	RBD ($n = 12$)	DLB ($n = 11$)	*P*-value
Age (years)	74.0 (5.2)	77.0 (5.3)	0.19
Sex (male/female)	10/ 2	4/ 7	0.036
Education (years)	12.8 (1.6)	12.1 (1.3)	0.236
Duration (years)	6.3 (3.3)	2.0 (1.2)	
MMSE (/30)	28.6 (1.5)	21.5 (3.7)	0.001
APOE ε4-allele present	2/11 (18%)	4/10 (40%)	0.361

Values are presented as mean (SD) or number (%).
Differences between groups were assessed using Student's t-test (age, education, and MMSE) and Fisher's exact test (sex and APOE ε4-allele).
APOE, apolipoprotein E; DLB, dementia with Lewy bodies; MMSE, Mini Mental State Examination; RBD, REM sleep behavior disorder.

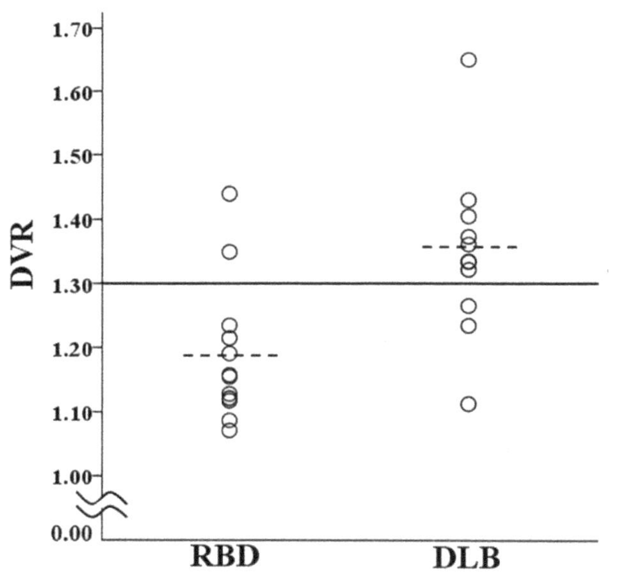

FIGURE 1 | Scatter plot of DVR for patients in the RBD group and DLB group. The solid line shows the cut off value (1.3) for discrimination between PiB-positive and PiB-negative. The dotted lines show the mean values of the RBD group (1.19) and DLB group (1.35). DLB, dementia with Lewy bodies; DVR, global cortical distribution volume ratio; PiB, Pittsburgh compound B; RBD, REM sleep behavior disorder.

DISCUSSION

In the present study, the amyloid-positive rate was 16.7% in RBD patients, while it was 72.7% in DLB patients. The result for DLB is in line with a previous systematic review reporting a 68% amyloid-positive rate in DLB (10).

In light of the high rate of concomitant AD-type pathology in DLB, it was expected that amyloid deposition in DLB is already observed in a considerable degree before onset of the disease. If this was the case, the amyloid-positive rate of the RBD group would have been similar to that of the DLB group. However, the amyloid-positive rate was unexpectedly low in the RBD group. Similar results were shown in an analysis of Alzheimer's biomarkers in cerebrospinal fluid, i.e., Aβ42 values were significantly higher in prodromal DLB patients than in those with DLB patients (14), indicating an apparently lower degree of amyloid accumulation in the former. In relation to this, according to a systematic review of amyloid PET in LBDs other than DLB, the amyloid-positive rate was 34% in the patient group of Parkinson's disease (PD) with dementia, while it was only 5% in that of PD with MCI (10). Namely, in the PD spectrum amyloid deposits are not likely to reach a plateau at the MCI stage. These findings along with our result suggest that amyloid deposition pathology in LBD, including DLB, does not start as early as in AD.

In the treatment of DLB, not only Lewy pathology but also the coexistence of complex AD-type pathology causes serious problems (9). Therefore, to clarify the time course of AD-type pathology in DLB is extremely important from a treatment perspective. The present study suggesting low amyloid deposition at the prodromal stage of DLB should be followed by studies attempting to elucidate the starting point of amyloid accumulation in the course of DLB. Those studies may provide valuable information on the time to begin the treatment for amyloid pathology in DLB.

There are several limitations in the present study. First, although the patients of the RBD group were screened by the RBDSQ-J with high sensitivity and specificity, they did not receive polysomnography and, therefore, remained "patients with probable RBD." Second, the patients of the RBD group might be in the prodromal stage of α-synucleinopathies other than DLB. However, a previous report showed that RBD patients have the highest risk of developing DLB among neurodegenerative disorders during follow-up (5), suggesting that our RBD patients include a high proportion of patients who later develop DLB. In either case, it is necessary to conduct a follow-up examination of our RBD patients to confirm phenoconversion to DLB. Third, males were over-presented in the RBD group, which was inevitable because of the known sex difference in the frequency of this disorder (4, 6). As far as we know, there have been no data suggesting sex differences in the rate and degree of amyloid positivity in DLB, the possibility that the skewed sex distribution was involved in the present result cannot be excluded entirely. Fourth, we suggested that amyloid accumulation does not occur in the RBD group based on the amyloid-positive rate of 16.7%, but to be exact it should be confirmed that this rate is comparable to that in a healthy control group, which was not included in this study. Fifth, the confirmation of the absence of dementia in the RBD group was based exclusively on the MMSE. Finally, the present study was a pilot study with a relatively few number of subjects, necessitating a replication study with a larger number of subjects.

In conclusion, the prevalence of amyloid deposition in RBD as a prodromal symptom of DLB was significantly lower than that in DLB. This result suggests that amyloid accumulation does not always precede the onset of cognitive decline in patients with DLB.

AUTHOR CONTRIBUTIONS

RK conceptualized the study, conducted neuropsychological examinations, analyzed the data, and drafted the manuscript. HH and SK conducted neuropsychological examinations and revised the manuscript. NO analyzed the data and drafted the manuscript. MY conducted neuroradiological examinations and was involved in drafting the manuscript. KO encouraged the study and revised the manuscript. All authors have read and approved the final version of this manuscript.

FUNDING

This study was supported by Grant-in-Aid for Scientific Research (C) (16K09228) from the Ministry of Education, Culture, Sports, Science, and Technology of Japan.

REFERENCES

McKeith IG, Boeve BF, Dickson DW, Halliday G, Taylor JP, Weintraub D, et al. Diagnosis and management of dementia with Lewy bodies: fourth consensus report of the DLB Consortium. *Neurology*. (2017) 89:88– 100. doi: 10.1212/WNL.0000000000004058

Mueller C, Ballard C, Corbett A, Aarsland D. The prognosis of dementia with Lewy bodies. *Lancet Neurol*. (2017) 16:390– 8. doi: 10.1016/S1474-4422(17)30074-1

Fujishiro H, Nakamura S, Sato K, Iseki E. Prodromal dementia with Lewy bodies. *Geriatr Gerontol Int*. (2015) 15:817–26. doi: 10.1111/ggi.12466

Miyamoto T, Miyamoto M, Iwanami M, Kobayashi M, Nakamura M, Inoue Y, et al. The REM sleep behavior disorder screening questionnaire: validation study of a Japanese version. *Sleep Med*. (2009) 10:1151–4. doi: 10.1016/j.sleep.2009.05.007

Miyamoto T, Miyamoto M, Inoue Y, Usui Y, Suzuki K, Hirata K. Reduced cardiac 123I-MIBG scintigraphy in idiopathic REM sleep behavior disorder. *Neurology*. (2006) 67:2236–38. doi: 10.1212/01.wnl.0000249313.25627.2e

Iranzo A, Fernandez-Arcos A, Tolosa E, Serradell M, Molinuevo JL, Valldeoriola F, et al. J. Neurodegenerative disorder risk in idiopathic REM sleep behavior disorder: study in 174 patients. *PLoS ONE*. (2014) 9:e89741. doi: 10.1371/journal.pone.0089741

Ballard C, Ziabreva I, Perry R, Larsen JP, O'Brien J, McKeith I, et al. Differences in neuropathologic characteristics across the Lewy body dementia spectrum. *Neurology*. (2006) 67:1931–4. doi: 10.1212/01.wnl.0000249130.63615.cc

Irwin DJ, Grossman M, Weintraub D, Hurtig HI, Duda JE, Xie SX, et al. Neuropathological and genetic correlates of survival and dementia onset in synucleinopathies: a retrospective analysis. *Lancet Neurol*. (2017) 16:55–65. doi: 10.1016/S1474-4422(16)30291-5

Lemstra AW, de Beer MH, Teunissen CE, Schreuder C, Scheltens P, van der Flier WM, et al. Concomitant AD pathology affects clinical manifestation and survival in dementia with Lewy bodies. *J Neurol Neurosurg Psychiatry*. (2017) 88:113–8. doi: 10.1136/jnnp-2016-313775

Petrou M, Dwamena BA, Foerster BR, MacEachern MP, Bohnen NI, Müller ML, et al. Amyloid deposition in Parkinson's disease and cognitive impairment: a systematic review. *Mov Disord*. (2015) 30:928–35. doi: 10.1002/ mds.26191

Jack CR Jr., Knopman DS, Jagust WJ, Shaw LM, Aisen PS, Weiner MW, et al. Hypothetical model of dynamic biomarkers of the Alzheimer's pathological cascade. *Lancet Neurol*. (2010) 9:119–28. doi: 10.1016/S1474-4422(09)70299-6

Nakajima K, Matsumoto N, Kasai T, Matsuo S, Kiso K, Okuda K. Normal values and standardization of parameters in nuclear cardiology: Japanese Society of Nuclear Medicine working group database. *Ann Nucl Med*. (2016) 30:188–99. doi: 10.1007/s12149-016-1065-z

Gomperts SN, Rentz DM, Moran E, Becker JA, Locascio JJ, Klunk WE, et al. Imaging amyloid deposition in Lewy body diseases. *Neurology*. (2008) 71:903–10. doi: 10.1212/01.wnl.0000326146.60732.d6

Bousiges O, Bombois S, Schraen S, Wallon D, Quillard MM, Gabelle A, et al. Cerebrospinal fluid Alzheimer biomarkers can be useful for discriminating dementia with Lewy bodies from Alzheimer's disease at the prodromal stage. *J Neurol Neurosurg Psychiatry*. (2018) 89:467–75. doi: 10.1136/jnnp-2017-316385

8

Association of Blood Pressure Variability and Intima-Media Thickness with White Matter Hyperintensities in Hypertensive Patients

*Xin Chen, Yingqian Zhu, Shasha Geng, Qingqing Li and Hua Jiang**

Department of Geriatrics, Shanghai East Hospital, Tongji University School of Medicine, Shanghai, China

***Correspondence:**
Hua Jiang
huajiang2013@tongji.edu.cn

Background and Purpose: Ambulatory blood pressure variability (ABPV), ABP, and carotid intima-media thickness (IMT) are closely associated with white matter hyperintensities (WMH), and few studies focused on establishing effective models based on ABP, ABPV, and IMT to predict the WMH burden. We aimed to evaluate the value of a predictive model based on the metrics of ABP, ABPV, and IMT, which were independently associated with the WMH burden.

Methods: We retrospectively enrolled 140 hypertensive inpatients for physical examinations in Shanghai East Hospital, Tongji University School of Medicine between February 2018 and January 2019. The basic clinical information of all subjects was recorded, and we also collected the metrics of ABP, ABPV, and IMT. Patients with Fazekas scale grade $\geq$2 were classified into heavy burden of WMH group. Then, we analyzed the association between all characteristics and the WMH burden. Multivariate analysis was performed to assess whether the metrics of ABP, ABPV, and IMT were independently associated with WMH, and we used receiver operating characteristic (ROC) to evaluate the value of predictive model based on the metrics of ABP, ABPV, and IMT.

Results: Higher WMH grade was associated with increasing age, diabetes mellitus, higher total cholesterol (TC), higher low-density lipoprotein (LDL), higher IMT, higher 24-h systolic blood pressure (SBP), higher daytime SBP, higher nocturnal SBP, 24-h and daytime standard deviation (SD) of SBP, and 24-h SBP weight SD; 24-h SBP, 24-h SBP-SD, and IMT were independently related to the burden of WMH even after adjusting for the clinical variables. In addition, we also established a model that has a higher predictive capacity using 24-h SBP, 24-h SBP-SD, and IMT in the ROC analysis to assess the WMH burden in hypertensive patients.

Conclusions: Higher 24-h SBP, higher 24-h SBP-SD, and larger IMT were independently associated with a greater burden of WMH among elderly primary hypertension Asian patients. Establishing a model based on these factors might provide a new approach for enhancing the accuracy of diagnosis of WMH using metrics in 24-h ABPM and carotid ultrasound.

Keywords: white matter hyperintensities, carotid intima-media thickness, ambulatory blood pressure, ambulatory blood pressure variability, hypertension

INTRODUCTION

White matter hyperintensities (WMH), also named white matter lesions, are commonly observed in the elderly, usually detected on magnetic resonance imaging (MRI) with hyperintense signal appearances on T2-weighted MRI (Fazekas et al., 1993). WMH are considered as a manifestation of cerebral small vessel disease (CSVD; Wardlaw et al., 2013), and its extensive lesions are highly related to the risk of cognitive decline (Altamura et al., 2016), stroke (Fazekas et al., 1993; Jeerakathil et al., 2004), and gait disturbance (Polvikoski et al., 2010). As the pathogenesis of WMH has not been completely understood, it might be in the subclinical stage for long before the onset of the first clinical manifestations (Pantoni, 2010). Therefore, early detection of patients with subclinical CSVD may be effective in preventing future adverse prognosis.

WMH have been identified to be more prevalent in people with hypertension (Jiménez-Balado et al., 2019). Twenty-four-hour ambulatory blood pressure (ABP) monitoring (24-h ABPM) has been conformed as a more scientific method to predict blood pressure-related brain damage than office blood pressure measurement (Ohkubo et al., 2000). Previous studies have proven that increased 24-h ABP variability (ABPV) and higher 24-h ABP levels are closely associated with WMH (Yamaguchi et al., 2014; Filomena et al., 2015). In addition, subclinical atherosclerotic changes have been reported to be related to CSVD and WMH burden (Rundek et al., 2017). Intima-media thickness (IMT) is not only an effective marker of subclinical atherosclerosis but also a predictive factor of cardiocerebrovascular disease (Lorenz et al., 2007). A recent study has shown that increased IMT is independently associated with a heavier burden of WMH among elderly and Hispanic people (Della-Morte et al., 2018). However, to our knowledge, only a few studies focused on establishing effective models based on ABP, ABPV, and IMT to predict the burden of WMH among Asian primary hypertension patients. In this study, we investigated the association of the ABP, ABPV, and IMT metrics with the burden of WMH, Moreover, we also evaluated the value of predictive model based on the metrics of ABP, ABPV, and IMT, which were independently associated with the WMH burden.

MATERIALS AND METHODS

Participants

This was a retrospective, cross-sectional study. We recorded information of 140 hypertensive inpatients for physical examinations due to headache or dizziness in Shanghai East Hospital, Tongji University School of Medicine between February 2018 and January 2019. Hypertension was defined as systolic blood pressure (SBP) $\geq$140 mm Hg and/or diastolic blood pressure (DBP) $\geq$90 mmHg. The inclusion criteria were: (1) patients with primary hypertension diagnosed $\geq$1 year; (2) age $\geq$40 years old; and (3) underwent 24-h ABPM, carotid IMT (cIMT) measurements, and MRI scan within 30 days. The exclusion conditions were: (1) with secondary hypertension; (2) with history of stroke or dementia; (3) with large-vessel cerebrovascular diseases; and (4) with severe infections, severe nephrosis or liver diseases, or tumors. We recorded the basic information of all patients: age, sex, disease history, smoking history, body mass index, C-reactive protein (CRP), glucose, triglyceride (TG), total cholesterol (TC), high-density lipoprotein (HDL) cholesterol, and low-density lipoprotein (LDL) cholesterol. This study was approved by the Ethics Committee of Shanghai East Hospital, Tongji University School of Medicine.

Twenty-Four-Hour ABPM

All participants underwent 24-h ABPM with an automated device (TM-2430, AND, Tokyo, Japan), which has been verified in accordance with the protocol of the British Hypertension Society (Palatini et al., 1998). Patients underwent ABPM during their hospital stay. They were asked to follow their usual activities without physical exercise or excessive movement on the non-dominant arm during ABPM recordings. Blood pressure was measured every 30 min between 6:00 am and 10:00 pm (day time), and every 60 min between 10:00 pm and 6:00 am (night time). We recorded mean SBP, mean DBP, blood pressure variability (BPV) [which included average real variability (ARV), coefficient of variation (CV), and weighted standard deviation (SD) of SBP and DBP].

ARV was defined as the absolute differences of consecutive measurements and was calculated according to the following formula: $\text{ARV} = 1/\sum w \times \sum_{k=1}^{N-1} w \times |\text{BP}_{k+1} - \text{BP}_k|$ (Cretu et al., 2016). CV was defined as the ratio between the SD and the mean SBP or DBP at the same period and was calculated by the following formula: CV = SD/mean BP (Bilo et al., 2007; Filomena et al., 2015). Weighted SD (wSD) was defined as the mean of day and night SD values corrected for the number of hours included in each of these periods, it was calculated by the following formula: $\text{wSD} = (\text{SD}_{\text{day time}} \times T_{\text{day time}} + \text{SD}_{\text{night time}} \times T_{\text{night time}})/T_{\text{day time+night time}}$ (Bilo et al., 2007; Filomena et al., 2015). In addition, we also calculated nocturnal systolic dip status according to the following formula: $[(SBP_{day\ time} - SBP_{night\ time})/SBP_{day\ time}] \times 100\%$ to assess the circadian variation, and normal status was considered as the value between 10% and 20% dip (O'Brien et al., 2013).

Carotid Ultrasound

Carotid ultrasound was performed in accordance with the standard scanning and reading protocols by a well-trained physician. cIMT was automatedly measured using a high-resolution B-mode ultrasound system (SSA-250A, Toshiba, Tokyo, Japan), which can improve precision and reduce variance of the measurements. We scanned arteries to visualize the IMT on the posterior or distal wall of the artery, and the measurements were made outside the areas of plaque (Touboul et al., 2007). All measurements were performed on frozen images. The two best-quality images were selected for analysis of each artery. IMT was defined as the distance from the anterior margin of the first echogenic line to the anterior margin of the second line. The first line represents the intima–lumen interface, and the second line represents the collagen-containing top layer of adventitia. All IMT values were calculated as the average of six measurements. We defined the carotid artery segments like the Northern Manhattan Study (Della-Morte et al., 2018): (1) near and far wall of the segment extending from 10 to 20 mm proximal to the tip of the flow divider into the common carotid artery; (2) near and far wall of the carotid bifurcation beginning at the tip of the flow divider and extending 10 mm proximal to the flow divider tip; and (3) near and far wall of the proximal 10 mm of the internal carotid artery. We recorded the mean cIMT by calculating the means of the near and far wall IMT of all carotid segments (Rundek et al., 2002; Della-Morte et al., 2018; Koç and Sümbül, 2019). These were previously reported with excellent reliability in the Northern Manhattan Study (Della-Morte et al., 2018).

MRI Data and Measurement of WMH

Brain MRI was measured using 1.5-Tesla MRI (Philips Medical Systems, Best, Netherlands), which included diffusion-weighted, T1-weighted, and T2-weighted imaging, fluid-attenuated inversion recovery (FLAIR), and susceptibility-weighted imaging (SWI). The sections were 5 mm thick. WMH were rated in FLAIR sequences in accordance with the Fazekas scale. Imaging markers of WMH were defined as follows: for periventricular: grade 0 (absent lesions), grade 1 (caps or pencilthin lining), 2 grade (smooth halo), and grade 3 (irregular periventricular lesions extending into the deep white matter); and for deep white matter: grade 0 (absent), grade 1 (punctuate foci), grade 2 (beginning of confluent foci), and grade 3 (large confluent areas; Fazekas et al., 1987). We classified patients into heavy burden of WMH group when their grade is ≥2 in either the periventricular or in the deep white matter according to the Fazekas scale. All MRI examinations were independently assessed by two experienced neurologists who were blind to other clinical variables. In case of disagreement, lesions were ascertained by consensus. An intrarater reliability test was performed in 140 subjects. Interreader- and intrareader-intraclass correlation coefficients for periventricular WMH scores were 0.88 and 0.83, respectively. In addition, the interreader- and intrareader-intraclass correlation coefficients for subcortical WMH scores were 0.86 and 0.89, respectively. Pearson's correlation coefficient between periventricular and subcortical WMHs was 0.74.

Statistical Analysis

The statistical analyses were performed using SPSS22.0 software (IBM SPSS, Armonk, NY, USA). The categorical variables of clinical features were expressed as number and percentage and analyzed with the chi-square test. The Mann–Whitney *U*-test or Student's *t*-test was used to comparing continuous variables of clinical characteristics, which were expressed as mean ± SD. Potential risk markers and variables for which the $P < 0.05$ in univariate analysis were included in the multivariate logistic regression analysis. Forward elimination multivariate logistic regression analyses were performed. Parameters of ABP, ABPV, and IMT with $P < 0.05$ were included in receiver operating characteristic (ROC) analysis to show their evaluated values and establish a combination. $P < 0.05$ was considered to be statistically significant.

RESULTS

A total of 140 patients were enrolled in this study. The average age was 69.24 ± 10.54 years, and 54.29% were male. Seventy-five percent of them were treated with BP-lowering agents (**Table 1**).

According to the MRI images, 94 patients were classified into 0–1 WMH grades, and 46 patients were classified into 2–3 WMH grades. In the univariate analysis (**Table 1**), the burden of WMH was associated with increasing age, diabetes mellitus, higher CH, higher LDL, higher IMT, higher 24-h SBP, higher daytime SBP, and higher nocturnal SBP (all $p < 0.05$). We also calculated the metrics of BPV in all periods and found that 24-h and daytime SD of SBP, and 24-h SBP weight SD significantly increased in those with 2–3 WMH grades (all $p < 0.05$; **Table 2**).

We used multivariate analysis to assess whether IMT, SBP levels (24-h SBP, daytime SBP, and nocturnal SBP), and BPV metrics (24-h and daytime SD of SBP, 24-h SBP weight SD) were independently associated with 2–3 WMH grades after adjustment by clinical variables (age, sex, diabetes mellitus, TC, LDL cholesterol, use of anti-hypertensive treatment, and the parameters of ABP, ABPV, and IMT with $P < 0.05$ in univariate analysis). We found higher 24-h SBP [odds ratio (OR): 1.063, 95% CI: 1.033–1.135, $P = 0.036$], 24-h SBP-SD (OR: 1.280, 95% CI: 1.117–1.552, $P = 0.014$), and IMT (OR: 1.207, 95% CI: 1.135–1.492, $P = 0.002$) were independent predictors of heavy burden of WMH (**Table 3**).

We performed ROC analysis to show the predictive capacity of the 24-h SBP [area under curve (AUC): 0.688, 95% CI: 0.594–0.783, $P = 0.020$], 24-h SBP-SD (AUC: 0.742, 95% CI: 0.653–0.830, $P = 0.001$), and IMT (AUC: 0.711, 95% CI: 0.622–0.819, $P = 0.001$). We saved probabilities of 24-h SBP, 24-h SBP-SD, and IMT in multivariate analysis and obtained the predictive model (AUC: 0.785, 95% CI: 0.705–0.865,

TABLE 1 | Baseline factors associated with the burden of WMH.

Characteristics	All Subjects n = 140	0–1 grade n = 94	2–3 grade n = 46	P-value
Age (years)	69.24 ± 10.54	66.47 ± 10.12	74.89 ± 9.09	0.001*
Male (%)	76 (54.29%)	47 (50.00%)	29 (63.00%)	0.146
Diabetes mellitus (%)	51 (36.43%)	27 (28.72%)	24 (52.17%)	0.007*
Smoking habit (%)	37 (26.43%)	25 (26.60%)	12 (26.09%)	0.949
Central obesity (%)	98 (70.00%)	65 (69.15%)	33 (71.74%)	0.753
Body mass index	28.75 ± 4.22	28.71 ± 4.34	28.81 ± 4.26	0.831
CRP	4.96 ± 1.51	4.05 ± 1.57	6.73 ± 1.46	0.153
Glucose	5.74 ± 1.63	5.61 ± 1.51	6.02 ± 1.84	0.163
TG	1.69 ± 1.13	1.78 ± 1.24	1.49 ± 0.85	0.143
TC	4.68 ± 1.22	4.83 ± 1.20	4.38 ± 1.23	0.041*
HDL	1.15 ± 0.28	1.17 ± 0.28	1.13 ± 0.27	0.494
LDL	2.48 ± 0.91	2.60 ± 0.88	223 ± 0.93	0.025*
IMT (mm)	0.711 ± 0.17	0.689 ± 0.17	0.77 ± 0.19	0.026*
Duration of hypertension (year)	8.33 ± 4.15	8.12 ± 4.96	3.45 ± 4.38	0.325
Nocturnal dipping of SBP	0.043 ± 0.081	0.052 ± 0.074	0.025 ± 0.094	0.067
Dipper status (%)	33 (23.57%)	23 (24.47%)	10 (21.74)	0.721
24-h SBP (mmHg)	128.76 ± 17.47	126.56 ± 17.51	133.24 ± 16.68	0.033*
24-h DBP (mmHg)	73.46 ± 9.54	73.89 ± 9.77	72.59 ± 9.09	0.448
Daytime SBP (mmHg)	131.65 ± 16.28	129.90 ± 16.67	135.22 ± 15.02	0.070*
Daytime DBP (mmHg)	75.75 ± 9.94	76.39 ± 10.15	74.43 ± 9.46	0.275
Nocturnal SBP (mmHg)	126.10 ± 19.80	123.27 ± 19.42	131.89 ± 19.50	0.015*
Nocturnal DBP (mmHg)	71.30 ± 9.93	71.51 ± 10.11	70.87 ± 9.64	0.721
BP-lowing treatment (%)	105 (75.00%)	69 (73.40%)	36 (78.26%)	0.533
No. of BP-lowing agents				
No treatment (%)	35 (25.00%)	25 (26.60%)	10 (21.74%)	0.533
1 BP-lowing agent (%)	78 (55.71%)	53 (56.38%)	25 (54.35%)	0.820
≥2 BP-lowing agents (%)	26 (18.57%)	16 (17.02%)	10 (21.74%)	0.500
Class of BP-lowing drugs				
ACEIs (%)	5 (3.57%)	2 (2.13%)	3 (6.52%)	0.188
ARB (%)	44 (31.43%)	30 (31.91%)	15 (32.61%)	0.934
β-Blockers (%)	3 (2.14%)	2 (2.13%)	1 (2.17%)	0.986
Dihydropyridinic CCB (%)	71 (50.71%)	47 (48.96%)	23 (50.00%)	0.989
Npnloop diuretics (%)	10 (7.14%)	7 (7.45%)	3 (6.52%)	0.842

*WMH, white matter hyperintensities; CRP, C-reactive protein, glucose; TG, triglyceride; TC, total cholesterol; HDL, high-density lipoprotein cholesterol; LDL, low-density lipoprotein cholesterol; IMT, intima-media thickness; SBP, systolic blood pressure; DBP, diastolic blood pressure; ACEI, indicate angiotensin-converting enzyme inhibitor; ARB, angiotensin receptor blockers; CCB, calcium-channel block, *P < 0.05.*

P = 0.001) in the ROC analysis; the AUC of the model was higher than any of the 24-h SBP, 24-h SBP-SD, and IMT (**Table 4**; **Figure 1**).

DISCUSSION

The major findings in our study were that: (1) higher WMH grade was associated with increasing age, diabetes mellitus, higher TC, higher LDL, higher IMT, higher 24-h SBP, higher daytime SBP, higher nocturnal SBP, 24-h and daytime SD of SBP, and 24-h SBP weight SD; and (2) 24-h SBP, 24-h SBP-SD, and IMT independently related to the burden of WMH even after adjusting for the clinical variables. (3) In addition, we established a model with a higher predictive capacity using 24-h SBP, 24-h SBP-SD, and IMT in the ROC analysis to assess the WMH burden in hypertensive patients.

In this study, we found higher 24-h SBP level was the only ABP metric that was independently associated with the higher grade of WMH (2–3 grades). This result was consistent with previous studies suggesting the necessity of measurement of ABP among hypertensive patients for predicting the burden of WMH (Stewart et al., 2009; Filomena et al., 2015). The Rotterdam study showed that not only higher SBP but also higher DBP were independent predictive factors of the progression of periventricular WM disease (van Dijk et al., 2008). In a recent study, increased DBP was demonstrated to be associated with the brain WMH score, but the role of SBP was less clear (McNeil et al., 2018). Similarly, another study also found no significant relationship between SBP and WMH, whereas the 2-year change from baseline to year 2 in ambulatory SBP predicted the 2-year WMH change (Wolfson et al., 2013). The differences in results might due to the different included criteria and different ethnicity, but all these results emphasize the essentiality of considering individual different BP components with regard to WMH. In this study, we found 24-h SBP-SD was the only independent factor that related to the burden of WMH among all the ABPV metrics, and consistent findings could be found in several other studies (Wardlaw et al., 2013; Yamaguchi et al., 2014; Yang et al., 2018). However, 24-h SBP-wSD was not independently associated with the burden of WMH after adjusting all clinical variables; this may be caused by the sample size and inclusion criteria. In addition, a Chinese study found that SD and CV of SBP, CV of DBP in 24 h,

TABLE 2 | Association between ABPV measurements and the burden of WMH.

BPV Measures	All Subjects *n* = 140	0–1 grade *n* = 94	2–3 grade *n* = 46	*P*-value
Systolic BP				
24-h ARV	10.34 ± 3.27	9.97 ± 2.75	11.22 ± 2.31	0.064
Awake ARV	10.81 ± 3.11	10.61 ± 3.15	11.44 ± 3.78	0.102
Asleep ARV	9.98 ± 3.46	9.87 ± 3.28	11.10 ± 3.27	0.057
24-h SD	13.41 ± 3.31	12.87 ± 2.88	14.54 ± 3.85	0.005*
24-h wSD	12.21 ± 3.22	11.59 ± 2.94	13.23 ± 3.43	0.008*
Awake SD	12.41 ± 3.72	11.61 ± 3.20	14.04 ± 4.18	0.001*
Asleep SD	11.79 ± 3.69	11.67 ± 3.12	12.03 ± 4.07	0.589
24-h CV	10.56 ± 2.66	10.28 ± 2.32	11.13 ± 3.21	0.077
Awake CV	9.49 ± 2.87	9.01 ± 2.54	10.47 ± 3.27	0.104
Asleep CV	9.58 ± 3.15	9.68 ± 2.60	9.37 ± 4.06	0.582
Diastolic BP				
24-h ARV	7.13 ± 2.16	7.25 ± 1.87	7.02 ± 2.03	0.557
Awake ARV	7.78 ± 2.63	7.89 ± 2.21	7.64 ± 2.01	0.476
Asleep ARV	6.53 ± 2.59	6.71 ± 2.24	6.49 ± 2.51	0.318
24-h SD	9.36 ± 2.06	9.33 ± 1.99	9.44 ± 2.23	0.757
24-h wSD	8.79 ± 2.11	8.70 ± 2.17	8.83 ± 2.45	0.746
Awake SD	8.88 ± 2.24	8.71 ± 2.02	9.24 ± 2.01	0.186
Asleep SD	8.53 ± 2.68	8.71 ± 2.31	8.19 ± 3.31	0.288
24-h CV	12.88 ± 2.99	12.76 ± 2.90	13.11 ± 3.18	0.516
Awake CV	11.86 ± 3.15	11.55 ± 2.97	12.48 ± 3.42	0.099
Asleep CV	12.18 ± 4.12	12.38 ± 3.59	11.75 ± 5.07	0.401

*ABPV, ambulatory blood pressure variability; WMH, white matter hyperintensities; BPV, blood pressure variability; BP, blood pressure; ARV, average real variability; CV, coefficient of variation; SD, standard deviation; wSD, weighted standard deviation, *P < 0.05.*

TABLE 3 | Association of 24-h SBP, 24-h SBP-SD, and IMT with WMH.

Characteristics	OR (95% CI)	*P*-value
24-h SBP (mmHg)	1.063 (1.033–1.135)	0.036*
24-h SBP-SD (mmHg)	1.280 (1.117–1.552)	0.014*
IMT (mm)	1.207 (1.135–1.492)	0.002*

*Models are adjusted by age, sex, diabetes mellitus, total cholesterol, low-density lipoprotein cholesterol, use of antihypertensive treatment, and the parameters of ABP, ABPV and IMT with P < 0.05 in univariate analysis. SBP, systolic blood pressure; SD, standard deviation; IMT, intima-media thickness; WMH, white matter hyperintensities; OR, odd ratio; CI, confidence interval, *P < 0.05.*

TABLE 4 | Receiver operating characteristic model and the predictive values.

Characteristics	AUC (95% CI)	*P*-Value
24-h SBP (mmHg)	0.688 (0.594–0.783)	0.020*
24-h SBP-SD (mmHg)	0.742 (0.653–0.830)	0.001*
IMT (mm)	0.711 (0.622–0.819)	0.001*
Model	0.785 (0.705–0.865)	0.001*

*AUC, Area Under Curve; CI, confidence interval; SBP, systolic blood pressure; SD, standard deviation; IMT, intima-media thickness, *P < 0.05.*

daytime and nighttime and SD of DBP in nighttime were positively associated with the degree of enlarged perivascular spaces (EPVSs), which was closely related to WMH (Yang et al., 2017a,b). In the same year, this team also indicated that higher SBP levels were independently associated with EPVSs in basal ganglia but not in center semioval, which supported EPVSs to be a marker of CSVD (Yang et al., 2017a,b). In another study, higher variability in SBP that was self-measured at home (HBP) was also shown to be related to the progression of brain WMH (Liu et al., 2016). In contrast, Filomena et al. (2015) found that among all the ABPV metrics, short-term ARV of SBP was independently related to the presence of CSVD, but not SD of SBP. The different results might be attributed to the differences in scoring methods.

The underlying pathologic mechanisms of the association between BP and ABPV levels and WMH burden have not been fully understood. Increased permeability of the small vessel walls and damage of the blood brain barrier (BBB) have been demonstrated to contribute to the development of WMH. A previous study found that contrast agents leaked much more in the area of perforating arterial in patients with WMH than in normal people (Starr et al., 2003). Another study used the ratio of CSF and serum albumin to show BBB permeability and discovered that the burden of WMH was associated with the permeability of BBB (Wallin et al., 1990). Increased BP levels and ABPV would cause more stress on vessel walls, which might further cause endothelial injuries and arterial stiffness (Schillaci et al., 2012; Diaz et al., 2013). Thus, it is likely that higher levels of BP and ABPV could lead to the development of WMH through endothelial injuries. Furthermore, WMH was thought to originate from ischemic injury. Yao et al. (1992) found that ischemia in white matter regions could be observed by the increased proportion of oxygen uptake in those regions. In recent studies, researchers found that changes in hemodynamics might contribute to the ischemia of white matter regions (Mok et al., 2012; Poels et al., 2012). The impairment of cerebral blood flow (CBF) has been considered as the most common type of hemodynamic change. Increased ABPV levels with sudden changes in BP might lead to cerebral hypoperfusion and development of WMH. Moreover, WMH could contribute to higher 24-h ABPV. The results in this

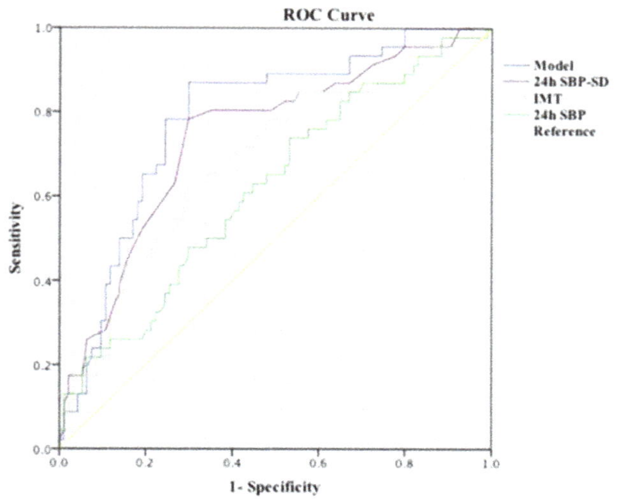

FIGURE 1 | Curves of receiver operating characteristic.

study showed that 24-h SBP and 24-h SBP-SD, but not that of DBP, were independently related to the burden of WMH. Further studies are still needed to explore the underlying mechanisms.

In this study, we also reported a significant association between IMT and WMH. cIMT has been reported to be closely related to brain MRI changes (Pico et al., 2002). In a cardiovascular health study, researchers found increased IMT was strongly associated with WMH (Manolio et al., 1999). Similarly, other researchers reported in elderly hypertensive patients with memory disorder, in elderly patients with Alzheimer's disease (AD), or vascular dementia patients a significant association between IMT and leukoaraiosis on MRI could be observed (Kearney-Schwartz et al., 2009; Altamura et al., 2016). In addition, increased IMT has been demonstrated as a risk factor of lacunar infarction, and lacunar infarction might result in increased WMH grade (Manolio et al., 1999; Tsivgoulis et al., 2005). These findings were consistent with the results in our study, and all these results revealed that increased IMT might be a useful marker of WMH.

Even though the exact pathophysiological changes are still unclear, some molecular mechanisms have been proposed as the link between IMT and WMH. In a postmortem study, WMH was found to be related to the impairment of arterioles (e.g., cellular wall thickening), revealing that cerebral arteriosclerosis might be one of the important factors in the development of WMH (Pantoni and Garcia, 1995). Moreover, changes in the large arterial wall might alter the cerebral microcirculation and lead to chronic brain hypoxia, which in turn contributes to the development of WMH. A previous study has indicated that the cerebral microcirculation was especially sensitive to increased pulsatile stress that might ultimately cause microvascular damage and WMH (Gutierrez et al., 2015). The molecular mechanisms of this process were likely mediated by the upregulation of proinflammatory and pro-growth factors leading to increased IMT Della-Morte and Rundek (2016). Furthermore, WMH could be caused by lower CBF, and lower CBF velocity, in turn, was associated with the increased IMT; atherosclerosis was considered to play a major role in this process (Appelman et al., 2008; Kwater et al., 2014).

To our best knowledge, although many studies have demonstrated ABPV, ABP, and IMT were closely associated with WMH (Filomena et al., 2015; Yang et al., 2017a,b), few studies established predictive model of the WMH burden using ABP level, ABPV level, and IMT. We established a model with a higher predictive capacity using 24-h SBP, 24-h SBP-SD, and IMT in ROC analysis to evaluate the WMH burden in patients with hypertension. This could enhance the accuracy of evaluating WMH burden in clinical application. Moreover, both 24-h ABPM and carotid ultrasound are noninvasive tests with easy operation and low cost. They can be effective in predicting the WMH burden in hypertensive patients. This study might provide a measuring method of discrimination of metrics in 24-h ABPM and carotid ultrasound to diagnose WMH.

This study has not only strengths but also limitations. As this was a retrospective, single-center, and small-scale study, this might cause higher selection biases. In addition, no classification of hypertension grade was recorded, which might influence the results. Moreover, the 24-h ABPM was performed during the hospital stay, and so the results of this study may not necessarily applicable to outpatients. Therefore, In the future, multicenter, prospective, and large-scale studies are still needed to clarify these problems.

In conclusion, results obtained from this study showed that 24-h SBP, 24-h SBP-SD, and IMT were independently associated with the WMH burden. Meanwhile, we established a model using 24-h SBP, 24-h SBP-SD, and IMT in ROC analysis to assess the WMH burden in patients with hypertension. This study might provide a new approach for enhancing the accuracy of diagnosis of WMH using metrics in 24-h ABPM and carotid ultrasound.

AUTHOR CONTRIBUTIONS

HJ designed the study. XC collected information and wrote the article. YZ, SG, and QL reviewed and revised the article before the submission. They also made a great contribution to search literature during the process of Interactive Review. Moreover, they gave a lot of useful advices.

FUNDING

This study was funded by the Important Weak Subject Construction Project of Pudong Health and Family Planning Commission of Shanghai (grant no. PWZbr2017-06).

REFERENCES

Altamura, C., Scrascia, F., Quattrocchi, C. C., Errante, Y., Gangemi, E., Curcio, G., et al. (2016). Regional MRI diffusion, white-matter hyperintensities and cognitive function in Alzheimer's disease and vascular dementia. *J. Clin. Neurol.* 12, 201–208. doi: 10.3988/jcn.2016.12.2.201

Appelman, A. P., van der Graaf, Y., Vincken, K. L., Tiehuis, A. M., Witkamp, T. D., Mali, W. P., et al. (2008). Total cerebral blood flow, white matter lesions and brain atrophy: the SMART-MR study. *J. Cereb. Blood Flow Metab.* 28, 633–639. doi: 10.1038/sj.jcbfm.9600563

Bilo, G., Giglio, A., Styczkiewicz, K., Caldara, G., Maronati, A., Kawecka-Jaszcz, K., et al. (2007). A new method for assessing 24-h blood pressure variability after excluding the contribution of nocturnal blood pressure fall. *J. Hypertens.* 25, 2058–2066. doi: 10.1097/hjh.0b013e32829c6a60

Cretu, D. E., Japie, C., Weiss, E., Bunea, M., Frunza, S., Daraban, A. M., et al. (2016). From clinical considerations to theory—blood pressure variability profiles and patterns. *Maedica* 11, 101–108.

Della-Morte, D., Dong, C., Markert, M. S., Elkind, M. S. V., Sacco, R. L., Wright, C. B., et al. (2018). Carotid intima-media thickness is associated with white matter hyperintensities: the Northern Manhattan Study. *Stroke* 49, 304–311. doi: 10.1161/strokeaha.117.018943

Della-Morte, D., and Rundek, T. (2016). Erratum: the role of shear stress and arteriogenesis in maintaining vascular homeostasis and preventing cerebral atherosclerosis. *Brain Circ.* 2:104. doi: 10.4103/2394-8108.186288

Diaz, K. M., Veerabhadrappa, P., Kashem, M. A., Thakkar, S. R., Feairheller, D. L., Sturgeon, K. M., et al. (2013). Visit-to-visit and 24-h blood pressure variability: association with endothelial and smooth muscle function in African Americans. *J. Hum. Hypertens.* 27, 671–677. doi: 10.1038/jhh.2013.33

Fazekas, F., Chawluk, J. B., Alavi, A., Hurtig, H. I., and Zimmerman, R. A. (1987). MR signal abnormalities at 1.5 T in Alzheimer's dementia and normal aging. *AJR Am. J. Roentgenol.* 149, 351–356. doi: 10.2214/ajr.149.2.351

Fazekas, F., Kleinert, R., Offenbacher, H., Schmidt, R., Kleinert, G., Payer, F., et al. (1993). Pathologic correlates of incidental MRI white matter signal hyperintensities. *Neurology* 43, 1683–1689. doi: 10.1212/wnl.43.9.1683

Filomena, J., Riba-Llena, I., Vinyoles, E., Tovar, J. L., Mundet, X., Castañé, X., et al. (2015). Short-term blood pressure variability relates to the presence of subclinical brain small vessel disease in primary hypertension. *Hypertension* 66, 634–640; discussion 445. doi: 10.1161/hypertensionaha.115.05440

Gutierrez, J., Elkind, M. S., Cheung, K., Rundek, T., Sacco, R. L., and Wright, C. B. (2015). Pulsatile and steady components of blood pressure and subclinical cerebrovascular disease: the Northern Manhattan Study. *J. Hypertens.* 33, 2115–2122. doi: 10.1097/hjh.0000000000000686

Jeerakathil, T., Wolf, P. A., Beiser, A., Massaro, J., Seshadri, S., D'Agostino, R. B., et al. (2004). Stroke risk profile predicts white matter hyperintensity volume: the Framingham Study. *Stroke* 35, 1857–1861. doi: 10.1161/01.str.0000135226.53499.85

Jiménez-Balado, J., Riba-Llena, I., Abril, O., Garde, E., Penalba, A., Ostos, E., et al. (2019). Cognitive impact of cerebral small vessel disease changes in patients with hypertension. *Hypertension* 73, 342–349. doi: 10.1161/HYPERTENSIONAHA.118.12090

Kearney-Schwartz, A., Rossignol, P., Bracard, S., Felblinger, J., Fay, R., Boivin, J. M., et al. (2009). Vascular structure and function is correlated to cognitive performance and white matter hyperintensities in older hypertensive patients with subjective memory complaints. *Stroke* 40, 1229–1236. doi: 10.1161/strokeaha.108.532853

Koç, A. S., and Sümbül, H. E. (2019). Age should be considered in cut-off values for increased carotid intima-media thickness. *Turk Kardiyol. Dern. Ars.* 47, 301–311. doi: 10.5543/tkda.2018.94770

Kwater, A., Gąsowski, J., and Grodzicki, T. (2014). Intima-media thickness of carotid artery and aortic pulse wave velocity as determinants of cerebral blood flow velocity. *J. Hum. Hypertens.* 28, 384–387. doi: 10.1038/jhh.2013.123

Liu, Z., Zhao, Y., Zhang, H., Chai, Q., Cui, Y., Diao, Y., et al. (2016). Excessive variability in systolic blood pressure that is self-measured at home exacerbates the progression of brain white matter lesions and cognitive impairment in the oldest old. *Hypertens. Res.* 39, 245–253. doi: 10.1038/hr.2015.135

Lorenz, M. W., Markus, H. S., Bots, M. L., Rosvall, M., and Sitzer, M. (2007). Prediction of clinical cardiovascular events with carotid intima-media thickness: a systematic review and meta-analysis. *Circulation* 115, 459–467. doi: 10.1161/circulationaha.106.628875

Manolio, T. A., Burke, G. L., O'leary, D. H., Evans, G., Beauchamp, N., Knepper, L., et al. (1999). Relationships of cerebral MRI findings to ultrasonographic carotid atherosclerosis in older adults: the Cardiovascular Health Study. CHS Collaborative Research Group. *Arterioscler. Thromb. Vasc. Biol.* 19, 356–365. doi: 10.1161/01.atv.19.2.356

McNeil, C. J., Myint, P. K., Sandu, A. L., Potter, J. F., Staff, R., Whalley, L. J., et al. (2018). Increased diastolic blood pressure is associated with MRI biomarkers of dementia-related brain pathology in normative ageing. *Age Ageing* 47, 95–100. doi: 10.1093/ageing/afx102

Mok, V., Ding, D., Fu, J., Xiong, Y., Chu, W. W., Wang, D., et al. (2012). Transcranial Doppler ultrasound for screening cerebral small vessel disease: a community study. *Stroke* 43, 2791–2793. doi: 10.1161/strokeaha.112.665711

O'Brien, E., Parati, G., Stergiou, G., Asmar, R., Beilin, L., Bilo, G., et al. (2013). European society of hypertension position paper on ambulatory blood pressure monitoring. *J. Hypertens.* 31, 1731–1768. doi: 10.1097/HJH.0b013e328363e964

Ohkubo, T., Hozawa, A., Nagai, K., Kikuya, M., Tsuji, I., Ito, S., et al. (2000). Prediction of stroke by ambulatory blood pressure monitoring versus screening blood pressure measurements in a general population: the Ohasama study. *J. Hypertens.* 18, 847–854. doi: 10.1097/00004872-200018070-00005

Palatini, P., Frigo, G., Bertolo, O., Roman, E., Da Cortà, R., and Winnicki, M. (1998). Validation of the A&D TM-2430 device for ambulatory blood pressure monitoring and evaluation of performance according to subjects' characteristics. *Blood Press. Monit.* 3, 255–260.

Pantoni, L. (2010). Cerebral small vessel disease: from pathogenesis and clinical characteristics to therapeutic challenges. *Lancet Neurol.* 9, 689–701. doi: 10.1016/s1474-4422(10)70104-6

Pantoni, L., and Garcia, J. H. (1995). The significance of cerebral white matter abnormalities 100 years after Binswanger's report. A review. *Stroke* 26, 1293–1301. doi: 10.1161/01.str.26.7.1293

Pico, F., Dufouil, C., Levy, C., Besançon, V., de Kersaint-Gilly, A., Bonithon-Kopp, C., et al. (2002). Longitudinal study of carotid atherosclerosis and white matter hyperintensities: the EVA-MRI cohort. *Cerebrovasc. Dis.* 14, 109–115. doi: 10.1159/000064741

Poels, M. M., Zaccai, K., Verwoert, G. C., Vernooij, M. W., Hofman, A., van der Lugt, A., et al. (2012). Arterial stiffness and cerebral small vessel disease: the Rotterdam Scan Study. *Stroke* 43, 2637–2642. doi: 10.1161/STROKEAHA.111.642264

Polvikoski, T. M., Van Straaten, E. C., Barkhof, F., Sulkava, R., Aronen, H. J., Niinistö, L., et al. (2010). Frontal lobe white matter hyperintensities and neurofibrillary pathology in the oldest old. *Neurology* 75, 2071–2078. doi: 10.1212/wnl.0b013e318200d6f9

Rundek, T., Della-Morte, D., Gardener, H., Dong, C., Markert, M. S., Gutierrez, J., et al. (2017). Relationship between carotid arterial properties and cerebral white matter hyperintensities. *Neurology* 88, 2036–2042. doi: 10.1212/WNL.0000000000003951

Rundek, T., Elkind, M. S., Pittman, J., Boden-Albala, B., Martin, S., Humphries, S. E., et al. (2002). Carotid intima-media thickness is associated with allelic variants of stromelysin-1, interleukin-6, and hepatic lipase genes: the Northern Manhattan Prospective Cohort Study. *Stroke* 33, 1420–1423. doi: 10.1161/01.str.0000015558.63492.b6

Schillaci, G., Bilo, G., Pucci, G., Laurent, S., Macquin-Mavier, I., Boutouyrie, P., et al. (2012). Relationship between short-term blood pressure variability and large-artery stiffness in human hypertension: findings from 2 large databases. *Hypertension* 60, 369–377. doi: 10.1161/hypertensionaha.112.197491

Starr, J. M., Wardlaw, J., Ferguson, K., MacLullich, A., Deary, I. J., and Marshall, I. (2003). Increased blood-brain barrier permeability in type II diabetes demonstrated by gadolinium magnetic resonance imaging. *J. Neurol. Neurosurg. Psychiatry* 74, 70–76. doi: 10.1136/jnnp.74.1.70

Stewart, R., Xue, Q. L., Masaki, K., Petrovitch, H., Ross, G. W., White, L. R., et al. (2009). Change in blood pressure and incident dementia: a 32-year prospective study. *Hypertension* 54, 233–240. doi: 10.1161/hypertensionaha.109.128744

Touboul, P. J., Hennerici, M. G., Meairs, S., Adams, H., Amarenco, P., Bornstein, N., et al. (2007). Mannheim carotid intima-media thickness consensus (2004–2006). An update on behalf of the Advisory Board of the 3rd and 4th Watching the Risk Symposium, 13th and 15th European

Stroke Conferences, Mannheim, Germany, 2004 and Brussels, Belgium, 2006. *Cerebrovasc. Dis.* 23, 75–80. doi: 10.1159/000097034

Tsivgoulis, G., Vemmos, K. N., Spengos, K., Papamichael, C. M., Cimboneriu, A., Zis, V., et al. (2005). Common carotid artery intima-media thickness for the risk assessment of lacunar infarction versus intracerebral haemorrhage. *J. Neurol.* 252, 1093–1100. doi: 10.1007/s00415-005-0821-0

van Dijk, E. J., Prins, N. D., Vrooman, H. A., Hofman, A., Koudstaal, P. J., and Breteler, M. M. (2008). Progression of cerebral small vessel disease in relation to risk factors and cognitive consequences: Rotterdam Scan study. *Stroke* 39, 2712–2719. doi: 10.1161/strokeaha.107.513176

Wallin, A., Blennow, K., Fredman, P., Gottfries, C. G., Karlsson, I., and Svennerholm, L. (1990). Blood brain barrier function in vascular dementia. *Acta Neurol. Scand.* 81, 318–322. doi: 10.1111/j.1600-0404.1990.tb01562.x

Wardlaw, J. M., Smith, C., and Dichgans, M. (2013). Mechanisms of sporadic cerebral small vessel disease: insights from neuroimaging. *Lancet Neurol.* 12, 483–497. doi: 10.1016/s1474-4422(13)70060-7

Wolfson, L., Wakefield, D. B., Moscufo, N., Kaplan, R. F., Hall, C. B., Schmidt, J. A., et al. (2013). Rapid buildup of brain white matter hyperintensities over 4 years linked to ambulatory blood pressure, mobility, cognition and depression in old persons. *J. Gerontol. A Biol. Sci. Med. Sci.* 68, 1387–1394. doi: 10.1093/gerona/glt072

Yamaguchi, Y., Wada, M., Sato, H., Nagasawa, H., Koyama, S., Takahashi, Y., et al. (2014). Impact of ambulatory blood pressure variability on cerebral small vessel disease progression and cognitive decline in community-based elderly Japanese. *Am. J. Hypertens.* 27, 1257–1267. doi: 10.1093/ajh/hpu045

Yang, S., Qin, W., Yang, L., Fan, H., Li, Y., Yin, J., et al. (2017a). The relationship between ambulatory blood pressure variability and enlarged perivascular spaces: a cross-sectional study. *BMJ Open* 7:e015719. doi: 10.1136/bmjopen-2016-015719

Yang, S., Yuan, J., Zhang, X., Fan, H., Li, Y., Yin, J., et al. (2017b). Higher ambulatory systolic blood pressure independently associated with enlarged perivascular spaces in basal ganglia. *Neurol. Res.* 39, 787–794. doi: 10.1080/01616412.2017.1324552

Yang, S., Yuan, J., Qin, W., Yang, L., Fan, H., Li, Y., et al. (2018). Twenty-four-hour ambulatory blood pressure variability is associated with total magnetic resonance imaging burden of cerebral small-vessel disease. *Clin. Interv. Aging* 13, 1419–1427. doi: 10.2147/cia.s171261

Yao, H., Sadoshima, S., Ibayashi, S., Kuwabara, Y., Ichiya, Y., and Fujishima, M. (1992). Leukoaraiosis and dementia in hypertensive patients. *Stroke* 23, 1673–1677. doi: 10.1161/01.str.23.11.1673

9

Altered Static and Temporal Dynamic Amplitude of Low-Frequency Fluctuations in the Background Network During Working Memory States in Mild Cognitive Impairment

Pengyun Wang[1], Rui Li[1], Bei Liu[2], Cheng Wang[3], Zirui Huang[4], Rui Dai[5], Bogeng Song[6], Xiao Yuan[7], Jing Yu[8] and Juan Li[1]**

[1]CAS Key Laboratory of Mental Health, Center on Aging Psychology, Institute of Psychology, Chinese Academy of Sciences, Beijing, China, [2]Department of Human Resources, Institute of Disaster Prevention, Beijing, China, [3]Department of Psychology, Zhejiang Normal University, Jinhua, China, [4]Department of Anesthesiology and Center for Consciousness Science, University of Michigan, Ann Arbor, MI, United States, [5]State Key Laboratory of Brain and Cognitive Science, Institute of Biophysics, Chinese Academy of Sciences, Beijing, China, [6]School of Psychology, Capital Normal University, Beijing, China, [7]School of Sociology, China University of Political Science and Law, Beijing, China, [8]Faculty of Psychology, Southwest University, Chongqing, China

***Correspondence:**
Jing Yu
helen12@swu.edu.cn
Juan Li
lijuan@psych.ac.cn

Previous studies investigating working memory performance in patients with mild cognitive impairment (MCI) have mainly focused on the neural mechanisms of alterations in activation. To date, very few studies have investigated background network alterations in the working memory state. Therefore, the present study investigated the static and temporal dynamic changes in the background network in MCI patients during a working memory task. A hybrid delayed-match-to-sample task was used to examine working memory performance in MCI patients. Functional magnetic resonance imaging (fMRI) data were collected and the marker of amplitude of low-frequency fluctuations (ALFF) was used to investigate alterations in the background network. The present study demonstrated static and dynamic alterations of ALFF in MCI patients during working memory tasks, relative to the resting state. Traditional static analysis revealed that ALFF decreased in the right ventrolateral prefrontal cortex (VLPFC), right dorsolateral PFC (DLPFC), and left supplementary motor area for normal controls (NCs) in the working memory state. However, the same regions showed increased ALFF in MCI patients. Furthermore, relative to NCs, MCI patients demonstrated altered performance-related functional connectivity (FC) patterns, with the right VLPFC and right DLPFC as ROIs. In terms of temporal dynamic analysis, the present study found that in the working memory state dynamic ALFF of bilateral thalamus regions was increased in NCs but decreased in MCI patients. Additionally, MCI patients demonstrated altered performance-related coefficient of variation patterns; the regions in MCI patients were larger and more widely distributed in the parietal and temporal lobes, relative to NCs. This is the first study to examine static and temporal dynamic alterations of

ALFF in the background network of MCI patients in working memory states. The results extend previous studies by providing a new perspective on the neural mechanisms of working memory deficits in MCI patients.

Keywords: mild cognitive impairment, working memory, amplitude of low-frequency fluctuations, background network, temporal dynamics

INTRODUCTION

Mild cognitive impairment (MCI) is a syndrome where individuals display certain forms of cognitive dysfunction, but the ability to perform basic daily activities remains intact (Petersen, 2004). Working memory, delayed recall, and spatial memory rapidly decline in the 6 years following MCI diagnosis (Cloutier et al., 2015). Many studies have focused on the deficit in working memory displayed by MCI patients (Klekociuk and Summers, 2014; Kirova et al., 2015) and the corresponding neural mechanisms, including altered activation during working memory tasks (Bokde et al., 2010; Lou et al., 2015; Migo et al., 2015). More recently, several studies have investigated the background network in MCI patients during working memory tasks. For example, previous studies found altered local synchronization (indexed by regional homogeneity, ReHo; Wang et al., 2016) and distant synchronization (indexed by degree of centrality, DC; Wang et al., 2017) of the background network in MCI patients during a working memory task. Additionally, Lou et al. (2015) found that MCI patients showed increased background network efficiency, which might compensate for the decreased activity and maintain the working memory state. However, the methods used to characterize the background network during the working memory state in MCI patients are generally at a network level, rather than at an individual voxel level. Specifically, ReHo employs the Kendall's coefficient of concordance to measure the coordination of activity between voxels within a region, reflecting intra-regional synchronization [i.e., functional connectivity (FC; Zang et al., 2004)]. Similarly, the DC reflects the properties of the whole brain connectivity network. For a binary graph, DC is the number of edges connecting to a node. In a previous study, we distinguished local connectivity and distant connectivity and found only distant synchronization of the background network was changed in MCI patients (Wang et al., 2017). Thus, whether the oscillation of an individual voxel in the background network is altered in MCI patients during a working memory task is still unknown.

As early as 1995, Biswal et al. (1995) demonstrated that spontaneous low-frequency oscillations (<0.08 Hz) in the human brain during the resting state are physiologically meaningful. Amplitude of low-frequency fluctuations (ALFF) measures the total power of oscillations within a specific frequency range during a given time course (Zang et al., 2007). ALFF reflects individual voxel characteristics rather than the properties of the brain network because ALFF is calculated in each single voxel without the consideration of relationships with any other voxels. ALFF is physiologically meaningful in reflecting the function of brain network for both healthy and pathological populations, and have been used in various resting state functional magnetic resonance imaging (fMRI) studies. For example, ALFF is higher and dominant in the regions of default mode network than in other regions (Yang et al., 2007; Zang et al., 2007; Zou et al., 2008). Moreover, ALFF is significantly higher in bilateral visual cortices when scans conducted with eyes open than eyes closed (Yang et al., 2007). These measures also have implications for pathological populations. Abnormalities have been shown in ALFF in a number of regions implicated in the disorders in children with attention deficit hyperactivity (Zang et al., 2007), patients with major depressive (Liu et al., 2013), patients with Mesial temporal lobe epilepsy (Zhang et al., 2010), and in MCI patients (Han et al., 2011). More importantly, ALFF in some brain regions showed transformational pattern as the disease burden got heavy [from healthy older adults, to older adults with subjective cognitive decline, to MCI patients, to Alzheimer's disease (AD; Yang et al., 2018)]. In the present study, we used this index to investigate whether the oscillations of individual voxels in the background network were altered in MCI patients during a working memory task.

In addition, in conventional resting state studies, FC and other properties (such as ReHo, DC, and ALFF) are assumed to be temporally stationary during a typical resting fMRI session of approximately 5–10 min. Based on this assumption, these measures are typically calculated over the entire duration of the resting fMRI session. However, this assumption may underestimate the complex and dynamic changes in interaction patterns (Chen et al., 2017), which have been demonstrated to contain valuable information (Smith et al., 2012; Allen et al., 2014). Given the increasing evidence of dynamic FC during resting states and its importance for characterizing the brain's intrinsic functional organization, some studies have explored the temporal dynamics of FC during resting state in MCI patients. These studies have revealed that by combining evidence from the dynamic FC with that from traditional static FC, the diagnostic accuracy for MCI patients can be significantly improved (Wee et al., 2016; Chen et al., 2017; Zhang et al., 2017). However, these studies focus on dynamic changes during the resting state. To date, there are no studies exploring the dynamic network during a working memory task in MCI patients. Therefore, using the index of ALFF, the present study investigated the temporal dynamic changes in oscillations in the background network of MCI patients during a working memory task.

MATERIALS AND METHODS

Participants

Participants were recruited from a community-based screening data pool in Beijing (healthy older adults, $n = 865$; MCI, $n = 115$;

Dementia, $n = 21$; Yu et al., 2012, 2014; Yin et al., 2015). All the participants were asked to complete a neuropsychological battery and clinical assessment. Subsequently, some of the participants were selected to participate in the neuroimaging investigations. Experienced psychiatrists performed clinical diagnoses based on the results of previous tests and MCI patients were diagnosed according to the diagnostic criteria for MCI (Petersen et al., 1999, 2001). The psychiatrists' clinical experience and scores on the Montreal Cognitive Assessment (MoCA; Nasreddine et al., 2005), the Mini-Mental Status Examination (MMSE; Folstein et al., 1975), and the Clinical Dementia Rating (CDR; Morris, 1993) were also used for the clinical diagnoses. Seventeen MCI patients and 16 healthy, age-matched control subjects (normal control, NC) participated in this study. See **Table 1** for participants' demographics and performance of neuropsychological tests and working memory task, which were also presented in our previous study (Wang et al., 2016). This study was approved by the research ethics committees of the Institute of Psychology, Chinese Academy of Science (H11036). Written informed consent was obtained from each participant.

Working Memory Task: A Hybrid Delayed-Match-to-Sample Task (DMST)

Participants performed a modified DMST working memory task within the fMRI scanner (Jiang et al., 2000; Guo et al., 2008) as described in our previous study (Wang et al., 2016). In brief, the working memory task consisted of 32 trials separated into four blocks of eight trials. On each trial, two sample objects with green borders were presented side by side on the screen. Participants were asked to remember these two objects within 3,500 ms. Following this, test objects were presented. The test objects were selected from two groups: matching targets (the same as the sample objects) or non-matching distracter objects (new objects which differed from the sample objects). Target objects were presented two, three, or four times, and distractor objects were presented two, three, or four times, up to a total of 12 (or 13) test objects per trial. Each test object was presented for 1,000 ms separated by jitters of 800/900/1,000/1,100/1,200 ms. All test objects were pseudo-randomized and counter-balanced. During the test, participants were instructed to determine whether each test object matched the previously presented sample objects by pressing one of two buttons using their left or right thumb. The hand used for indicating a matching outcome was counterbalanced among participants. To avoid the effect of visual processing capacity, scrambled picture blocks (using the actual objects images) were presented alternatively with the DMST test trials, providing a baseline for each participant. Each of the scrambled picture blocks consisted of five pictures (2,000 ms for each picture). Participants were instructed to press both buttons when they perceived the scrambled pictures. Note that half of the test objects had been studied prior to scanning, whilst the other half were novel; however, this was not the focus of the present study.

TABLE 1 | Summary of participants' demographic information and performance of neuropsychological tests and working memory task.

	NC	MCI	*p*-value
N	16	17	-
Sex (male/female)	8/8	9/8	0.866
Age (years)	68.56 ± 5.76	70.53 ± 4.54	0.283
Education (years)	11.75 ± 3.17	9.82 ± 4.63	0.176
Self-rating anxiety scale	25.25 ± 4.51	29.08 ± 6.13	0.063
ADL	14.19 ± 0.54	15.15 ± 2.30	0.115
MMSE	28.25 ± 1.39	24.47 ± 3.88	<0.010
MoCA	26.19 ± 1.52	19.18 ± 4.45	<0.001
CDR	0	0.5	-
Accuracy	$91.12 \pm 4.64\%$	$77.50 \pm 17.98\%$	0.007
Response time	609.76 ± 56.09	692.86 ± 86.36	0.003
Working memory performance	1.51 ± 0.15 ($\times 10^{-3}$)	1.16 ± 0.36 ($\times 10^{-3}$)	0.001

Note: NC, normal control; MCI, mild cognitive impairment; ADL, the Activities of Daily Life; MMSE, the Mini-Mental Status Examination; MoCA, the Montreal Cognitive Assessment; CDR, the Clinical Dementia Rating. To account for the tradeoff between accuracy and response time, working memory performance was measured using response accuracy divided by response time.

Image Acquisition

Participants were scanned using a Siemens Trio 3.0 tesla scanner (Erlangen, Germany) at the Beijing MRI Center for Brain Research. Images collected included during resting state, T1-weighted structural images, and during the working memory task. Both the resting and working state images were collected using the following parameters: repetition time (TR) = 2,000 ms, time echo (TE) = 30 ms, flip angle = 90°, field of view (FOV) = 200 × 200 mm^2, 33 axial slices, thickness = 3.0 mm, gap = 0.6 mm, acquisition matrix = 64 × 64, and in-plane resolution = 3.125 × 3.125. During resting and working memory states, 200 and 652 (four runs) functional volumes were collected, respectively. During the resting state scanning, participants were instructed to keep their eyes closed, and not to think of anything in particular. T1-weighted structural images were acquired with the following parameters: 176 slices, acquisition matrix = 256 × 256, voxel size = 1 × 1 × 1 mm^3, TR = 1,900 ms, TE = 2.2 ms, and flip angle = 9°. Full details of the scanning parameters have been published previously (Yu et al., 2016).

Behavioral Data Analysis

The response accuracy on the working memory task was calculated according to the total hit rate (correct target detection) minus the total false alarm rate (false report for distractors). Response times (RTs) were calculated as the mean response time for all test stimuli (targets and distractors). As described in our previous study (Wang et al., 2016), to account for the tradeoff between accuracy and response time, working memory performance was further measured using response accuracy divided by response time, which is the reciprocal of the "inverse efficiency score" previously reported (Kennett et al., 2001; Spence et al., 2001).

Image Preprocessing

Functional MRI data were preprocessed using the Statistical Parametric Mapping program (SPM8[1]) and the toolbox for Data

[1] http://www.fil.ion.ucl.ac.uk/spm

Processing and Analysis of Brain Imaging[2] (Yan and Zang, 2010). To acquire equal volumes of resting and working memory states, the second run of task data were selected to compare with the resting state. The first nine volumes of the working memory task data were discarded to allow for equilibration of the magnetic field, and the first 46 volumes of resting state data were discarded accordingly. All 154 volumes of both resting and working memory states were corrected for intra-volume acquisition time differences between slices using Sinc interpolation. A high-pass filter (128 s cut-off period) was used to remove low-frequency confounds. Spatial smoothing was then performed using a 4 mm full-width at half-maximum (FWHM) Gaussian kernel. Full details of the parameters used in the pre-processing have been published previously (Wang et al., 2016; Yu et al., 2016).

It should be noted that, in order to make the resting and working memory states comparable, for the working memory run an additional variable of task condition was included e.g., targets and distracters present vs. absent trials; response vs. no response trials. The rationale for removing task-load effects has been discussed previously (Jones et al., 2010; Gordon et al., 2012). By including this pre-processing step, the resting and task data differed only in the subjects' cognitive state.

Static ALFF

A whole-brain wise ALFF was calculated for each subject using the DPABI program. In brief, after pre-processing, the time series for each voxel was filtered (bandpass, 0.01–0.1 Hz) to remove the effects of very low-frequency drift and high-frequency noise (Biswal et al., 1995; Lowe et al., 1998). Subsequently, for each given voxel, the time series was converted to the frequency domain by a fast Fourier transform (parameters: taper percent = 0, length = shortest). The square root of the power spectrum was computed and averaged across a predefined frequency interval (0.01–0.1 Hz). This average square root value was defined as ALFF at the given voxel (Zang et al., 2007). For standardization purposes, all individual ALFFs were computed and standardized into ALFF z-values by subtracting the mean voxel-wise ALFF obtained for the entire brain (i.e., global ALFF), and then dividing by the standard deviation (SD; Zuo et al., 2013). This subject-wise ALFF normalization has been demonstrated to improve both normality and reliability across subjects (Zuo et al., 2013).

Temporal Dynamic ALFF (TD-ALFF)

Dynamic ALFF was generated using sliding time window analysis by DPABI. First, rectangular windows (length of 32 TRs, overlapping by four TRs) were applied to BOLD signals to obtain a windowed time series. Rectangular windows (length of 64 and 128 TRs, overlapping by four TRs) were also applied to check that whether the patterns change with the length of rectangular windows. Second, the ALFF was calculated, as described above, within each window. Third, the mean, SD, and coefficient of variation (CV, SD/mean) maps were calculated across the time windows. The CV maps were then transformed to standardized z-scores, relative to the mean and SD across all voxels.

Between-Group Comparisons of ALFF in the Resting State and the Background Network of the Working Memory State

To explore any interaction effects of group and cognitive state on ALFF, we performed a two-way repeated measures analysis of variance (ANOVA) using SPM8, with group (MCI vs. NC) as a between-subject factor and cognitive state (resting vs. working memory state) as a repeated measure. *Post hoc* two-sample t-tests were performed on clusters showing significant group × state interactions. The statistical threshold was set at $p < 0.001$ using the AlphaSim correction for multiple comparisons with a threshold of $p < 0.01$ at the voxel level (using DPABI). All coordinates are reported in the MNI format.

Functional Connectivity (FC) Analysis

To examine the performance-related alterations in FC of the background network in MCI patients during a working memory task, we conducted a seed-based connectivity analysis using regions showing group × state interactions as seeds. First, for the background network during a working memory task for each individual, voxel-wise FC maps to a given seed were computed as maps of temporal correlation coefficients between the BOLD time course of each voxel and the averaged BOLD time course across voxels in the seed region. FC maps from individual subjects were then transformed using Fisher's z transformation. Second, we calculated Pearson correlation coefficients ($p < 0.05$) to explore the relationship between the FC map and working memory performance in both the MCI and NC group. Bootstrap results were based on 1,000 bootstrap samples, and 95% confidence intervals are reported.

Performance Related CV Maps During Working Memory State in MCI and NC

To explore which brain regions showed dynamic variation of ALFF related to working memory performance during the working memory state. Pearson correlation coefficients were calculated for both MCI and NC groups. The statistical threshold was set at $p < 0.001$ using the AlphaSim correction for multiple comparisons with a threshold of $p < 0.05$ at the voxel level.

RESULTS

Alteration of Static ALFF Across Resting and Working Memory States in MCI and NC

We observed significant interactions between group and state in the right ventrolateral prefrontal cortex (VLPFC; peak MNI coordinates: $x = 45$, $y = 39$, $z = 6$, cluster size = 10; average statistical coefficients of this region: $F_{(1,31)} = 19.14$, $p < 0.001$, $\eta_p^2 = 0.38$), right dorsolateral PFC (DLPFC; peak

[2]http://rfmri.org/dpabi

MNI coordinates: $x = 36$, $y = 39$, $z = 21$; cluster size = 15; average statistical coefficients of this region: $F_{(1,31)} = 18.42$, $p < 0.001$, $\eta_p^2 = 0.37$), and a region of the left supplementary motor area peak (MNI coordinates: $x = -3$, $y = -9$, $z = 57$; cluster size = 16; average statistical coefficients of this region: $F_{(1,31)} = 26.71$, $p < 0.001$, $\eta_p^2 = 0.46$; **Figure 1**). For all of the three clusters, further *post hoc t*-tests revealed that the value of ALFF was decreased in the resting state relative to the working memory state in MCI patients, but unchanged in NCs (**Figure 1**). Additionally, for all of the three clusters, *post hoc t*-tests showed that the value of ALFF was higher in MCI patients than in NCs during the resting state, while there was no difference between two groups during the working memory state.

Since these interaction effects were mainly due to abnormal hyperactivity in MCI patients during the resting state, the Pearson correlations between the brain ALFF activity and working memory performance in MCI patients was calculated to examine whether the hyperactivity was a compensatory process due to the reduced functionality of these brain regions. No significant correlation was found in MCI patients ($p > 0.10$).

Performance-Related Functional Connectivity of Regions Showing Group × State Interactions During a Working Memory Task

To examine performance-related FC alterations of the background network in MCI patients during a working memory task, we conducted a seed-based connectivity analysis using regions that showed group × state interactions as seeds. Subsequently, we calculated Pearson correlation coefficients to explore the relationship between the FC map and working memory performance in both MCI and NC groups. The results demonstrate altered performance-related FC patterns in MCI patients when compared to NCs. In NC subjects, the working memory performance was related to FC between

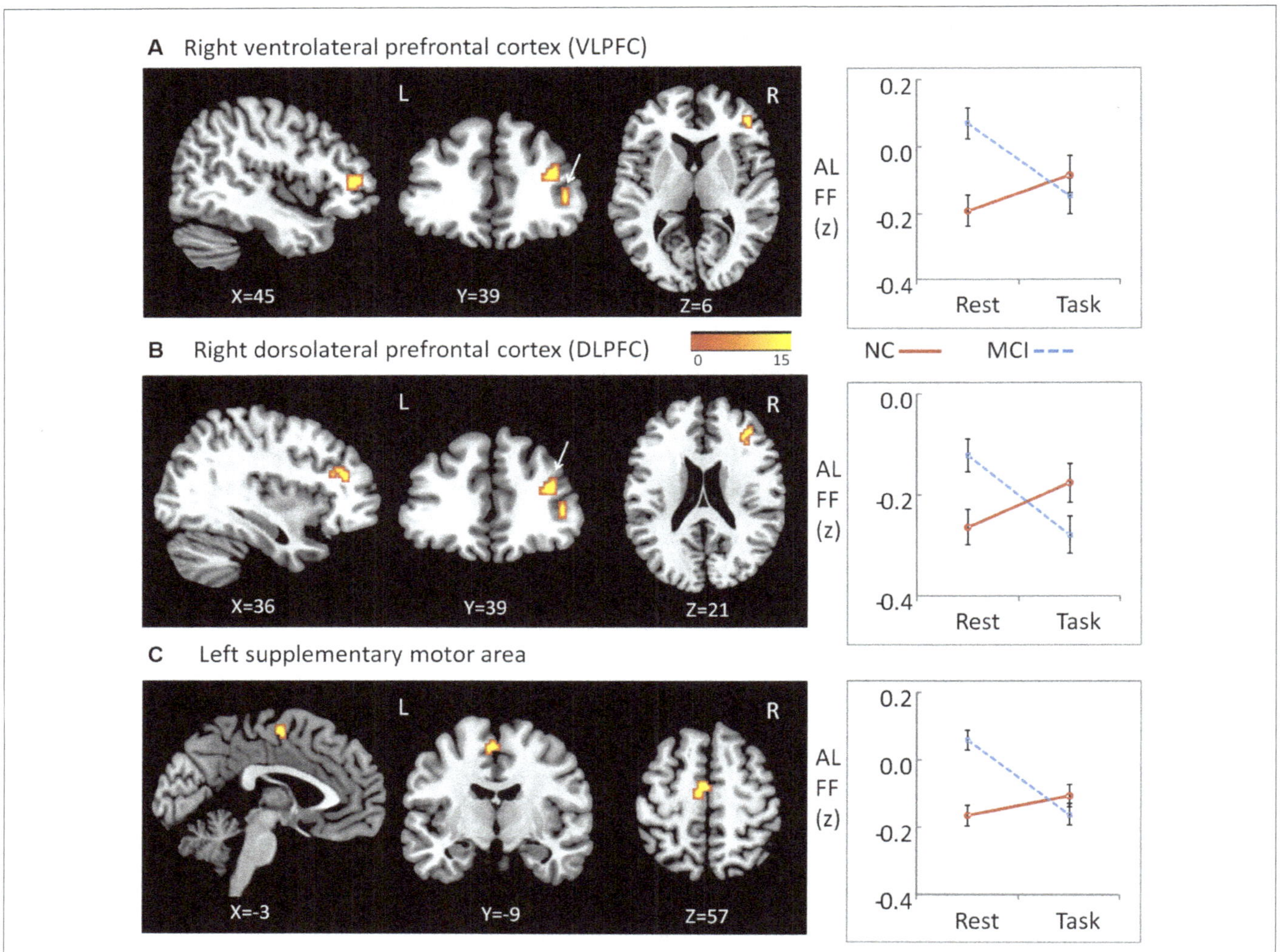

FIGURE 1 | Regions showing Group × State interactions for amplitude of low-frequency fluctuations (ALFF) and the patterns of interaction. **(A)** Region in right ventrolateral prefrontal cortex (VLPFC), **(B)** region in right dorsolateral PFC (DLPFC), **(C)** regions in left supplementary motor area.

the right VLPFC and regions in the left inferior occipital gyrus (peak MNI coordinates: $x = -45$, $y = -69$, $z = -12$; cluster size = 257; $r = 0.85$, $p < 0.001$, Cohen's $d = 3.23$), regions in the right inferior occipital gyrus (peak MNI coordinates: $x = 30$, $y = -96$, $z = -9$; cluster size = 402; $r = 0.86$, $p < 0.001$, Cohen's $d = 3.37$), and the conjunction area of the limbic and occipital lobes (peak MNI coordinates: $x = -18$, $y = -69$, $z = 6$, cluster size = 170; $r = 0.85$, $p < 0.001$, Cohen's $d = 3.23$). Also, working memory performance was related to FC between the right DLPFC and regions of the right middle occipital gyrus (peak MNI coordinates: $x = 24$, $y = -90$, $z = 6$; cluster size = 138; $r = 0.87$, $p < 0.001$, Cohen's $d = 3.53$).

In contrast, working memory performance in MCI patients was positively correlated with FC between the right VLPFC and regions of the right medial parietal cortex (peak MNI coordinates: $x = 9$, $y = -30$, $z = 48$; cluster size = 446; $r = 0.86$, $p < 0.001$, Cohen's $d = 3.37$) and the right superior parietal lobule (peak MNI coordinates: $x = 27$, $y = -69$, $z = 54$; cluster size = 319; $r = 0.91$, $p < 0.001$, Cohen's $d = 4.39$). No regions showed performance-related FC with the DLPFC in MCI patients. When regions in the left supplementary motor area were used as ROIs, we found no performance-related FC in either NCs or MCI patients (**Figure 2**).

Alteration of Temporal Dynamic ALFF Across Resting and Working Memory States in MCI and NC Groups

To explore the interaction effects of group and cognitive state on CV of dynamic ALFF, we performed a two-way repeated ANOVA, with group (MCI vs. NC) as a between-subject factor and cognitive state (resting vs. working memory) as a repeated measure. Significant interactions between group and state were found in regions located in the bilateral thalamus (peak MNI coordinates: $x = 3$, $y = -18$, $z = 12$; cluster size = 52; average statistical coefficients of this region: $F_{(1,31)} = 25.18$, $p < 0.001$, $\eta_p^2 = 0.45$). Further *post hoc t*-tests revealed that the CV of dynamic ALFF was increased in the working memory state relative to the resting state in NCs but decreased in MCI patients (**Figure 3A**). It was noted that the patterns of the results were the same when used length of rectangular windows as 64 and 128 TRs.

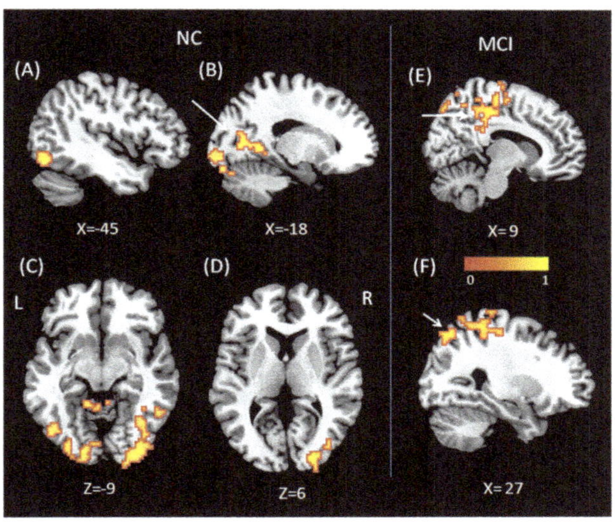

FIGURE 2 | Regions showing performance related functional connectivity (FC) with right VLPFC **(A–C)** and right DLPFC **(D)** for normal control (NC). Regions showing performance related FC with right VLPFC **(E,F)** for mild cognitive impairment (MCI). **(A)** Region in left inferior occipital gyrus, **(B)** conjunction area of left limbic lobe and occipital lobe, **(C)** regions in right inferior occipital gyrus, **(D)** regions in right middle occipital gyrus, **(E)** right medial parietal cortex, **(F)** right superior parietal lobule.

Performance Related CV Maps During the Working Memory State in MCI and NC

To explore which brain regions showed dynamic variation of ALFF in relation to the behavioral performance during the working memory state, Pearson correlation coefficients were calculated for both MCI and NC groups. Performance-related CV maps during the working memory state in MCI and NC groups are shown in **Figure 3B**. Two salient features were observed. First, the coefficients of correlation were negative in the majority of the regions, showing significant correlations with working memory performance in both groups. Second, relative to NCs, the regions in MCI patients were larger, and widely distributed in the parietal and temporal lobes.

DISCUSSION

The present study demonstrated alterations of static ALFF in MCI patients from the resting state to the working memory state. Specifically, the values of ALFF in the right VLPFC, right DLPFC, and left supplementary motor area decreased in the working memory state in MCI patients, but were unchanged in NCs. It should be noted that, compared to our previous study, which focused on the difference between MCI patients and NCs during the resting state, the main purpose of the current study was to uncover the alterations in MCI patients from resting state to working memory state. Therefore, the brain regions that showed interaction effects were the focus of this study. We found that relative to NCs, the brain ALFF activation in the right VLPFC, right DLPFC, and left supplementary motor area was decreased from the resting to the working memory state in MCI patients. These interaction effects were mainly due to abnormal hyperactivity in MCI patients during the resting state. In the resting state, two regions in the lateral PFC (in both the VLPFC and DLPFC) showed higher ALFF in MCI patients, compared to NCs. These results are in agreement with some previous studies but in disagreement with others. On the one hand, some previous studies have found the inverse pattern of results to the present study. Han et al. (2011) found that MCI patients had decreased ALFF/fALFF activity in several lateral prefrontal regions. Similarly, using independent component analysis (ICA), Sorg et al. (2007) also found that MCI patients had reduced spontaneous activity in the lateral prefrontal regions. On the other hand, however, other studies have

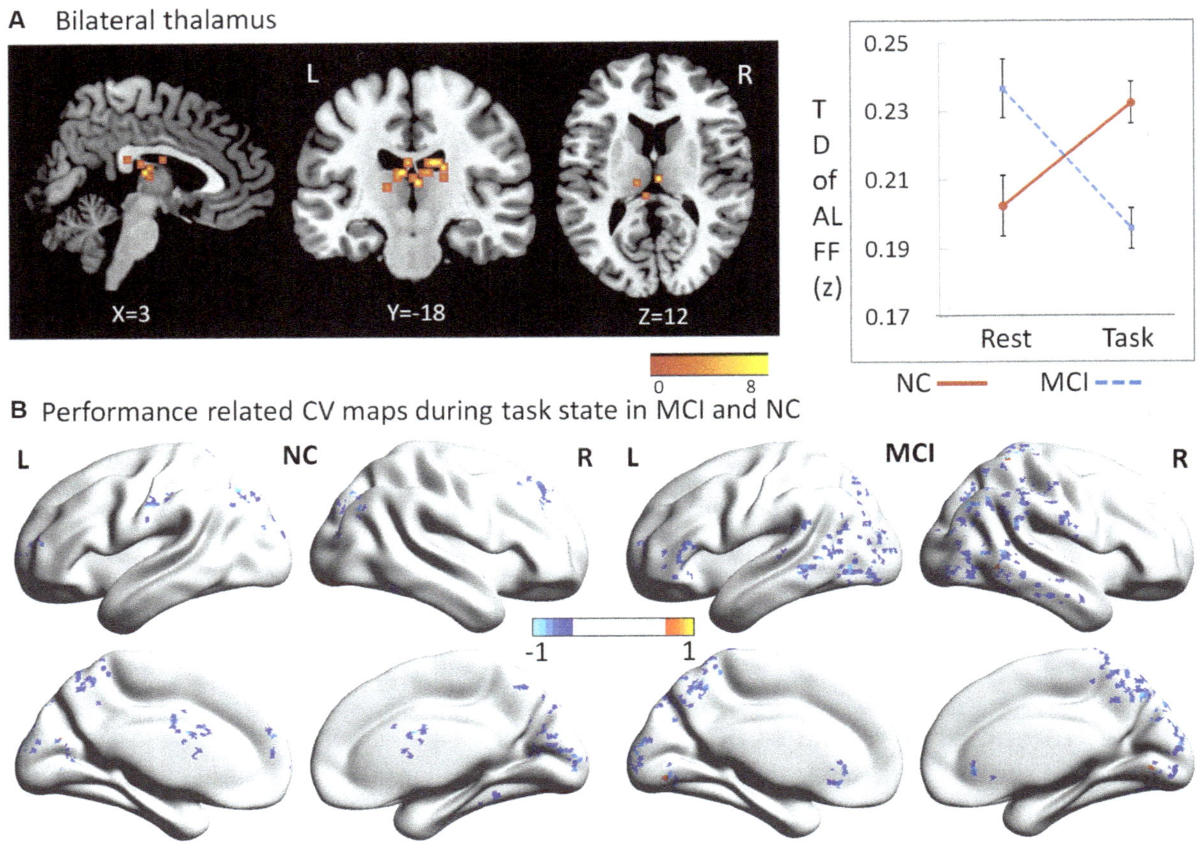

FIGURE 3 | Regions showing alteration of temporal dynamic ALFF across resting and working memory states in MCI and NC groups. **(A)** Regions in bilateral thalamus, **(B)** performance related CV maps during the working memory state in MCI and NC.

demonstrated similar results to our experiments. Using ReHo, our previous study revealed that MCI patients had higher ReHo than NCs in the lateral prefrontal regions during the resting state (Wang et al., 2016). Using the index of ICA, Qi et al. (2010) also found that MCI patients had increased brain activity in lateral prefrontal regions, thought to be compensatory hyperactivity. Based on the current evidence, it is not certain whether these changes (decrease or increase) in MCI patients are damaging or compensatory. Cabeza et al. (2018) have suggested that for hyper activation to be considered compensative, it ought to be positively related with cognitive performance. No direct evidence of a correlation has been provided by previous studies and no significant correlation was found in either MCI or NC groups in the current study. An alternative explanation is that the changes represent a deficit of function. The DLPFC and VLPFC are part of the executive network, whereas the left supplementary motor area belongs to the motor network (Yeo et al., 2011). These networks are quieter during the resting state in contrast to the default mode network in normal adults (Yeo et al., 2011). Therefore, the hyperactivity of these networks in MCI patients in the present study is more likely to be a deficit of inhibitive function.

The next question relates to the FC between abnormal brain regions and other parts of the brain, and how this is related to the behavioral performance during a working memory task. Using FC analysis with right VLPFC and right DLPFC as ROIs, the present study found that MCI patients demonstrated altered performance-related FC patterns as compared to NCs. For NCs, the FC between VLPFC, DLPFC, and regions in the bilateral inferior occipital gyrus and limbic lobe might facilitate working memory performance. For MCI patients, those with higher FC between VLPFC and regions in the right medial parietal cortex and right superior parietal lobule showed better working memory performance.

The delayed-match-to-sample task requires participants to judge continuously whether the present picture is the same as the previous one. Thus, the task requires the use of the executive component in order to access images maintained in the "visuospatial sketchpad" (Baddeley, 1992). Therefore, the communication between the central executive system and the "visuospatial sketchpad" is critical for successful working memory performance. Regions of the PFC, including the DLPFC and VLPFC, have been suggested as key components of the central executive system (Nee et al., 2013; D'Esposito and

Postle, 2015), whereas regions in the bilateral occipital lobe have been described as critical for visual image representation. For example, it has been found that short-term retention of complex visuospatial patterns (Christophel et al., 2012), objects, faces, houses, scenes, and body stimuli (Han et al., 2013; Lee et al., 2013; Sreenivasan et al., 2014), relies on the occipital cortex and other areas in the parietal and temporal cortices. The occipital cortex has also been implicated in processes related to reconstructed images and observed images (Ishai et al., 2000; Rissman and Wagner, 2012). Therefore, our finding, that the FC between the PFC and the occipital lobe was positively correlated with working memory performance in NCs, demonstrates that efficient information transfer between the central executive system and the visuospatial sketchpad in the background network is necessary for efficient working memory function. However, this critical neural pathway was not found in MCI patients. Instead, higher FC between the right VLPFC and regions in the right medial parietal cortex and the right superior parietal lobule facilitated working memory performance in MCI patients. This pathway has been considered as critical for the right frontoparietal network, which is important for working memory function, especially involving the executive component (Yeo et al., 2011). This is a more fundamental neural pathway for the performance of successful working memory. The two distinct neuronal pathways in MCI patients and NCs may suggest that for MCI patients, the fundamental pathway of working memory is impaired. Subsequently, the individual differences observed in working memory performance in MCI patients depend on the functionality of this pathway. For NCs, however, the fundamental neural structure for working memory is intact, thus their individual differences mainly result from the superior neural circuit, such as the pathway between the PFC and occipital areas. As the frontoparietal network is a fundamental pathway for working memory, we suggest that the hyperactivity observed in MCI patients is not compensatory, as suggested by Cabeza et al. (2018).

Recent studies have demonstrated that dynamic changes in neural interactions contain valuable information (Smith et al., 2012; Allen et al., 2014). To characterize the brain's intrinsic functional organization more deeply, we explored the dynamic changes during resting and working memory states in MCI patients and NCs. We found that the dynamic ALFF of bilateral thalamus regions was increased in NCs but decreased in MCI patients during the working memory state, relative to resting state. These results provide further evidence that the thalamus plays a key role in working memory. Previous work has shown that working memory capacity and executive function share a common underlying executive attention component (McCabe et al., 2010). Additionally, long-range communication of information between brain regions also likely plays an important role in working memory function (Sauseng et al., 2005; Crespo-Garcia et al., 2013). For example, in a human MEG study, synchronized oscillations in the alpha, beta, and gamma bands were observed between frontoparietal and visual areas during the retention interval of a visual working memory task. These synchronized oscillations were memory load-dependent and correlated with an individual's working memory capacity, suggesting a mechanism for effective communication between brain regions involved in the temporary maintenance of relevant visual information (Palva et al. 2010). Critically, the thalamus has been suggested to be not only key in attentional selection, but more generally in regulating information transmission across the cortex (Saalmann et al., 2012). In the present study, the dynamic ALFF in bilateral thalamus regions was increased from the resting to the working memory state in NCs, which suggests that the thalamus works as an executive attention component and an effective communication regulator during the working memory task. For MCI patients, however, this mechanism was inversed. The dynamic ALFF in these regions was decreased in the working memory state, which may result in a weakened ability of attentional selection and information regulation, resulting in an impairment of working memory function.

Next, we investigated in which regions the dynamic variation of ALFF was related to the behavioral performance during the working memory state. As outlined in the "Results" section, two salient features were observed in the performance-related CV maps. First, the coefficients of correlation were negative in the majority of the regions that showed significant correlations with working memory performance in both groups, which suggests the dynamic variation of ALFF in these regions reduced performance on the ongoing behavioral task. Second, MCI patients demonstrated altered performance-related CV patterns relative to NCs. The altered regions in MCI patients were larger, and widely distributed in the parietal and temporal lobes. Given the negative effect on the working memory task, these results indicate that MCI patients exhibit widespread and varied low-frequency fluctuations in the parietal and temporal lobes, which reduce their working memory function.

It has been found that some regions in frontal, parietal and temporal lobes can be modulated noninvasively to improve neural networks and eventually memory tasks (Wang et al., 2014; Koch et al., 2018). From a translation point of view, the altered brain regions in MCI patients found in the present study (such as VLPFC, DLPFC, and supplementary motor area) may be identified as target areas for that are precociously altered in the degenerative process leading to dementia.

One of the limitations of the present study was that no biomarker (such as cerebrospinal fluid, or amyloid positron-emission tomography scan) was included during the clinical diagnosis of MCI patients. Therefore it was impossible to identify subtypes of MCI patients according to the intrinsic pathological mechanism. Considering the high pathological heterogeneity of clinically diagnosed MCI patients, each subtypes may exhibit different patterns in the issues of the present study, which should be explore further in the following studies.

To the best of our knowledge, this is the first study to examine alterations of static and dynamic ALFF in the background network of MCI patients during working memory states. The results provide a new perspective regarding the neural mechanisms of working memory deficits in MCI patients and extend our knowledge of altered brain patterns in resting and task-evoked states.

AUTHOR CONTRIBUTIONS

PW conceived the idea, designed the study, analyzed and interpreted data, drafted part of the manuscript. RL, CW, RD, and ZH assisted to analyze and interpret the data. BL, BS, and XY assisted to analyze the data, make charts, and drafted part of the manuscript. JY carried out the experiment and drafted part of the manuscript. JL conceived the idea, designed the study, and participated in writing up and revising the manuscript.

FUNDING

This work was supported by the National Key Research and Development Program of China (2017YFB1401203, 2018YFC2000303, 2018YFC2001701, and 2016YFC1305900), Beijing Municipal Science & Technology Commission (Z171100000117006, Z171100008217006), International cooperation project of the Chinese Academy of Sciences (153111KYSB20180024), and National Natural Science Foundation of China (31671157, 31711530157, 31470998, 31861133011, 31400895, and 31871123).

REFERENCES

Allen, E. A., Damaraju, E., Plis, S. M., Erhardt, E. B., Eichele, T., and Calhoun, V. D. (2014). Tracking whole-brain connectivity dynamics in the resting state. *Cereb. Cortex* 24, 663–676. doi: 10.1093/cercor/bhs352

Baddeley, A. (1992). Working memory. *Science* 255, 556–559. doi: 10.1126/science.1736359

Biswal, B., Yetkin, F. Z., Haughton, V. M., and Hyde, J. S. (1995). Functional connectivity in the motor cortex of resting human brain using echo-planar mri. *Magn. Reson. Med.* 34, 537–541. doi: 10.1002/mrm.1910340409

Bokde, A. L., Karmann, M., Born, C., Teipel, S. J., Omerovic, M., Ewers, M., et al. (2010). Altered brain activation during a verbal working memory task in subjects with amnestic mild cognitive impairment. *J. Alzheimers Dis.* 21, 103–118. doi: 10.3233/jad-2010-091054

Cabeza, R., Albert, M., Belleville, S., Craik, F. I., Duarte, A., Grady, C. L., et al. (2018). Maintenance, reserve and compensation: the cognitive neuroscience of healthy ageing. *Nat. Rev. Neurosci.* 19, 701–710. doi: 10.1038/s41583-018-0068-2

Chen, X., Zhang, H., Zhang, L., Shen, C., Lee, S. W., and Shen, D. (2017). Extraction of dynamic functional connectivity from brain grey matter and white matter for MCI classification. *Hum. Brain Mapp.* 38, 5019–5034. doi: 10.1002/hbm.23711

Christophel, T. B., Hebart, M. N., and Haynes, J. D. (2012). Decoding the contents of visual short-term memory from human visual and parietal cortex. *J. Neurosci.* 32, 12983–12989. doi: 10.1523/JNEUROSCI.0184-12.2012

Cloutier, S., Chertkow, H., Kergoat, M.-J., Gauthier, S., and Belleville, S. (2015). Patterns of cognitive decline prior to dementia in persons with mild cognitive impairment. *J. Alzheimers Dis.* 47, 901–913. doi: 10.3233/JAD-142910

Crespo-Garcia, M., Pinal, D., Cantero, J. L., Diaz, F., Zurron, M., and Atienza, M. (2013). Working memory processes are mediated by local and long-range synchronization of alpha oscillations. *J. Cogn. Neurosci.* 25, 1343–1357. doi: 10.1162/jocn_a_0037

D'Esposito, M., and Postle, B. R. (2015). The cognitive neuroscience of working memory. *Annu. Rev. Psychol.* 66, 115–142. doi: 10.1146/annurev-psych-010814-015031

Folstein, M. F., Folstein, S. E., and McHugh, P. R. (1975). "Mini-mental state": a practical method for grading the cognitive state of patients for the clinician. *J. Psychiatr. Res.* 12, 189–198. doi: 10.1016/0022-3956(75)90026-6

Gordon, E. M., Stollstorff, M., and Vaidya, C. J. (2012). Using spatial multiple regression to identify intrinsic connectivity networks involved in working memory performance. *Hum. Brain Mapp.* 33, 1536–1552. doi: 10.1002/hbm.21306

Guo, C., Lawson, A. L., Zhang, Q., and Jiang, Y. (2008). Brain potentials distinguish new and studied objects during working memory. *Hum. Brain Mapp.* 29, 441–452. doi: 10.1002/hbm.20409

Han, X., Berg, A. C., Oh, H., Samaras, D., and Leung, H. C. (2013). Multi-voxel pattern analysis of selective representation of visual working memory in ventral temporal and occipital regions. *Neuroimage* 73, 8–15. doi: 10.1016/j.neuroimage.2013.01.055

Han, Y., Wang, J., Zhao, Z., Min, B., Lu, J., Li, K., et al. (2011). Frequency-dependent changes in the amplitude of low-frequency fluctuations in amnestic mild cognitive impairment: a resting-state fMRI study. *Neuroimage* 55, 287–295. doi: 10.1016/j.neuroimage.2010.11.059

Ishai, A., Ungerleider, L. G., Martin, A., and Haxby, J. V. (2000). The representation of objects in the human occipital and temporal cortex. *J. Cogn. Neurosci.* 12, 35–51. doi: 10.1162/089892900564055

Jiang, Y., Haxby, J. V., Martin, A., Ungerleider, L. G., and Parasuraman, R. (2000). Complementary neural mechanisms for tracking items in human working memory. *Science* 287, 643–646. doi: 10.1126/science.287.5453.643

Jones, T. B., Bandettini, P. A., Kenworthy, L., Case, L. K., Milleville, S. C., Martin, A., et al. (2010). Sources of group differences in functional connectivity: an investigation applied to autism spectrum disorder. *Neuroimage* 49, 401–414. doi: 10.1016/j.neuroimage.2009.07.051

Kennett, S., Eimer, M., Spence, C., and Driver, J. (2001). Tactile-visual links in exogenous spatial attention under different postures: convergent evidence from psychophysics and ERPs. *J. Cogn. Neurosci.* 13, 462–478. doi: 10.1162/08989290152001899

Kirova, A.-M., Bays, R. B., and Lagalwar, S. (2015). Working memory and executive function decline across normal aging, mild cognitive impairment, and Alzheimer's disease. *Biomed Res. Int.* 2015:748212. doi: 10.1155/2015/748212

Klekociuk, S. Z., and Summers, M. J. (2014). Lowered performance in working memory and attentional sub-processes are most prominent in multi-domain amnestic mild cognitive impairment subtypes. *Psychogeriatrics* 14, 63–71. doi: 10.1111/psyg.12042

Koch, G., Bonni, S., Pellicciari, M. C., Casula, E. P., Mancini, M., Esposito, R., et al. (2018). Transcranial magnetic stimulation of the precuneus enhances memory and neural activity in prodromal Alzheimer's disease. *Neuroimage* 169, 302–311. doi: 10.1016/j.neuroimage.2017.12.048

Lee, S.-H., Kravitz, D. J., and Baker, C. I. (2013). Goal-dependent dissociation of visual and prefrontal cortices during working memory. *Nat. Neurosci.* 16, 997–999. doi: 10.1038/nn.3452

Liu, F., Guo, W., Liu, L., Long, Z., Ma, C., Xue, Z., et al. (2013). Abnormal amplitude low-frequency oscillations in medication-naive, first-episode patients with major depressive disorder: a resting-state fMRI study. *J. Affect. Disord.* 146, 401–406. doi: 10.1016/j.jad.2012.10.001

Lou, W., Shi, L., Wang, D., Tam, C. W., Chu, W. C., Mok, V. C., et al. (2015). Decreased activity with increased background network efficiency in amnestic MCI during a visuospatial working memory task. *Hum. Brain Mapp.* 36, 3387–3403. doi: 10.1002/hbm.22851

Lowe, M., Mock, B., and Sorenson, J. (1998). Functional connectivity in single and multislice echoplanar imaging using resting-state fluctuations. *Neuroimage* 7, 119–132. doi: 10.1006/nimg.1997.0315

McCabe, D. P., Roediger, H. L., McDaniel, M. A., Balota, D. A., and Hambrick, D. Z. (2010). The relationship between working memory capacity and executive functioning: evidence for a common executive attention construct. *Neuropsychology* 24, 222–243. doi: 10.1037/a0017619

Migo, E. M., Mitterschiffthaler, M., O'Daly, O., Dawson, G. R., Dourish, C. T., Craig, K. J., et al. (2015). Alterations in working memory networks in amnestic mild cognitive impairment. *Neuropsychol. Dev. Cogn. B Aging Neuropsychol. Cogn.* 22, 106–127. doi: 10.1080/13825585.2014.894958

Morris, J. C. (1993). The clinical dementia rating (CDR): current version and scoring rules. *Neurology* 43, 2412–2414. doi: 10.1212/wnl.43.11.2412-a

Nasreddine, Z. S., Phillips, N. A., Bédirian, V., Charbonneau, S., Whitehead, V., Collin, I., et al. (2005). The Montreal Cognitive Assessment, MoCA: a brief screening tool for mild cognitive impairment. *J. Am. Geriatr. Soc.* 53, 695–699. doi: 10.1111/j.1532-5415.2005.53221.x

Nee, D. E., Brown, J. W., Askren, M. K., Berman, M. G., Demiralp, E., Krawitz, A., et al. (2013). A meta-analysis of executive components of working memory. *Cereb. Cortex* 23, 264–282. doi: 10.1093/cercor/bhs007

Palva, J. M., Monto, S., Kulashekhar, S., and Palva, S. (2010). Neuronal synchrony reveals working memory networks and predicts individual memory capacity. *Proc. Natl. Acad. Sci. U S A* 107, 7580–7585. doi: 10.1073/pnas.0913113107

Petersen, R. C. (2004). Mild cognitive impairment as a diagnostic entity. *J. Intern. Med.* 256, 183–194. doi: 10.1111/j.1365-2796.2004.01388.x

Petersen, R. C., Doody, R., Kurz, A., Mohs, R. C., Morris, J. C., Rabins, P. V., et al. (2001). Current concepts in mild cognitive impairment. *Arch. Neurol.* 58, 1985–1992. doi: 10.1001/archneur.58.12.1985

Petersen, R. C., Smith, G. E., Waring, S. C., Ivnik, R. J., Tangalos, E. G., and Kokmen, E. (1999). Mild cognitive impairment: clinical characterization and outcome. *Arch. Neurol.* 56, 303–308. doi: 10.1001/archneur.56.3.303

Qi, Z., Wu, X., Wang, Z., Zhang, N., Dong, H., Yao, L., et al. (2010). Impairment and compensation coexist in amnestic MCI default mode network. *Neuroimage* 50, 48–55. doi: 10.1016/j.neuroimage.2009.12.025

Rissman, J., and Wagner, A. D. (2012). Distributed representations in memory: insights from functional brain imaging. *Annu. Rev. Psychol.* 63:101. doi: 10.1146/annurev-psych-120710-100344

Saalmann, Y. B., Pinsk, M. A., Wang, L., Li, X., and Kastner, S. (2012). The pulvinar regulates information transmission between cortical areas based on attention demands. *Science* 337, 753–756. doi: 10.1126/science.1223082

Sauseng, P., Klimesch, W., Schabus, M., and Doppelmayr, M. (2005). Fronto-parietal EEG coherence in theta and upper alpha reflect central executive functions of working memory. *Int. J. Psychophysiol* 57, 97–103. doi: 10.1016/j.ijpsycho.2005.03.018

Smith, S. M., Miller, K. L., Moeller, S., Xu, J., Auerbach, E. J., Woolrich, M. W., et al. (2012). Temporally-independent functional modes of spontaneous brain activity. *Proc. Natl. Acad. Sci. U S A* 109, 3131–3136. doi: 10.1073/pnas.1121329109

Sorg, C., Riedl, V., Mühlau, M., Calhoun, V. D., Eichele, T., Läer, L., et al. (2007). Selective changes of resting-state networks in individuals at risk for Alzheimer's disease. *Proc. Natl. Acad. Sci. U S A* 104, 18760–18765. doi: 10.1073/pnas.0708803104

Spence, C., McGlone, F. P., Kettenmann, B., and Kobal, G. (2001). Attention to olfaction. A psychophysical investigation. *Exp. Brain Res.* 138, 432–437. doi: 10.1007/s002210100713

Sreenivasan, K. K., Vytlacil, J., and D'Esposito, M. (2014). Distributed and dynamic storage of working memory stimulus information in extrastriate cortex. *J. Cogn. Neurosci.* 26, 1141–1153. doi: 10.1162/jocn_a_00556

Wang, P., Li, R., Yu, J., Huang, Z., and Li, J. (2016). Frequency-dependent brain regional homogeneity alterations in patients with mild cognitive impairment during working memory state relative to resting state. *Front. Aging Neurosci.* 8:60. doi: 10.3389/fnagi.2016.00060

Wang, P., Li, R., Yu, J., Huang, Z., Yan, Z., Zhao, K., et al. (2017). Altered distant synchronization of background network in mild cognitive impairment during an executive function task. *Front. Behav. Neurosci.* 11:174. doi: 10.3389/fnbeh.2017.00174

Wang, J. X., Rogers, L. M., Gross, E. Z., Ryals, A. J., Dokucu, M. E., Brandstatt, K. L., et al. (2014). Targeted enhancement of cortical-hippocampal brain networks and associative memory. *Science* 345, 1054–1057. doi: 10.1126/science.1252900

Wee, C.-Y., Yang, S., Yap, P.-T., Shen, D., and Alzheimer's Disease Neuroimaging Initiative. (2016). Sparse temporally dynamic resting-state functional connectivity networks for early MCI identification. *Brain Imaging Behav.* 10, 342–356. doi: 10.1007/s11682-015-9408-2

Yang, H., Long, X.-Y., Yang, Y., Yan, H., Zhu, C.-Z., Zhou, X.-P., et al. (2007). Amplitude of low frequency fluctuation within visual areas revealed by resting-state functional MRI. *Neuroimage* 36, 144–152. doi: 10.1016/j.neuroimage.2007.01.054

Yang, L., Yan, Y., Wang, Y., Hu, X., Lu, J., Chan, P., et al. (2018). Gradual disturbances of the amplitude of low-frequency fluctuations (ALFF) and fractional ALFF in Alzheimer spectrum. *Front. Neurosci.* 12:975. doi: 10.3389/fnins.2018.00975

Yan, C., and Zang, Y. (2010). DPARSF: a MATLAB toolbox for "pipeline" data analysis of resting-state fMRI. *Front. Syst. Neurosci.* 4:13. doi: 10.3389/fnsys.2010.00013

Yeo, B. T., Krienen, F. M., Sepulcre, J., Sabuncu, M. R., Lashkari, D., Hollinshead, M., et al. (2011). The organization of the human cerebral cortex estimated by intrinsic functional connectivity. *J. Neurophysiol.* 106, 1125–1165. doi: 10.1152/jn.00338.2011

Yin, S., Zhu, X., Huang, X., and Li, J. (2015). Visuospatial characteristics of an elderly Chinese population: results from the WAIS-R Block Design Test. *Front. Aging Neurosci.* 7:17. doi: 10.3389/fnagi.2015.00017

Yu, J., Li, J., and Huang, X. (2012). The Beijing version of the montreal cognitive assessment as a brief screening tool for mild cognitive impairment: a community-based study. *BMC Psychiatry* 12:156. doi: 10.1186/1471-244x-12-156

Yu, J., Li, R., Jiang, Y., Broster, L. S., and Li, J. (2016). Altered brain activities associated with neural repetition effects in mild cognitive impairment patients. *J. Alzheimers Dis.* 53, 693–704. doi: 10.3233/jad-160086

Yu, J., Su, T., Zhou, T., He, Y., Lu, J., Li, J., et al. (2014). Uric formaldehyde levels are negatively correlated with cognitive abilities in healthy older adults. *Neurosci. Bull.* 30, 172–184. doi: 10.1007/s12264-013-1416-x

Zang, Y.-F., He, Y., Zhu, C.-Z., Cao, Q.-J., Sui, M.-Q., Liang, M., et al. (2007). Altered baseline brain activity in children with ADHD revealed by resting-state functional MRI. *Brain Dev.* 29, 83–91. doi: 10.1016/j.braindev.2006.07.002

Zang, Y., Jiang, T., Lu, Y., He, Y., and Tian, L. (2004). Regional homogeneity approach to fMRI data analysis. *Neuroimage* 22, 394–400. doi: 10.1016/j.neuroimage.2003.12.030

Zhang, Z., Lu, G., Zhong, Y., Tan, Q., Chen, H., Liao, W., et al. (2010). fMRI study of mesial temporal lobe epilepsy using amplitude of low-frequency fluctuation analysis. *Hum. Brain Mapp.* 31, 1851–1861. doi: 10.1002/hbm.20982

Zhang, Y., Zhang, H., Chen, X., Lee, S.-W., and Shen, D. (2017). Hybrid high-order functional connectivity networks using resting-state functional MRI for mild cognitive impairment diagnosis. *Sci. Rep.* 7:6530. doi: 10.1038/s41598-017-06509-0

Zuo, X.-N., Xu, T., Jiang, L., Yang, Z., Cao, X.-Y., He, Y., et al. (2013). Toward reliable characterization of functional homogeneity in the human brain: preprocessing, scan duration, imaging resolution and computational space. *Neuroimage* 65, 374–386. doi: 10.1016/j.neuroimage.2012.10.017

Zou, Q.-H., Zhu, C.-Z., Yang, Y., Zuo, X.-N., Long, X.-Y., Cao, Q.-J., et al. (2008). An improved approach to detection of amplitude of low-frequency fluctuation (ALFF) for resting-state fMRI: fractional ALFF. *J. Neurosci. Methods* 172, 137–141. doi: 10.1016/j.jneumeth.2008.04.012

10

HIV-Associated Neurocognitive Impairment in the Modern ART Era: Are we Close to Discovering Reliable Biomarkers in the Setting of Virological Suppression?

Alessandra Bandera[1,2], Lucia Taramasso[1,3], Giorgio Bozzi[1], Antonio Muscatello[1], Jake A. Robinson[4], Tricia H. Burdo[4†] and Andrea Gori[1,2†]*

[1]Infectious Disease Unit, Department of Internal Medicine, Fondazione IRCCS Ca' Granda Ospedale Maggiore Policlinico, Milan, Italy, [2]Department of Pathophysiology and Transplantation, University of Milano, Milan, Italy, [3]Infectious Diseases Clinic, Department of Health Sciences, School of Medical and Pharmaceutical Sciences, Policlinico Hospital San Martino, University of Genova (DISSAL), Genova, Italy, [4]Department of Neuroscience, Lewis Katz School of Medicine at Temple University, Philadelphia, PA, United States

***Correspondence:**
Alessandra Bandera
alessandra.bandera@unimi.it

† These authors have contributed equally to this work

The prevalence of the most severe forms of HIV-associated neurocognitive disorders (HAND) is decreasing due to worldwide availability and high efficacy of antiretroviral treatment (ART). However, several grades of HIV-related cognitive impairment persist with effective ART and remain a clinical concern for people with HIV (PWH). The pathogenesis of these cognitive impairments has yet to be fully understood and probably multifactorial. In PWH with undetectable peripheral HIV-RNA, the presence of viral escapes in cerebrospinal fluid (CSF) might explain a proportion of cases, but not all. Many other mechanisms have been hypothesized to be involved in disease progression, in order to identify possible therapeutic targets. As potential indicators of disease staging and progression, numerous biomarkers have been used to characterize and implicate chronic inflammation in the pathogenesis of neuronal injuries, such as certain phenotypes of activated monocytes/macrophages, in the context of persistent immune activation. Despite none of them being disease-specific, the correlation of several CSF cellular biomarkers to HIV-induced neuronal damage has been investigated. Furthermore, recent studies have been evaluating specific microRNA (miRNA) profiles in the CSF of PWH with neurocognitive impairment (NCI). The aim of the present study is to review the body of evidence on different biomarkers use in research and clinical settings, focusing on PWH on ART with undetectable plasma HIV-RNA.

Keywords: marker, neurocognitive impairment, HIV, Art, ANI, HAND, AIDS, dementia

INTRODUCTION

Thirty-seven million people are currently living with HIV infection in the world, according to World Health Organization estimates. A variable proportion of people with HIV (PWH), suggested up to 60%, might develop some form of HIV-associated neurocognitive disorder (HAND) in the course of their life (Schouten et al., 2011). HAND is categorized as three main conditions based on the severity of neurocognitive deficits: asymptomatic neurocognitive impairment (ANI), HIV-associated mild neurocognitive disorder (MND), and HIV-associated dementia (HAD; Antinori et al., 2007).

The neurocognitive impairment (NCI) underlying these conditions has a multifactorial etiopathogenesis, with many contributing factors. One of the most studied contributing factors is the uncontrolled replication of HIV in cerebrospinal fluid (CSF) and brain tissue, causing direct central nervous system (CNS) damage, further complicating the global picture of HAND. However, a certain grade of NCI has been found in PWH on stable antiretroviral treatment (ART) with persistently undetectable viremia, highlighting ongoing brain volume loss and white matter injury without association to HIV viral load (McMurtray et al., 2008; Cardenas et al., 2009; Gongvatana et al., 2009). These data suggest that the direct role of the virus alone cannot explain the presence of HAND and that other factors, such as chronic inflammation, cytokine release and cellular damage, could all be involved in the pathological process. Specifically, common autopsy findings in ART-treated PWH included brain endothelial cell activation and alterations in neurochemical synaptic transmission with a lymphocyte infiltrate rather than the monocyte dominant encephalitis observed in advanced pre-ART HIV disease.

Many factors have been studied so far to determine the risk of developing HIV-associated NCI, but, until now, a single marker has not been identified that effectively differentiates PWH with or without NCI. In PWH with uncontrolled HIV replication and HAND, therapy is optimized for controlling viral replication; however, there is no standardized consensus on therapy targeting HAND for PWH with optimal viral suppression. The identification of biomarkers with the potential for predicting or stratifying the risk for NCI could be pivotal for the early diagnosis of HAND and long-term management of chronically infected PWH, assessing the efficacy of therapeutic interventions along time. However, as ART-mediated viral suppression limits the role of HIV as a mechanism of CNS injury, potential biomarkers should be investigated between inflammation-linked or neuronal damage markers that could be influenced by different individual host characteristics, such as the genetic likelihood of Alzheimer's, age, and comorbidities.

In this review article, we analyzed the current body of evidence concerning biomarkers of NCI in PWH on ART and with controlled HIV replication, investigating their applicability in the context of clinical practice. The aim of this review is to investigate which mechanisms are currently studied and possibly correlated to NCI, and whether some markers of neuronal damage or immune activation could be used for diagnostic purposes or even in the longitudinal follow-up of ART-treated PWH.

METHODS

This review article is based on the literature analyzing the markers of NCI in the course of ART-treated HIV infection. Our review examined all articles published in English and available on PubMed database until December 16, 2018. No restriction criteria based on year of publication were used. Online publications ahead of print were also included. The PubMed database was screened using the search terms: {(HIV) [AND NCI] AND marker} NOT review [Publication Type]. One-hundred and eleven articles published between August 1996 and December 2018 were initially selected and screened for eligibility based on title and abstract. With the aim of eliminating the confounding factor of uncontrolled CSF viral replication and viral escapes, we excluded studies performed in ART naïve subject. *In vitro* studies, post-mortem studies, and animal studies were also excluded. The remaining manuscripts were thereafter read in whole, and included in the review article, if they reported data on at least one possible marker of NCI, studied in PWH (at least partly) on ART.

Forty-three articles were excluded because they did not focus on any biomarker or only concerned viral markers; four because the studies were performed on animals; two were *in vitro* studies; four were post-mortem studies; eight were performed in ART-naïve PWH or PWH with CSF replicating HIV; four were reviews (**Figure 1**).

Forty-six articles were included in the final version of the review, encompassing 201 distinct hypotheses of correlation between different biomarkers and NCI.

References cited in the studies were also checked to identify other relevant articles not found in our initial search.

Technical Limitations

One of the major issues linked to identification of reliable biomarkers of NCI is the reproducibility of the results. In fact, the techniques that are used to measure different biomarkers in different studies are often not fully comparable. ELISA-based assays, which are commonly used to detect and dose many biomarkers, have been originally developed to measure a single analyte and later developed as multiplex assays, allowing measurement of multiple analytes from a single sample. However, many different sources and kits from different manufacturers are now available and they might provide different results, while the same analyte can be measured differently in multiplex or single determinations. In addition, different kits can be designed for different ranges of values with different software and require different dilutions of the CSF or plasma, which can confound the data between studies. Also, the modern omics approach has similar limitations as well. The results of an omics study can vary with the manufacturer, the platform, and which version is used, owing to low overlap of results when the same samples are run on different platforms. In addition, the omics approach requires correction for multiple comparisons and discussion of fold change definitions, both of which are controversial within the fields.

Finally, statisticians often advocate log transformation of results that may be appropriate for some biomarkers but is problematic for others. Indeed, log transformation of results may obscure the marginal values of more labile analytes, whose values can be at the margin of detection, and leads to publication of findings driven by a very few positive values.

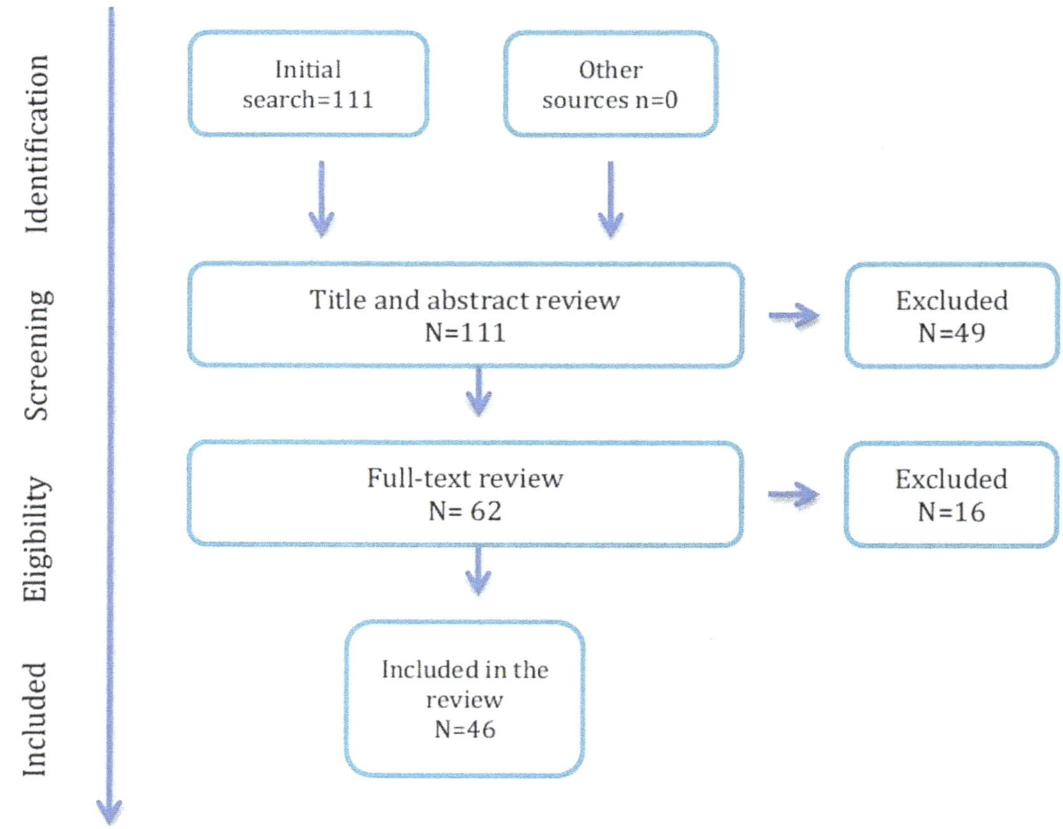

FIGURE 1 | Flowchart for study selection.

All those technical issues must be considered in the final considerations on the significance of the various analytes that have been studied in CNS.

MARKERS OF NEURONAL DAMAGE AND ALTERATION OF SIGNALING

Key events that follow invasion of CNS by HIV and contribute to HAND include direct neuronal apoptosis, dysregulation of neuronal support cells, and loss of synaptodendritic signaling. Identifying sensitive CSF biomarkers of HIV-induced neuronal damage seems essential for HIV/neuroAIDS staging, evaluation of response to treatment, and clarifying possible mechanisms of neural damage. We summarized data on available neuronal damage and alteration of signaling biomarkers, underlying the main strengths and limitations of the available literature on the topic (**Table 1**).

β-Amyloid 42

β-Amyloid 42 (Aβ42) is the major component of brain amyloid plaques in the course of Alzheimer's disease, and may activate mast cells, which could play an important role in Alzheimer's disease pathogenesis (Niederhoffer et al., 2009). Patients without clinical cognitive impairment with Aβ42 pathology are considered at high risk of preclinical Alzheimer's disease (Sperling et al., 2011), cognitive decline (Petersen et al., 2016), and progression to mild cognitive impairment (Knopman et al., 2012). Aβ42 levels in CNS have been previously linked to HIV-RNA load, indicating that HIV replication in the brain could be an active driver of neuroinflammation and of abnormal protein clearance (Levine et al., 2016). However, few studies have focused on Aβ42 levels with successful suppression of HIV replication. CSF levels of Aβ42 from ART-naïve PWH have been previously correlated with average white matter hyperintensities ($\rho = 0.319$, $p = 0.045$; Trentalange et al., 2018) that, in turn, have been associated with cognitive impairment (Mok and Kim, 2015). However, such correlation was not confirmed in ART-treated PWH (Trentalange et al., 2018), and a study conducted in 94 PWH (72% with HIV-RNA undetectable) did not find a correlation between CSF Aβ42 levels and abnormalities in the periventricular white matter (Steinbrink et al., 2013). In the same study, the CSF Aβ42 was correlated to scores of different neuropsychological tests, and Aβ42 correlated significantly with HIV Memorial Sloan–Kettering scale (MSKS) score but not with HIV dementia scale (HDS) and the Mosaic test (MT) scores (Steinbrink et al., 2013). Moreover, in ART-treated PWH with undetectable HIV RNA in their plasma or CSF, CSF Aβ42 levels

TABLE 1 | Biomarkers of neuronal damage and correlation with neurocognitive impairment (NCI) in people living with HIV.

Biomarker	Body fluid	Findings	Research gaps	Reference
β-Amyloid 42				
	CSF	No correlation with white matter hyperintensity in ART-treated PWH.	Lack of randomized trials; Lack of longitudinal data; little data in course of ART	Trentalange et al. (2018)
	CSF	No correlation with abnormalities in the periventricular white matter.		Steinbrink et al. (2013)
	CSF	Significant correlation with neuropsychological tests score: -HIV Memorial Sloan–Kettering scale score -Not with HIV dementia scale (HDS) and the Mosaic test (MT) scores		Steinbrink et al. (2013)
	CSF	NO correlation with GDS.		Cysique et al. (2015)
ε4 APOE carriage		Association with lower CSF Aβ1-42 concentrations. NO correlation with NCI.	Association with NCI not proven in HIV	Bertram et al. (2008)
ε4 APOE carriage		No association with HAND in HIV.		Bora et al. (2014) and Cysique et al. (2015)
Neurofilament proteins				
	Plasma	Higher concentration in worse cognitive performance.	No data in correlation with experimental neuroprotective therapies. Lack of randomized trials.	Anderson et al. (2018)
	CSF	Independent biomarker of baseline NCI status.		Guha et al. (2019)
	CSF	Negative association with cognitive performance.		Jessen Krut et al. (2014) and Anderson et al. (2018)
	CSF	Trend towards higher levels in aviremic PWH with NCI compared to others.		Edén et al. (2016)
	CSF	Higher levels in NCI vs. unimpaired PWH.		Guha et al. (2019)
	CSF	High levels in untreated neuroasymptomatic PWH.		Jessen Krut et al. (2014)
	CSF	Predictive of HAD development in neuroasymptomatic PWH.		Gisslén et al. (2007)
	CSF	Low levels in ART-treated PWH and in PWH.		Jessen Krut et al. (2014)
	CSF	Levels decline after starting ART.		Jessen Krut et al. (2014)
	CSF	Levels remain stable in course of stable ART.		Sacktor et al. (2018)
	CSF	Similar levels in course of ART in early treated PWH compared to others.		Oliveira et al. (2017)
	CSF	Correlation with neopterin levels.		Edén et al. (2016)
	CSF	Direct correlation with C1q in CSF.		McGuire et al. (2016)
Calcium binding protein B (S100B)				
	CSF	Higher levels in NCI compared to unimpaired subjects.	Little data, lack of longitudinal studies. Lack of randomized trials.	Yuan et al. (2017) and Guha et al. (2019)
Tau protein				
	CSF	Higher mean values in PWH with moderate or severe abnormalities of periventricular white matter.	Little longitudinal data, absence of a defined cut-off for defining NCI, little use in the follow-up of PWH on ART. Lack of randomized trials.	Steinbrink et al. (2013)
	CSF	No correlation with white matter hyperintensities in ART, weak correlation off ART.		Trentalange et al. (2018)
	CSF	Significant correlation with neuropsychological test score: -Memorial Sloan–Kettering scale score -HIV dementia scale score -Mosaic test score		Steinbrink et al. (2013)

(Continued)

TABLE 1 | (Continued)

Biomarker	Body fluid	Findings	Research gaps	Reference
	CSF	Normalization after improvement of neurocognitive function in a single case report.		Andersson et al. (2006)
	CSF	No changes in virologically suppressed PWH after switch to ART regimens with enhanced central nervous system penetrability.		Tiraboschi et al. (2015)
Phospho-tau	CSF	Significant correlation with GDS.		Cysique et al. (2015)
LIPIDS				
Sphingomyelin:ceramide ratio	CSF	Greater sphingomyelin:ceramide ratios for acyl chain lengths of C16:0, C18:0, C22:0, and C24:0 were associated with worse performance on several indices of memory.	Lack of randomized trials; Lack of longitudinal data	Mielke et al. (2010)
Sphingomyelin:cholesterol ratios	CSF	Higher sphingomyelin:cholesterol ratios were significantly associated with worse performance on the Rey Auditory Verbal Learning Test trail 5 score ($p = 0.018$) and delayed recall.		Mielke et al. (2010)
Extracellular vesicles				
	CSF	Higher in HIV + that in uninfected subjects.	Little studied, still no longitudinal data, absence of solid correlations in ART-treated PWH. Lack of randomized trials	Guha et al. (2019)
	CSF	Higher levels in NCI compared to unimpaired subjects.		Guha et al. (2019)
	CSF	Direct correlation with S100B.		Guha et al. (2019)
Wnt pathway				
DKK1	Plasma	Higher levels in NCI compared to unimpaired subjects, particularly in PWH taking ART with HIV RNA levels $\leq$50 copies/mL.	Little studied, still no longitudinal data, absence of solid correlations in ART-treated PWH. Lack of randomized trials.	Yu et al. (2017)
Mitochondrial DNA				
	CSF	Higher levels in NCI compared to unimpaired subjects.	Contradictory data, lack of reliable data in ART-treated PWH; lack of longitudinal data. Lack of randomized trials.	Pérez-Santiago et al. (2016)
	CSF	Higher levels in better neurocognitive performance.		Pérez-Santiago et al. (2017)
	CSF	Inverse correlation with NFL levels.		Pérez-Santiago et al. (2017)
	CSF	Association with biomarkers of inflammation (IP-10 in CSF and MCP-1 in plasma).		Pérez-Santiago et al. (2016)
	CSF	Higher levels in individuals with detectable CSF HIV RNA and in the absence of ART.		Mehta et al. (2017)
	CSF	Higher levels in PWH with mild NCI than in asymptomatic subjects.		Mehta et al. (2017)
	CSF	Direct association with IL-6; inverse association with ceruloplasmin, transferrin, and VEGF.		Mehta et al. (2017)
	CSF	Direct association with MCP-1 in CSF, TNF-α and IL-8 in plasma.		Pérez-Santiago et al. (2017)
Different mitochondrial haplogroup carriage		No correlation with IL-6, IL-8, IP-10, and TNF-α in CSF in African and Hispanic ancestry. Haplogroup H had significantly lower CSF TNF-α levels in European ancestry with suppressed plasmatic HIV-RNA viremia.		Samuels et al. (2016)

Abbreviations: ART, antiretroviral treatment; GDS, global deficit score, CSF, cerebrospinal fluid; PWH, people with HIV.

did not correlate with clinically relevant levels of impairment, defined in accordance with the Global Deficit Score (GDS) method, or with past diagnosis of HAND (Cysique et al., 2015). Also, the ε4 allele of Apolipoprotein E (APOE), an apolipoprotein thought to be partially responsible for amyloid clearance in the CNS and a risk factor for late-onset sporadic Alzheimer's disease (Bertram et al., 2008), showed no association with HAND in HIV (Cysique et al., 2015).

Although Aβ42 could probably be used in other settings, including cognitive impairment in HIV viremic PWH, current evidences on its use in controlled HIV infection are still limited and do not offer additional information on cognitive evaluation and staging in the clinical practice.

Neurofilament Proteins

The light subunit of the neurofilament protein (NFL) is a major structural element of myelinated axons that is crucial for maintaining the axonal caliber and facilitating an effective nerve conduction (Hoffman et al., 1987). Elevated NFL levels are found in CSF of PWH when this structural component is released during neuronal and axonal injury, which has been reported in several neurological disorders including HAND (Abdulle et al., 2007; Jessen Krut et al., 2014; Peterson et al., 2014; McGuire et al., 2015; Gisslén et al., 2016; Yilmaz et al., 2017). In HIV-infected adults, higher plasma NFL concentration has been significantly associated with worse neuropsychological performance, after adjustment for possible confounding factors including age, CD4+ T cell count, and plasma HIV RNA levels (Anderson et al., 2018). High NFL concentration in CSF was found to be an independent biomarker of baseline NCI status in multivariable linear regression models adjusted for age, race, and plasma viral load (Guha et al., 2019). CSF NFL levels were also found to correlate with C1q concentrations in CSF in ART naïve PWH. The complement system (C1q/C3) is a key mediator of synaptic pruning during normal development and HIV inappropriately induces C1q and C3 production in the brain. In a 2016 study of 40 PWH with 58% of PWH on ART, a nearly significant elevation of CSF C1q expression was observed in cognitively impaired subjects between 18 and 24 years old compared to cognitively normal subjects, and within the PWH group, CSF C1q correlated with CSF NFL levels (McGuire et al., 2016). However, the association between GDSs and CSF NFL has been observed mostly in individuals not receiving ART, in which plasma NFLs are higher compared to PWH receiving ART and usually decline over time after ART initiation (Andersson et al., 2006; Jessen Krut et al., 2014; Anderson et al., 2018). A trend towards higher CSF NFL was also seen in aviremic PWH with NCI compared to others (Edén et al., 2016) and, in a work including mostly ART-treated PWH (67 PWH of which 67% aviremic), CSF NFL levels were higher in PWH with NCI compared to unimpaired HIV-infected subjects ($p < 0.05$; Guha et al., 2019). In the same study, CSF NFL was higher in NCI ($p = 0.009$) and HAND ($p = 0.007$) but not in unimpaired HIV-infected subjects compared to HIV-uninfected controls (Guha et al., 2019). In another interesting study, high levels of CSF NFL were consistently found in HAD subjects and in untreated asymptomatic PWH, especially those with lower counts of CD4+ T lymphocytes, suggesting a subclinical axonal injury also in neuroasymptomatic PWH and not on treatment (Jessen Krut et al., 2014). Importantly, higher CSF NFL levels were found in neuroasymptomatic PWH compared to CD4-matched controls in a previous study, in which enrolled PWH were not on ART or, in some cases, treated with old drug combinations, which would now be considered suboptimal, and had with elevated median CSF HIV-RNA levels in both cases and controls (Gisslén et al., 2007). In a cross-sectional comparison between ART-treated PWH and HIV-uninfected subjects, only a minority of subjects [7/85 (8%) and 4/204 (2%), respectively] had high CSF NFL levels (Jessen Krut et al., 2014), and similar NFL concentrations were found in PWH under combined ART and in HIV-negative subjects 3.9 years older (Jessen Krut et al., 2014). While ART usually reduces CSF NFL concentrations in naïve subjects (Jessen Krut et al., 2014) in PWH with NCI and on stable ART, NFL does not seem to change significantly after 24 weeks (Sacktor et al., 2018). Moreover, ART-treated HIV aviremic subjects had similar CSF NFL concentrations either if treated early or late (after median 1.8 vs. 17.2 months) for HIV infection (Oliveira et al., 2017). In conclusion, NFL is a sensitive biomarker for axonal injury in several neurological disorders including HAND (Abdulle et al., 2007; Gisslén et al., 2007, 2016; Yilmaz et al., 2017), and the correlation found between CSF NFL and neopterin in NCI subjects suggests an association between NCI, CNS inflammation, and neuronal damage (Edén et al., 2016). NFL is one of the markers with a more consistent correlation with NCI in HIV; however, a longitudinal evaluation of NFL in ART-treated aviremic PWH seems not to be informative.

Calcium Binding Protein B

Calcium binding protein B (S100B) is secreted by astrocytes and oligodendrocytes and can enter the extracellular space or bloodstream after spilling from injured cells. For this reason, S100B is considered a peripheral marker of CNS damage and blood-brain barrier permeability (Blyth et al., 2009; Kazmierski et al., 2012; Wu et al., 2016). Glial responses in HIV-infected individuals can be detected by elevation of CSF S100B (Green et al., 1999; Pemberton and Brew, 2001; Du Pasquier et al., 2013; Abassi et al., 2017) and its levels have been found to be higher in the CSF of PWH with NCI compared to unimpaired HIV-infected subjects ($p < 0.05$; Guha et al., 2019). In particular, CSF S100B was higher in NCI ($p = 0.023$) and HAND ($p = 0.002$) but not in unimpaired HIV-infected subjects compared to uninfected controls in a recent study conducted by Guha et al. (2019). However, in that study, SB100 was not confirmed as an independent biomarker of baseline NCI status in multivariable linear regression models adjusted for age, race, and plasma viral load (Guha et al., 2019). In another study, significantly higher levels of S100B were found in CSF of PWH with NCI compared with PWH without impairment ($p = 0.0023$); however, the analysis was unadjusted for possible confounding factors (Yuan et al., 2017). Definitive studies confirming the role of SB100 in the evaluation of NCI in the course of aviremic HIV infection are still lacking.

Tau Protein

Total-tau and phospho-tau are considered reliable markers of clinically relevant neurodegeneration. Tau is a protein implicated in the assembly and stability of microtubules, while phospho-tau, its hyper-phosphorylated form, is produced in the course of inflammation and detaches from microtubules, forming neurofibrillary tangles (Calcagno et al., 2016). In a previous study performed in PWH (72% with HIV-RNA <200 copies/ml), higher mean values of total tau have been found in PWH with moderate or severe abnormalities of periventricular white matter than in PWH with no or mild abnormalities ($p < 0.001$ and $p = 0.006$, respectively; Steinbrink et al., 2013). The same findings were also confirmed in PWH with white matter abnormalities in the area of the basal ganglia, who showed significantly higher total tau levels ($p = 0.0013$) compared to PWH with no, or mild, abnormalities ($p = 0.027$; Steinbrink et al., 2013). On the other side, in ART-treated PWH, tau CSF levels did not correlate with the presence of hyperintensities in the white matter, which has been in turn associated with NCI, while a weak correlation was seen in naive PWH (Trentalange et al., 2018). The correlation among total tau level in CSF and scores of different neuropsychological tests has also been evaluated. Total tau correlated with the MSKS score ($r = 0.252$; $p = 0.018$), HDS score ($r = 0.268$; $p = 0.015$), and the MT score ($r = 0.229$; $p = 0.036$). Interestingly, none of those scores correlated with phospho-tau levels (Steinbrink et al., 2013). On the other hand, greater levels of NCI, evaluated by the GDS, were associated with higher CSF levels of phospho-tau ($r = 0.10$; $p = 0.03$), but NCI showed only borderline association at the univariate analysis ($p = 0.05$) to CSF total-tau levels, not confirmed at multivariable analysis (Cysique et al., 2015).

Although the normalization of CSF-tau has been correlated to improvement of neurocognitive function in a single case of a person initiating ART (Andersson et al., 2006), no changes in tau levels were found in studies of switch therapy in virologically suppressed PWH switching to ART regimens with enhanced CNS penetrability (Tiraboschi et al., 2015). In summary, tau CNS levels showed good correlation with both neuroimaging features and neuropsychological tests evocative of NCI in different studies. Data are still lacking on the possibility of use of this marker in the follow up of NCI.

Lipid Biomarkers

During the course of CNS disorders, a disruption in the lipid metabolism may occur in the CNS, resulting in elevated CSF levels or brain accumulation of lipid biomarkers. Indeed, levels of ceramide and sphingomyelin are significantly increased in brain tissues and CSF of PWH with dementia (Haughey et al., 2004). This could be due to an induction of the lipid metabolism caused by the cytokines produced by glial cells. Moreover, an overproduction of ceramide, resulting from oxidative assault on lipid membranes in the CNS, can be implicated in brain accumulation of lipids and increased ceramide in the CSF of HIV/neuroAIDS subjects (Haughey et al., 2004; Farooqui et al., 2007). CSF levels of sphingomyelin, ceramide, and sterol species have been studied and compared with performance on standard neurological tests in 31 PWH (80% on ART; Mielke et al., 2010). Greater sphingomyelin/ceramide ratios for acyl chain lengths of C16:0, C18:0, C22:0, and C24:0 were associated with poorer performance on memory testing (Mielke et al., 2010). Moreover, higher sphingomyelin:cholesterol ratios were found in PWH with lower scores on the Rey Auditory Verbal Learning Test trail 5 and delayed recall tests (Mielke et al., 2010). Ceramide C16:0 and ceramide C22:0 levels were also evaluated in a prospective double-blind trial, in which PWH were treated with fluconazole, paroxetine or placebo. The study failed to prove a significant improvement in plasma and CSF lipid levels. However, in PWH treated with paroxetine, plasma ceramide C22:0 levels were reduced more than in those treated with placebo and also a cognitive improvement was noticed in the same group, although not consistent across all cognitive domains (Sacktor et al., 2018). In conclusion, data on lipid biomarkers trend in the course of suppressive ART are still lacking, and little is known on the potential use for diagnosis and follow-up of aviremic PWH.

Extracellular Vesicles

Extracellular vesicles (EVs) are generated from most cell types and released into blood and CSF to carry and deliver cellular products to other neighboring or distant cells, including proteins, lipids, and nucleic acids (Thery et al., 2002; Rashed et al., 2017), but also, in the course of viral infection, viral proteins (Kadiu et al., 2012) and pro- or anti-inflammatory factors (Li et al., 2013). EVs can be classified as exosomes (50–150 nm, originate from multivesicular bodies) or microvesicles (200 nm to 1 μm, originate from plasma membrane), depending on their origin and particle size, and have been studied as possible markers of many neurologic disorders and neuroinflammatory and neurodegenerative diseases (Gupta and Pulliam, 2014; Coleman and Hill, 2015; Madison and Okeoma, 2015; Welton et al., 2017). Few studies have characterized their role and function in the course of HIV infection (Sun et al., 2017; Chettimada et al., 2018; Guha et al., 2019).

In a work including HIV-uninfected and HIV-infected subjects (67% aviremic), CSF EVs were more abundant in HIV-infected compared to HIV-uninfected subjects, regardless of NCI status ($p < 0.0001$) and were more abundant in NCI ($p = 0.04$ and $p = 0.011$ for EVs and CSF, respectively) or HAND ($p < 0.0001$ and $p = 0.02$ for EVs and CSF, respectively) compared to unimpaired HIV-infected subjects (Guha et al., 2019). CSF EV concentrations also showed a positive correlation with NFL levels, while no correlations were found with S100B and neopterin (Guha et al., 2019). Although the study of EV seems promising, evidence to support their use in clinical practice is still missing.

Wnt Pathway

Wnts are a family of 19 highly conserved, small secreted glycoproteins that bind to the seven-transmembrane Frizzeled receptors and its co-receptor, LDL receptor-related proteins 5 and 6, to engage a signaling cascade that culminates in β-catenin-dependent or -independent signaling. The

Wnt pathway plays a critical role in cell communication, differentiation, and survival (Al-Harthi, 2012; Clevers and Nusse, 2012), and its dysregulation has been linked to neurodegenerative diseases, including Alzheimer's disease, Parkinson's disease, and amyotrophic lateral sclerosis (Al-Harthi, 2012; Purro et al., 2014). To date, few data are available on the signaling and regulation of Wnt pathway in the course of HIV infection and HAND. Previous studies found that Wnt/β-catenin was a restriction factor for HIV in astrocytes (Li et al., 2011; Narasipura et al., 2012; Richards et al., 2015), and inhibition of Wnt/β-catenin signaling influenced the glutamate uptake and metabolism in astrocytes (Lutgen et al., 2016). The Dickkopf-related protein 1 (DKK1) is a secreted soluble antagonist of the Wnt pathway that induces the rapid disassembly of synapses in mature neurons, and it mediates synaptic loss induced by Aβ (Purro et al., 2012). In HIV-infected subjects, DKK1 levels did differ with NCI (mean 813 pg/ml vs. 549 pg/ml, $p < 0.05$), particularly in PWH taking ART with HIV RNA levels ≤50 c/ml (Yu et al., 2017). Even if studies are still lacking in HIV, Wnt pathway regulates synaptic transmission and plasticity, and its study could provide a new understanding of some neuropathological processes in the course of HAND.

Mitochondrial DNA

Copy number of mtDNA in the brain and mitochondrial damage and mtDNA copy number within brain tissue have been correlated with a variety of neurodegenerative pathologies and aging. Moreover, considering the similarities of mtDNA with bacterial genomes, it acts as a "damage-associated molecular pattern" molecule, triggering toll-like receptor-9 activation and consequent inflammation. For all these reasons, quantity of mtDNA in CSF recently emerged as a biomarker of mitochondrial alteration and has been correlated with brain inflammation. Pérez-Santiago et al. (2016) first described an association between mtDNA levels in CSF and neurocognitive deficits in a group of 28 HIV+ subjects, most of which were not virologically suppressed neither in plasma nor in CSF at time of this cross-sectional analysis. Interestingly, a strong association was demonstrated between mtDNA in CSF and inflammatory markers, specifically IP-10 in CSF and Monocyte Chemo-Attractant Protein-1 (MCP-1) in plasma, in individuals with NCI, thus leading to the hypothesis that PWH with NCI may have inflammatory responses that differ from PWH without NCI and may also respond differently to the presence of mtDNA. A similar analysis was performed in the CHARTER population to determine the relationship between CSF mtDNA with CSF inflammatory markers, angiogenesis, iron transport, and HAND (Mehta et al., 2017). Interestingly, Mehta et al. (2017) found higher cell-free mtDNA levels in untreated PWH with detectable CSF HIV RNA. Even if these markers did not distinguish between PWH with or without NCI, mtDNA levels were higher in PWH with mild NCI as compared to asymptomatic subjects. There was also an association between CSF mtDNA and levels of interleukin-6 (IL-6) within the PWH group, even after adjustment for HIV RNA and CSF WBC. Moreover, levels of mtDNA correlated with lower levels of ceruloplasmin and transferrin, and the angiogenesis marker VEGF, after adjusting for the presence of HIV RNA and WBCs in CSF.

In a subsequent wok, Pérez-Santiago et al. (2017) analyzed the association between CSF, inflammation, and neurocognitive performance in PWH on long-term ART with persistent viral suppression in plasma. In this work, cell-free mtDNA in CSF samples has been inversely associated with peripheral and CSF inflammation [MCP-1 in CSF, and tumor necrosis factor-α (TNF-α) and IL-8 in plasma] under virologically effective ART (also after adjustment for past AIDS diagnosis). Indeed, contrary to the previous study, in this cohort of virally suppressed individuals, higher cell-free mtDNA levels within CSF supernatant were associated with better neurocognitive performance, as measured by the summary *T* score. Additionally, lower mtDNA in the CSF correlated with higher levels of NFL. Thus, in ART-treated PWH, a disequilibrium in cellular and mitochondrial function, similar to other neurodegenerative diseases such as Alzheimer's disease and Parkinson's disease, is recognized, which leads to mtDNA depletion, neuronal damage, and worse neurocognitive outcomes. Well-defined longitudinal studies will be needed to clarify the relationship between free mtDNA and neurocognitive outcomes during HIV suppression.

Another study approach focused on mtDNA is to define mitochondrial haplogroups, which have been shown to affect a range of HIV disease characteristics, including those potentially related to inflammation. Indeed, *in vitro* studies have shown that European mitochondrial haplogroups differ in expression and methylation of inflammation pathway genes. An analysis performed by Samuels et al. (2016) on participants from the CHARTER study who had genetic data and CSF samples showed no significant associations of any of the four measured CSF cytokines (IL-6, IL-8, IP-10, and TNF-α) with mitochondrial haplogroup in participants of African or Hispanic ancestry. However, in the subgroup of participants of European ancestry with suppressed plasmatic HIV-RNA viremia, the common haplogroup H had significantly lower CSF TNF-α levels (Samuels et al., 2016).

MARKERS OF INFLAMMATION

During ART-mediated viral suppression, the dominant hypothesis for ongoing brain dysfunction has been linked to persistent inflammation. Following the introduction of ART, a sharp decrease of systemic inflammation has been demonstrated but not with resolution to normal levels. We summarized increasing evidence of the association between markers of inflammation and NCI (**Table 2**).

Monocyte Chemo-Attractant Protein (MCP-1)

Among the most studied biomarkers of inflammation, MCP-1 is a chemokine produced by a number of cells constitutively or after oxidative stress (including activated microglia and astrocytes) and, by regulating migration and infiltration of monocytes/macrophages, contributes to neuroinflammation and

TABLE 2 | Biomarkers of inflammation and correlation with NCI in people living with HIV.

Biomarker	Body fluid	Findings	Research gaps	Reference
MCP-1	CSF	Shown to correlate with change in NCI performance in mostly treated PWH; found to be higher in PWH with NCI compared to non-NCI; shown to be higher than plasma MCP-1 in PWH with NCI; elevated at baseline in HIV suppressed individuals with NCI switching therapy.	Lack of randomized trials; Lack of strong longitudinal data; Lack of studies conducted on large numbers of HIV suppressed individuals.	Marcotte et al. (2013), Yuan et al. (2013), Tiraboschi et al. (2015) and Yuan et al. (2015)
	PLASMA	MRI studies show correlation with subcortical injury; shown to be lower than CSF MCP-1 in PWH with NCI and shown not to correlate with NCI.	Inconclusive data; Lack of randomized trials; Lack of studies conducted on large numbers of HIV suppressed individuals.	Ragin et al. (2006)
TNF alpha	CSF	Shown to decrease in 24 weeks in suppressed PWH with NCI after switch to an ART regimen with high neuropenetration; Levels found to be slightly lower in PWH having started ART early compared to late ART.	Lack of randomized trials; Limited population numbers.	Tiraboschi et al. (2015) and Oliveira et al. (2017)
IL-6	CSF	Levels found to be slightly lower in PWH having started ART early compared to late ART; showed by one study to correlate to a reduced likelihood of NCI in PWH, both naïve and on ART.	Inconclusive data; Lack of randomized trials; Lack of longitudinal studies; Lack of studies conducted on large numbers of HIV suppressed individuals	Oliveira et al. (2017) and Kallianpur et al. (2018)
IP-10/CXCL10	CSF	Found to be higher in PWH with NCI compared to non-NCI; higher levels in ART-treated PWH with NCI than in untreated PWH with NCI.	Lack of randomized trials; Lack of longitudinal studies.	Yuan et al. (2013) and Yuan et al. (2015)
	PLASMA	Found to be higher in PWH with NCI compared to non-NCI; plasma levels shown to decrease in a study investigating the use of paroxetine and fluconazole for the treatment of HAND.	Lack of longitudinal studies; viability as a biomarker in clinical practice has yet to be tested.	Yuan et al. (2015) and Sacktor et al. (2018)
IL-8 or CXCL-8	CSF	Found to be higher in PWH with NCI compared to non-NCI; shown to be higher than plasma IL-8 in PWH with NCI; CSF levels shown to increase in a study investigating the use of paroxetine and fluconazole for the treatment of HAND.	Inconclusive data; Lack of longitudinal studies; Lack of studies conducted on large numbers of HIV suppressed individuals	Yuan et al. (2013) and Sacktor et al. (2018)
IFN-α	CSF	Found to negatively correlate with several individual and composite neuropsychological tests, despite lack of correlation with treatment status.	Lack of randomized trials; Lack of strong longitudinal data; Lack of studies conducted on large numbers of HIV suppressed individuals.	Anderson et al. (2017)
IL-16	Serum	Found to be associated with slower processing speed.	Lack of randomized trials; Lack of strong longitudinal data; Lack of studies conducted on large numbers of HIV suppressed individuals.	Okafor et al. (2017)
ICAM5	CSF	Found to be higher in PWH with NCI compared to non-NCI, and to correlate with disease progression in a small number of PWH.	Lack of randomized trials; Lack of strong longitudinal data; Lack of studies conducted on large numbers of HIV suppressed individuals.	Yuan et al. (2017)
	Plasma	Found to be higher in PWH with NCI compared to non-NCI, and to correlate with disease progression in a small number of subjects.		

TABLE 2 | (Continued)

Biomarker	Body fluid	Findings	Research gaps	Reference
Microbial translocation markers	PLASMA	LPS levels found to correlate with HAND in a subset of HCV-positive participants; LPS found to be a significant predictor of lower processing speed in ART suppressed heavy drinkers; BDG levels found to correlate to worse neurocognitive performance.	Lack of randomized trials; Lack of strong longitudinal data; Lack of studies conducted on large numbers of HIV suppressed individuals.	Vassallo et al. (2013), Hoenigl et al. (2016) and Monnig et al. (2017)
Growth factors	CSF	G-CSF found to be higher in PWH with NCI compared to non-NCI.	Lack of randomized trials; Lack of strong longitudinal data; Lack of studies conducted on large numbers of HIV suppressed individuals.	Yuan et al. (2015)
	PLASMA	CSF VEGF showed to have borderline association with GDS-defined NCI; ceruloplasmin and CSF haptoglobin levels associated to likelihood to develop NCI; G-CSF found to be higher in PWH with NCI compared to non-NCI.		Yuan et al. (2015) and Kallianpur et al. (2018)

Abbreviations: NCI, neurocognitive impairment; ART, antiretroviral therapy; CSF, cerebrospinal fluid; GDS, global deficit score; PWH, people with HIV.

injury (Deshmane et al., 2009; Rahimian and He, 2016). A work from 2006 investigated the relationship between biomarkers and MRI diffusion tensor imaging measurements of centrum semiovale, caudate, and putamen, which have been shown to correlate with cognitive status. In 11 ART-treated HIV-infected subjects, plasma MCP-1 levels correlated with subcortical injury (Ragin et al., 2006). A 2013 work aimed at investigating biomarkers within 98 HIV-infected individuals categorized according to neurocognitive performance (including "stably impaired" and "worsening"), of which 73% of PWH were on ART and 54% were virally suppressed. Linear regression identified that, among markers, only MCP-1 in CSF was associated with neurocognitive change. Models constructed with the aim of diagnosis showed that a combination of MCP-1 and TNF-α allowed classifying 100% of the subjects with stable impairment (Marcotte et al., 2013). In a 2013 preliminary study, Yuan et al. (2013) measured cytokine levels in the CSF of 107 HIV-infected PWH (43% of whom were on ART) with and without NCI through quantification bioassays. Cases with NCI demonstrated significantly higher levels of MCP-1 (along with IL-8 and IP-10; Yuan et al., 2013). In 2015, Yuan et al. (2015) compared cytokine levels in paired CSF and plasma samples from 85 HIV+ individuals (43% of whom were on ART) with or without NCI. The expression of MCP-1 was significantly higher in CSF compared to plasma, and more importantly, CSF MCP-1 was significantly higher among subjects with NCI, while plasma MCP-1 did not correlate with cognitive impairment (Yuan et al., 2015). In a 2015 prospective, single-arm pilot study by Tiraboschi et al. (2015), 12 ART suppressed PWH with NCI on a regimen including TDF/FTC/EFV were switched to ABC/3TC/MVC. All participants showed elevated MCP-1 levels (along with neopterin) in CSF at baseline, although no significant change in MCP-1 levels was detected after week 24 from switch to the regimen with high neuropenetration (Tiraboschi et al., 2015). In summary, CSF MCP-1 showed promising correlation to NCI in multiple independent studies with distinct endpoints and designs. However, most studies encompassed both untreated and treated PWH (with some of the latter still being viremic); therefore, the role of CSF MCP-1 as a viable biomarker for NCI in ART-suppressed PWH is yet to be assessed.

Tumor Necrosis Factor Alpha (TNF-α)

TNF-α is a proinflammatory cytokine that exerts homeostatic and pathophysiological roles in the CNS. TNF-α is released in large amounts by microglia in pathological conditions, and this production constitutes part of the neuroinflammatory response and has been associated with a number of neurological disorders (Olmos and Lladó, 2014). In the aforementioned 2015 prospective, single-arm pilot switch study by Tiraboschi et al. (2015), a statistically significant reduction in median TNF-α concentration in CSF was observed after a 24-week switch to an ART regimen with high neuropenetration; no significant differences were observed, taking other inflammatory markers into exam. Of note, median CSF HIV RNA decreased as well (all participants had suppressed plasma HIV RNA; Tiraboschi et al., 2015). In a study by Oliveira et al. (2017), paired blood and

CSF samples were collected from 16 HIV-infected individuals on suppressive "early" or "late" ART. Median CSF TNF-α levels were slightly but significantly lower in individuals on early ART compared to those who had initiated ART later. No difference was detected among groups for blood TNF-α (Oliveira et al., 2017).

In conclusion, there is limited but promising evidence in favor of TNF-α being associated with inflammation due to uncontrolled/residual viremia. Further studies are warranted.

Interleukin-6

IL-6, a mediator of the acute phase response, can be produced by astrocytes exposed to HIV (Nitkiewicz et al., 2017). Lower IL-6 levels in CSF have been observed in individuals who had started ART early compared to those who had initiated ART later in a work by Oliveira et al. (2017). No difference was detected among groups for plasma IL-6 concentration. These data supported the concept that early ART initiation reduces at least some inflammation mediators in CSF. A possible effect of IL-6 on CSF HIV DNA molecular diversity was also explored but no mediation effect was observed (Oliveira et al., 2017). In a 2017 work investigating the relationship between CSF levels of proteins involved in iron transport and/or angiogenesis and neuropsychiatric impairment in 405 HIV-positive individuals (73% of subjects on ART, 46% of PWH were virally suppressed), CSF levels of IL-6 were not found to correlate with HAND. Of note, CSF IL-6 was shown to correlate to a reduced likelihood of impairment in 135 patients with mild-moderate comorbidity (Kallianpur et al., 2018). Despite promising reports, data concerning a possible role of CSF IL-6 in NCI of PWH are inconsistent. Further studies are needed to expand the current knowledge.

Interferon-γ-Inducible Protein (IP-10 or CXCL10)

IP-10 is a CXC or α-chemokine that acts on its receptor, CXCR3, to attract activated T cells, NK cells, and blood monocytes. A potent chemoattractant, it has been proposed to enhance retroviral infection and mediate neuronal injury. CSF IP-10 levels are known to correlate with CSF HIV-RNA and to decrease in subjects starting ART (Cinque et al., 2005). In the aforementioned 2013 preliminary study by Yuan et al. (2013) on 107 HIV-infected individuals, significantly higher levels of IP-10 (along with IL-8 and MCP-1) were found in the CSF of individuals with NCI compared to those without NCI. Interestingly, IP-10 was the only marker found to be associated with ART treatment, as CSF IP-10 was found to be higher in ART-treated PWH with NCI than in untreated PWH with NCI (Yuan et al., 2013). Again, in 2015, Yuan et al. (2015) compared cytokine levels in paired CSF and plasma samples from 85 HIV-infected individuals with or without NCI. Both CSF and plasma IP-10 were found to correlate with each other in the PWH cohort (Yuan et al., 2015). In 2018, Sacktor et al. (2018) published the results of a double-blind, placebo-controlled trial evaluating paroxetine and fluconazole for the treatment of HAND. Paroxetine was associated with improvement in a summary neuropsychological test measure, and in some—but not all—distinct neuropsychological tests. The authors investigated changes in biomarkers of cellular stress, inflammation, and neuronal injury over 24 weeks in response to treatment. Both paroxetine treatment alone and combined paroxetine/fluconazole treatment showed a decrease in plasma IP-10 levels compared to placebo (Sacktor et al., 2018).

In conclusion, a small number of independent studies with distinct designs and endpoints correlate IP-10 to NCI, interestingly, both as a plasma and CSF marker. IP-10 seems to be a reliable marker for NCI during ART, and correlation to a novel treatment for HAND has been described. However, viability as a biomarker in clinical practice has yet to be tested.

Interleukin-8 (IL-8 or CXCL-8)

Produced by macrophages and other cell types, IL-8 is the primary cytokine involved in neutrophil chemotaxis. In the cited 2013 and 2015 studies by Yuan et al. (2013, 2015). CSF levels of IL-8 were significantly higher in HIV-infected individuals with NCI compared to those without NCI. IL-8 levels were significantly higher in CSF than plasma levels (Yuan et al., 2013, 2015). On the other hand, while the 2018 paroxetine/fluconazole trial by Sacktor et al. (2018) suggest a beneficial effect of paroxetine on HAND, both paroxetine treatment alone and combined paroxetine/fluconazole treatment showed an increase in CSF IL-8/CXCL-8 levels compared to placebo. Therefore, despite promising reports, data concerning a possible role of CSF IL-8 in NCI of ART suppressed PWH is inconsistent.

Interferon Alpha

A renowned antiviral cytokine, interferon α (IFNα) has been found to be elevated in CSF of individuals with advanced HAD since the pre-combined ART era.

A 2016 cross-sectional study investigated the association between IFNα and neurocognitive performance, measured by an eight-test neuropsychological battery. Of 15 PWH, 60% were ART-experienced and 20% had undetectable viral load; CSF and plasma IFNα levels did not differ between treated and untreated or suppressed and non-suppressed PWH. CSF IFNα was found to negatively correlate with three individual tests and the composite test. Additionally, CSF IFNα correlated strongly with CSF NFL. Plasma IFNα did not show a significant correlation to cognitive performance (Anderson et al., 2017). While these results strongly suggest that CSF IFNα continues to play a role in HAND pathogenesis during the cART era, they pertain to a single study. Further works are needed to establish the correlation of IFNα and NCI in ART-suppressed PWH.

Interleukin-16

IL-16 is a pleiotropic cytokine acting as a chemoattractive and modulating factor of T cell activation. In a 2017 work aimed at determining the relationship between body mass index (BMI), HIV-associated NCI, and the potential mediating effects of inflammatory cytokines, 90 HIV-infected PWH (86.7% of whom were virally suppressed) were evaluated. Serum concentrations of IL-16 were significantly associated with slower processing speed, independently of BMI (Okafor et al., 2017). None of the other studies taken into consideration in the present review showed a significant correlation between IL-16 and NCI.

Further studies are needed to establish such a correlation in ART-suppressed PWH.

Intercellular Adhesion Molecule-5

Intercellular adhesion molecule-5 (ICAM5) is an ICAM expressed on neurons that may inhibit CNS T cell activation. Elevated levels of ICAM5 have been previously found in patients with brain injury (Guo et al., 2000; Di Battista et al., 2015).

Only one previous study, according to the selection criteria chosen for the present review article, addressed changes in ICAM5 in the HIV-infected population (Yuan et al., 2017). In that study, higher ICAM5 concentrations were found in PWH with NCI compared to PWH without impairment. Plasma and CSF ICAM5 levels showed a significant correlation to each other, and plasma ICAM5 significantly correlated with CSF S100B (Yuan et al., 2017). Moreover, high concentrations of plasma and CSF ICAM5 were found in PWH who developed NCI while levels did not change in individuals who did not develop any form of impairment. The change of plasma ICAM5 levels always corresponded with that in CSF (Yuan et al., 2017). Future studies will clarify the applicability of these preliminary findings in the HIV-infected population.

Eotaxin

Eotaxin is a chemokine that acts as a potent eosinophil chemoattractant and that, according to recent studies, may also contribute to degenerative processes in the CNS (Huber et al., 2018). However, only one study, among those selected for the present review article, addressed the evaluation of this biomarker, failing to determine any significant findings. In 85 HIV-infected subjects (43% of whom were on ART), eotaxin levels did not correlate with the diagnosis of NCI, neither in CSF nor in plasma (Yuan et al., 2015).

Microbial Translocation Markers

Chronic inflammation after ART introduction has been associated with microbial translocation with bacterial and fungal antigens across damaged gastrointestinal tract to drive systemic and CNS inflammation.

A component of the cell wall of gram-negative bacteria, lipopolysaccharide (LPS), can reach high plasma levels with translocation of microbial products across the intestinal mucosa into the peripheral circulation. LPS is suspected to trigger monocyte activation and to increase trafficking of infected cells into the brain (Epple et al., 2009). However, LPS measure is not easy to perform, as LPS assays are problematic because of blocking factors in bio-fluids and different types of LPS. Therefore, LPS cannot be measured in the standard ELISA format, and results of bioassays provide measures that are not fully comparable between different sites. In a work by Vassallo et al. (2013), LPS plasma levels were compared between 179 PWH with HAND and those with no HAND (87% of subjects on ART and 67% virally suppressed). A clear association was found between LPS levels and HAND in a subset of HCV-positive participants, while the association was non-significant among the HCV-negative group (LPS had previously been shown to be elevated in hepatitis C co-infection; Vassallo et al., 2013). LPS, along with its ligand sCD14, was also found to be a significant predictor of lower processing speed in a 2017 randomized clinical trial focused on alcohol intervention on ART-suppressed heavy drinkers living with HIV (Monnig et al., 2017).

1,3-β-D-glucan (BDG) is a component of most fungal cell walls and therefore is thought to be another useful indicator of gut mucosal barrier impairment. In a 2016 cross-sectional cohort study, levels of BDG were measured in plasma and CSF in 21 adults with acute/early HIV infection, started on ART during the earliest phase of infection with HIV RNA suppression. Higher plasma BDG levels were significantly related to higher GDSs, reflecting worse neurocognitive performance. Interestingly, CSF BDG was only found to be elevated in two individuals, those with the highest GDSs (Hoenigl et al., 2016).

In light of the wide body of work supporting the gut–brain barrier as a novel target in the ART era, LPS is a promising biomarker. LPS correlates with processing speed at least in a very specific subset of HIV-positive, ART-suppressed PWH. However, HCV co-infection represents a significant confounding factor and further studies on LPS and BDG are warranted in ART-suppressed PWH.

Growth Factors

Iron Transporters and VEGF

Iron is necessary for mitochondrial function, and its transport is thought to influence immune activation and angiogenesis (Cherayil, 2010; Saghiri et al., 2015); iron availability can be both related to HAND and neurodegenerative diseases (Bhatia and Chow, 2016; Edén et al., 2016). Altered angiogenesis, in particular, may lead to disruption of blood-brain barrier integrity in PWH, with consequent possibility of migration of activated immune cells into the CNS and development of inflammation and infection (Nightingale et al., 2014). In one single study satisfying inclusion criteria for the present review, VEGF levels and iron transporters (i.e., ceruloplasmin and aptoglobin) have been studied in relation to NCI in HIV (Kallianpur et al., 2018). Elevated CSF VEGF levels were associated with higher GDSs and with NCI, defined by GDS (Kallianpur et al., 2018). Moreover, aviremic PWH without neurological comorbidities and with higher ceruloplasmin levels were more likely to have GDS impairment. The same results were also found in PWH with higher CSF haptoglobin levels (Kallianpur et al., 2018). Despite those preliminary results, the authors of the study highlighted that the associations they found were not adjusted for multiple testing and required thus replication and further investigation (Kallianpur et al., 2018).

Fibroblast Growth Factors

Fibroblast growth factors (FGFs) are implicated in brain development and in neuroprotective functions. An alteration of FGF levels in CSF may be linked to neuronal injury and has been previously described in the course of amyotrophic lateral sclerosis (Johansson et al., 2003), moyamoya (Yoshimoto et al., 1997), and Alzheimer's disease (Mashayekhi et al., 2010).

FGF levels in CSF have been poorly studied in humans and, in particular, in the setting of HIV-infected subjects (Bharti et al., 2016). However, one study performed among 100 PWH (37% of whom were aviremic) failed to prove a consistent correlation between FGF-2 levels and cognitive disorders, while finding a correlation between lower FGF-1 levels and NCI (Bharti et al., 2016). The body of evidence regarding this marker in the clinical practice or in studies focused on NCI in the course of HIV is thus still scarce.

Granulocyte Colony-Stimulating Factor

Granulocyte colony-stimulating factor (G-CSF) is a hematopoietic growth factor that stimulates proliferation and differentiation of myeloid cells. However, G-CSF and its receptor are also expressed by neurons in many brain regions and recent studies suggested its role as a neurotrophic factor, as G-CSF has an anti-apoptotic function and stimulates neuronal differentiation in the brain (Schneider et al., 2005). In the context of HIV-related NCI, few studies have evaluated G-CSF levels. In a previous study performed in 85 HIV-infected subjects (43% of participants were on ART; Yuan et al., 2015), G-CSF levels did not differ significantly in plasma and CSF, indicating a possible reliability of blood measurement of this marker without the need of lumbar puncture. However, G-CSF levels were significantly higher in PWH with NCI compared to those who had no impairment, in both CSF (p = 0.0079) and plasma (p = 0.0191; Yuan et al., 2015). In another study evaluating a total of 107 CSF samples from PWH, G-CSF levels in the CSF were not different between ART-treated and untreated PWH but were higher in PWH with impaired cognition (Yuan et al., 2013).

Those preliminary results may suggest specificity in G-CSF levels in identifying PWH with HAND, also in the context of ART. However, no longitudinal studies are available to date and the evidence for its use remains very scarce.

IMMUNE ACTIVATION MARKERS

T Cell Activation

Considering the emerging role of inflammation as a contributing factor in neurological damage in the setting of ART-mediated virological suppression, well-characterized immune activation drivers have been explored as potential biomarkers of NCI during ART. Low CD4/CD8 ratio despite suppressive ART has been linked to immune activation and used to identify PWH with accelerated aging at risks of clinical events, including NCI. By evaluating the association of LPS levels with NCI, Vassallo et al. (2013) also considered CD4/CD8 ratio, which was significantly associated with NCI in HCV-negative subjects in univariate analysis. However, after considering age, proviral DNA, CD8 T cell count, and CD4/CD8 ratio in a logistic regression model, only age and proviral HIV-DNA resulted independently associated to NCI. In a subsequent work, Vassallo et al. (2013) explored the association between CD4/CD8 ratio, T-lymphocyte activation, and NCI in a large cohort (200 PWH) of virologically suppressed individuals on ART. They found that in ART-treated PWH on stable therapy for at least 3 years with virological suppression, a CD4/CD8 <1 resulted in an independent risk factor for symptomatic HAND (Vassallo et al., 2013). Moreover, a significant correlation between CD4/CD8 ratio and T-cell activation (measured by the number of CD4+CD38+HLADR+ T lymphocytes) was found, contributing to the evidence that CD4/CD8 ratio can be considered as a marker of chronic immune activation. A similar analysis was performed in MSM (men who have sex with men) Neurocog Study, in which 200 HIV-infected MSM PWH were screened for NCI and, after excluding people suffering from anxiety, depression or previous diagnosis of mood disorders, 20 were identified as potentially having NCI (Rawson et al., 2015). In this study, no significant difference in current, nadir or peak CD4 and CD8 counts, CD4/CD8 ratios, CD4/CD8 ratio inversion (<1), plasma viral load detectability, and peak plasma viral load were identified between subjects with NCI and the control group. Thus, until now, no definitive demonstration has been reached to define any significant benefit in monitoring CD8 T cells or CD4/CD8 T cell ratio inversion as an indicator of NCI.

Recently, Merlini and coauthors evaluated the effects of 12 months of virally suppressive ART on the peripheral and CSF pro-inflammatory milieu (Merlini et al., 2018). As expected, they found a decline in both plasma and CSF viral replication after 12 months of ART, and a simultaneous reduction in peripheral and CSF immune activation, measured by CD38+CD8+ cells, sCD14, IL-6, MCP-1, and IP-10. Interestingly, subjects with high pre-ART CSF/plasma HIV-RNA ratio maintained a skewed T cell homeostasis toward more effector/exhausted phenotype after ART introduction. In contrast, HIV people with low CSF/plasma HIV-RNA at baseline displayed a trend toward recovered peripheral CD4+ and CD8+ T cells phenotypes, thus suggesting that a lower pre-ART CSF viral burden and a subsequent viral suppression can prevent CNS invasion by HIV and consequent detrimental immune activation.

Monocyte/Macrophage Activation

Considering the role of the monocyte–macrophage lineage in the HIV-associated CNS disease, activation specifically involving these cells has been studied as a potential marker of neurocognitive damage during ART-mediated viral suppression.

Neopterin

Neopterin is a metabolite of guanosine triphosphate catabolism, and its increase in CSF is considered a marker of macrophage and microglial activation (Rahimian and He, 2016) and an independent predictor of CSF NFL levels (Jessen Krut et al., 2014). CSF neopterin levels are usually high in PWH who do not receive ART (Fuchs et al., 1989) and may decrease after ART initiation, possibly in parallel with improvement of neurocognitive function in the course of ART (Andersson et al., 2006). However, in certain individuals, some levels of immune activation may persist in the CNS also after the achievement of undetectable HIV-RNA levels, and the concentrations of CSF neopterin remain elevated for a long time also after having started ART (Edén et al., 2007; Yilmaz et al., 2013). In ART-treated PWH, neopterin level correlates with white matter hyperintensities that are in turn associated with neurological complications, including cognitive impairment (ρ = 0.321, p = 0.064; Trentalange et al., 2018). However, the direct correlation between neopterin levels and NCI in HIV-infected aviremic subjects is not univocal. In a recent work including 112 subjects (67% aviremic), neopterin was not an independent biomarker of baseline NCI status in multivariable linear regression models, adjusted for age, race, and plasma viral load (Guha et al., 2019). These findings corroborated the results of two previous studies, in which no correlation was found between CSF neopterin and GDS (Bharti et al., 2016; Pérez-Santiago et al., 2016). Both studies were limited by a relatively small sample size, and a large part of the study population had detectable HIV viremia. However, CSF neopterin levels were not found to be significantly different between neurocognitively normal, ANI, and MND PWH in another study conducted on a population of aviremic PWH (n = 37; Burdo et al., 2013). On the other hand, in that same study, higher levels of neopterin were found in PWH who were more impaired by GDS criteria than in those without cognitive impairment, and higher levels were also found in people with an executive domain impairment compared to others (Burdo et al., 2013). Similar results were reported in another recent study performed in aviremic PWH, in which CSF neopterin was higher in aviremic PWH with NCI compared to others (p = 0.04; Edén et al., 2016).

However, a study performed on 99 aviremic PWH followed up longitudinally did not prove a difference in the proportion of abnormal neopterin levels between PWH with or without a decline in the neurocognitive function (Edén et al., 2016). In another longitudinal evaluation, after persistent undetectable viremia, CSF neopterin at second visit was significantly higher than at first visit after a median of 16 months, despite ART use and long-term viral suppression (p = 0.05, paired t-test; Burdo et al., 2013). Furthermore, no changes in neopterin levels were found in a longitudinal study evaluating ART switch to regimens with enhanced CNS penetrability (Tiraboschi et al., 2015), neither in PWH initiating paroxetine in a double-blind trial, in which paroxetin use correlated with improvement in neurocognitive function (Sacktor et al., 2018). The correlation of CSF neopterin levels and scores of different neuropsychological tests has also been evaluated in aviremic PWH. Higher levels of neopterin were correlated with poorer results on forward Corsi Block Tapping Test (r = −0.474; p = 0.004), backward Corsi Block Tapping Test (r = −0.468; p = 0.005), forward Digit test (r = -0.480; p = 0.004), Verbal Fluency test (r = −0.361; p = 0.033), Raven's Standard Progressive Matrices test (r = −0.308; p = 0.071), the time estimation during the Test of Weights and Measures Estimation (r = −0.295; p = 0.085) and the Test of Weights and Measures total score (r = −0.294; p = 0.087; Ceccarelli et al., 2017). In conclusion, while neopterin CSF levels might be considered a reliable marker of macrophage and microglial activation and a predictor of worse performance in some cognitive domains, its use in the longitudinal follow-up of aviremic PWH is not sustained by current evidence. Further studies, possibly combining the evaluation of many biomarkers of immune activation and neuronal injury, could help improve its utility in the definition and diagnosis of neurologic disorders in the course of HIV.

Soluble CD14

Soluble CD14 (sCD14) is the soluble form of the monocyte LPS receptor, cleaved and released from the membrane after monocyte activation (McGuire et al., 2015). In a 2011 study by Lyons et al. (2011), relationships between plasma sCD14, CCL2, and LPS levels and neurocognitive test scores were investigated in 97 HIV-infected subjects. Plasma sCD14 levels were higher in subjects with test scores indicating global impairment, particularly in attention and learning domains, regardless of HAND diagnosis. The authors suggest such results imply the involvement of cortical and limbic pathways by inflammatory processes in the cART era. Of note, individuals in the study population were on ART in 74% cases, of which 39% had undetectable plasma HIV RNA (Lyons et al., 2011). In 2017, a secondary analysis on a randomized clinical trial focused on alcohol intervention was published by Monnig et al. (2017) investigating the relationship between the gut–brain axis, HIV infection, and alcohol consumption. Blood samples and cognitive scores were obtained at baseline and 3-month follow-up of the trial from 21 HIV-positive, ART-suppressed, heavy drinkers. sCD14 (along with LPS) was found to be a significant predictor of lower processing speed (Monnig et al., 2017). In a 2018 work evaluating MRI white matter hyperintensity (WMH) in naive compared to treated HIV-infected individuals (n = 107), plasma sCD14 levels were weakly associated with WMH score; however, no consistent associations between plasma biomarkers, CSF biomarkers, and WMH scores were found. Of note, sCD14 levels were lower in treated PWH compared to naive individuals (Trentalange et al., 2018). In conclusion, there is evidence that plasma sCD14, a well-studied monocyte activation marker, correlates with processing speed at least in a very specific subset of ART-suppressed PWH. Promising data suggest a correlation with global impairment and MRI signal, but new studies are warranted involving aviremic PWH exclusively.

Soluble CD163

One of the most promising pathways, CD163, is released from macrophage surface and shed as soluble CD163 (sCD163) following activation and differentiation of monocyte and macrophages. It has been hypothesized that virologically suppressed PWH would show persistent activation of monocytes, which could be assessed by measuring sCD163 in blood, which would correlate with HAND. A 2013 longitudinal study by Burdo et al. (2013) on 34 ART-suppressed individuals showed that PWH with NCI by GDS metrics had higher plasma sCD163 than those who were not impaired. Interestingly, CSF sCD163 did not correlate to GDS. Such results were discussed to be consistent with persistent monocyte/macrophage activation in neurophysiologically impaired HIV-infected individuals despite virally suppressive ART (Burdo et al., 2013). In a 2015 study, the relationship between cell-free mtDNA in CSF and neurocognitive performance during HIV infection, CSF sCD163 was the sole soluble inflammatory biomarker whose levels trended toward being higher in PWH with NCI compared to those without NCI. Of note, only 45% PWH were on ART (33% with viremia below the threshold of detectability; Pérez-Santiago et al., 2016). Bryant et al. (2017) conducted a study in 2017 evaluating sCD163 levels in ante mortem plasma (n = 54) and CSF (n = 32) samples from 74 HIV-infected participants who donated their brains to research at autopsy. Higher plasma sCD163 was found to be associated with greater synaptodendritic damage and microglial activation in cortical and subcortical brain regions at autopsy. Despite this, interestingly, plasma sCD163 was showed not to have any correlation to HAND diagnosis and neuropsychological test performance. On another note, CSF sCD163 was not associated with any histological feature (Bryant et al., 2017). In conclusion, a group of diverse studies suggest that plasma sCD163 correlates with NCI in virologically suppressed ART-treated individuals and to neural damage in PWH, regardless of symptoms, and CSF sCD163 tends to be higher in PWH with NCI. Such results, albeit partly inconsistent, are promising and warrant further investigation.

Monocyte Phenotypes

A number of studies focused on different monocyte phenotypes in blood that may drive HAND neuropathogenesis. Specifically, HIV infection has been correlated to an expansion of CD14+ monocytes expressing CD16+: CD14++CD16+ (intermediate) and CD14+CD16++ (nonclassic) monocytes, reaching variable levels depending on the stage of disease and use of ART. As CD16+ monocytes express higher levels of cell migration markers (i.e., CXCR5, CXCR1, and integrin CD11b) and transmigrate across the blood-brain barrier more efficiently than CD16− cells, it has been suggested that such cells can be involved HAND pathogenesis. In a recent study, a trend toward lower proportions of circulating intermediate monocytes in PWH who displayed a significant decline in memory performance during ART-mediated viral suppression was shown, suggesting an increase of transmigration of this cell subset in the CNS (Fabbiani et al., 2017). In addition, PWH with a significant decline in memory performance over time had lower expression of surface CD163 on the subset of intermediate monocytes/macrophages, corresponding to a higher release of sCD163 (Fabbiani et al., 2017).

As activated macrophages secrete soluble factors potentially toxic to neurons, some authors focused on the measurement of cytokines, proteases, and other factors produced by these cells after stimulation. Cathepsin B, a factor secreted by macrophages, has been described as a protease linked to neuronal apoptosis and inflammation. Moreover, cathepsin B, together with cystatins B and C has been shown to be overexpressed by HIV-infected monocyte-derived macrophages (MDMs). In a study conducted on a population of mostly ART-treated (>80%) HIV women, Cantres-Rosario et al. (2013) showed a significantly higher proportion of intracellular cathepsin-B and cystatin B in CD14+ cells of HIV+ subjects with HAD compared to subjects without neurological impairment. Additional analyses on the same study evaluating cathepsin B levels and activity together with cystatin C levels on monocytes did not reveal any difference between HAD subjects and controls. Taken together, these studies suggest a role for monocyte subpopulation as candidate biomarkers and suggest new opportunities to target viral reservoirs within the CNS, thus reducing neuroinflammation, neuronal damage, and cognitive impairment.

OMICS APPROACH TO NCI MARKERS RESEARCH

Genomics

Considering that not all HIV-infected subjects develop some form of neurocognitive disorder, the study of genetic factors that could possibly predispose to neurologic disease has attracted increasing interest and some studies aimed at characterizing the genetic profile of HIV-infected individuals at increased risk for HAND. CCL3L1, a potent ligand for CCR5 receptor and chemoattractant for macrophages, displays significant copy number differences among different ethnic groups. In this regard, Gonzalez et al. (2005) reported that the risk of AIDS events, including NCI, was higher when CCL3L1 chemokine gene copy was lower than the average of the same ethnic group, together with CCR5 detrimental alleles. A subsequent study performed by Brown et al. (2012) confirmed previous data about differences in CCL3L1 median copy number between various ethnicities; however, CCL3L1 copy number was similar in patients infected with HIV who had any form of HAND and in those who did not. Levine et al. (2016) in a very comprehensive study quantified multiple histopathological markers, genotyped genes associated with risk of NCI, and measured HIV-RNA in brain tissues. In this multilevel analysis, they found that MAP2 and SYP, which are two markers of synaptodendritic integrity, showed the more robust correlation with HAND with global pre-mortem cognitive function and with HIV-RNA viral load in the same regions. Moreover, a concomitant increase of Aβ and Iba-1 (ionized calcium-binding adaptor molecule-1) was evidenced as HIV-RNA increased, suggesting dysfunctional protein clearance and neuroinflammation. Genetic markers that predicted histopathology included MIP1-α and DRD3 genotype that are predictors of Iba-1 immunoreactivity, IL1-α genotype that predicted GFAP (glial fibrillary acidic protein) immunoreactivity, and ApoE genotype that predicted Aβ immunoreactivity. These data seem to support a pathogenetic model in which CNS HIV replication represents one of the main drivers for neuroinflammation and abnormal clearance. As a consequence, synaptodendritic degeneration occurs, leading to NCI of proteins. Genetic polymorphisms in genes encoding cytokines and chemokines and neuronal protein clearance pathways could influence histopathological degeneration.

Transcriptomics

Levine et al. (2013) in the last years applied a new research approach by examining the comprehensive gene expression of blood monocytes, with the aim of identifying the transcriptional changes possibly linked to HIV-associated NCI. Specifically aiming to describe peripheral molecular genetic mechanisms favoring the development of HAND, they firstly described that dysregulation of Kelch-like ECH-associated protein-1 (KEAP1), hypoxia upregulated-1, and IL-6 receptor, implicating oxidative stress, constituted a possible underlying pathogenic process. In a recent work published in 2018 (Quach et al., 2018), they further expanded these observations by validating the original findings in an independent sample of participants from the Multicenter AIDS Cohort Study (MACS) and determined whether gene expression changes evaluated at baseline could predict NCI at 2-years of follow-up. Contrary to what is expected, results from this new study did not replicate observation from their previous analysis and gene expression profiles at baseline were not predictive of neurocognitive decline in the following 2 years. Considering the inconsistency of these two observations, we have no evidence that gene expression profiles of monocytes can constitute a reliable biomarker of HAND.

Proteomics and Metabolomics

Multiplex mass spectrometry-based approaches allow the analysis of multiple samples in a single experiment. MS techniques make it possible to study a multitude of proteins and their differential level of expression at the same time in the course of CNS diseases. PWH with HAND have been compared to PWH without HAND and to uninfected controls (Bora et al., 2014) using proteomics approach, studying 193 different proteins. A cut-off of 1.5-fold was used to define protein upregulation. Five proteins among those previously described as HIV-interacting proteins were found to be upregulated in PWH with HAND: endoplasmin, mitochondrial damage mediator-BH3-interacting domain death agonist, orosomucoid, APOE, and metalloproteinase inhibitor 2. On the contrary, using a cut-off of 0.6-fold to measure downregulation, peroxiredoxin-2 isoform, a ruvB-like 2 protein, had lower expression in HAND (Bora et al., 2014). Untargeted CSF metabolite profiling was also used with the aim of identifying an altered metabolic path that can be linked to HAND. Neurotransmitter production, mitochondrial function, oxidative stress, and metabolic waste were studied (Cassol et al., 2014). CSF metabolites of ART-treated PWH with HAND were compared to unimpaired patients with similar demographic characteristics. Despite the metabolite expression being similar in the two groups after multiple testing correction, recursive support vector machine (SVM) classification models identified eight metabolites (including glutamate, myo-inositol, beta-hydroxybutyric acid, 1,2-propanediol) capable of discriminating the presence of HAND with an accuracy that exceeded 85%. Glutamate and N-acetylaspartate of myo-inositol and ketone bodies (beta-hydroxybutyric acid, 1,2-propanediol) showed increased levels in HAND and also had a correlation with lower scores in neurocognitive tests, plasmatic markers of inflammation, and intrathecal interferon responses (Cassol et al., 2014). The profile of the biomarkers that have been delineated in this study highlights how, also in the absence of detectable HIV-RNA, an abnormal synthesis of neurotransmitters, glial activation, altered mitochondrial function, and accumulation of metabolic waste products may all be driving forces for the development of HAND. While further validation is needed, proteomics and metabolomics studies show the potential of identifying new biomarkers and cluster of biomarker expression in different neurocognitive disorders that could potentially give new evidence about this new promising approach.

MicroRNA

MicroRNAs (miRNAs) have been abundantly demonstrated in the brain, where they regulate synaptic plasticity and brain development, implying that miRNA dysregulation may parallel neurocognitive dysfunction. First, a study on HIV subjects compared miRNA profiling on tissue from frontal cortex and CSF in PWH with or without HAND to healthy controls (Pacifici et al., 2013). In this article, the authors showed a different expression of 66 miRNA in CSF, of which 35 were also found in the frontal cortex. Specifically, they identified four miRNA with identical expression in tissue in CSF and one miRNA 20-fold higher expressed in CSF compared to brain tissue. Analysis of significantly altered miRNA showed their role in remodeling of cytoskeleton, cellular adhesion, expression of chemokine, neurogenesis, axonal guidance, notch signaling, synaptogenesis, and nerve impulses.

In a pilot study by Kadri et al. (2015), a plasma miRNA signature was associated with NCI in a cohort of PWH cared at LSU Health Sciences Center (LSUHSC) HIV Outpatient Clinic (HOP). As they did not consider alcohol consumption in this study, they later analyzed the miRNA profiling in the setting of alcohol use disorders in newly recruited PLWHA at the LSUHSC HOP clinic (Wyczechowska et al., 2017). They found that alcohol use disorders can represent a confounding factor for miRNA profile linked to HAND. Moreover, they confirmed their previous analysis using plasma samples from the CHARTER study and, also considering differences in the two, they validated a miRNA profile including 15 miRNA pairs that differentiate cognitively impaired PWH in both sites, LSUHSC and CHARTER.

Evidence from these studies, despite the many variables affecting circulating miRNA and thus encoding as potential confounders, could serve as a rationale for the development of novel tools for diagnosis and monitoring of HAND.

CONCLUSIONS

In the modern ART era, considering the benefit in life expectancy of PWH, it is crucial to reassess the pathogenesis of HAND and the influence of age, ART, and comorbidities. Several studies have been performed to identify quantitative CSF/blood biomarkers for HAND; however, many gaps remain to be addressed: (i) most studies are cross-sectional, thus lacking to demonstrate a predictive role for the biomarkers associated with NCI; (ii) NCI classification is often analyzed as classical categories (ANI, MND, and HAD), thus losing the possibility to define markers associated with the evolution of individual cognitive performance; (iii) a minority of works evaluated the effect of optimized ART on possible CSF/blood biomarkers associated to different neurocognitive behavior, thus lacking information on the potential use of these markers to guide ART use and selection.

Use of an approach aimed to explore multiple biomarkers could help clarify the most critical gaps in current HIV research, and it is likely that omics approaches (transcriptomics, proteomics, and metabolics) will accelerate HAND biomarker discovery and validation with a possible impact on the development of adjunctive treatment and monitoring of CNS disease.

AUTHOR CONTRIBUTIONS

AB, LT and GB: conception and design of study, database creation, acquisition of data, drafting of article and critical revision of the final manuscript. AM, JR, TB and AG: drafting of article and critical revision of the manuscript. All authors gave final approval to the submitted manuscript.

FUNDING

This research did not receive any specific grant from funding agencies in the public, commercial, or not-for-profit sectors.

REFERENCES

Abassi, M., Morawski, B. M., Nakigozi, G., Nakasujja, N., Kong, X., Meya, D. B., et al. (2017). Cerebrospinal fluid biomarkers and HIV-associated neurocognitive disorders in HIV-infected individuals in Rakai, Uganda. *J. Neurovirol.* 23, 369–375. doi: 10.1007/s13365-016-0505-9

Abdulle, S., Mellgren, A., Brew, B. J., Cinque, P., Hagberg, L., Price, R. W., et al. (2007). CSF neurofilament protein (NFL)—A marker of active HIV-related neurodegeneration. *J. Neurol.* 254, 1026–1032. doi: 10.1007/s00415-006-0481-8

Al-Harthi, L. (2012). Wnt/β-catenin and its diverse physiological cell signaling pathways in neurodegenerative and neuropsychiatric disorders. *J. Neuroimmune Pharmacol.* 7, 725–730. doi: 10.1007/s11481-012-9412-x

Anderson, A. M., Easley, K. A., Kasher, N., Franklin, D., Heaton, R. K., Zetterberg, H., et al. (2018). Neurofilament light chain in blood is negatively associated with neuropsychological performance in HIV-infected adults and declines with initiation of antiretroviral therapy. *J. Neurovirol.* 24, 695–701. doi: 10.1007/s13365-018-0664-y

Anderson, A. M., Lennox, J. L., Mulligan, M. M., Loring, D. W., Zetterberg, H., Blennow, K., et al. (2017). Cerebrospinal fluid interferon α levels correlate with neurocognitive impairment in ambulatory HIV-Infected individuals. *J. Neurovirol.* 23, 106–112. doi: 10.1007/s13365-016-0466-z

Andersson, L. M., Hagberg, L., Rosengren, L., Fuchs, D., Blennow, K., and Gisslén, M. (2006). Normalisation of cerebrospinal fluid biomarkers parallels improvement of neurological symptoms following HAART in HIV dementia—Case report. *BMC Infect. Dis.* 6:141. doi: 10.1186/1471-2334-6-141

Antinori, A., Arendt, G., Becker, J. T., Brew, B. J., Byrd, D. A., Cherner, M., et al. (2007). Updated research nosology for HIV-associated neurocognitive disorders. *Neurology* 69, 1789–1799. doi: 10.1212/01.WNL.0000287431.88658.8b

Bertram, L., Lange, C., Mullin, K., Parkinson, M., Hsiao, M., Hogan, M. F., et al. (2008). Genome-wide association analysis reveals putative Alzheimer's disease susceptibility loci in addition to APOE. *Am. J. Hum. Genet.* 83, 623–632. doi: 10.1016/j.ajhg.2008.10.008

Bharti, A. R., Woods, S. P., Ellis, R. J., Cherner, M., Rosario, D., Potter, M., et al. (2016). Fibroblast growth factors 1 and 2 in cerebrospinal fluid are associated with HIV disease, methamphetamine use, and neurocognitive functioning. *HIV AIDS* 8, 93–99. doi: 10.2147/hiv.s93306

Bhatia, N. S., and Chow, F. C. (2016). Neurologic complications in treated HIV-1 infection. *Curr. Neurol. Neurosci. Rep.* 16:62. doi: 10.1007/s11910-016-0666-1

Blyth, B. J., Farhavar, A., Gee, C., Hawthorn, B., He, H., Nayak, A., et al. (2009). Validation of serum markers for blood-brain barrier disruption in traumatic brain injury. *J. Neurotrauma* 26, 1497–1507. doi: 10.1089/neu.2008-0738

Bora, A., Ubaida Mohien, C., Chaerkady, R., Chang, L., Moxley, R. IV., Sacktor, N., et al. (2014). Identification of putative biomarkers for HIV-associated neurocognitive impairment in the CSF of HIV-infected patients under cART therapy determined by mass spectrometry. *J. Neurovirol.* 20, 457–465. doi: 10.1007/s13365-014-0263-5

Brown, A., Sacktor, N., Marder, K., Cohen, B., Schifitto, G., Skolasky, R. L., et al. (2012). CCL3L1 gene copy number in individuals with and without HIV-associated neurocognitive disorder. *Curr. Biomark. Find.* 2012, 1–6. doi: 10.2147/cbf.s27685

Bryant, A. K., Moore, D. J., Burdo, T. H., Lakritz, J. R., Gouaux, B., Soontornniyomkij, V., et al. (2017). Plasma soluble CD163 is associated with postmortem brain pathology in human immunodeficiency virus infection. *AIDS* 31, 973–979. doi: 10.1097/qad.0000000000001425

Burdo, T. H., Weiffenbach, A., Woods, S. P., Letendre, S., Ellis, R. J., and Williams, K. C. (2013). Elevated sCD163 in plasma but not cerebrospinal fluid is a marker of neurocognitive impairment in HIV infection. *AIDS* 27, 1387–1395. doi: 10.1097/qad.0b013e32836010bd

Calcagno, A., Atzori, C., Romito, A., Vai, D., Audagnotto, S., Stella, M. L., et al. (2016). Blood brain barrier impairment is associated with cerebrospinal fluid markers of neuronal damage in HIV-positive patients. *J. Neurovirol.* 22, 88–92. doi: 10.1007/s13365-015-0371-x

Cantres-Rosario, Y., Plaud-Valentin, M., Gerena, Y., Skolasky, R. L., Wojna, V., and Melendez, L. M. (2013). Cathepsin B and cystatin B in HIV-seropositive women are associated with infection and HIV-1-associated neurocognitive disorders. *AIDS* 27, 347–356. doi: 10.1097/qad.0b013e32835b3e47

Cardenas, V., Meyerhoff, D., Studholme, C., Kornak, J., Rothlind, J., Lampiris, H., et al. (2009). Evidence for ongoing brain injury in human immunodeficiency virus- positive patients treated with antiretroviral therapy. *J. Neurovirol.* 15, 324–333. doi: 10.1080/13550280902973960

Cassol, E., Misra, V., Dutta, A., Morgello, S., and Gabuzda, D. (2014). Cerebrospinal fluidmetabolomics reveals altered waste clearance and accelerated aging in HIV patients with neurocognitive impairment. *AIDS* 28, 1579–1591. doi: 10.1097/qad.0000000000000303

Ceccarelli, G., Brenchley, J. M., Cavallari, E. N., Scheri, G. C., Fratino, M., Pinacchio, C., et al. (2017). Impact of high-dose multi-strain probiotic supplementation on neurocognitive performance and central nervous system immune activation of HIV-1 infected individuals. *Nutrients* 9:E1269. doi: 10.3390/nu9111269

Cherayil, B. J. (2010). Iron and immunity: immunological consequences of iron deficiency and overload. *Arch. Immunol. Ther. Exp.* 58, 407–415. doi: 10.1007/s00005-010-0095-9

Chettimada, S., Lorenz, D. R., Misra, V., Dillon, S. T., Reeves, R. K., Manickam, C., et al. (2018). Exosome markers associated with immune activation and oxidative stress in HIV patients on antiretroviral therapy. *Sci. Rep.* 8:7227. doi: 10.1038/s41598-018-25515-4

Cinque, P., Bestetti, A., Marenzi, R., Sala, S., Gisslen, M., Hagberg, L., et al. (2005). Cerebrospinal fluid interferon-γ-inducible protein 10 (IP-10, CXCL10) in HIV-1 infection. *J. Neuroimmunol.* 168, 154–163. doi: 10.1016/j.jneuroim.2005.07.002

Clevers, H., and Nusse, R. (2012). Wnt/β-catenin signaling and disease. *Cell* 149, 1192–1205. doi: 10.1016/j.cell.2012.05.012

Coleman, B. M., and Hill, A. F. (2015). Extracellular vesicles—Their role in the packaging and spread of misfolded proteins associated with neurodegenerative diseases. *Semin. Cell Dev. Biol.* 40, 89–96. doi: 10.1016/j.semcdb.2015.02.007

Cysique, L. A., Hewitt, T., Croitoru-Lamoury, J., Taddei, K., Martins, R. N., Chew, C. S., et al. (2015). APOE ε4 moderates abnormal CSF-aβ-42 levels, while neurocognitive impairment is associated with abnormal CSF tau levels in HIV+ individuals—A cross-sectional observational study. *BMC Neurol.* 15:51. doi: 10.1186/s12883-015-0298-0

Deshmane, S. L., Kremlev, S., Amini, S., and Sawaya, B. E. (2009). Monocyte chemoattractant protein-1 (MCP-1): an overview. *J. Interferon Cytokine Res.* 29, 313–326. doi: 10.1089/jir.2008.0027

Di Battista, A. P., Buonora, J. E., Rhind, S. G., Hutchison, M. G., Baker, A. J., Rizoli, S. B., et al. (2015). Blood biomarkers in moderate-to-severe traumatic brain injury: potential utility of a multi-marker approach in characterizing outcome. *Front. Neurol.* 6:110. doi: 10.3389/fneur.2015.00110

Du Pasquier, R. A., Jilek, S., Kalubi, M., Yerly, S., Fux, C. A., Gutmann, C., et al. (2013). Marked increase of the astrocytic marker S100B in the cerebrospinal fluid of HIV-infected patients on LPV/r-monotherapy. *AIDS* 27, 203–210. doi: 10.1097/qad.0b013e32835a9a4a

Edén, A., Marcotte, T. D., Heaton, R. K., Nilsson, S., Zetterberg, H., Fuchs, D., et al. (2016). Increased intrathecal immune activation in virally suppressed HIV-1 infected patients with neurocognitive impairment. *PLoS One* 11:e0157160. doi: 10.1371/journal.pone.0157160

Edén, A., Price, R. W., Spudich, S., Fuchs, D., Hagberg, L., and Gisslen, M. (2007). Immune activation of the central nervous system is still present after >4 years of effective highly active antiretroviral therapy. *J. Infect. Dis.* 196, 1779–1783. doi: 10.1086/523648

Epple, H. J., Schneider, T., Troeger, H., Kunkel, D., Allers, K., Moos, V., et al. (2009). Impairment of the intestinal barrier is evident in untreated but absent in suppressively treated HIV-infected patients. *Gut* 58, 220–227. doi: 10.1136/gut.2008.150425

Fabbiani, M., Muscatello, A., Perseghin, P., Bani, M., Incontri, A., Squillace, N., et al. (2017). Brief report: peripheral monocyte/macrophage phenotypes associated with the evolution of cognitive performance in HIV-infected patients. *J. Acquir. Immune Defic. Syndr.* 76, 219–224. doi: 10.1097/qai.0000000000001480

Farooqui, A. A., Horrocks, L. A., and Farooqui, T. (2007). Modulation of inflammation in brain: a matter of fat. *J. Neurochem.* 101, 577–599. doi: 10.1111/j.1471-4159.2006.04371.x

Fuchs, D., Chiodi, F., Albert, J., Asjö, B., Hagberg, L., Hausen, A., et al. (1989). Neopterin concentrations in cerebrospinal fluid and serum of individuals infected with HIV-1. *AIDS* 3, 285–288. doi: 10.1097/00002030-198905000-00006

Gisslén, M., Hagberg, L., Brew, B. J., Cinque, P., Price, R. W., and Rosengren, L. (2007). Elevated cerebrospinal fluid neurofilament light protein concentrations predict the development of AIDS dementia complex. *J. Infect. Dis.* 195, 1774–1778. doi: 10.1086/518043

Gisslén, M., Price, R. W., Andreasson, U., Norgren, N., Nilsson, S., Hagberg, L., et al. (2016). Plasma concentration of the neurofilament light protein (NFL) is a biomarker of CNS injury in HIV infection: a cross-sectional study. *EBioMedicine* 3, 135–140. doi: 10.1016/j.ebiom.2015.11.036

Gongvatana, A., Schweinsburg, B. C., Taylor, M. J., Theilmann, R. J., Letendre, S. L., Alhassoon, O. M., et al. (2009). White matter tract injury and cognitive impairment in human immunodeficiency virus-infected individuals. *J. Neurovirol.* 15, 187–195. doi: 10.1080/13550280902769756

Gonzalez, E., Kulkarni, H., Bolivar, H., Mangano, A., Sanchez, R., Catano, G., et al. (2005). The influence of CCL3L1 gene-containing segmental duplication on HIV-1/AIDS susceptibility. *Science* 307, 1434–1440. doi: 10.1126/science.1101160

Green, A. J., Giovannoni, G., Miller, R. F., Harrison, M. J., and Thompson, E. J. (1999). Cerebrospinal fluid S-100b concentrations in patients with HIV infection. *AIDS* 13, 139–140.

Guha, D., Mukerji, S. S., Chettimada, S., Misra, V., Lorenz, D. R., Morgello, S., et al. (2019). CSF extracellular vesicles and neurofilament light protein as biomarkers of CNS injury in HIV-infected patients on antiretroviral therapy. *AIDS* 33, 615–625. doi: 10.1097/qad.0000000000002121

Guo, H., Tong, N., Turner, T., Epstein, L. G., McDermott, M. P., Kilgannon, P., et al. (2000). Release of the neuronal glycoprotein ICAM-5 in serum after hypoxic-ischemic injury. *Ann. Neurol.* 48, 590–602. doi: 10.1002/1531-8249(200010)48:4<590::aid-ana5>3.3.co;2-z

Gupta, A., and Pulliam, L. (2014). Exosomes as mediators of neuroinflammation. *J. Neuroinflammation* 11:68. doi: 10.1186/1742-2094-11-68

Haughey, N. J., Cutler, R. G., Tamara, A., McArthur, J. C., Vargas, D. L., Pardo, C. A., et al. (2004). Perturbation of sphingolipid metabolism and ceramide production in HIV-dementia. *Ann. Neurol.* 55, 257–267. doi: 10.1002/ana.10828

Hoenigl, M., de Oliveira, M. F., Pérez-Santiago, J., Zhang, Y., Morris, S., McCutchan, A. J., et al. (2016). (1→3)-β-D-Glucan levels correlate with neurocognitive functioning in HIV-infected persons on suppressive antiretroviral therapy: a cohort study. *Medicine* 95:e3162. doi: 10.1097/MD.0000000000003162

Hoffman, P. N., Cleveland, D. W., Griffin, J. W., Landes, P. W., Cowan, N. J., and Price, D. L. (1987). Neurofilament gene expression: a major determinant of axonal caliber. *Proc. Natl. Acad. Sci. U S A* 84, 3472–3476. doi: 10.1073/pnas.84.10.3472

Huber, A. K., Giles, D. A., Segal, B. M., and Irani, D. N. (2018). An emerging role for eotaxins in neurodegenerative disease. *Clin. Immunol.* 189, 29–33. doi: 10.1016/j.clim.2016.09.010

Jessen Krut, J., Mellberg, T., Price, R. W., Hagberg, L., Fuchs, D., Rosengren, L., et al. (2014). Biomarker evidence of axonal injury in neuroasymptomatic HIV-1 patients. *PLoS One* 9:e88591. doi: 10.1371/journal.pone.0088591

Johansson, A., Larsson, A., Nygren, I., Blennow, K., and Askmark, H. (2003). Increased serum and cerebrospinal fluid FGF-2 levels in amyotrophic lateral sclerosis. *Neuroreport* 14, 1867–1869. doi: 10.1097/00001756-200310060-00022

Kadiu, I., Narayanasamy, P., Dash, P. K., Zhang, W., and Gendelman, H. E. (2012). Biochemical and biologic characterization of exosomes and microvesicles as facilitators of HIV-1 infection in macrophages. *J. Immunol.* 189, 744–754. doi: 10.4049/jimmunol.1102244

Kadri, F., LaPlante, A., De Luca, M., Doyle, L., Velasco-Gonzalez, C., Patterson, J. R., et al. (2015). Defining plasma microRNAs associated with cognitive impairment in HIV-infected patients. *J. Cell. Physiol.* 231, 829–836. doi: 10.1002/jcp.25131

Kallianpur, A. R., Gittleman, H., Letendre, S., Ellis, R., Barnholtz-Sloan, J. S., Bush, W. S., et al. (2018). Cerebrospinal fluid ceruloplasmin, haptoglobin and vascular endothelial growth factor are associated with neurocognitive impairment in adults with HIV infection. *Mol. Neurobiol.* 6, 3808–3818. doi: 10.1007/s12035-018-1329-9

Kazmierski, R., Michalak, S., Wencel-Warot, A., and Nowinski, W. L. (2012). Serum tight-junction proteins predict Hemorrhagic transformation in ischemic stroke patients. *Neurology* 79, 1677–1685. doi: 10.1212/wnl.0b013e31826e9a83

Knopman, D. S., Jack, C. R., Wiste, H. J., Weigand, S. D., Vemuri, P., Lowe, V., et al. (2012). Short-term clinical outcomes for stages of NIA-AA preclinical Alzheimer disease. *Neurology* 78, 1576–1582. doi: 10.1212/WNL.0b013e3182563bbe

Levine, A. J., Horvath, S., Miller, E. N., Singer, E. J., Shapshak, P., Baldwin, G. C., et al. (2013). Transcriptome analysis of HIV-infected peripheral blood monocytes: gene transcripts and networks associated with neurocognitive functioning. *J. Neuroimmunol.* 26, 96–105. doi: 10.1016/j.jneuroim.2013.09.016

Levine, A. J., Soontornniyomkij, V., Achim, C. L., Masliah, E., Gelman, B. B., Sinsheimer, J. S., et al. (2016). Multilevel analysis of neuropathogenesis of neurocognitive impairment in HIV. *J. Neurovirol.* 22, 431–441. doi: 10.1007/s13365-015-0410-7

Li, W., Henderson, L. J., Major, E. O., and Al-Harthi, L. (2011). IFN-γ mediates enhancement of HIV replication in astrocytes by inducing an antagonist of the β-catenin pathway (DKK1) in a STAT 3-dependent manner. *J. Immunol.* 186, 6771–6778. doi: 10.4049/jimmunol.1100099

Li, J., Liu, K., Liu, Y., Xu, Y., Zhang, F., Yang, H., et al. (2013). Exosomes mediate the cell-to-cell transmission of IFN-α-induced antiviral activity. *Nat. Immunol.* 14, 793–803. doi: 10.1038/ni.2647

Lutgen, V., Narasipura, S. D., Sharma, A., Min, S., and Al-Harthi, L. (2016). β-Catenin signaling positively regulates glutamate uptake and metabolism in astrocytes. *J. Neuroinflammation* 13:242. doi: 10.1186/s12974-016-0691-7

Lyons, J. L., Uno, H., Ancuta, P., Kamat, A., Moore, D. J., Singer, E. J., et al. (2011). Plasma sCD14 is a biomarker associated with impaired neurocognitive test performance in attention and learning domains in HIV infection. *J. Acquir. Immune Defic. Syndr.* 57, 371–379. doi: 10.1097/qai.0b013e3182237e54

Madison, M. N., and Okeoma, C. M. (2015). Exosomes: implications in HIV-1 pathogenesis. *Viruses* 7, 4093–4118. doi: 10.3390/v7072810

Marcotte, T. D., Deutsch, R., Michael, B. D., Franklin, D., Cookson, D. R., Bharti, A. R., et al. (2013). A concise panel of biomarkers identifies neurocognitive functioning changes in HIV-infected individuals. *J. Neuroimmune Pharmacol.* 8, 1123–1135. doi: 10.1007/s11481-013-9504-2

Mashayekhi, F., Hadavi, M., Vaziri, H. R., and Naji, M. (2010). Increased acidic fibroblast growth factor concentrations in the serum and cerebro-spinal fluid of patients with Alzheimer's disease. *J. Clin. Neurosci.* 17, 357–359. doi: 10.1016/j.jocn.2009.05.037

McGuire, J. L., Gill, A. J., Douglas, S. D., Kolson, D. L., and CNS HIV Anti-Retroviral Therapy Effects Research (CHARTER) group. (2015). Central and peripheral markers of neurodegeneration and monocyte activation in HIV-associated neurocognitive disorders. *J. Neurovirol.* 21, 439–448. doi: 10.1007/s13365-015-0333-3

McGuire, J. L., Gill, A. J., Douglas, S. D., Kolson, D. L., and CNS HIV Antiretroviral Therapy Effects Research (CHARTER) Group. (2016). The complement system, neuronal injury and cognitive function in horizontally-acquired HIV-infected youth. *J. Neurovirol.* 22, 823–830. doi: 10.1007/s13365-016-0460-5

McMurtray, A., Nakamoto, B., Shikuma, C., and Valcour, V. (2008). Cortical atrophy and white matter hyperintensities in HIV: the Hawaii Aging with HIV Cohort Study. *J. Stroke Cerebrovasc. Dis.* 17, 212–217. doi: 10.1016/j.jstrokecerebrovasdis.2008.02.005

Mehta, S. R., Pérez-Santiago, J., Hulgan, T., Day, T. R., Barnholtz-Sloan, J., Gittleman, H., et al. (2017). Cerebrospinal fluid cell-free mithocondrial DNA is associated with HIV replication, iron transport, and mild HIV-associated neurocognitive impairment. *J. Neuroinflammation* 14:72. doi: 10.1186/s12974-017-0848-z

Merlini, E., Iannuzzi, F., Calcagno, A., Bai, F., Trunfio, M., d'Arminio Monforte, A., et al. (2018). Peripheral and cerebrospinal fluid immune activation and inflammation in chronically HIV-infected patients before and after virally suppressive combination antiretroviral therapy (cART). *J. Neurovirol.* 24, 679–694. doi: 10.1007/s13365-018-0661-1

Mielke, M. M., Bandaru, V. V., McArthur, J. C., Chu, M., and Haughey, N. J. (2010). Disturbance in cerebral spinal fluid sphingolipid content is associated with memory impairment in subjects infected with the human immunodeficiency virus. *J. Neurovirol.* 16, 445–456. doi: 10.3109/13550284.2010.525599

Mok, V., and Kim, J. S. (2015). Prevention and management of cerebral small vessel disease. *J. Stroke* 17, 111–122. doi: 10.5853/jos.2015.17.2.111

Monnig, M. A., Kahler, C. W., Cioe, P. A., Monti, P. M., Mayer, K. H., Pantalone, D. W., et al. (2017). Markers of microbial translocation and immune activation predict cognitive processing speed in heavy-drinking men living with HIV. *Microorganisms* 5:E64. doi: 10.3390/microorganisms5040064

Narasipura, S. D., Henderson, L. J., Fu, S. W., Chen, L., Kashanchi, F., and Al-Harthi, L. (2012). Role of β-catenin and TCF/LEF family members in transcriptional activity of HIV in astrocytes. *J. Virol.* 86, 1911–1921. doi: 10.1128/jvi.06266-11

Niederhoffer, N., Levy, R., Sick, E., Andre, P., Coupin, G., Lombard, Y., et al. (2009). Amyloid β peptides trigger CD47-dependent mast cell secretory and phagocytic responses. *Int. J. Immunopathol. Pharmacol.* 22, 473–483. doi: 10.1177/039463200902200224

Nightingale, S., Winston, A., Letendre, S., Michael, B. D., McArthur, J. C., Khoo, S., et al. (2014). Controversies in HIV-associated neurocognitive disorders. *Lancet Neurol.* 13, 1139–1151. doi: 10.1016/S1474-4422(14)70137-1

Nitkiewicz, J., Borjabad, A., Morgello, S., Murray, J., Chao, W., Emdad, L., et al. (2017). HIV induces expression of complement component C3 in astrocytes by NF-κB-dependent activation of interleukin-6 synthesis. *J. Neuroinflammation* 14:23. doi: 10.1186/s12974-017-0794-9

Okafor, C. N., Kelso, N. E., Bryant, V., Burrell, L. E. II., Míguez, M. J., Gongvatana, A., et al. (2017). Body mass index, inflammatory biomarkers and neurocognitive impairment in HIV-infected persons. *Psychol. Health Med.* 22, 289–302. doi: 10.1080/13548506.2016.1199887

Oliveira, M. F., Chaillon, A., Nakazawa, M., Vargas, M., Letendre, S. L., Strain, M. C., et al. (2017). Early antiretroviral therapy is associated with lower HIV DNA molecular diversity and lower inflammation in cerebrospinal fluid but does not prevent the establishment of compartmentalized HIV DNA populations. *PLoS Pathog.* 13:e1006112. doi: 10.1371/journal.ppat.1006112

Olmos, G., and Lladó, J. (2014). Tumor necrosis factor α: a link between neuroinflammation and excitotoxicity. *Mediators Inflamm.* 2014:861231. doi: 10.1155/2014/861231

Pacifici, M., Delbue, S., Ferrante, P., Jeansonne, D., Kadri, F., Nelson, S., et al. (2013). Cerebrospinal fluid miRNA profile in HIV-encephalitis. *J. Cell. Physiol.* 228, 1070–1075. doi: 10.1002/jcp.24254

Pemberton, L. A., and Brew, B. J. (2001). Cerebrospinal fluid S-100β and its relationship with AIDS dementia complex. *J. Clin. Virol.* 22, 249–253. doi: 10.1016/s1386-6532(01)00196-2

Pérez-Santiago, J., De Oliveira, M. F., Var, S. R., Day, T. R. C., Woods, S. P., Gianella, S., et al. (2017). Increased cell-free mitochondrial DNA is a marker of ongoing inflammation and better neurocognitive function in virologically suppressed HIV-infected individuals. *J. Neurovirol.* 23, 283–289. doi: 10.1007/s13365-016-0497-5

Pérez-Santiago, J., Schrier, R. D., de Oliveira, M. F., Gianella, S., Var, S. R., Day, T. R., et al. (2016). Cell-free mitochondrial DNA in CSF is associated with early viral rebound, inflammation and severity of neurocognitive deficits in HIV infection. *J. Neurovirol.* 22, 191–200. doi: 10.1007/s13365-015-0384-5

Petersen, R. C., Wiste, H. J., Weigand, S. D., Rocca, W. A., Roberts, R. O., Mielke, M. M., et al. (2016). Association of elevated amyloid levels with cognition and biomarkers in cognitively normal people from the community. *JAMA Neurol.* 73, 85–92. doi: 10.1001/jamaneurol.2015.3098

Peterson, J., Gisslen, M., Zetterberg, H., Fuchs, D., Shacklett, B. L., Hagberg, L., et al. (2014). Cerebrospinal fluid (CSF) neuronal biomarkers across the spectrum of HIV infection: hierarchy of injury and detection. *PLoS One* 9:e116081. doi: 10.1371/journal.pone.0116081

Purro, S. A., Dickins, E. M., and Salinas, P. C. (2012). The secreted Wnt antagonist Dickkopf-1 is required for amyloid β-mediated synaptic loss. *J. Neurosci.* 32, 3492–3498. doi: 10.1523/JNEUROSCI.4562-11.2012

Purro, S. A., Galli, S., and Salinas, P. C. (2014). Dysfunction of Wnt signaling and synaptic disassembly in neurodegenerative diseases. *J. Mol. Cell Biol.* 6, 75–80. doi: 10.1093/jmcb/mjt049

Quach, A., Horvath, S., Nemanim, N., Vatakis, D., Witt, M. D., Miller, E. N., et al. (2018). No reliable gene expression biomarkers of current or impending neurocognitive impairment in peripheral blood monocytes of persons living with HIV. *J. Neurovirol.* 24, 350–361. doi: 10.1007/s13365-018-0625-5

Ragin, A. B., Wu, Y., Storey, P., Cohen, B. A., Edelman, R. R., and Epstein, L. G. (2006). Monocyte chemoattractant protein-1 correlates with subcortical brain injury in HIV infection. *Neurology* 66, 1255–1257. doi: 10.1212/01.wnl.0000208433.34723.65

Rahimian, P., and He, J. J. (2016). HIV/neuroAIDS biomarkers. *Prog. Neurobiol.* 157, 117–132. doi: 10.1016/j.pneurobio.2016.04.003

Rashed, H., Bayraktar, E., Helal, K., Abd-Ellah, M. F., Amero, P., Chavez-Reyes, A., et al. (2017). Exosomes: from garbage bins to promising therapeutic targets. *Int. J. Mol. Sci.* 18:E538. doi: 10.3390/ijms18030538

Rawson, T. M., Dubb, S., Pozniak, A., Kelleher, W. P., Mandalia, S., Gazzard, B., et al. (2015). Assessing the role of peripheral CD8 T cells in neurocognitive impairment in HIV-infected men who have sex with men: data from the MSM Neurocog Study. *Int. J. STD AIDS* 26, 128–132. doi: 10.1177/0956462414531934

Richards, M. H., Narasipura, S. D., Kim, S., Seaton, M. S., Lutgen, V., and Al-Harthi, L. (2015). Dynamic interaction between astrocytes and infiltrating PBMCs in context of neuroAIDS. *Glia* 63, 441–451. doi: 10.1002/glia.22763

Sacktor, N., Skolasky, R. L., Moxley, R., Wang, S., Mielke, M. M., Munro, C., et al. (2018). Paroxetine and fluconazole therapy for HIV-associated neurocognitive impairment: results from a double-blind, placebo-controlled trial. *J. Neurovirol.* 24, 16–27. doi: 10.1007/s13365-017-0587-z

Saghiri, M. A., Asatourian, A., Orangi, J., Sorenson, C. M., and Sheibani, N. (2015). Functional role of inorganic trace elements in angiogenesis—Part I: N, Fe, Se, P, Au, and Ca. *Crit. Rev. Oncol. Hematol.* 96, 129–142. doi: 10.1016/j.critrevonc.2015.05.010

Samuels, D. C., Kallianpur, A. R., Ellis, R. J., Bush, W. S., Letendre, S., Franklin, D., et al. (2016). European mitochondrial DNA haplogroups are associated with cerebrospinal fluid biomarkers of inflammation in HIV infection. *Pathog. Immun.* 1, 330–351. doi: 10.20411/pai.v1i2.156

Schneider, A., Kuhn, H. G., and Schäbitz, W. R. (2005). A role for G-CSF (granulocyte-colony stimulating factor) in the central nervous system. *Cell Cycle* 4, 1753–1757. doi: 10.4161/cc.4.12.2213

Schouten, J., Cinque, P., Gisslen, M., Reiss, P., and Portegies, P. (2011). HIV-1 infection and cognitive impairment in the cART era: a review. *AIDS* 25, 561–575. doi: 10.1097/qad.0b013e3283437f9a

Sperling, R. A., Aisen, P. S., Beckett, L. A., Bennett, D. A., Craft, S., Fagan, A. M., et al. (2011). Toward defining the preclinical stages of Alzheimer's disease:

recommendations from the national institute on aging and the Alzheimer's association workgroup. *Alzheimers Dement.* 7, 1–13. doi: 10.1016/j.jalz.2011.03.003

Steinbrink, F., Evers, S., Buerke, B., Young, P., Arendt, G., Koutsilieri, E., et al. (2013). Cognitive impairment in HIV infection is associated with MRI and CSF pattern of neurodegeneration. *Eur. J. Neurol.* 20, 420–428. doi: 10.1111/ene.12006

Sun, B., Dalvi, P., Abadjian, L., Tang, N., and Pulliam, L. (2017). Blood neuron-derived exosomes as biomarkers of cognitive impairment in HIV. *AIDS* 31, F9–F17. doi: 10.1097/qad.0000000000001595

Thery, C., Zitvogel, L., and Amigorena, S. (2002). Exosomes: composition, biogenesis and function. *Nat. Rev. Immunol.* 2, 569–579. doi: 10.1038/nri855

Tiraboschi, J. M., Muñoz-Moreno, J. A., Puertas, M. C., Alonso-Villaverde, C., Prats, A., Ferrer, E., et al. (2015). Viral and inflammatory markers in cerebrospinal fluid of patients with HIV-1-associated neurocognitive impairment during antiretroviral treatment switch. *HIV Med.* 16, 388–392. doi: 10.1111/hiv.12243

Trentalange, A., Prochet, A., Imperiale, D., Cusato, J., Tettoni, M., Nunnari, G., et al. (2018). Cerebral white matter hyperintensities in HIV-positive patients. *Brain Imaging Behav.* doi: 10.1007/s11682-018-9966-1 [Epub ahead of print].

Vassallo, M., Dunais, B., Durant, J., Carsenti-Dellamonica, H., Harvey-Langton, A., Cottalorda, J., et al. (2013). Relevance of lipopolysaccharide levels in HIV-associated neurocognitive impairment: the Neuradapt study. *J. Neurovirol.* 19, 376–382. doi: 10.1007/s13365-013-0181-y

Welton, J. L., Loveless, S., Stone, T., von Ruhland, C., Robertson, N. P., and Clayton, A. (2017). Cerebrospinal fluid extracellular vesicle enrichment for protein biomarker discovery in neurological disease; multiple sclerosis. *J. Extracell. Vesicles* 6:1369805. doi: 10.1080/20013078.2017.1369805

Wu, H., Brown, E. V., Acharya, N. K., Appelt, D. M., Marks, A., Nagele, R. G., et al. (2016). Age-dependent increase of blood-brain barrier permeability and neuron- binding autoantibodies in S100B knockout mice. *Brain Res.* 1637, 154–167. doi: 10.1016/j.brainres.2016.02.026

Wyczechowska, D., Lin, H.-Y., LaPlante, A., Jeansonne, D., Lassak, A., Parsons, C. H., et al. (2017). A miRNA signature for cognitive deficits and alcohol use disorder in persons living with HIV/AIDS. *Front. Mol. Neurosci.* 10:385. doi: 10.3389/fnmol.2017.00385

Yilmaz, A., Blennow, K., Hagberg, L., Nilsson, S., Price, R. W., Schouten, J., et al. (2017). Neurofilament light chain protein as a marker of neuronal injury: review of its use in HIV-1 infection and reference values for HIV-negative controls. *Expert Rev. Mol. Diagn.* 17, 761–770. doi: 10.1080/14737159.2017.1341313

Yilmaz, A., Yiannoutsos, C. T., Fuchs, D., Price, R. W., Crozier, K., Hagberg, L., et al. (2013). Cerebrospinal fluid neopterin decay characteristics after initiation of antiretroviral therapy. *J. Neuroinflammation* 10:62. doi: 10.1186/1742-2094-10-62

Yoshimoto, T., Houkin, K., Takahashi, A., and Abe, H. (1997). Evaluation of cytokines in cerebrospinal fluid from patients with moyamoya disease. *Clin. Neurol. Neurosurg.* 99, S218–S220. doi: 10.1016/s0303-8467(97)00047-4

Yu, C., Seaton, M., Letendre, S., Heaton, R., and Al-Harthi, L. (2017). Plasma Dickkopf-related protein 1, an antagonist of the Wnt pathway, is associated with HIV-associated neurocognitive impairment. *AIDS* 31, 1379–1385. doi: 10.1097/qad.0000000000001481

Yuan, L., Liu, A., Qiao, L., Sheng, B., Xu, M., Li, W., et al. (2015). The relationship of CSF and plasma cytokine levels in HIV infected patients with neurocognitive impairment. *Biomed. Res. Int.* 2015:506872. doi: 10.1155/2015/506872

Yuan, L., Qiao, L., Wei, F., Yin, J., Liu, L., Ji, Y., et al. (2013). Cytokines in CSF correlate with HIV-associated neurocognitive disorders in the post-HAART era in China. *J. Neurovirol.* 19, 144–149. doi: 10.1007/s13365-013-0150-5

Yuan, L., Wei, F., Zhang, X., Guo, X., Lu, X., Su, B., et al. (2017). Intercellular adhesion molecular-5 as marker in HIV associated neurocognitive disorder. *Aging Dis.* 8, 250–256. doi: 10.14336/ad.2016.0918

11

Moderating Effect of Cortical Thickness on BOLD Signal Variability Age-Related Changes

Daiana R. Pur[1], Roy A. Eagleson[1,2], Anik de Ribaupierre[3], Nathalie Mella[3] and Sandrine de Ribaupierre[1,4]*

[1] School of Biomedical Engineering, Western University, London, ON, Canada, [2] Department of Electrical and Computer Engineering, Western University, London, ON, Canada, [3] Department of Psychology, University of Geneva, Geneva, Switzerland, [4] Department of Clinical Neurological Sciences, Schulich School of Medicine, Western University, London, ON, Canada

Correspondence:
Daiana R. Pur
dpur@uwo.ca

The time course of neuroanatomical structural and functional measures across the lifespan is commonly reported in association with aging. Blood oxygen-level dependent signal variability, estimated using the standard deviation of the signal, or "$BOLD_{SD}$," is an emerging metric of variability in neural processing, and has been shown to be positively correlated with cognitive flexibility. Generally, $BOLD_{SD}$ is reported to decrease with aging, and is thought to reflect age-related cognitive decline. Additionally, it is well established that normative aging is associated with structural changes in brain regions, and that these predict functional decline in various cognitive domains. Nevertheless, the interaction between alterations in cortical morphology and $BOLD_{SD}$ changes has not been modeled quantitatively. The objective of the current study was to investigate the influence of cortical morphology metrics [i.e., cortical thickness (CT), gray matter (GM) volume, and cortical area (CA)] on age-related $BOLD_{SD}$ changes by treating these cortical morphology metrics as possible physiological confounds using linear mixed models. We studied these metrics in 28 healthy older subjects scanned twice at approximately 2.5 years interval. Results show that $BOLD_{SD}$ is confounded by cortical morphology metrics. Respectively, changes in CT but not GM volume nor CA, show a significant interaction with $BOLD_{SD}$ alterations. Our study highlights that CT changes should be considered when evaluating $BOLD_{SD}$ alternations in the lifespan.

Keywords: signal variability, BOLD fMRI, structural alterations, cortical morphology, aging, cortical thickness, neural processing, biomarker

INTRODUCTION

Normal aging is associated with marked functional and structural neuroanatomical alterations in cortical thickness (CT), gyrification, cortical surface area (CA), gray (GM), and white matter volume (WM) (Salat et al., 2009; Thambisetty et al., 2010; McGinnis et al., 2011; Hogstrom et al., 2013). Importantly, magnetic resonance imaging studies (MRI) show that the magnitude and rate of change of these cortical morphometry metrics is not constant across the cortex but rather it varies with age and brain region (Raz, 2005; Jiang et al., 2014; Storsve et al., 2014; Dotson et al., 2016), and is reported to accelerate with increasing age (Driscoll et al., 2009; Jiang et al., 2014). For example, a longitudinal study of alterations in cortical morphometry in older adults found accelerated changes with increasing age in temporal and occipital cortices (Storsve et al., 2014). Furthermore, other studies report that the temporal lobes are most vulnerable to age-related morphometric changes, and that these changes reflect age-related cognitive impairment (Singh et al., 2006; Fjell et al., 2009; Pacheco et al., 2015). There is considerable evidence that neuroanatomical alterations reflect underlying functional alterations, especially in cognition (Fjell et al., 2006; Rossini et al., 2007; Ziegler et al., 2010; Achiron et al., 2013). In fact, functional magnetic resonance imaging (fMRI) studies, which rely on the blood oxygen level-dependent (BOLD) signal as a correlate of neuronal activity, report that changes in cortical morphology across adult lifespan impact the hemodynamic properties of the brain. For example, there are cortical laminar differences in BOLD signal (Tian et al., 2010; Huber et al., 2015), thicker cortical regions were reported to have a lower relative oxygen extraction fraction (Zhao et al., 2016). Therefore, since aging is associated with significant neuroanatomical alterations, these should be considered when assessing function (i.e., cognitive ability) using the BOLD signal.

The Standard Deviation of the BOLD signal can be used to estimate variability (hereafter, "$BOLD_{SD}$"), and is believed to reflect the brain's dynamic ability to undergo fast moment-to-moment switching through network reconfigurations (Garrett et al., 2010, 2014; Grady and Garrett, 2014). It is an emerging index of cognitive health in aging, with higher regional $BOLD_{SD}$ being associated with enhanced performance on certain cognitive tasks (i.e., task switching) but not on others (i.e., distractor inhibition) (Armbruster-Genc et al., 2016; Guitart-Masip et al., 2016). Generally, increased $BOLD_{SD}$ is associated with younger age, faster and more consistent performance on cognitive tasks, and cognitive flexibility (Garrett et al., 2013a; Armbruster-Genc et al., 2016). The physiological mechanisms underlying $BOLD_{SD}$ remain largely unknown. For instance, decreased dopaminergic transmission is proposed to be associated with decreased $BOLD_{SD}$ in subcortical areas in older adults compared to younger ones (Guitart-Masip et al., 2016). Another study reported that higher $BOLD_{SD}$ is associated with superior pain coping capabilities (Rogachov et al., 2016). However, there are few studies investigating the interaction between age-related alterations in cortical morphology and $BOLD_{SD}$. One study reported that increased microstructural integrity of WM pathways is associated with greater $BOLD_{SD}$ (Burzynska et al., 2015). Given that neuroanatomical alterations associated with normative aging are known to influence cognitive performance, and that they influence the BOLD signal, their impact as physiological confounds to $BOLD_{SD}$ should be investigated. This is particularly relevant because there is a considerable degree of inconsistency of methods used and results across studies investigating $BOLD_{SD}$. In fact, some studies report greater regional $BOLD_{SD}$ in older adults (Garrett et al., 2010, 2011; Nomi et al., 2017), individuals with stroke (Kielar et al., 2016), multiple sclerosis (Petracca et al., 2017), Alzheimer disease (Makedonov et al., 2013, 2016; Scarapicchia et al., 2018) and other neurological disorders (Zöller et al., 2017).

The objective of this study is to investigate the contribution of cortical morphology (i.e., CT, CA, and GM volume) to age-related $BOLD_{SD}$ changes in older adults. A longitudinal framework, consisting of two scan points, should help reduce some of the inter-individual variance in neuroanatomy by accounting for external factors such as lifestyle, and various socio-economic and demographic factors. To this end, we investigated global and regional differences in $BOLD_{SD}$ in a group of older adults scanned twice at an interval of approximately 2.5 years, and regressed the effect of cortical morphology by introducing CT, CA, and GM as covariates. We hypothesized that cortical morphology metrics show an interaction with $BOLD_{SD}$. We predict that age-related neuroanatomical alterations in CT, CA, GM are physiological confounds to $BOLD_{SD}$ measures, and that consequently adjusting for these metrics may help "unmask" the functional relevance of $BOLD_{SD}$.

MATERIALS AND METHODS

Participants

All data obtained for the present study were obtained from the longitudinal Geneva Aging Study, after approval by the ethics committee of the Faculty of Psychology and Educational Sciences of the University of Geneva and the Swiss Ethic committee. Older subjects were initially recruited either from the University of the Third Age of Geneva or through newspaper and association advertisements for pensioners, as part of a larger longitudinal study. All participants gave written informed consent and older adults received a small amount of money as a compensation for their transportation fees.

Our initial sample consisted of 31 older adults scanned twice (mean age at first scan = 71.65 ± 6.03 years, mean age at second scan = 74.06 ± 5.99 years; 9 males). These subjects were chosen, within our pool, because they were the only ones that had undergone two T1 structural images and task fMRI scans, as well as other cognitive tests. Participants were screened for health problems with a questionnaire. The structural MRIs were inspected to rule out severe abnormalities (white matter changes, ventricular enlargement, tumors etc.). Three of the participants showed signs of Parkinson or lesion on their anatomical MRI, so they were excluded from the final sample (n = 28). All models and results in this current paper thus reflect 28 older adults (mean age at first scan = 71.61 ± 6.21 years, mean age at second scan = 74.07 ± 6 15 years; 7 males). The scans were 2.46 ± 0.69 years apart.

MRI Data Acquisition

Participants were scanned in a Siemens Trio 3T magnet. A BOLD fMRI task-rest sequence was administered using a reaction time paradigm, where the participant had to indicate on which side a cross was changing into a square, as fast as possible (Mella et al., 2013). The task consisted of eight experimental blocks, interspersed with eight resting blocks (respectively, 52–20 s). The BOLD activity was obtained using an echo planar imaging acquisition (echo time, TE = 30 ms, time repetition, TR = 2100 ms, flip angle = 80°, field of view, FOV = 205 mm). Then, a structural T1-weighted MRI was acquired (TE = 2.27 ms, TR = 1900 ms, FOV = 256 mm, voxel size 1.0 mm × 1.0 mm × 1.0 mm).

Structural Data Processing

Structural T1-weighted MR images were analyzed using Freesurfer version 6.0, a widely used and freely available automated processing pipeline[1], which allows surface-based three dimensional reconstruction and quantification of cortical morphology. The standard steps for analysis were implemented (using "recon-all" pipeline with the default set of parameters). Regional measures of GM, CT, and CA for each hemisphere were obtained using the automated anatomic parcellation procedure. Technical details are found in prior publications (Dale et al., 1999; Fischl et al., 1999a,b, 2001; Fischl and Dale, 2000; Zhang et al., 2001; Salat et al., 2004; Winkler et al., 2012). In brief, T1-weighted images underwent preprocessing steps including motion correction, brain extraction, intensity normalization, and Talairach transformation (Sled et al., 1998; Smith, 2002; Ségonne et al., 2004; Reuter et al., 2010). GM and WM surface boundaries were reconstructed to estimate the distance between them across the cortex (Fischl and Dale, 2000). The generated cortical models were inflated into spheres to be registered to a spherical atlas and parcellated into regions of interest using Destrieux atlas (Fischl and Dale, 2000; Segonne et al., 2007; Destrieux et al., 2010).

Functional Data Processing

Processing of the functional data were performed using FSL version 5.0 (Analysis Group, FMRIB, Oxford, United Kingdom (Smith et al., 2004). Standard preprocessing were followed using FSL's FEAT and FSL's Melodic for functional data (Jenkinson et al., 2012). Briefly, for each participant preprocessing steps included motion correction, slice timing, spatial normalization, highpass temporal filtering (100 s), smoothing (kernel 5 mm FWHM), and linear registration (12 degrees of freedom) of the functional data to the high-resolution T1 structural image, and from T1 to 1 mm standard space (MNI 152). Additionally, FSL's Melodic was used to correct each functional image for artifacts using automatic dimensionality estimation via independent component analysis (ICA) (Beckmann and Smith, 2004). Change in cortical morphology between the two scanning sessions was determined as cortical morphology metrics GM (delta.volume), CT (delta.thickness), CA (delta.area) at timepoint 2–at timepoint 1.

BOLD Signal Variability Calculation

As part of the Geneva Dataset, the subjects were performing different cognitive tasks, and for the current study, only the fixation/rest blocks from the block design task fMRI were selected to calculate BOLD$_{SD}$, as previously described (Garrett et al., 2010). BOLD$_{SD}$ analysis was restricted to the GM using participant specific GM mask obtained from FSL's FAST. First, fixation blocks were normalized so that the overall four-dimensional mean across brain and block was 100. Next, for each voxel, the block mean was subtracted to remove block-wise drift, followed by concatenation of all blocks. The standard deviation of the normalized mean of the concatenated fixation blocks was used to obtain BOLD$_{SD}$ values for each brain region (n = 148) of each subject, as defined by the Destrieux Atlas (Destrieux et al., 2010), using in-house MATLAB code. Change (delta.variability) in variability between the two scanning sessions was calculated as variability at timepoint 2–variability at timepoint 1. BOLD$_{SD}$ encompassing both timepoints was introduced as "variability" (see section "Regional Model").

Statistical Analysis

Linear mixed effects models (LMMs) were used to investigate the potential confounding effect of cortical morphology, GM, CT, CA on BOLD$_{SD}$ (Bates, 2005; Zuur et al., 2011).The LMMs allow estimation of the effects of explanatory variables ("fixed effects") and their interactions on the dependent variable (i.e., BOLD$_{SD}$), while statistically controlling for the effects of randomly selected participants ("random effects") on the dependent variable (BOLD$_{SD}$). Multiple models were run and the likelihood-ratio test was used to (1) investigate if introducing subjects as random effects improves the fit of the model (2) to select the optimal combination of fixed effects fitted with maximum likelihood, while keeping the random effects structure the same. Therefore, the likelihood-ratio test via ANOVA was used to compare the goodness of fit of different models. R statistical software package (R Core Team, 2013)[2] was used for all statistical analyses. Correlation between cortical morphology measures were computed using cor function in R. All models were fitted using the "lmer" or "lm" function in R. "lmerTest" R package was used to obtain summary table and p-values for linear mixed models via Satterthwaite's degrees of freedom method (Kuznetsova et al., 2017). A spatio-temporal approach to LMMs allowed characterization of regionally specific variation across the brain (Bernal-Rusiel et al., 2013). This approach was implemented to investigate if there is a significant change in BOLD variability across time (1) all cortical regions (2) region specific. Random effect structure with subjects varying in their "baseline" BOLD variability was retained (random intercept, 1| ID). Additionally, to model a different rate of change in the expected response levels, time varying predictors were introduced by random slopes (i.e., thickness, time) ("Regional Model"). To reduce spatial correlation issues an LMM model with the described structure was applied at each spatial location (i.e., region of interest) independently. Each model produced a parameter which quantifies the mean change in BOLD variability (delta.variability) for that region. P-values were corrected for multiple comparisons using false discovery rate (FDR) at $q = 0.05$ (Benjamini and Yekutieli, 2001).

Models

Model 1 < lm (delta.variability~ region).

Model 2 < - lmer [delta.variability~ region+(1| ID), REML = F].

Model 3 < - lmer [delta.variability ~ delta.thickness + region+(1| ID), REML = F].

Model 4 < - lmer [delta.variability ~ delta.area + region + (1| ID), REML = F].

---

[1] http://surfer.nmr.mgh.harvard.edu/

[2] www.R-project.org

Model 5 < - lmer [delta.variability ~ delta.thickness + delta.area + region+(1| ID), REML = F].
Model 6 < - delta.variability ~ delta.volume + region + (1 | ID).

Final Model
lmer [delta.variability~ delta.thickness + region+(1| ID)].

Regional Model
lmer [variability~ time + thickness + (1+thickness + time| ID)].

RESULTS

Relations Between Cortical Thickness and BOLD Signal Variability Age-Related Changes

The functional and structural data of 28 participants was assessed. As expected, our study showed that CA and GM are highly correlated $r = 0.904$, $p < 0.001$ (95% Cl 0.901–0.908) and consequently collinearity was suspected. Multiple LMMs were utilized to assess the effect of neuroanatomical metrics CT, CA, and GM on $BOLD_{SD}$ age-related changes. Results from the linear mixed effect models run with likelihood-ratio test via ANOVA, are presented in **Table 1**. (A) indicates that subject intercept should be introduced as a random effect, while (B–E) show the steps that have led to the final model. Specifically, **Table 1**. (B,C) indicate that introducing CT or CA as covariates, separately, each significantly improve the fit of the model $p < 0.0001$, $p < 0.05$, respectively. However, from (D) it is apparent that adding CA to a model that already has CT as a covariate does not improve the fit of the model, meaning that CT only should be included in the final model (see section "Final Model"). (E) indicates that introducing GM as a covariate does not improve the fit of the model. Neither CT, GM, nor CA mean changes were significant as tested with LMMs. Regional Model LMM indicated that neither overall nor regionally specific mean $BOLD_{SD}$ change was significant after FDR correction.

DISCUSSION

Cortical Thickness and Its Association With $BOLD_{SD}$

In this study we aimed at determining the contribution of cortical morphology to $BOLD_{SD}$ in order to better understand

TABLE 1 | Results from likelihood-ratio test via ANOVA for model comparison (fit with "lmer" function in R).

	Df	AIC	BIC	logLik	Deviance	Chisq Chi	Df.	Pr > Chisq
(A) Determine if random effects for subject intercept should be introduced								
Model 1	Delta.variability ~ Region							
Model 2	Delta.variability ~ Region + (1| ID)							
Model 1	149	−2771.9	−1828.8	1534.9	−3069.9			
Model 2	150	−3744.8	−3744.8	2022.4	−4044.8	974.97	1	< 2.2e − 16
(B) Determine if introducing thickness as a covariate improves the goodness-of-fit								
Model 2	Delta.variability ~ Region + (1| ID)							
Model 3	Delta.variability ~ Delta.thickness + Region + (1| ID)							
Model 2	150	−3744.8	−2795.4	2022.4	−4044.8			
Model 3	151	−3765.5	−2809.8	2033.8	−4067.5	22.691	1	1.903e − 06
(C) Determine if introducing area as a covariate improves the goodness-of-fit								
Model 2	Delta.variability ~ Region + (1| ID)							
Model 4	Delta.variability ~ Delta.area + Region + (1| ID)							
Model 2	150	−3744.8	−2795.4	2022.4	−4044.8			
Model 4	151	−3749.0	−2793.3	2025.5	−4051.0	6.2025	1	0.01276
(D) Determine if introducing both area and thickness as covariates as compared to just one improves the goodness-of-fit								
Model 3	Delta.variability ~ Delta.thickness + Region + (1| ID)							
Model 5	Delta.variability ~ Delta.thickness + Delta.area + Region + (1| ID)							
Model 3	151	−3765.5	−2809.8	2033.8	−4067.5			
Model 5	152	−3766.7	−2804.7	2035.4	−4070.7	3.2151	1	0.07296
(E) Determine if introducing gray matter volume as covariate improves the goodness-of-fit								
Model 2	Delta.variability ~ Region + (1| ID)							
Model 6	Delta.variability ~ Delta.volume + Region + (1| ID)							
Model 2	150	−3744.8	−2795.4	2022.4	−4044.8			
Model 6	151	−3743.1	−2787.3	2022.5	−4045.1	0.2245	1	0.6357

AIC, akaike information criterion; BIC, Bayesian information criterion; Chisq Chi, chi-square test statistic; Df, degrees of freedom; logLik, log-likelihood; Pr > Chisq. P < 0.05. ID represents subject identification number.

the physiological nature of brain function capture by $BOLD_{SD}$. $BOLD_{SD}$ changes across the lifespan have been shown to be robust to certain vascular factor such as cerebral blood flow, BOLD cerebrovascular reactivity, maximal BOLD signal change (Garrett et al., 2017), as well as GM volume changes (Nomi et al., 2017). However, using LMMs, we found that functional alterations in aging as captured by $BOLD_{SD}$ are confounded by the structural metric CT. This is not surprising, considering that it is well known that BOLD signal change/activation is dependent on the laminar organization of the cortex, and consequently is influenced by its depth or thickness (Koopmans et al., 2010; Tian et al., 2010; Bandettini, 2012). In fact, neurovascular coupling is reported to vary by cortical depth and layer (Goense et al., 2012).

In a longitudinal study investigating CT, GM volume, CA across the lifespan, Storsve et al. (2014) reported cortical morphology metric specific and region specific rates of mean annual percentage change (APC) in healthy adults aged 23–87 years. In most regions, GM volume has a mean APC of −0.51, CT of −0.35, and CA of −0.19. Other longitudinal studies in older adults, report similar reductions: in GM volume, mean APC ranging from −0.5 to −2.1 ± 1.6% (Tang et al., 2001; Fjell et al., 2009), in CT, mean APC −0.3% (Shaw et al., 2016), in WM tracts, mean APC ranging from −0.20 to −0.65 depending on the tract location (Storsve et al., 2015). In our sample, the change in cortical morphology from scan 1 to scan 2 (2.5 years apart) was not statistically significant. However, the findings reported by these longitudinal studies suggest that while the neuroanatomical alterations may be too subtle to reach statistically significance in the investigated timespan of 2.5 years, they may still contribute to $BOLD_{SD}$ age-related findings. Particularly, accounting for CT age-related changes may help "unmask" the functional value of $BOLD_{SD}$.

While the relationship between cortical morphology metrics in aging is dynamic, GM volume changes were largely accounted by changes in CT rather than CA, highlighting the importance of tracking changes in CT (Storsve et al., 2014). In fact, studies show that CT and CA are genetically independent (Panizzon et al., 2009). Their neurodevelopment in the lifespan is largely independent of each other suggesting that they should be considered as separate metrics with different contributions to cortical volume (Im et al., 2008; Winkler et al., 2010; Eyler et al., 2011; Lemaitre et al., 2012; Storsve et al., 2014). Furthermore, studies show that that some cortices experience decrease in cortical morphology metrics at a higher rate than others (Storsve et al., 2014).

The hemodynamic properties of each brain region are highly correlated with its cortical structure (Ulrich and Yablonskiy, 2016; Wen et al., 2018). Studies based on quantitative gradient recalled echo (qGRE) analysis use the GRE signal decay rate parameter (R2t*) to gather information on tissue-specific contributions to the fMRI signal. Regional R2t* metric variations are associated with variations in neuronal density and myelination (positive correlation), as well as glial cells and synapses concentration (i.e., negative correlation) (Wen et al., 2018). In normal aging R2t* increases in all cortical regions (Zhao et al., 2016). Thicker regions show the opposite pattern, respectively, decreased neuronal density, and higher concentration of glial cells and synapses relative to neurons. Thicker areas also tend to extract less oxygen from the blood, as measured by oxygen extraction ratios (i.e., expressed as local-to-global ratio). These findings indicate that laminar differences in cellular content impact neurovascular coupling mechanisms, which in turn may compromise the power of $BOLD_{SD}$ measurements to detect "real" changes in neuronal variability processing (Harris et al., 2011). Although, laminar differences in $BOLD_{SD}$ remain rather elusive, our study suggests the that CT should be considered in BOLD variability studies.

Age-Related Changes in $BOLD_{SD}$

In our study, we did not find a significant change in $BOLD_{SD}$, likely due to the low timespan between scans (2.5 years), and relatively low sample (n = 28). Overall, most studies reporting a decrease in $BOLD_{SD}$ suggest that this finding may indicate structural reductions in synaptic complexity and integrity, as well as functional decline in neural optimization and flexibility (Garrett et al., 2010). Burzynska et al. (2015) reported a positive correlation between increased microstructural integrity of WM and $BOLD_{SD}$ in healthy adults, consequently warranting the consideration of structural alterations in variability studies. Nomi et al. (2017) found increases in variability in bilateral anterior insula, anterior cingulate and ventral temporal cortex, and decreases in $BOLD_{SD}$ in sensory brain regions and other subcortical areas, in participants with ages ranging from 6 to 86 years. In their study they accounted for GM volume but not CT or CA. Two seminal studies investigated $BOLD_{SD}$ differences in aging alone (Garrett et al., 2010) and in relation to performance on cognitive tasks (Garrett et al., 2011) between a young group of participants (20–30 years) and an older one (56–85 years) and found both increases and decreases in regional variability with younger age alone, and younger age and better performance (Garrett et al., 2011) making it rather difficult to isolate specific key contributing regions. Most regions in these two studies showed the same trend but there were some inconsistencies. For example, superior frontal gyrus was reported to show greater variability with younger age and better performance (Garrett et al., 2011) in one study, while another one reported that its variability increases with age (Garrett et al., 2010). CT was not considered in any of these studies. The relationship between cognitive performance and/or flexibility and $BOLD_{SD}$ is definitely complex and task dependent. Behavioral studies indicate age-related differences in intra-individual variability on cognitive performance tests involving reaction time, and working memory. Older adults showing higher intra-individual variability on reaction time tests than younger adults, while the opposite is observed on working memory tests (Fagot et al., 2018). Additionally, the relationship between $BOLD_{SD}$ change, aging and cognitive health has not been a consistent finding. Some studies have found increased BOLD in healthy older adults (Baum and Beauchamp, 2014), Alzheimer's (Scarapicchia et al., 2018), attention deficit hyperactivity disorder (ADHD) (Nomi et al., 2018), and other neurological disorders (Zöller et al., 2017).

Other Possible Confounds in $BOLD_{SD}$ Studies

Most studies investigating BOLD variability utilized a cross-sectional design while we used a within-subject design. This design is a highlight of our study because it allows for the investigation of normative age-related differences, specifically intra-individual effects of the processing of aging on cortical morphology and $BOLD_{SD}$, rather than process of aging simply age differences across groups. Importantly, the within-subject design helps account for numerous sources of individual differences that may affect BOLD variability such as differences in dopaminergic neurotransmission (Guitart-Masip et al., 2016; Alavash et al., 2018), significant differences in vascular features, pain sensitivity and coping (Rogachov et al., 2016), clinical symptomology (Ke et al., 2015; Nomi et al., 2018; Zöller et al., 2018), and even differences in tendency for financial risk taking (Samanez-Larkin et al., 2010). Given that in our study the participants were scanned at an interval of approximately 2.5 years, we were able to at least partially account for such factors. Furthermore, it is clear from the literature that there are numerous environmental factors [i.e., socioeconomic status, education (Chan et al., 2018)] that may contribute to individual neuroanatomical alterations, which in turn may confound BOLD variability studies. This further supports the findings of our study, specifically that CT is a neuroanatomical metric that should be accounted for.

Lastly, there may be inconsistency in results between studies due to: (1) using task-fMRI and resting-state fMRI, (2) calculation of BOLD signal variability using standard deviation vs. mean-square successive difference) (for review, Garrett et al., 2013b), (3) type of statistical analysis performed (e.g., partial least squares method, LMM, general linear model), and (4) not accounting for contribution of CT and the other mentioned sources of individual differences.

STUDY LIMITATIONS

The main limitations, as discussed above and further addressed by Garrett et al. (2013b); Scarapicchia et al. (2018), are the lack of standardization in acquiring and analyzing the fMRI data. Additionally, the sample used in our study consists of a relatively small sample of older adults and rather short scan-rescan time, consequently this limits our ability to make strong generalization to other age groups or longer time spans, respectively. Nevertheless, since studies show that the brain undergoes extensive annual structural alterations across the lifespan at different rates, our finding that CT contributes to $BOLD_{SD}$ alterations, remains an important consideration.

CONCLUSION

In conclusion, contrary to a view that BOLD variability is just "noise," we consider it to be emerging as an important metric of normal aging. Keeping in mind that across the lifespan there are considerable cortical morphometry alterations and that cortical depth affects the BOLD signal, we reported that CT contributes to BOL_{DSD} changes, in an older sample of health adults. An increasing number of studies are considering healthy regional $BOLD_{SD}$ changes in the context of functional networks (Rogachov et al., 2016; Nomi et al., 2017). Pursuing this direction while accounting for CT and other possible confounding factors such as dopaminergic neurotransmission, socioeconomic background etc., should reveal new insights into the mechanisms behind age-related neural processes.

AUTHOR CONTRIBUTIONS

DP, RE, and SR conceived and designed this specific project on the data collected by NM and AR. DP analyzed the data. All co-authors participated in writing of the manuscript.

FUNDING

This work was supported by the SNF (Swiss National Foundation, Grant Nos. 100014_135410, PMPDP1 171335, and PMPDP1 158319).

ACKNOWLEDGMENTS

We thank the participants of the Geneva Aging Study. We also thank the Department of Statistical and Actuarial Sciences at Western University for helpful discussions and advice on data analysis and statistical modeling.

REFERENCES

Achiron, A., Chapman, J., Tal, S., Bercovich, E., Gil, H., and Achiron, A. (2013). Superior temporal gyrus thickness correlates with cognitive performance in multiple sclerosis. *Brain Struct. Funct.* 218, 943–950. doi: 10.1007/s00429-012-0440-3

Alavash, M., Lim, S. J., Thiel, C., Sehm, B., Deserno, L., and Obleser, J. (2018). Dopaminergic modulation of hemodynamic signal variability and the functional connectome during cognitive performance. *Neuroimage* 172, 341–356. doi: 10.1016/j.neuroimage.2018.01.048

Armbruster-Genc, D. J. N., Ueltzhoffer, K., and Fiebach, C. J. (2016). Brain signal variability differentially affects cognitive flexibility and cognitive stability. *J. Neurosci.* 36, 3978–3987. doi: 10.1523/JNEUROSCI.2517-14.2016

Bandettini, P. A. (2012). The BOLD plot thickens: sign- and layer-dependent hemodynamic changes with activation. *Neuron* 76, 468–469. doi: 10.1016/j.neuron.2012.10.026

Bates, D. (2005). Fitting linear mixed models in R. *R News* 5, 27–30. doi: 10.1159/300323281

Baum, S. H., and Beauchamp, M. S. (2014). Greater BOLD variability in older compared with younger adults during audiovisual speech perception. *PLoS One* 9:e111121. doi: 10.1371/journal.pone.011121

Beckmann, C. F., and Smith, S. M. (2004). Probabilistic independent component analysis for functional magnetic resonance imaging. *IEEE Trans. Med. Imaging* 23, 137–152. doi: 10.1109/TMI.2003.822821

Benjamini, Y., and Yekutieli, D. (2001). The control of the false discovery rate in multiple testing under dependency. *Ann. Stat.* 29, 1165–1188. doi: 10.1214/aos/1013699998

Bernal-Rusiel, J. L., Reuter, M., Greve, D. N., Fischl, B., and Sabuncu, M. R. (2013). Spatiotemporal linear mixed effects modeling for the mass-univariate analysis of longitudinal neuroimage data. *Neuroimage* 81, 358–370. doi: 10.1016/j.neuroimage.2013.05.049

Burzynska, A. Z., Wong, C. N., Voss, M. W., Cooke, G. E., McAuley, E., and Kramer, A. F. (2015). White matter integrity supports BOLD signal variability and cognitive performance in the aging human brain. *PLoS One* 10:e0120315. doi: 10.1371/journal.pone.0120315

Chan, M. Y., Na, J., Agres, P. F., Savalia, N. K., Park, D. C., and Wig, G. S. (2018). Socioeconomic status moderates age-related differences in the brain's functional network organization and anatomy across the adult lifespan. *Proc. Natl. Acad. Sci. U.S.A.* 115, E5144–E5153. doi: 10.1073/pnas.1714021115

Dale, A. M., Fischl, B., and Sereno, M. I. (1999). Cortical surface-based analysis. I. segmentation and surface reconstruction. *Neuroimage* 9, 179–194. doi: 10.1006/nimg.1998.0395

Destrieux, C., Fischl, B., Dale, A., and Halgren, E. (2010). Automatic parcellation of human cortical gyri and sulci using standard anatomical nomenclature. *Neuroimage* 53, 1–15. doi: 10.1016/j.neuroimage.2010.06.010

Dotson, V. M., Szymkowicz, S. M., Sozda, C. N., Kirton, J. W., Green, M. L., O'Shea, A., et al. (2016). Age differences in prefrontal surface area and thickness in middle aged to older adults. *Front. Aging Neurosci.* 7:250. doi: 10.3389/fnagi.2015.00250

Driscoll, I., Davatzikos, C., An, Y., Wu, X., Shen, D., Kraut, M., et al. (2009). Longitudinal pattern of regional brain volume change differentiates normal aging from MCI. *Neurology* 72, 1906–1913. doi: 10.1212/WNL.0b013e3181a82634

Eyler, L. T., Prom-Wormley, E., Panizzon, M. S., Kaup, A. R., Fennema-Notestine, C., Neale, M. C., et al. (2011). Genetic and environmental contributions to regional cortical surface area in humans: a magnetic resonance imaging twin study. *Cereb. Cortex* 21, 2313–2321. doi: 10.1093/cercor/bhr013

Fagot, D., Mella, N., Borella, E., Ghisletta, P., Lecerf, T., and de Ribaupierre, A. (2018). Intra-individual variability from a lifespan perspective: a comparison of latency and accuracy measures. *J. Intell.* 6, 1–18. doi: 10.3390/jintelligence6010016

Fischl, B., and Dale, A. M. (2000). Measuring the thickness of the human cerebral cortex from magnetic resonance images. *Proc. Natl. Acad. Sci. U.S.A.* 97, 11050–11055. doi: 10.1073/pnas.200033797

Fischl, B., Liu, A., and Dale, A. M. (2001). Automated manifold surgery: constructing geometrically accurate and topologically correct models of the human cerebral cortex. *IEEE Trans. Med. Imaging* 20, 70–80. doi: 10.1109/42.906426

Fischl, B., Sereno, M. I., and Dale, A. M. (1999a). Cortical surface-based analysis. II: inflation, flattening, and a surface-based coordinate system. *Neuroimage* 9, 195–207. doi: 10.1006/nimg.1998.0396

Fischl, B. Sereno, M. I., Tootell, R. B., and Dale, A. M. (1999b). High-resolution intersubject averaging and a coordinate system for the cortical surface. *Hum. Brain Mapp.* 8, 272–284.

Fjell, A. M., Walhovd, K. B., Fennema-Notestine, C., McEvoy, L. K., Hagler, D. J., Holland, D., et al. (2009). One-year brain atrophy evident in healthy aging. *J. Neurosci.* 29, 15223–15231. doi: 10.1523/JNEUROSCI.3252-09.2009

Fjell, A. M., Walhovd, K. B., Reinvang, I., Lundervold, A., Salat, D., Quinn, B. T., et al. (2006). Selective increase of cortical thickness in high-performing elderly - structural indices of optimal cognitive aging. *Neuroimage* 29, 984–994. doi: 10.1016/j.neuroimage.2005.08.007

Garrett, D. D., Kovacevic, N., McIntosh, A. R., and Grady, C. L. (2010). Blood oxygen level-dependent signal variability is more than just noise. *J. Neurosci.* 30, 4914–4921. doi: 10.1523/JNEUROSCI.5166-09.2010

Garrett, D. D., Kovacevic, N., McIntosh, A. R., and Grady, C. L. (2011). The importance of being variable. *J. Neurosci.* 31, 4496–4503. doi: 10.1523/JNEUROSCI.5641-10.2011

Garrett, D. D., Kovacevic, N., McIntosh, A. R., and Grady, C. L. (2013a). The modulation of BOLD variability between cognitive states varies by age and processing speed. *Cereb. Cortex* 23, 684–693. doi: 10.1093/cercor/bhs055

Garrett, D. D., Samanez-Larkin, G. R., MacDonald, S. W. S., Lindenberger, U., McIntosh, A. R., and Grady, C. L. (2013b). Moment-to-moment brain signal variability: a next frontier in human brain mapping? *Neurosci. Biobehav. Rev.* 37, 610–624. doi: 10.1016/j.neubiorev.2013.02.015

Garrett, D. D., Lindenberger, U., Hoge, R. D., and Gauthier, C. J. (2017). Age differences in brain signal variability are robust to multiple vascular controls. *Sci. Rep.* 7:10149. doi: 10.1038/s41598-017-09752-7

Garrett, D. D., McIntosh, A. R., and Grady, C. L. (2014). Brain signal variability is parametrically modifiable. *Cereb. Cortex* 24, 2931–2940. doi: 10.1093/cercor/bht150

Goense, J., Merkle, H., and Logothetis, N. K. (2012). High-resolution FMRI reveals laminar differences in neurovascular coupling between positive and negative BOLD responses. *Neuron* 76, 629–639. doi: 10.1016/j.neuron.2012.09.019

Grady, C. L., and Garrett, D. D. (2014). Understanding variability in the BOLD signal and why it matters for aging. *Brain Imaging Behav.* 8, 274–283. doi: 10.1007/s11682-013-9253-0

Guitart-Masip, M., Salami, A., Garrett, D., Rieckmann, A., Lindenberger, U., and Bäckman, L. (2016). BOLD variability is related to dopaminergic neurotransmission and cognitive aging. *Cereb. Cortex* 26, 2074–2083. doi: 10.1093/cercor/bhv029

Harris, J. J., Reynell, C., and Attwell, D. (2011). The physiology of developmental changes in BOLD functional imaging signals. *Dev. Cogn. Neurosci.* 1, 199–216. doi: 10.1016/j.dcn.2011.04.001

Hogstrom, L. J., Westlye, L. T., Walhovd, K. B., and Fjell, A. M. (2013). The structure of the cerebral cortex across adult life: age-related patterns of surface area, thickness, and gyrification. *Cereb. Cortex* 23, 2521–2530. doi: 10.1093/cercor/bhs231

Huber, L., Goense, J., Kennerley, A. J., Trampel, R., Guidi, M., Reimer, E., et al. (2015). Cortical lamina-dependent blood volume changes in human brain at 7 T. *Neuroimage* 107, 23–33. doi: 10.1016/j.neuroimage.2014.11.046

Im, K., Lee, J. M., Lyttelton, O., Kim, S. H., Evans, A. C., and Kim, S. I. (2008). Brain size and cortical structure in the adult human brain. *Cereb. Cortex* 18, 2181–2191. doi: 10.1093/cercor/bhm244

Jenkinson, M., Beckmann, C. F., Behrens, T. E. J., Woolrich, M. W., and Smith, S. M. (2012). FSL. *Neuroimage* 62, 782–790. doi: 10.1016/j.neuroimage.2011.09.015

Jiang, J., Sachdev, P., Lipnicki, D. M., Zhang, H., Liu, T., Zhu, W., et al. (2014). A longitudinal study of brain atrophy over two years in community-dwelling older individuals. *Neuroimage* 86, 203–211. doi: 10.1016/j.neuroimage.2013.08.022

Ke, J., Zhang, L., Qi, R., Xu, Q., Li, W., Hou, C., et al. (2015). Altered blood oxygen level-dependent signal variability in chronic post-traumatic stress disorder during symptom provocation. *Neuropsychiatr. Dis. Treat.* 11, 1805–1815. doi: 10.2147/NDT.S87332

Kielar, A., Deschamps, T., Chu, R. K., Jokel, R., Khatamian, Y. B., Chen, J. J., et al. (2016). Identifying dysfunctional cortex: dissociable effects of stroke and aging on resting state dynamics in MEG and fMRI. *Front. Aging Neurosci.* 8:40. doi: 10.3389/fnagi.2016.00040

Koopmans, P. J., Barth, M., and Norris, D. G. (2010). Layer-specific BOLD activation in human V1. *Hum. Brain Mapp.* 31, 1297–1304. doi: 10.1002/hbm.20936

Kuznetsova, A., Brockhoff, P. B., and Christensen, R. H. B. (2017). LmerTest package: tests in linear mixed effects models. *J. Stat. Softw.* 82, 1–26. doi: 10.18637/jss.v082.i13

Lemaitre, H., Goldman, A. L., Sambataro, F., Verchinski, B. A., Meyer-Lindenberg, A., Weinberger, D. R., et al. (2012). Normal age-related brain morphometric changes: nonuniformity across cortical thickness, surface area and gray matter volume? *Neurobiol. Aging* 33, 617.e1–617.e9. doi: 10.1016/j.neurobiolaging.2010.07.013

Makedonov, I., Black, S. E., and MacIntosh, B. J. (2013). BOLD FMRI in the white matter as a marker of aging and small vessel disease. *PLoS One* 8:e67652. doi: 10.1371/journal.pone.0067652

Makedonov, I., Chen, J. J., Masellis, M., and MacIntosh, B. J. (2016). Physiological fluctuations in white matter are increased in Alzheimer's disease and correlate with neuroimaging and cognitive biomarkers. *Neurobiol. Aging* 37, 12–18. doi: 10.1016/j.neurobiolaging.2015.09.010

McGinnis, S. M., Brickhouse, M., Pascual, B., and Dickerson, B. C. (2011). Age-related changes in the thickness of cortical zones in humans. *Brain Topogr.* 24, 279–291. doi: 10.1007/s10548-011-0198-6

Mella, N., de Ribaupierre, S., Eagleson, R., and de Ribaupierre, A. (2013). Cognitive intraindividual variability and white matter integrity in aging. *ScientificWorldJournal* 2013:350623. doi: 10.1155/2013/350623

Nomi, J. S., Bolt, T. S., Chiemeka Ezie, C. E., Uddin, L. Q., and Heller, A. S. (2017). Moment-to-moment BOLD signal variability reflects regional changes in neural flexibility across the lifespan. *J. Neurosci.* 37, 5539–5548. doi: 10.1523/JNEUROSCI.3408-16.2017

Nomi, J. S., Schettini, E., Voorhies, W., Bolt, T. S., Heller, A. S., and Uddin, L. Q. (2018). Resting-state brain signal variability in prefrontal cortex is associated with ADHD symptom severity in children. *Front. Hum. Neurosci.* 12:90. doi: 10.3389/fnhum.2018.00090

Pacheco, J., Goh, J. O., Kraut, M. A., Ferrucci, L., and Resnick, S. M. (2015). Greater cortical thinning in normal older adults predicts later cognitive impairment. *Neurobiol. Aging* 36, 903–908. doi: 10.1016/j.neurobiolaging.2014.08.031

Panizzon, M. S., Fennema-Notestine, C., Eyler, L. T., Jernigan, T. L., Prom-Wormley, E., Neale, M., et al. (2009). Distinct genetic influences on cortical surface area and cortical thickness. *Cereb. Cortex* 19, 2728–2735. doi: 10.1093/cercor/bhp026

Petracca, M., Saiote, C., Bender, H. A., Arias, F., Farrell, C., Magioncalda, P., et al. (2017). Synchronization and variability imbalance underlie cognitive impairment in primary-progressive multiple sclerosis. *Sci. Rep.* 7:46411. doi: 10.1038/srep46411

R Core Team (2013). *R: A Language and Environment for Statistical Computing.* Vienna: R Foundation for Statistical Computing. Available at: https://www.R-project.org/

Raz, N. (2005). Regional brain changes in aging healthy adults: general trends, individual differences and modifiers. *Cereb. Cortex* 15, 1676–1689. doi: 10.1093/cercor/bhi044

Reuter, M., Rosas, H. D., and Fischl, B. (2010). Highly accurate inverse consistent registration: a robust approach. *Neuroimage* 53, 1181–1196. doi: 10.1016/j.neuroimage.2010.07.020

Rogachov, A., Cheng, J. C., Erpelding, N., Hemington, K. S., Crawley, A. P., and Davis, K. D. (2016). Regional brain signal variability: a novel indicator of pain sensitivity and coping. *Pain* 157, 2483–2492. doi: 10.1097/j.pain.0000000000000665

Rossini, P. M., Rossi, S., Babiloni, C., and Polich, J. (2007). Clinical neurophysiology of aging brain: from normal aging to neurodegeneration. *Prog. Neurobiol.* 83, 375–400. doi: 10.1016/j.pneurobio.2007.07.010

Salat, D. H., Buckner, R. L., Snyder, A. Z., Greve, D. N., Desikan, R. S. R., Busa, E., et al. (2004). Thinning of the cerebral cortex in aging. *Cereb. Cortex* 14, 721–730. doi: 10.1093/cercor/bhh032

Salat, D. H., Lee, S. Y., van der Kouwe, A. J., Greve, D. N., Fischl, B., and Rosas, H. D. (2009). Age-associated alterations in cortical gray and white matter signal intensity and gray to white matter contrast. *Neuroimage* 48, 21–28. doi: 10.1016/j.neuroimage.2009.06.074

Samanez-Larkin, G. R., Kuhnen, C. M., Yoo, D. J., and Knutson, B. (2010). Variability in nucleus accumbens activity mediates age-related suboptimal financial risk taking. *J. Neurosci.* 30:1426. doi: 10.1523/JNEUROSCI.4902-09.2010

Scarapicchia, V., Mazerolle, E. L., Fisk, J. D., Ritchie, L. J., and Gawryluk, J. R. (2018). Resting state BOLD variability in Alzheimer's disease: a marker of cognitive decline or cerebrovascular status? *Front. Aging Neurosci.* 10:39. doi: 10.3389/fnagi.2018.00039

Ségonne, F., Dale, A. M., Busa, E., Glessner M., Salat, D., Hahn, H. K., et al. (2004). A hybrid approach to the skull stripping problem in MRI. *Neuroimage* 22, 1060–1075. doi: 10.1016/j.neuroimage.2004.03.032

Segonne, F., Pacheco, J., and Fischl, B. (2007). Geometrically accurate topology-correction of cortical surfaces using nonseparating loops. *IEEE Trans. Med. Imaging* 26, 518–529. doi: 10.1109/TMI.2006.887364

Shaw, M. E., Sachdev, P. S., Anstey, K. J., and Cherbuin, N. (2016). Age-related cortical thinning in cognitively healthy individuals in their 60s: the path through life study. *Neurobiol. Aging* 39, 202–209. doi: 10.1016/j.neurobiolaging.2015.12.009

Singh, V., Chertkow, H., Lerch, J. P., Evans, A. C., Dorr, A. E., and Kabani, N. J. (2006). Spatial patterns of cortical thinning in mild cognitive impairment and Alzheimer's disease. *Brain* 129(Pt 11), 2885–2893. doi: 10.1093/brain/awl256

Sled, J. G., Zijdenbos, A. P., and Evans, A. C. (1998). A nonparametric method for automatic correction of intensity nonuniformity in MRI data. *IEEE Trans. Med. Imaging* 17, 87–97. doi: 10.1109/42.663698

Smith, S. M. (2002). Fast robust automated brain extraction. *Hum. Brain Mapp.* 17, 143–155. doi: 10.1002/hbm.10062

Smith, S. M., Jenkinson, M., Woolrich, M. W., Beckmann, C. F., Behrens, T. E. J., Johansen-Berg, H., et al. (2004). Advances in functional and structural MR image analysis and implementation as FSL. *Neuroimage* 23(Suppl. 1), S208–S219. doi: 10.1016/j.neuroimage.2004.07.051

Storsve, A. B., Fjell, A. M., Tamnes, C. K., Westlye, L. T., Overbye, K., Aasland, H. W., et al. (2014). Differential longitudinal changes in cortical thickness, surface area and volume across the adult life span: regions of accelerating and decelerating change. *J. Neurosci.* 34, 8488–8498. doi: 10.1523/JNEUROSCI.0391-14.2014

Storsve, A. B., Fjell, A. M., Yendiki, A., and Walhovd, K. B. (2016). Longitudinal changes in white matter tract integrity across the adult lifespan and its relation to cortical thinning. *PLoS One* 11:e0156770. doi: 10.1371/journal.pone.0156770

Tang, Y., Whitman, G. T., Lopez, I., and Baloh, R. W. (2001). Brain volume changes on longitudinal magnetic resonance imaging in normal older people. *J. Neuroimaging* 11, 393–400. doi: 10.1111/j.1552-6569.2001.tb00068.x

Thambisetty, M., Wan, J., Carass, A., An, Y., Prince, J. L., and Resnick, S. M. (2010). Longitudinal changes in cortical thickness associated with normal aging. *Neuroimage* 52, 1215–1223. doi: 10.1016/j.neuroimage.2010.04.258

Tian, P., Teng, I. C., May, L. D., Kurz, R., Lu, K., Scadeng, M., et al. (2010). Cortical depth-specific microvascular dilation underlies laminar differences in blood oxygenation level-dependent functional MRI signal. *Proc. Natl. Acad. Sci. U.S.A.* 107, 15246–15251. doi: 10.1073/pnas.1006735107

Ulrich, X., and Yablonskiy, D. A. (2016). Separation of cellular and BOLD contributions to T2* signal relaxation. *Magn. Reson. Med.* 75, 606–615. doi: 10.1002/mrm.25610

Wen, J., Goyal, M. S., Astafiev, S. V., Raichle, M. E., and Yablonskiy, D. A. (2018). Genetically defined cellular correlates of the baseline brain MRI signal. *Proc. Natl. Acad. Sci. U.S.A.* 115, E9727–E9736. doi: 10.1073/pnas.1808121115

Winkler, A. M., Kochunov, P., Blangero, J., Almasy, L., Zilles, K., Fox, P. T., et al. (2010). Cortical thickness or grey matter volume? The importance of selecting the phenotype for imaging genetics studies. *Neuroimage* 53, 1135–1146. doi: 10.1016/j.neuroimage.2009.12.028

Winkler, A. M., Sabuncu, M. R., Yeo, B. T. T., Fischl, B., Greve, D. N., Kochunov, P., et al. (2012). Measuring and comparing brain cortical surface area and other areal quantities. *Neuroimage* 61, 1428–1443. doi: 10.1016/j.neuroimage.2012.03.026

Zhang, Y., Brady, M., and Smith, S. (2001). Segmentation of brain MR images through a hidden markov random field model and the expectation-maximization algorithm. *IEEE Trans. Med. Imaging* 20, 45–57. doi: 10.1109/42.906424

Zhao, Y., Wen, J., Cross, A. H., and Yablonskiy, D. A. (2016). On the relationship between cellular and hemodynamic properties of the human brain cortex throughout adult lifespan. *Neuroimage* 133, 417–429. doi: 10.1016/j.neuroimage.2016.03.022

Ziegler, D. A., Piguet, O., Salat, D. H., Prince, K., Connally, E., and Corkin, S. (2010). Cognition in healthy aging is related to regional white matter integrity, but not cortical thickness. *Neurobiol. Aging* 31, 1912–1926. doi: 10.1016/j.neurobiolaging.2008.10.015

Zöller, D., Padula, M. C., Sandini, C., Schneider, M., Scariati, E., Van De Ville, D., et al. (2018). Psychotic symptoms influence the development of anterior cingulate BOLD variability in 22q11.2 deletion syndrome. *Schizophr. Res.* 193, 319–328. doi: 10.1016/j.schres.2017.08.003

Zöller, D., Schaer, M., Scariati, M., Padula, C. M., Eliez, S., and Van De Ville, D. (2017). Disentangling resting-state BOLD variability and PCC functional connectivity in 22q11.2 deletion syndrome. *Neuroimage* 149, 85–97. doi: 10.1016/j.neuroimage.2017.01.064

Zuur, A. F., Leno, E. N., Walker, N. J., Saveliev, A. A., and Smith, G. M. (2011). *Mixed Effects Models and Extensions in Ecology with R.* New York, NY: Springer.

12

Exosome Determinants of Physiological Aging and Age-Related Neurodegenerative Diseases

Marianna D'Anca[1], Chiara Fenoglio[1], Maria Serpente[1], Beatrice Arosio[2], Matteo Cesari[2,3], Elio Angelo Scarpini[1,4] and Daniela Galimberti[4,5]*

[1]Department of Pathophysiology and Transplantation, Dino Ferrari Center, Faculty of Medicine and Surgery, University of Milan, Milan, Italy, [2]Department of Clinical Sciences and Community Health, Faculty of Medicine and Surgery, University of Milan, Milan, Italy, [3]Geriatrics Unit, Fondazione IRCCS Ca' Granda, Ospedale Maggiore Policlinico, Milan, Italy, [4]Neurodegenerative Diseases Unit, Fondazione IRCCS Ca' Granda, Ospedale Maggiore Policlinico, Milan, Italy, [5]Department of Biomedical, Surgical and Dental Sciences, Dino Ferrari Center, Faculty of Medicine and Surgery, University of Milan, Milan, Italy

***Correspondence:**
Chiara Fenoglio
chiara.fenoglio@unimi.it

Aging is consistently reported as the most important independent risk factor for neurodegenerative diseases. As life expectancy has significantly increased during the last decades, neurodegenerative diseases became one of the most critical public health problem in our society. The most investigated neurodegenerative diseases during aging are Alzheimer disease (AD), Frontotemporal Dementia (FTD) and Parkinson disease (PD). The search for biomarkers has been focused so far on cerebrospinal fluid (CSF) and blood. Recently, exosomes emerged as novel biological source with increasing interest for age-related neurodegenerative disease biomarkers. Exosomes are tiny Extracellular vesicles (EVs; 30–100 nm in size) released by all cell types which originate from the endosomal compartment. They constitute important vesicles for the release and transfer of multiple (signaling, toxic, and regulatory) molecules among cells. Initially considered with merely waste disposal function, instead exosomes have been recently recognized as fundamental mediators of intercellular communication. They can move from the site of release by diffusion and be retrieved in several body fluids, where they may dynamically reflect pathological changes of cells present in inaccessible sites such as the brain. Multiple evidence has implicated exosomes in age-associated neurodegenerative processes, which lead to cognitive impairment in later life. Critically, consolidated evidence indicates that pathological protein aggregates, including Aβ, tau, and α-synuclein are released from brain cells in association with exosomes. Importantly, exosomes act as vehicles between cells not only of proteins but also of nucleic acids [DNA, mRNA transcripts, miRNA, and non-coding RNAs (ncRNAs)] thus potentially influencing gene expression in target cells. In this framework, exosomes could contribute to elucidate the molecular mechanisms underneath neurodegenerative diseases and could represent a promising source of biomarkers. Despite the involvement of exosomes in age-associated neurodegeneration, the study of exosomes and their genetic cargo in physiological aging and in neurodegenerative diseases is still in its infancy. Here, we review, the current knowledge on protein and ncRNAs cargo of exosomes in normal aging and in age-related neurodegenerative diseases.

Keywords: exosomes, aging, non-coding RNA, Alzheimer's disease, frontotemporal dementia, Parkinson's disease

INTRODUCTION

The growing increase of lifespan has implemented the research in aging processes and in age related pathologies like Alzheimer's Disease (AD), Frontotemporal Dementia (FTD) and Parkinson's disease (PD). Aging encloses multiple and complex processes where cellular senescence is the critical one. Senescent phenotype is characterized by three phenomena: the permanent cell growth arrest; the resistance to apoptosis; the acquisition of altered and differentiated functions (Campisi and d'Adda Di Fagagna, 2007; Campisi, 2012). Several evidence associates senescence to an increase in exosome release introducing a new phenotype named Senescence-Associated Secretory Phenotype (SASP) observed *in vitro* after genotoxic stress in different kinds of cells (Lehmann et al., 2008; Takasugi et al., 2017). Exosomes are tiny Extracellular vesicles (EVs) sizing from 30 nm to 100 nm, shed from almost all the cells, including the nervous ones (Zhang and Yang, 2018). Exosomes were thought to serve as cellular garbage but now there are many evidence that support their role in the intercellular communication (Rashed et al., 2017) pouring their content, through different mechanisms, to the recipient cells in the neighborhood as well as in the periphery even passing through the blood brain barrier (BBB; Alvarez-Erviti et al., 2011; Ridder et al., 2014). Indeed exosomes were detected in many biological fluids as in serum, plasma, urine, cerebrospinal fluid (CSF) and others (Caby et al., 2005; Franzen et al., 2015; Yagi et al., 2016). The growing interest in the last decade on exosome research is linked to their composition that represents a "mirror" of the physiological as well as the pathological state of the donor cells (Willms et al., 2016). Exosome cargo consists of lipid, proteins, mRNAs and ncRNAs, mostly microRNAs, whose sorting is regulated from the cell of origin with complex mechanisms that are not fully understood (Simons and Raposo, 2009). Instead, it is not clear, if the recipient cell can have an active role to select the exosome cargo or if it depends only from the parental cell. Not only their content but also markers on their membrane surface reflect their origin. Therefore, besides general exosome markers useful to discriminate exosomes from other EVs (e.g., CD81, CD9, ALIX, TSG101), the detection of neural derived exosomes (NDEs) is possible due to the presence of L1CAM (L1- cell adhesion molecule), that is a Central Nervous System (CNS)-specific exosome marker (Kenwrick, 2002; Fauré et al., 2006; Lachenal et al., 2010). Therefore, the investigation of the impressive variety of NDEs cargoes, especially proteins and microRNAs, could open a "window into the brain" creating a direct thread between the CNS and the periphery (Shi et al., 2019). To support this assumption, more and more findings have reported the presence of proteins and microRNAs critical for age-related disorders inside NDEs (Rajendran et al., 2014; Soria et al., 2017). This review article, is intended to explore the current understanding on the exosome's role in physiological aging comparing to pathological aging in the most relevant elderly neurological disorders, such as AD, FTD and PD emphasizing the emerging discoveries on proteins and ncRNAs inside exosomes.

EXTRACELLULAR VESICLES (EVs)

EVs are membrane surrounded structures released outside the cells. To date, these vesicles have been cataloged-based on their dimension and origin. Among those exosomes, originating from the endosomal compartment, are the most investigated. They have small dimensions (30–100 nm) and round shape (Mashouri et al., 2019). The biochemical content of exosomes consists of lipid, proteins but also microRNA and mRNAs. Several studies reported that mRNAs delivered by exosomes to target cells were translated in functional proteins (Pegtel et al., 2010); in the same way miRNAs regulated gene expression in recipient cells (**Figure 1**; Hu et al., 2019). Moreover, it has been reported the presence of genomic and mitochondrial DNA (Hough et al., 2018). Exosome contents not only reflect the donor cell composition but also reflect a sophisticated sorting mechanism. Analysis of exosome proteome revealed that some proteins specifically arise from cell and tissue of origin, and some are characterisitic for all exosomes (**Figure 2A**; Mashouri et al., 2019). The lipid content of exosomes is cell-specific or conserved. Indeed lipids protect exosome shape, take part in exosome biogenesis, and regulate homeostasis in the recipient cells (Vidal et al., 1989). Noteworthy, exosomes are present in several body fluids such as blood, urine, breast milk, saliva and also CSF (Urbanelli et al., 2016). Given that, they appear potentially useful biomarkers for the diagnosis of several diseases, including neurodegenerative diseases.

Exosomes in Aging and Cellular Senescence

The increasing number of aged individuals in the global population will likely lead to an increase of costs accounting on health care system. Thus, it is of crucial importance improving the comprehension of the mechanisms underneath ageing processes and developing new therapeutic strategies in order to reduce the effects of age-related morbidities. The goal standard will promote an improvement in health lifespan and a reduction of age-related co-morbidities conditions.

Aging is defined as a loss of physiological function during the time and is regulated by specific molecular pathways (Xu and Sun, 2015). Aging process leads to an increased risk of several chronic diseases such as cancer, cardiovascular disease, and autoimmune disease, but also dementia. It is associated with the body's altered capacity to face up stress caused by metabolism, infection, and damage to cellular macromolecules. The comprehension of molecular mechanisms driving aging will help the scientific community to figure out why aged individuals are more vulnerable to those diseases and why they may be less stress-resistant (Panagiotou et al., 2018).

Aging is considered conserved across *taxia* and it is characterized by nine hallmarks comprising: genomic instability, telomere shortening, epigenetic alterations, loss of proteostasis, deregulated nutrient sensing, mitochondrial dysfunction, senescence, stem cell exhaustion and alteration in intercellular communication (Shiels et al., 2017). Moreover, the so-called "inflammaging," a chronic inflammatory status, represents the main feature of aging process (Salvioli et al., 2013).

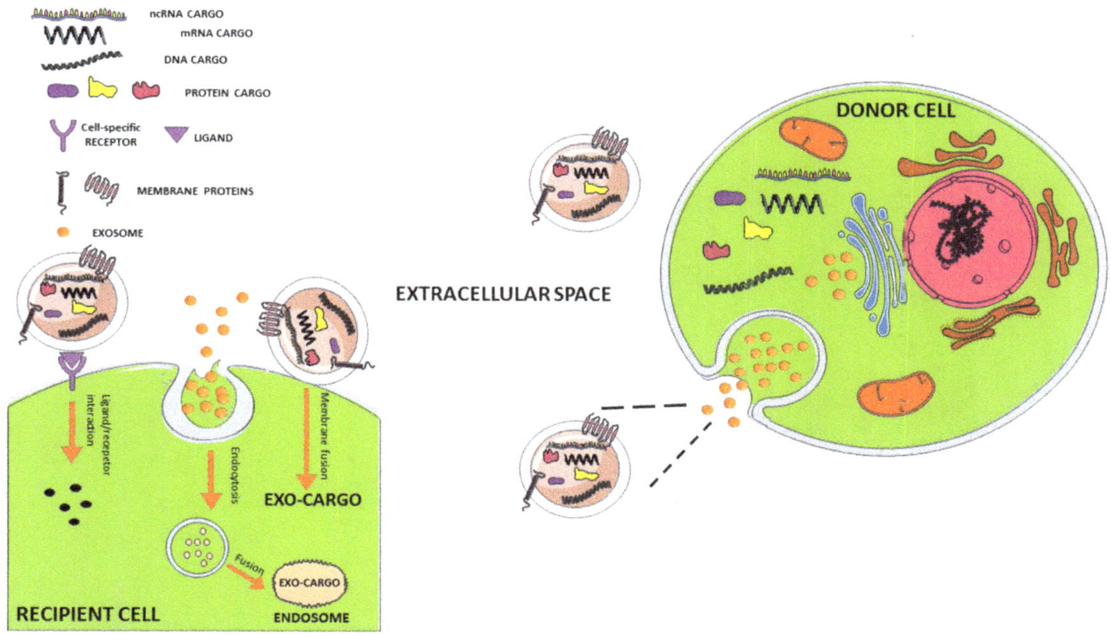

FIGURE 1 | Interaction mechanisms between exosome and recipient cell. Exosomes secreted from a donor cell can move through biological fluids to reach the recipient cell close or distant to the site of their origin. The interaction mechanisms with recipient cell are various: (1) membrane fusion with transfer of exosomal cargo to recipient cell; (2) internalization of whole exosome by endocytosis and release of the cargo by fusion with endosomal membrane; (3) activation of signaling pathways through ligand/receptor interaction. For more details, see review by Jan et al. (2017, 2019).

While aging involves the entire organism, not all cell types age at the same rate and it is conceivable that senescent cells may contribute to spread senescence to young cells (Olivieri et al., 2015).

Senescence is a particular phenotype of eukaryotic cells leading to a loss of replication ability in response to several stimuli that induce DNA damage (Campisi and d'Adda Di Fagagna, 2007).

The major component in the signal transmission from senescent cells to the surrounding tissue is the SASP that can facilitate the removal of senescent and remodeling of tissue by attraction of phagocytic immune cells (Urbanelli et al., 2016). Beside previously known SASP components, many Wnt ligands have been counted. Wnt is a secreted signaling molecule extremely conserved playing critical roles in many processes including stem cell proliferation and maintenance of homeostasis in the canonical pathway (β-catenin dependent) and transcriptional and non-transcriptional cellular responses in the non-canonical ones (β-catenin independent) triggered by calcium or other Wnt ligands, as Frizzled receptors (Nusse, 2005). It should be noted that these two different pathways interact with each other and other multiple pathways, including the NF-κB, MAPK, and JNK pathways making Wnt signaling extremely complex and articulated (Zhang et al., 2014; Ma and Hottiger, 2016). It is not surprising that Wnt is involved in aging too (Nusse, 2005). Indeed some sources suggest that Wnt signaling decays with aging in brain impairing adult neurogenesis (Okamoto et al., 2011) and lung (Hofmann et al., 2014 but at the same time it may increase in an age-dependent manner (Brack et al., 2007; Liu et al., 2014). Furthermore, the key members of Wnt pathways involved in SASP are secreted in the extracellular space by exosomes. These vesicles carrying Wnt proteins on their surface have been reported to active Wnt signaling in target cells. These findings highlighted a new role of exosomes in mediating the cell-to-cell transmission of senescence signals, suggesting that exosomes represent a new SASP component (Urbanelli et al., 2016). For the first time in 2008, Lehmann et al. (2008) described an increase of exosomes secretion by senescent cells. This increase seems to be a general feature of cellular senescence and has been observed in fibroblasts, epithelial cells, and cancer cells (Takasugi, 2018). On the contrary, Eitan et al. (2017) in cross-longitudinal study showed that plasma exosomes concentration decreased with human age, at least from the early 30s to late 60s. Monocytes and B cells internalized more exosomes rather than T cells, even if these ones are the most representative kind of PBMC in bloodstream. In addition, exosomes were more incorporated in B cells and monocytes of aged donors suggesting that exosomes internalization not only is cell-specific but age-dependent. Moreover, aging can alter RNA and protein composition of exosomes. For example Galectin-3, which plays a role in osteoblast maturation, was reduced in the plasma exosomes of elderly people, presumably as consequence of the stem cell functionality loss in the skeleton, classical of aging process (Weilner et al., 2016). Plasma exosomes isolated from young but not elderly donors promoted the osteogenic

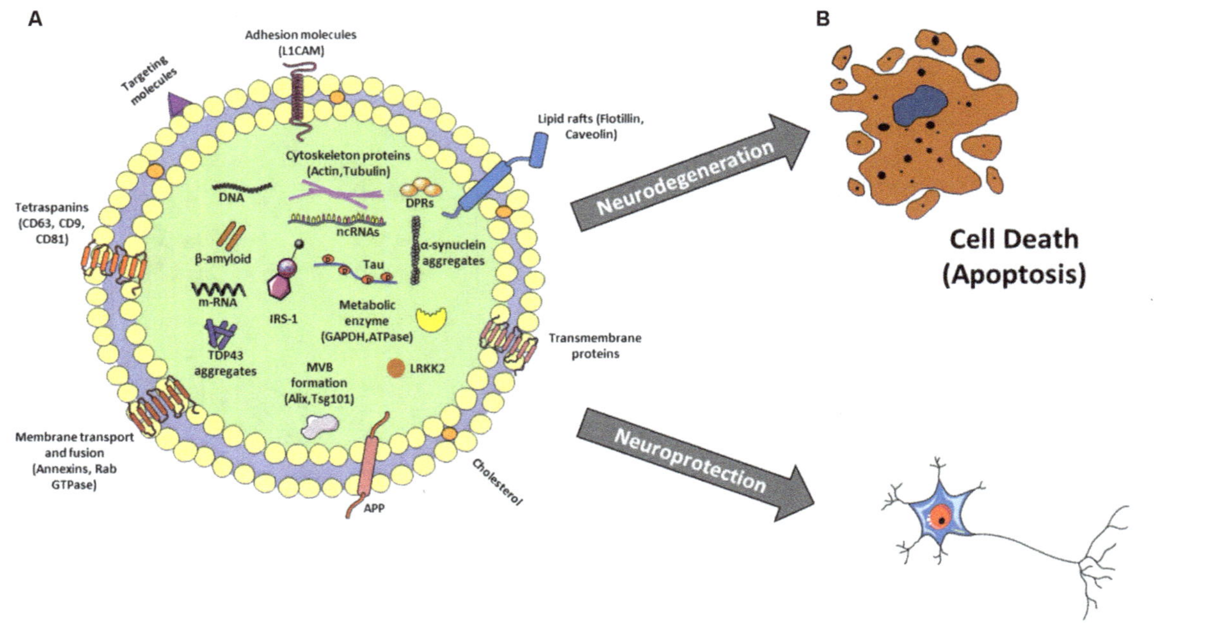

FIGURE 2 | (A) Exosome structure and cargo. Exosomes are surrounded by a phospholipid bilayer and their content reflects the cell of origin. So besides to generic molecules that identify all exosomes as Tetraspanins, Lipid rafts, MVB formation proteins, membrane transport and fusion proteins, there are other molecules specific to their origin, as L1CAM for neural exosomes as well as proteins related to aging and neurological diseases such as β-amyloid, p-Tau, LRKK2, insulin receptor substrate 1 (IRS-1), a-synuclein, amyloid precursor protein (APP), TDP-43, depeptide protein repeats (DPRs) and many others. In addition, there is also a nucleic component consisting of DNA, mRNA and different kinds of non-coding RNAs (ncRNAs; miRNAs, lncRNAs, circRNAs, piwi-RNA, etc. . .). **(B)** Exosomes: a double-edged sword in neurodegenerative disease. Exosomes could favorite and/or trigger the spreading of the disease leading to neurodegeneration or they could sequester neuro-toxic components from neural cells protecting them.

differentiation of mesenchymal stem cells in a galectin-3-dependent manner (Weilner et al., 2016). In particular, this protein, belonging to the lectin family, consists of carbohydrate recognition and collagen α-like domains. This chimeric structure allows Galectin-3 to interact with a multitude of intra-and extracellular proteins, in the nucleus as well as in the cytoplasm or on the membrane and in the extracellular space, after its secretion from different types of cells and tissues. Interacting with a myriad of proteins, Galectin-3 is involved in multiple biological processes, physiological and pathological, such as development, neuronal functions, immune reactions, endocytosis, neoplastic transformation and metastasis, and osteoblastogenesis, which impairing seems to contribute to age-related bone frailty (Dumic et al., 2006).

Exosomal miRNAs are also involved in brain aging (Pusic and Kraig, 2014). Peripheral exosomes isolated from young Wistar rats promoted differentiation in primary oligodendrocyte precursor cell (OPC) differentiation and remyelination in slice cultures. Moreover, nasal administration of EVs from young rats increased myelination in aged rat brain due to the presence of high levels of miR-219, which reduced the expression of inhibitory regulators of OPC differentiation (Pusic and Kraig, 2014). Recently, it has been described that the activity of acetylcholinesterase protein (AChE) was increased in young as well as old Wistar rats. An age-related increase was observed in CD63 levels in CSF exosomes but a decrease was observed in plasma vesicles of the older group. The authors showed that the young adult rats had significantly higher circulating IL-1β levels in the exosomes compared to the aged ones, without any effect on central content. These data suggest that the normal aging process caused different changes in the profiles of central and circulating exosomes. Altered IL-1β levels in circulating EVs could be linked, at least partly, to age-related inflammatory conditions, and a disruption of the CSF exosomes in aged rats, evaluated by CD63 levels, could be related to susceptibility to neurodegenerative disorders (Gomes de Andrade et al., 2018).

Cellular senescence triggered by specific conditions as irradiation, DNA-damaging reagents, and oncogenic RAS expression, all enhance exosomes secretion. This increase is mediated by p53 (Lehmann et al., 2008) and one of its targets, Tumor suppression-activated pathway 6 (TSAP6), but the mechanism whereby TSAP6 regulates exosomes secretion is not well understood. Nevertheless, it has been demonstrated that exosomes creating pro-inflammatory environment accelerate the aging process (Biran et al., 2017). Interestingly, exosomes contain various lengths of genomic DNA fragments and seem to be one of the major routes of DNA secretion (Fernando et al., 2017) and DNA secretion from exosomes increases upon cellular senescence (Takasugi, 2018). Intriguingly, cH2AX positive cytoplasmic chromatin fragments appear in senescent cultured cells (IMR90 and HEMa-LP); suggesting that damaged

DNA may be the major source of exosomes associated DNA in senescent cells (Ivanov et al., 2013). Exosomes are involved also in promoting genomic instability, another aging hallmark, thought the transfer of retrotransposons that are DNA elements able to create and insert multiple copies of themselves into host genomes. It is interesting to note that retrotransposons expression has been found to increase in senescent mouse cells (strain C57BL/6; De Cecco et al., 2013).

The deposition of toxic proteins is another event correlated with aging. To date, it is demonstrated that exosomes are involved in the transport of pathogenic proteins in the brain and in the progression of neurodegenerative diseases (Bellingham et al., 2012). Recently, the NDE levels of six neuronal proteins have been quantified in cognitively intact older subjects. Except for Phosphorylated tau-S396, the exosomal levels of Phosphorylated tau P-181, Beta Amyloid 42 (Aβ1–42), chatepsin D, repressor element 1-silencing transcription factor (REST) and neurogranin are significantly modified with aging (Goetzl et al., 2016).

The Role of Exosome miRNAs in Aging and Cellular Senescence

MicroRNAs are short non-coding RNAs that regulate negatively gene expression at post-transcriptional level. It has been reported that several miRNAs are involved in aging and cellular senescence (Urbanelli et al., 2016). The importance of exosomal miRNAs analysis lies in the fact that these molecules could potentially transmit signals to surrounding tissues with a good impact, but also with a detrimental role. Moreover, exosomal miRNAs are interesting in the context of aging biomarker search (Sprott, 2010). MiRNAs released from senescence cells in the extracellular environment by exosomes have been reported that are able to spread senescence in surrounding cells.

For example, miR-433 promoted the induction of senescence in ovarian cancer cells (A2780) and when overexpressed, miR-433 was released in association with exosomes (Weiner-Gorzel et al., 2015). MiR-34a and miR-29 can induce cell cycle arrest in colon carcinoma cell line (HCT116 cells) contributing to the stabilization of p53/p21 by targeting proteins relevant for its regulation such as Sirtuin 1 (SIRT1; Yamakuchi and Lowenstein, 2009). The miR17–92 cluster is down regulated in several cell aging models as endothelial cells, replicated CD8+ T cells, renal proximal tubular epithelial cells, and skin fibroblasts and they can target p53/p21 (Weilner et al., 2013). Another miRNA involved in cellular senescence is miR-146, whose expression was increased in senescent human fibroblasts (HCA2) when compared with proliferating quiescent ones. It is important to underlie that miRNA-146 targets IL-6 and IL-8, SASP components with pro-inflammatory function, suggesting a role for miR-146 as senescence-associated inflammation modulator (Bhaumik et al., 2009). On the other hand, miRNAs encapsulated in exosomes are able to suppress cellular senescence; this is the case of miR-214, involved in angiogenesis, that plays a role in vesicle-mediated signaling between endothelial cells. Exosomes derived from human microvascular endothelial cell line (HMEC-1) stimulated migration and angiogenesis in recipient cells, whereas exosomes from miR-214-depleted endothelial cells failed to stimulate these processes preventing senescence and allowing blood vessel formation (van Balkom et al., 2013). A recent microarray study performed on salivary exosomes miRNAs from young and old healthy subjects has identified mir-24-3p as a possible peripheral aging biomarker (Machida et al., 2015). Exosomes isolated from the bone marrow of young and aged C57BL/6 mice showed a similar concentration and size distribution. However, bioanalyzer data indicated that exosomes from young and aged mice were differently enriched in miRNAs. The amount of miR-183-5p was increased in aged bone marrow exosomes, and its overexpression detected also in bone marrow stromal cells, mimicked the effects of aged bone marrow exosomes (Davis et al., 2017).

EXOSOMES IN ELDERLY NEUROLOGICAL DISORDERS: NEUROPROTECTIVE OR NEURODEGENERATIVE ROLE?

Although there are, still few evidence on the role of exosome in the healthy aged brain, as we discussed before, it is known that exosomes have a role in the pathogenesis and in the progression of many neurodegenerative diseases (Soria et al., 2017). However, it is not established if they play a positive or negative role because the literature is controversial defining them like a double-edged sword in the neurodegenerative disease (Lee and Kim, 2017). The discovery that exosomes carry functional biomolecules as key pathogenic proteins (e.g., Aβ-amyloid, tau and α-synuclein) and miRNAs (**Figure 2A**) led to consider their involvement in neurological disorders (Thompson et al., 2016). Dysregulation of intercommunication between neurons or between neurons and glial cells mediated by exosomes could trigger the disease (Lee and Kim, 2017). On the contrary, exosomes could sequester neuro-toxic components from neural cells and flow neuro-protective ones (**Figure 2B**). This means that they can favorite the spreading of the disease or they can inhibit it (Lee and Kim, 2017). This section is intended to give an overview of the double roles of exosome proteins and microRNAs proposed for AD, FTD and PD.

Exosomes in Alzheimer's Disease (AD)

AD is considered the most frequent cause of dementia. It is characterized, clinically, by cognitive and behavioral disorders and, pathologically, by the extracellular deposit of insoluble Aβ-amyloid and intracellular neurofibrillary tangles (NFTs), consisting of tau fibrils. The amyloid plaques derived from impaired processing of the APP leading to the formation of the toxic Aβ-amyloid. APP is translocated into the endoplasmic reticulum (ER) and matures through Golgi apparatus. The mature form of APP is transported to the cell membrane where it undergoes to further proteolytic cleavage from β- and γ-secretases acting together to produce fibrils of the toxic Aβ-amyloid that accumulates with age in human AD brains (Busciglio et al., 1993; Takahashi et al., 2002). The dosage of Aβ-amyloid, total tau and phosphorylated tau in the CSF is recognized as the "core" of AD biomarkers in the clinical practice (Molinuevo et al., 2018). Interestingly, the first link between exosomes and AD proposed that Aβ-amyloid was released in association with exosomes. Moreover, the presence of other specific exosomal proteins as Alix and Flotillin-1 were also found accumulating into the AD brain (Rajendran et al., 2006; Sharples et al., 2008). A prion-like mechanism to explain how aggregates of Aβ-amyloid seem to self-propagate and spread to cells out of CNS is confirmed in AD mouse models. Seeding of Aβ was observed when extracts of AD human brain were injected in healthy mice that express the human wild-type APP gene causing the formation of the plaques in the site of injection and adjacent brain region (Morales et al., 2011). In addition, tauopathy was inducted in ALZ17 transgenic mice injecting aggregated of tau protein (Clavaguera et al., 2009). In the light of these findings, the hypothesis that exosomes could use a prion-like mechanism to disseminate toxic proteins associated with AD is taking hold (Coleman and Hill, 2015; Thompson et al., 2016). Exosomes could be involved in the trafficking of amyloid aggregates because Tg2576 mouse brain mice and post-mortem human AD brains were enriched in exosome markers within amyloid plaques (Kokubo et al., 2004; Rajendran et al., 2006). Phosphorylated tau was also detected in the exosomes from CSF of early-onset AD patients (Saman et al., 2012). ADAM10, Beta-secretase 1 (BACE1), nicastrin, and presenilin 1 and 2 (PSEN1 and 2) are other examples of AD pathogenic proteins found inside exosomes of transgenic mouse brain (Tg2576) and cell culture APP models, as CHO cell line (Sharples et al., 2008; Perez-Gonzalez et al., 2012). More recently, researchers have found that exosomes could stimulate aggregation of Aβ-amyloid and tau *in vivo* models, 5XFAD and rTg4510 transgenic mice (Dinkins et al., 2014; Polanco et al., 2016). In other words, exosomes, removing the excess of intracellular Aβ, shuttled it outside the cells concurring to plaque formation (Joshi et al., 2015). On the other hand, a neuroprotective role is also proposed. Neural exosomes could uptake Aβ-amyloid reducing the Aβ load in the brain as seen in the brains of mouse models (C57BL/6, KM670/671NL and V717F) where after the injection of exosomes, a decrease of Aβ and amyloid deposition was observed (Yuyama et al., 2015). Furthermore, extracellular tau could arise by secretion through exosomes in SH-SY5Y and COS-7 cell lines (Simón et al., 2012). Even if there is a body of literature arguing the role of exosomes in aggregate transmission, the fact remains that this theory assumes the presence of pathogenic proteins within exosomes about which the functional evidences are few or controversial (Lim and Lee, 2017). Nevertheless, the exosome hypothesis is appealing and partly explains the intercellular transmission of proteinopathies. Worth mentioning also, a research field that proposes exosomes as source of biomarkers for CNS disorders (**Figure 3**) due to their interesting characteristics suitable to the clinic (e.g., presence in many biological fluids, crossing the BBB, protection of the biomolecules inside them, etc.). Goetzl et al. (2015, 2018) measured the levels of different pathogenic proteins, Aβ-amyloid, total tau and p-tau isoforms inside NDEs immunoprecipitated with L1CAM to isolate specifically neuronal exosomes from blood of AD, Mild Cognitive Impairment (MCI) and controls (Kapogiannis et al., 2015). They found higher levels of these proteins vs. controls able to predict the development of AD 10 years before clinical onset (Fiandaca et al., 2015) or the progression from MCI to dementia (Winston et al., 2016). Instead, a contrary study showed no difference in NDEs total tau levels for AD patients (Shi et al., 2017). It is known that type-2 diabetes is an AD risk factor thus AD brains have markers of insulin resistance as Insulin Receptor Substrate-1 (IRS-1). Altered forms of IRS-1 were detected in NDEs of AD plasma patients and at lower levels compared to controls and to patients with type 2 diabetes with intermediate levels. This is interesting because NDEs IRS-1 protein levels could contribute to discriminate MCI/AD to controls and patients with type-2 diabetes at the same time (Kapogiannis et al., 2015). Pathological proteins were also found in exosomes extracted from CSF. In the work of Saman et al. (2012), the tau phosphorylated at threonine 181 (pT181) was more concentrated in CSF exosomes than in the total CSF and in early stage of AD, while it was absent in other dementing conditions as vascular or Lewy body diseases. This exosomal tau detected so early in AD suggests that CSF tau could be secreted, not shed from dead neurons (Saman et al., 2012).

The Role of Exosome miRNAs in AD

Not only proteins but also ncRNAs, mostly miRNAs, are detected within exosomes and are different from those of donor cell. These so named "exosomal RNAs" are shuttled between donor and recipient cells becoming "exosomal shuttle RNA" (esRNA). They are protected from the degradation and are functionally active suggesting the esRNAs as a novel mechanism of intercellular genetic transfer and communication (Valadi et al., 2007). Exosomal miRNAs have been isolated from exosomes derived from different kinds of cells (from C57BL6 primary cultures) including neurons and primary astrocytes (prepared using cortices obtained from neonatal rat) and fluids as blood and CSF (Caby et al., 2005; Guescini et al., 2010; Goldie et al., 2014; Liu et al., 2014; Cheng et al., 2015; Lugli et al., 2015). The relevance of miRNAs in the CNS is now widely documented with almost 70% of all miRNAs expressed in the human brain (Nowak and Michlewski, 2013) hypothesizing that neuronal miRNAs may regulate the transcription of more than a third of genes (Kosik, 2006). Therefore, it is not surprising that altered blood/CSF exosomal miRNAs signature could be related to neurodegenerative disease, in particular to AD (Cheng et al., 2015; Gui et al., 2015; Lugli et al., 2015). Cheng et al. (2015) profiled miRNAs from serum exosomes to determine a set of miRNAs differentially expressed in AD. They found a specific miRNAs signature consisting of 16 miRNAs, along with risk factors, and many of them were identified as implicated in AD pathogenesis in several mouse and cell models. In detail, mir-1306-5p, that targets ADAM10, was the microRNA with the best sensitivity and specificity to predict AD. Lugli et al. (2015) found another interesting microRNA signature in plasma exosomes using Illumina deep sequencing technology. The researchers identified 20 microRNAs downregulated among which the lowest expressed miRNA in AD group compared to controls was the miR-342-3p. This is a brain-enriched miRNAs and its expression was highly correlated across individuals. Interestingly, the failure of proteasomal machine in

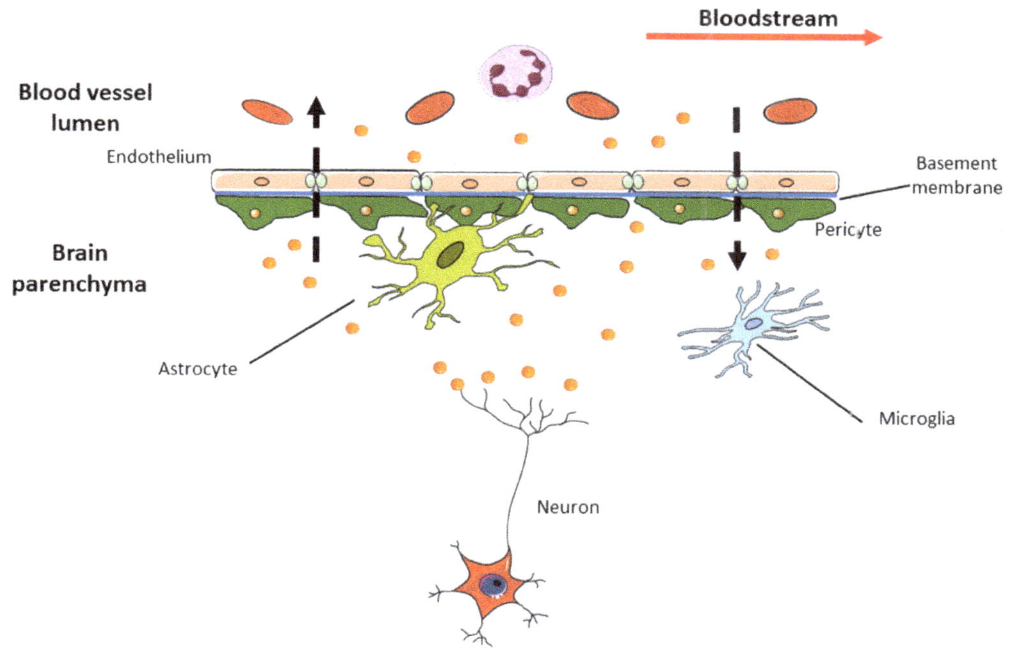

FIGURE 3 | Exosomes are able to pass through blood brain barrier (BBB) in both directions. This means that specific exosomes (i.e., the neural ones with L1CAM on their surface) detected in the cerebrospinal fluid (CSF) can be released into bloodstream and vice versa. This feature makes exosomes appealing in the research of new sources of biomarkers suitable for use in clinical practice, as liquid biopsy that could replace current invasive diagnostic methods.

tauopathies was supposed to be modulated by miRNA expression (Carrettiero et al., 2009). Indeed, hyperphosphorylation of tau was linked to up-regulation of ERK kinases after downregulation in AD brains of mir-15a, specifically dysregulated in AD (Hébert et al., 2010).

AD-related exosomal microRNAs were also investigated in the CSF. The overexpression of mir-193b in the hippocampus of AD C57BL/6J double transgenic mice could inhibit the expression of APP involving it in neurodegenerative process like an unique biomarker of AD (Liu et al., 2014). Gui et al. (2015) performed another study on exosomes from CSF. They isolated exosomes in CSF from AD patients and healthy controls, and used microarray analysis in order to identify microRNAs differentially abundant between AD, and normal group. AD exosomes showed fewer differences with healthy controls, with only six miRNAs showing significantly altered levels. In the same study, it was interesting to notice that also several mRNAs were differentially expressed in CSF exosomes in AD subjects. The levels of *APP* mRNA, *SNCA* (α-synuclein) mRNA, *DJ-1/PARK7* (Deglicase) mRNA, and *CX3CL1* (Fractalkine) mRNA were lower in AD exosomes, while the levels of neurofilamentL (*NEFL*) mRNA were higher. Interestingly, *MAPT* (Tau) mRNA was unchanged while the lncRNAs RP11- 462G22.1 and PCA3 were enriched in CSF exosomes from AD (**Figure 4**; Gui et al., 2015).

The potential therapeutic utility of exosomes is nowadays increasing. For example, siRNAs inside exosomes could use to target specific genes. Alvarez-Erviti et al. (2011) demonstrated that exosomes with exogenous siRNA anti-BACE1 were able to reduce the levels of BACE1 mRNA and protein in C57BL/6 mouse model brains. As well as the number of researches proposing one or more exosomal miRNAs as a potential biomarker to prognostic and/or diagnostic AD is growing. Recently, Yang et al. (2018) reported that serum exosome miR-135a and miR-384 were up-regulated while miR-193b was down-regulated in the serum of AD patients compared with normal controls, whereas exosomal miR-384 was the best among the three miRNAs to discriminate AD, Vascular Dementia (VaD), and PD with dementia (PDD). Receiver Operating Characteristic (ROC) curve to estimate the diagnostic utility of a biomarker or a set of them showed that the combination of miR-135a, -193b, and -384 was better than the single one to diagnose early-onset AD (Yang et al., 2018). Another study analyzed a limited subset of miRNAs involved in neuroinflammation, miR-137, miR-155 and miR-223 (**Figure 4**). They found that the median level of serum exosomal miR-223 was significantly reduced in patients with AD and was significantly correlated with Mini-Mental State Examination (MMSE) scores, Clinical Dementia Rating (CDR) scores, magnetic resonance spectroscopy (MRS) spectral ratios and serum concentrations of IL-1b, IL-6, TNF-a, and CRP. Authors concluded that exosomal miR-223 could be a promising biomarker for AD diagnosis although the sample size was limited and miRNAs screened are only three (Wei et al., 2018). Although both works are certainly interesting, they should be considered with attention because they lack the correlation with CSF values of β-amyloid, tau and P-tau. Anyway, they are pioneering for future studies.

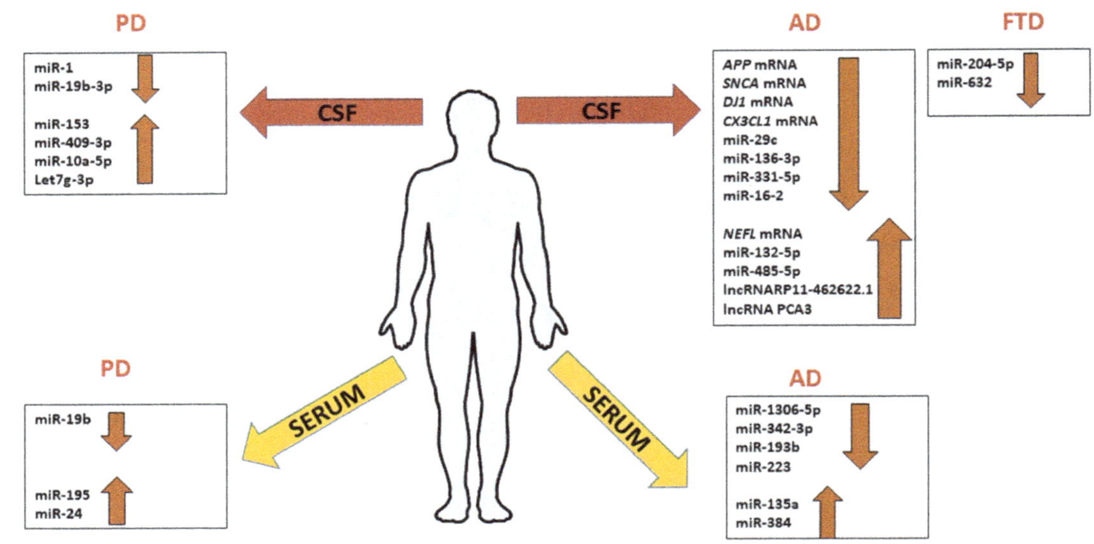

FIGURE 4 | Comprehensive expression profile patterns of ncRNAs differentially expressed in patients with Alzheimer's disease (AD), frontotemporal dementia (FTD) and Parkinson's disease (PD) extracted from serum or CSF exosomes.

It should be mentioned that exosomes have inside them other categories of ncRNA species as long noncoding RNAs (lncRNAs), circular RNAs (circRNAs), small nucleolar RNA (snoRNAs), small nuclear RNAs (snRNAs), transfer RNA (tRNAs), ribosomal RNAs (rRNAs), and piwi-interacting RNAs (piRNAs) identified comprehensively using high-throughput RNA-Seq (Kim et al., 2017). Although the role for some of them is emerging as critical for gene expression, their involvment in AD related to exosomes is still in the infancy.

Exosomes in Frontotemporal Dementia (FTD)

FTD is the most common form of dementia in the presenium accounting for up to 20% of patients with an onset before 65 years. Three clinically different syndromes characterize FTD: behavioral variant (bv) FTD, Progressive Non Fluent Aphasia (PNFA), and Semantic Dementia (SD). These different subtypes are related to different clinical features but mostly patients present a profound alteration in the behavior and personality, often associated with cognitive and executive impairment, except for PNFA and SD where the language impairment is prevalent (Snowden et al., 2007). All of these syndromes at pathological level are characterized by Frontotemporal lobar degeneration (FTLD). Histopathologically FTLD is defined on the type of protein depositing into FTLD-Tau, FTLD-TAR DNA Binding protein (TDP)-43, and FTLD-Fused in Sarcoma (FUS; Fenoglio et al., 2018).

Up to 40% of patients have a history of familial transmission with nearly 10% of patients showing an autosomal dominant inheritance pattern. The majority of familial FTLD account mutations in the microtubule associated protein tau (*MAPT*) and progranulin (*GRN*) genes, and the pathologic expansion of the hexanucleotide GGGGCC repeat in the first intron of *C9ORF72* gene (Rademakers and Hutton, 2007).

As discussed above for AD, also for FTD, the involving of exosomes in the pathology has been investigated although the current knowledge is still limited. FTD is characterized by TDP-43 aggregates accumulation throughout the nervous system. As for AD pathogenic proteins, also TDP-43 protein can be exchanged *via* exosomes between neuronal cells (Neuro2a cells and primary neurons) leading to propagation of TDP-43 proteinopathy in a "prion-like" manner (Iguchi et al., 2016). Indeed the uptake of exosomal TDP-43 oligomers from recipient cells induces higher toxicity than free TDP-43 in murine primary cortical neuron cell culture (C57Bl76J; Feiler et al., 2015). Furthermore, exosomes derived from ALS-FTD-CSF cell model showed a high concentration of full length and TDP-43 C-terminal fragments (CTFs). The latter lead to the formation of cytoplasmic inclusions within cells, so authors suggest that aberrant cleavage of TDP-43 in these exosomes acting as "seed" induces the formation of TDP-43 aggregates in the ALS-FTD-CSF-cultured cells (Ding et al., 2015). Not only TDP-43, but also dipeptide repeat proteins (DPRs) produced by aberrant translation of *C9ORF72* FTD patients throughout CNS seem to spread between cells *via* exosome-dependent pathways (Westergard et al., 2016).

As was the case for AD patients, levels of Aβ and pT181 were increased in FTD as well (Fiandaca et al., 2015). Interestingly, the levels of synaptophysin, synaptopodin, synaptotagmin-2, and neurogranin dosed in NDEs were decreased in patients with FTD compared to controls, probably because of reduced functionality of synaptic proteins in senile dementias. These levels were low years before dementia making synaptic NDEs proteins useful for preclinical diagnosis of dementia (Goetzl et al., 2016). Instead, the Repressor Element 1 Silencing Transcriptor factor (REST) was significantly high in FTD over controls and AD representing a potential marker to discriminate FTD patients from AD (Goetzl et al., 2015). The IRS-1 phosphorylated in serine 312 was able to distinguish at 84% of accuracy between FTD patients and controls (Kapogiannis et al., 2015).

Lastly, Benussi et al. (2016) studied human primary fibroblasts without GRN null mutations. They conclude that the glycosylated form of PGRN was released with exosomes and in the presence of mutation, the secretion of exosomes was extremely reduced and their composition changed enriching in Lamp1 protein. Overall, the GRN null mutations cause an alteration in the intercellular communication.

The Role of Exosome miRNAs in FTD

The current knowledge of exosomal miRNAs in the pathogenesis of FTLD is exiguous. The work of Schneider et al. (2018) is the only performed on exosomes from CSF of FTLD patients. MiRNA expression profiles of 23 presymptomatic and 15 symptomatic mutation carriers compared to 11 healthy non-mutation carriers were performed on the Genetic Frontotemporal Dementia Initiative (GENFI) cohort and sporadic FTD. They found that miR-204-5p and miR-632 significantly decreased in symptomatic respect to presymptomatic mutation carriers (**Figure 4**). In another cohort, the miR-632 was highly decreased in sporadic FTLD compared to sporadic AD and healthy controls. The authors, using *in silico* analysis, discovered a potential target of miR-204-5p and miR-632; HRK that encodes for HARAKIRI, a pro-apoptotic protein. Its aberrant increasing could contribute to the neuronal death in FTLD patients (Schneider et al., 2018). Although these findings open a new perspective in the FTLD research, they need further investigations.

Exosomes in Parkinson's Disease (PD)

PD is a chronic neurodegenerative disease characterized by motor impairments due to the selective death of dopaminergic neurons. Cognitive impairments can arise in the course of the disease at any time. The most of PD cases are sporadic but there are rare familial forms linked to mutations in several genes; *SNCA, parkin, DJ-1*, PTEN-induced kinase 1 (PINK-1) and Leucine-rich repeat kinase 2 (LRRK2; Thomas and Beal, 2007). Even if the molecular pathogenesis of PD is not fully understood, it's now universally accepted that α-synuclein plays a predominant role in PD accumulating in Lewy Bodies, a pathological hallmark of PD (Spillantini and Goedert, 2018). Indeed α-synuclein aggregates are responsible for synaptic pathology and neurodegeneration (Kramer and Schulz-Schaeffer, 2007). In addition, mutations that involve duplication or triplication of the wild-type *SNCA* are associated to autosomal dominant PD with a severity proportional to the degree of α-synuclein over-expression whereas missense mutations in *SNCA* (e.g., A53T) are linked to dominantly inherited forms of PD (Thomas and Beal, 2007). Therefore, it is not surprising that the spreading of pathology, already proposed for AD and demonstrated for PD involved α-synuclein. Several studies on murine primary cortical neurons and SH-SY5Y cell lines reported that α-synuclein was secreted from exosomes (Emmanouilidou et al., 2010; Danzer et al., 2012). Moreover, exosomes, providing environments for α-synuclein nucleation, catalyzed its aggregation in N2a cells and cultured hippocampal neurons (Olanow and Brundin, 2013; Grey et al., 2015). Another study in human H4 cell line demonstrated that the loss of function of P-type ATPase ion pump PARK9/ATP13A2 led to a decrease in secretion of α-synuclein into extracellular space, indeed the overexpression of PARK9/ATP13A2 caused the opposite effect, suggesting that PARK9/ATP13A2 was involved in the α-synuclein secretion at least in part *via* exosomes (Tsunemi et al., 2014). This consequence could have a neuroprotective effect. Probably because the increased release of exosomes containing α-synuclein reducing the intracellular levels of that protein, it could explain the surviving of neurons of substantia nigra in sporadic PD patients that overexpress PARK9/ATP13A2.

Furthermore, the biogenesis of α-synuclein exosomes seems to be modulated by zinc levels regulated from PARK9/ATP13A2 in SHSY5Y cells (Kong et al., 2014). Stuendl et al. (2016) measured the levels of CSF exosomal α-synuclein, and found differences among patients with PD and Lewy bodies. In accordance with previous studies in glioblastoma cell lines, the same group demonstrated that CSF exosomes derived from patients with PD and dementia with Lewy bodies induced the oligomerization of soluble α-synuclein in target cells in a dose-dependent manner (Stuendl et al., 2016). In this regard, Shi et al. (2014) were able to demonstrate in mouse models that CSF α-synuclein was promptly transported to blood, with a small portion within exosomes but CNS specific. An increased releasing of this protein to the blood of PD patients was explained discovering that in a large cohort of clinical samples (267 PD and 215 controls); the levels of plasma exosomal α-synuclein were significantly higher in PD patients. Another protein secreted from exosomes is LRRK2. Mutations in the *LRKK2* gene cause late-onset PD. LRKK2 secretion was regulated by 14-3-3 protein. Indeed, using 14-3-3 inhibitor, the LRRK2 secretion from exosomes was interrupted in mouse primary neurons and macrophages (Fraser et al., 2013).

The Role of Exosome miRNAs in PD

Concerning the involvement of exosomal miRNAs in PD, the literature is still scarce. Cao et al. (2017) profiled the expression of 24 candidate miRNAs, already dysregulated in previous studies, in the serum of 109 PD patients matched with healthy controls finding the downregulation of miR-19b and the upregulation of miR-195 and miR-24 compared to healthy controls. Instead, Gui et al. (2015) investigated the expression of 746 miRNAs in CSF of PD patients finding 16 miRNAs upregulated and 11 downregulated. In detail, miR-1 and miR-19b-3p were significantly reduced; miR-153, miR-409-3p, miR-10a-5p, and let-7g-3p were significantly overexpressed in PD CSF exosomes (**Figure 4**). With bioinformatics tools the predicted targets of these miRNAs were involved in critical pathways for PD; neurotrophin signaling, mTOR signaling, ubiquitin-mediated proteolysis, dopaminergic synapse, and glutamatergic synapse. To complete the study, authors analyzed exosomal miRNAs in AD too, as we mentioned before in this review article. They conclude that exosomal RNAs could be useful to distinguish accurately between PD and AD (Gui et al., 2015).

With respect to the research of new biomarkers for early diagnosis of PD, Dos Santos et al. (2018) combining an optimized technique of exosomal miRNA isolation with small RNA sequencing, they detected 1,683 exosomal miRNAs in the CSF on 40 early-stage PD patients and 40 well-matched controls. Then, using machine learning approach to find the best miRNA biomarkers for the accurate diagnosis of early-stage PD, they restricted analysis on a panel model of 5 microRNAs, let-7f-5p, miR-27a-3p, miR-125a-5p, miR-151a-3p, and miR-423-5p. Intriguingly, when combining miRNA profiles to protein analysis of the most studied PD related proteins as biomarkers, as DJ-1, UCHL1 and α-synuclein, the robustness of the generated model increased. This work was worth to be mentioned because it is the first study integrating the state-of-the-art microRNA sequencing with protein analysis and complex machine learning approach and obtained potential PD biomarkers in CSF exosomes able to discriminate early PD from healthy controls (Dos Santos et al., 2018). Unfortunately, studies are still scarce and need further investigations and validations although they are promising in the field of biomarker research.

CONCLUDING REMARKS

It is undeniable that last two decades have been characterized by an exponential increase in the number of publications regarding exosomes and their role in the pathogenesis of diseases as well as in the field of clinical biomarker research. Indeed due to their intrinsic ability to transfer biomolecules to other cells and to cross the BBB in both directions, they are becoming an attractive source of potential new biomarkers and/or reservoir of validated ones. The times when exosomes were considered full of junk are long gone. Indeed, new roles and functions for exosomes emerged to the point where these small EVs have been proposed with a double-edged sword role, "Trojan horses" of neurodegeneration or neuroprotective from neurodegeneration. This means that their involvement in neurodegenerative diseases is not totally understood. Some questions remain opened and the most interesting seem to be: (1) are exosomes carrier of disease propagating pathogenic molecules also *in vivo*; (2) can targeting the release of exosomes, or the release of their cargo have an inhibitor effect on the progression of diseases; and (3) can specific protein, or ncRNA signatures isolated from patients be used as biomarker of disease. Further investigations will clarify these aspects as well as the basic research on exosomes improving the comprehension on the role of exosomes in the etiology and progression of these pathologies.

AUTHOR CONTRIBUTIONS

MD and MS wrote the article. CF contributed to writing the article and supervised it. BA, MC, ES and DG supervised the final version of the manuscript.

FUNDING

This work was supported by grants from the Italian Ministry of Health (Ministero della Salute): NET-2011-02346784 and the Monzino Foundation.

REFERENCES

Alvarez-Erviti, L., Seow, Y., Yin, H., Betts, C., Lakhal, S., and Wood, M. J. A. (2011). Delivery of siRNA to the mouse brain by systemic injection of targeted exosomes. *Nat. Biotechnol.* 29, 341–345. doi: 10.1038/nbt.1807

Bellingham, S. A., Guo, B. B., Coleman, B. M., and Hill, A. F. (2012). Exosomes: vehicles for the transfer of toxic proteins associated with neurodegenerative diseases? *Front. Physiol.* 3:124. doi: 10.3389/fphys.2012.00124

Benussi, L., Ciani, M., Tonoli, E., Morbin, M., Palamara, L., Albani, D., et al. (2016). Loss of exosomes in progranulin-associated frontotemporal dementia. *Neurobiol. Aging* 40, 41–49. doi: 10.1016/j.neurobiolaging.2016.01.001

Bhaumik, D., Scott, G. K., Schokrpur, S., Patil, C. K., Orjalo, A. V., Rodier, F., et al. (2009). MicroRNAs miR-146a/b negatively modulate the senescence-associated inflammatory mediators IL-6 and IL-8. *Aging* 1, 402–411. doi: 10.18632/aging.100042

Biran, A., Zada, L., Abou Karam, P., Vadai, E., Roitman, L., Ovadya, Y., et al. (2017). Quantitative identification of senescent cells in aging and disease. *Aging Cell* 16, 661–671. doi: 10.1111/acel.12592

Brack, A. S., Conboy, M. J., Roy, S., Lee, M., Kuo, C. J., Keller, C., et al. (2007). Increased Wnt signaling during aging alters muscle stem cell fate and increases fibrosis. *Science* 317, 807–810. doi: 10.1126/science.1144090

Busciglio, J., Gabuzda, D. H., Matsudaira, P., and Yankner, B. A. (1993). Generation of beta-amyloid in the secretory pathway in neuronal and nonneuronal cells. *Proc. Natl. Acad. Sci. U S A* 90, 2092–2096. doi: 10.1073/pnas.90.5.2092

Caby, M. P., Lankar, D., Vincendeau-Scherrer, C., Raposo, G., and Bonnerot, C. (2005). Exosomal-like vesicles are present in human blood plasma. *Int. Immunol.* 17, 879–887. doi: 10.1093/intimm/dxh267

Campisi, J. (2012). Aging, cellular senescence and cancer. *Annu. Rev. Physiol.* 75, 685–705. doi: 10.1146/annurev-physiol-030212-183653

Campisi, J., and d'Adda Di Fagagna, F. (2007). Cellular senescence: when bad things happen to good cells. *Mol. Cell Biol.* 8, 729–740. doi: 10.1038/nrm2233

Cao, X. Y., Lu, J. M., Zhao, Z. Q., Li, M. C., Lu, T., An, X. S., et al. (2017). MicroRNA biomarkers of Parkinson's disease in serum exosome-like microvesicles. *Neurosci. Lett.* 644, 94–99. doi: 10.1016/j.neulet.2017.02.045

Carrettiero, D. C., Hernandez, I., Neveu, P., Papagiannakopoulos, T., and Kosik, K. S. (2009). The cochaperone BAG2 sweeps paired helical filament- insoluble tau from the microtubule. *J. Neurosci.* 29, 2151–2161. doi: 10.1523/JNEUROSCI

Cheng, L., Doecke, J. D., Sharples, R. A., Villemagne, V. L., Fowler, C. J., Rembach, A., et al. (2015). Prognostic serum miRNA biomarkers associated with Alzheimer's disease shows concordance with neuropsychological and neuroimaging assessment. *Mol. Psychiatry* 20, 1188–1196. doi: 10.1038/mp.2014.127

Clavaguera, F., Bolmont, T., Crowther, R. A., Abramowski, D., Frank, S., Probst, A., et al. (2009). Transmission and spreading of tauopathy in transgenic mouse brain. *Nat. Cell Biol.* 11, 909–913. doi: 10.1038/ncb1901

Coleman, B. M., and Hill, A. F. (2015). Extracellular vesicles—their role in the packaging and spread of misfolded proteins associated with neurodegenerative diseases. *Semin. Cell Dev. Biol.* 40, 89–96. doi: 10.1016/j.semcdb.2015.02.007

Danzer, K. M., Kranich, L. R., Ruf, W. P., Cagsal-Getkin, O., Winslow, A. R., Zhu, L., et al. (2012). Exosomal cell-to-cell transmission of α synuclein oligomers. *Mol. Neurodegener.* 7:42. doi: 10.1186/1750-1326-7-42

Davis, C., Dukes, A., Drewry, M., Helwa, I., Johnson, M. H., Isales, C. M., et al. (2017). MicroRNA-183-5p increases with age in bone-derived extracellular vesicles, suppresses bone marrow stromal (stem) cell proliferation and induces stem cell senescence. *Tissue Eng. Part A* 23, 1231–1240. doi: 10.1089/ten.TEA.2016.0525

De Cecco, M., Criscione, S. W., Peterson, A. L., Neretti, N., Sedivy, J. M., and Kreiling, J. A. (2013). Transposable elements become active and mobile in the genomes of aging mammalian somatic tissues. *Aging* 5, 867–883. doi: 10.18632/aging.100621

Ding, X., Ma, M., Teng, J., Teng, R. K. F., Zhou, S., Yin, J., et al. (2015). Exposure to ALS-FTD-CSF generates TDP-43 aggregates in glioblastoma cells through exosomes and TNTs-like structure. *Oncotarget* 6, 24178–24191. doi: 10.18632/oncotarget.4680

Dinkins, M. B., Dasgupta, S., Wang, G., Zhu, G., and Bieberich, E. (2014). Exosome reduction *in vivo* is associated with lower amyloid plaque load in the 5XFAD mouse model of Alzheimer's disease. *Neurobiol. Aging* 35, 1792–1800. doi: 10.1016/j.neurobiolaging.2014.02.012

Dos Santos, M. C. T., Barreto-Sanz, M. A., Correia, B. R. S., Bell, R., Widnall, C., Perez, L. T., et al. (2018). miRNA-based signatures in cerebrospinal fluid as potential diagnostic tools for early stage Parkinson's disease. *Oncotarget* 9, 17455–17465. doi: 10.18632/oncotarget.24736

Dumic, J., Dabelic, S., and Flögel, M. (2006). Galectin-3: an open-ended story. *Biochim. Biophys. Acta* 1760, 616–635. doi: 10.1016/j.bbagen.2005.12.020

Eitan, E., Green, J., Bodogai, M., Mode, N. A., Bæk, R., Jørgensen, M. M., et al. (2017). Age-related changes in plasma extracellular vesicle characteristics and internalization by leukocytes. *Sci. Rep.* 7:1342. doi: 10.1038/s41598-017-01386-z

Emmanouilidou, E., Melachroinou, K., Roumeliotis, T., Garbis, S. D., Ntzouni, M., Margaritis, L. H., et al. (2010). Cell-produced α-synuclein is secreted in a calcium-dependent manner by exosomes and impacts neuronal survival. *J. Neurosci.* 30, 6838–6851. doi: 10.1523/jneurosci.5699-09.2010

Fauré, J., Lachenal, G., Court, M., Hirrlinger, J., Chatellard-Causse, C., Blot, B., et al. (2006). Exosomes are released by cultured cortical neurones. *Mol. Cell. Neurosci.* 31, 642–648. doi: 10.1016/j.mcn.2005.12.003

Feiler, M. S., Strobel, B., Freischmidt, A., Helferich, A. M., Kappel, J., Brewer, B. M., et al. (2015). TDP-43 is intercellularly transmitted across axon terminals. *J. Cell Biol.* 211, 897–911. doi: 10.1083/jcb.201504057

Fenoglio, C., Scarpini, E., and Galimberti, D. (2018). Epigenetic regulatory modifications in genetic and sporadic frontotemporal dementia. *Expert Rev. Neurother.* 18, 469–475. doi: 10.1080/14737175.2018.1481389

Fernando, M. R., Jiang, C., Krzyzanowski, G. D., and Ryan, W. L. (2017). New evidence that a large proportion of human blood plasma cell-free DNA is localized in exosomes. *PLoS One* 12:e0183915. doi: 10.1371/journal.pone.0183915

Fiandaca, M. S., Kapogiannis, D., Mapstone, M., Boxer, A., Eitan, E., Schwartz, J. B., et al. (2015). Identification of preclinical Alzheimer's disease by a profile of pathogenic proteins in neurally derived blood exosomes: a case-control study. *Alzheimers Dement.* 11, 600.e1–607.e1. doi: 10.1016/j.jalz.2014.06.008

Franzen, C. A., Blackwell, R. H., Foreman, K. E., Kuo, P. C., Flanigan, R. C., and Gupta, G. N. (2015). Urinary exosomes: the potential for biomarker utility, intercellular signaling and therapeutics in urological malignancy. *J. Urol.* 195, 1331–1339. doi: 10.1016/j.juro.2015.08.115

Fraser, K. B., Moehle, M. S., Daher, J. P. L., Webber, P. J., Williams, J. Y., Stewart, C. A., et al. (2013). LRRK2 secretion in exosomes is regulated by 14-3-3. *Hum. Mol. Genet.* 22, 4988–5000. doi: 10.1093/hmg/ddt346

Goetzl, E. J., Abner, E. L., Jicha, G. A., Kapogiannis, D., and Schwartz, J. B. (2018). Declining levels of functionally specialized synaptic proteins in plasma neuronal exosomes with progression of Alzheimer's disease. *FASEB J.* 32, 888–893. doi: 10.1096/fj.201700731r

Goetzl, E. J., Boxer, A., Schwartz, J. B., Abner, E. L., Petersen, R. C., Miller, B. L., et al. (2015). Low neural exosomal levels of cellular survival factors in Alzheimer's disease. *Ann. Clin. Transl. Neurol.* 2, 769–773. doi: 10.1002/acn3.211

Goetzl, E. J., Kapogiannis, D., Schwartz, J. B., Lobach, I. V., Goetzl, L., Abner, E. L., et al. (2016). Decreased synaptic proteins in neuronal exosomes of frontotemporal dementia and Alzheimer's disease. *FASEB J.* 30, 4141–4148. doi: 10.1096/fj.201600816r

Goldie, B. J., Dun, M. D., Lin, M., Smith, N. D., Verrills, N. M., Dayas, C. V., et al. (2014). Activity-associated miRNA are packaged in Map1b-enriched exosomes released from depolarized neurons. *Nucleic Acids Res.* 42, 9195–9208. doi: 10.1093/nar/gku594

Gomes de Andrade, G., Reck Cechinel, L., Bertoldi, K., Galvão, F., Valdeci Worm, P., and Rodrigues Siqueira, I. (2018). The aging process alters IL-1β and CD63 levels differently in extracellular vesicles obtained from the plasma and cerebrospinal fluid. *Neuroimmunomodulation* 25, 18–22. doi: 10.1159/000488943

Grey, M., Dunning, C. J., Gaspar, R., Grey, C., Brundin, P., Sparr, E., et al. (2015). Acceleration of α-synuclein aggregation by exosomes. *J. Biol. Chem.* 290, 2969–2982. doi: 10.1074/jbc.M114.585703

Guescini, M., Genedani, S., Stocchi, V., and Agnati, L. F. (2010). Astrocytes and glioblastoma cells release exosomes carrying mtDNA. *J. Neural Transm.* 117, 1–4. doi: 10.1007/s00702-009-0288-8

Gui, Y., Liu, H., Zhang, L., Lv, W., and Hu, X. (2015). Altered microRNA profiles in cerebrospinal fluid exosome in Parkinson disease and Alzheimer disease. *Oncotarget* 6, 37043–37053. doi: 10.18632/oncotarget.6158

Hébert, S. S., Papadopoulou, A. S., Smith, P., Galas, M. C., Planel, E., Silahtaroglu, A. N., et al. (2010). Genetic ablation of dicer in adult forebrain neurons results in abnormal tau hyperphosphorylation and neurodegeneration. *Hum. Mol. Genet.* 19, 3959–3969. doi: 10.1093/hmg/ddq311

Hofmann, J. W., McBryan, T., Adams, P. D., and Sedivy, J. M. (2014). The effects of aging on the expression of Wnt pathway genes in mouse tissues. *Age* 36:9618. doi: 10.1007/s11357-014-9618-3

Hough, K. P., Trevor, J. L., Strenkowski, J. G., Wang, Y., Chacko, B. K., Tousif, S., et al. (2018). Exosomal transfer of mitochondria from airway myeloid-derived regulatory cells to T cells. *Redox Biol.* 18, 54–64. doi: 10.1016/j.redox.2018.06.009

Hu, H.-Y., Yu, C.-H., Zhang, H.-H., Zhang, S.-Z., Yu, W.-Y., Yang, Y., et al. (2019). Exosomal miR-1229 derived from colorectal cancer cells promotes angiogenesis by targeting HIPK2. *Int. J. Biol. Macromol.* 132, 470–477. doi: 10.1016/j.ijbiomac.2019.03.221

Iguchi, Y., Eid, L., Parent, M., Soucy, G., Bareil, C., Riku, Y., et al. (2016). Exosome secretion is a key pathway for clearance of pathological TDP-43. *Brain* 139, 3187–3201. doi: 10.1093/brain/aww237

Ivanov, A., Pawlikowski, J., Manoharan I., van Tuyn, J., Nelson, D. M., Rai, T. S., et al. (2013). Lysosome-mediated processing of chromatin in senescence. *J. Cell Biol.* 202, 129–143. doi: 10.1083/jcb.201212110

Jan, A. T., Azam, M., Rahman, S., Almigeiti, A. M. S., Choi, D. H., Lee, E. J., et al. (2017). Perspective insights into disease progression, diagnostics and therapeutic approaches in Alzheimer's disease: a judicious update. *Front. Aging Neurosci.* 9:356. doi: 10.3389/fnagi.2017.00356

Jan, A. T., Rahman, S., Khan, S., Tasduq, S. A., and Choi, I. (2019). Biology, pathophysiological role, and clinical implications of exosomes: a critical appraisal. *Cells* 8:E99. doi: 10.3390/cells8020099

Joshi, P., Benussi, L., Furlan, R., Ghidoni, R., and Verderio, C. (2015). Extracellular vesicles in Alzheimer's disease: friends or foes? focus on Aβ-vesicle interaction. *Int. J. Mol. Sci.* 16, 4800–4813. doi: 10.3390/ijms16034800

Kapogiannis, D., Boxer, A., Schwartz, J. B., Abner, E. L., Biragyn, A., Masharani, U., et al. (2015). Dysfunctionally phosphorylated type 1 insulin receptor substrate in neural-derived blood exosomes of preclinical Alzheimer's disease. *FASEB J.* 29, 589–596. doi: 10.1096/fj.14-262048

Kenwrick, S. (2002). Neural cell recognition molecule L1: relating biological complexity to human disease mutations. *Hum. Mol. Genet.* 9, 879–886. doi: 10.1093/hmg/9.6.879

Kim, K. M., Abdelmohsen, K., Mustapic, M., Kapogiannis, D., and Gorospe, M. (2017). RNA in extracellular vesicles. *Wiley Interdiscip. Rev. RNA* 8:e1413. doi: 10.1002/wrna.1413

Kokubo, H., Saido, T. C., Iwata, N., Helms, J. B., Shinohara, R., and Yamaguchi, H. (2004). Part of membrane-bound Aβ exists in rafts within senile plaques in Tg2576 mouse brain. *Neurobiol. Aging* 26, 409–418. doi: 10.1016/j.neurobiolaging.2004.04.008

Kong, S. M. Y., Chan, B. K. K., Park, J. S., Hill, K. J., Aitken, J. B., Cottle, L., et al. (2014). Parkinson's disease-linked human PARK9/ATP13A2 maintains zinc homeostasis and promotes α-Synuclein externalization *via* exosomes. *Hum. Mol. Genet.* 23, 2816–2833. doi: 10 1093/hmg/ddu099

Kosik, K. S. (2006). The neuronal microRNA system. *Nat. Rev. Neurosci.* 7, 911–920. doi: 10.1038/nrn2037

Kramer, M. L., and Schulz-Schaeffer, W. J. (2007). Presynaptic α-synuclein aggregates, not lewy bodies, cause neurodegeneration in dementia with lewy bodies. *J. Neurosci.* 27, 1405–1410. doi: 10.1523/jneurosci.4564-06.2007

Lachenal, G., Pernet-Gallay, K., Chivet, M., Hemming, F. J., Belly, A., Bodon, G., et al. (2010). Release of exosomes from differentiated neurons and its regulation by synaptic glutamatergic activity. *Mol. Cell. Neurosci.* 46, 409–418. doi: 10.1016/j.mcn.2010.11.004

Lee, J. Y., and Kim, H. S. (2017). Extracellular vesicles in neurodegenerative diseases: a double-edged sword. *Tissue Eng. Regen. Med.* 14, 667–678. doi: 10.1007/s13770-017-0090-x

Lehmann, B. D., Paine, M. S., Brooks, A. M., McCubrey, J. A., Renegar, R. H., Wang, R., et al. (2008). Senescence-associated exosome release from human prostate cancer cells. *Cancer Res.* 68, 7864–7871. doi: 10.1158/0008-5472.can-07-6538

Lim, Y. J., and Lee, S. J. (2017). Are exosomes the vehicle for protein aggregate propagation in neurodegenerative diseases? *Acta Neuropathol. Commun.* 5:64. doi: 10.1186/s40478-017-0467-z

Liu, C. G., Song, J., Zhang, Y. Q., and Wang, P. C. (2014). MicroRNA-193b is a regulator of amyloid precursor protein in the blood and cerebrospinal fluid derived exosomal microRNA- 193b is a biomarker of Alzheimer's disease. *Mol. Med. Rep.* 10, 2395–2400. doi: 10.3892/mmr.2014.2484

Lugli, G., Cohen, A. M., Bennett, D. A., Shah, R. C., Fields, C. J., Hernandez, A. G., et al. (2015). Plasma exosomal miRNAs in persons with and without Alzheimer disease: altered expression and prospects for biomarkers. *PLoS One* 10:e0139233. doi: 10.1371/journal.pone.0139233

Ma, B., and Hottiger, M. O. (2016). Crosstalk between Wnt/β-catenin and NF-κB signaling pathway during inflammation. *Front. Immunol.* 7:378. doi: 10.3389/fimmu.2016.00378

Machida, T., Tomofuji, T., Ekuni, D., Maruyama, T., Yoneda, T., Kawabata, Y., et al. (2015). MicroRNAs in salivary exosome as potential biomarkers of aging. *Int. J. Mol. Sci.* 16, 21294–21309. doi: 10.3390/ijms160921294

Mashouri, L., Yousefi, H., Aref, A. R., Ahadi, A. M., Molaei, F., and Alahari, S. K. (2019). Exosomes: composition, biogenesis, and mechanisms in cancer metastasis and drug resistance. *Mol. Cancer* 18:75. doi: 10.1186/s12943-019-0991-5

Molinuevo, J. L., Ayton, S., Batrla, R., Bednar, M. M., Bittner, T., Cummings, J., et al. (2018). *Current State of Alzheimer's Fluid Biomarkers.* Berlin: Springer.

Morales, R., Duran-Aniotz, C., Castilla, J., Estrada, L. D., and Soto, C. (2011). *De novo* induction of amyloid-β deposition *in vivo*. *Mol. Psychiatry* 17, 1347–1353. doi: 10.1038/mp.2011.120

Nowak, J. S., and Michlewski, G. (2013). miRNAs in development and pathogenesis of the nervous system: table 1. *Biochem. Soc. Trans.* 41, 815–820. doi: 10.1042/bst20130044

Nusse, R. (2005). Wnt signaling in disease and in development. *Cell Res.* 15, 28–32. doi: 10.1038/sj.cr.7290260

Okamoto, M., Inoue, K., Iwamura, H., Terashima, K., Soya, H., Asashima, M., et al. (2011). Reduction in paracrine Wnt3 factors during aging causes impaired adult neurogenesis. *FASEB J.* 25, 3570–3582. doi: 10.1096/fj.11-184697

Olanow, C. W., and Brundin, P. (2013). Parkinson's disease and alpha synuclein: is Parkinson's disease a prion-like disorder? *Mov. Disord.* 28, 31–40. doi: 10.1002/mds.25373

Olivieri, F., Albertini, M. C., Orciani, M., Ceka, A., Cricca, M., Procopio, A. D., et al. (2015). DNA damage response (DDR) and senescence: shuttled inflamma-miRNAs on the stage of inflamm-aging. *Oncotarget* 6, 35509–35521. doi: 10.18632/oncotarget.5899

Panagiotou, N., Neytchev, O., Selman, C., and Shiels, P. (2018). Extracellular vesicles, ageing, and therapeutic interventions. *Cells* 7:E110. doi: 10.3390/cells7080110

Pegtel, D. M., Cosmopoulos, K., Thorley-Lawson, D. A., van Eijndhoven, M. A. J., Hopmans, E. S., Lindenberg, J. L., et al. (2010). Functional delivery of viral miRNAs *via* exosomes. *Proc. Natl. Acad. Sci. U S A* 107, 6328–6333. doi: 10.1073/pnas.0914843107

Perez-Gonzalez, R., Gauthier, S. A., Kumar, A., and Levy, E. (2012). The exosome secretory pathway transports amyloid precursor protein carboxyl-terminal fragments from the cell into the brain extracellular space. *J. Biol. Chem.* 287, 43108–43115. doi: 10.1074/jbc.m112.404467

Polanco, J. C., Scicluna, B. J., Hill, A. F., and Götz, J. (2016). Extracellular vesicles isolated from the brains of rTg4510 mice seed tau protein aggregation in a threshold-dependent manner. *J. Biol. Chem.* 291, 12445–12466. doi: 10.1074/jbc.m115.709485

Pusic, A. D., and Kraig, R. P. (2014). Youth and environmental enrichment generate serum exosomes containing miR-219 that promote CNS myelination. *Glia* 62, 284–299. doi: 10.1002/glia.22606

Rademakers, R., and Hutton, M. (2007). The genetics of frontotemporal lobar degeneration. *Curr. Neurol. Neurosci. Rep.* 7, 434–442. doi: 10.1007/s11910-007-0067-6

Rajendran, L., Bali, J., Barr, M. M., Court, F. A., Kramer-Albers, E.-M., Picou, F., et al. (2014). Emerging roles of extracellular vesicles in the nervous system. *J. Neurosci.* 34, 15482–15489. doi: 10.1523/JNEUROSCI.3258-14.2014

Rajendran, L., Honsho, M., Zahn, T. R., Keller, P., Geiger, K. D., Verkade, P., et al. (2006). Alzheimer's disease β-amyloid peptides are released in association with exosomes. *Proc. Natl. Acad. Sci. U S A* 103, 11172–11177. doi: 10.1073/pnas.0603838103

Rashed, M. H., Bayraktar, E., Helal, G. K., Abd-Ellah, M. F., Amero, P., Chavez-Reyes, A., et al. (2017). Exosomes: from garbage bins to promising therapeutic targets. *Int. J. Mol. Sci.* 18:E538. doi: 10.3390/ijms18030538

Ridder, K., Keller, S., Dams, M., Rupp, A. K., Schlaudraff, J., Del Turco, D., et al. (2014). Extracellular vesicle-mediated transfer of genetic information between the hematopoietic system and the brain in response to inflammation. *PLoS Biol.* 12:e1001874. doi: 10.1371/journal.pbio.1001874

Salvioli, S., Monti, D., Lanzarini, C., Conte, M., Pirazzini, C., Bacalini, M. G., et al. (2013). Immune system, cell senescence, aging and longevity—inflamm-aging reappraised. *Curr. Pharm. Des.* 19, 1675–1679. doi: 10.2174/138161213805219531

Saman, S., Lee, N. C. Y., Hall, G. F., Saman, S., Visnick, Y., Jackson, B., et al. (2012). Exosome-associated tau is secreted in tauopathy models and is selectively phosphorylated in cerebrospinal fluid in early Alzheimer disease. *J. Biol. Chem.* 287, 3842–3849. doi: 10.1074/jbc.m111.277061

Schneider, R., McKeever, P., Kim, T., Graff, C., van Swieten, J. C., Karydas, A., et al. (2018). Downregulation of exosomal miR-204–5p and miR-632 as a biomarker for FTD: a GENFI study. *J. Neurol. Neurosurg. Psychiatry* 89, 851–858. doi: 10.1136/jnnp-2017-317492

Sharples, R., Vella, L. J., Nisbet, R. M., Naylor, R., Perez, K., Barnham, K. J., et al. (2008). Inhibition of γ-secretase causes increased secretion of amyloid precursor protein C-terminal fragments in association with exosomes. *FASEB J.* 22, 1469–1478. doi: 10.1096/fj.07-9357com

Shi, M., Kovac, A., Korff, A., Cook, T. J., Ginghina, C., Kristin, M., et al. (2017). CNS tau efflux *via* exosomes is likely increased in Parkinson's disease but not in Alzheimer's disease. *Alzheimers Dement.* 12, 1125–1131. doi: 10.1016/j.jalz.2016.04.003

Shi, M., Liu, C., Cook, T. J., Bullock, K. M., Zhao, Y., Ginghina, C., et al. (2014). Plasma exosomal α-synuclein is likely CNS-derived and increased in Parkinson's disease. *Acta Neuropathol.* 128, 639–650. doi: 10.1007/s00401-014-1314-y

Shi, M., Sheng, L., Stewart, T., Zabetian, C. P., and Zhang, J. (2019). New windows into the brain: central nervous system-derived extracellular vesicles in blood. *Prog. Neurobiol.* 175, 96–106. doi: 10.1016/j.pneurobio.2019.01.005

Shiels, P. G., Stenvinkel, P., Kooman, J. P., and McGuinness, D. (2017). Circulating markers of ageing and allostatic load: a slow train coming. *Pract. Lab. Med.* 7, 49–54. doi: 10.1016/j.plabm.2016.04.002

Simón, D., García-García, E., Gómez-Ramos, A., Falcón-Pérez, J. M., Díaz-Hernández, M., Hernández, F., et al. (2012). Tau overexpression results in its secretion *via* membrane vesicles. *Neurodegener. Dis.* 10, 73–75. doi: 10.1159/000334915

Simons, M., and Raposo, G. (2009). Exosomes—vesicular carriers for intercellular communication. *Curr. Opin. Cell Biol.* 21, 575–581. doi: 10.1016/j.ceb.2009.03.007

Snowden, J., Neary, D., and Mann, D. (2007). Frontotemporal lobar degeneration: clinical and pathological relationships. *Acta Neuropathol.* 114, 31–38. doi: 10.1007/s00401-007-0236-3

Soria, F. N., Pampliega, O., Bourdenx, M., Meissner, W. G., Bezard, E., and Dehay, B. (2017). Exosomes, an unmasked culprit in neurodegenerative diseases. *Front. Neurosci.* 11:26. doi: 10.3389/fnins.2017.00026

Spillantini, M. G., and Goedert, M. (2018). Neurodegeneration and the ordered assembly of α-synuclein. *Cell Tissue Res.* 373, 137–148. doi: 10.1007/s00441-017-2706-9

Sprott, R. L. (2010). Biomarkers of aging and disease: introduction and definitions. *Exp. Gerontol.* 45, 2–4. doi: 10.1016/j.exger.2009.07.008

Stuendl, A., Kunadt, M., Kruse, N., Bartels, C., Moebius, W., Danzer, K. M., et al. (2016). Induction of α-synuclein aggregate formation by CSF exosomes from patients with Parkinson's disease and dementia with Lewy bodies. *Brain* 139, 481–494. doi: 10.1093/brain/awv346

Takasugi, M. (2018). Emerging roles of extracellular vesicles in cellular senescence and aging. *Aging Cell* 17:2. doi: 10.1111/acel.12734

Takasugi, M., Okada, R., Takahashi, A., Virya Chen, D., Watanabe, S., and Hara, E. (2017). Small extracellular vesicles secreted from senescent cells promote cancer cell proliferation through EphA2. *Nat. Commun.* 8:15729. doi: 10.1038/ncomms15728

Takahashi, R. H., Milner, T. A., Li, F., Nam, E. E., Edgar, M. A., Yamaguchi, H., et al. (2002). Intraneuronal Alzheimer Aβ42 accumulates in multivesicular bodies and is associated with synaptic pathology. *Am. J. Pathol.* 161, 1869–1879. doi: 10.1016/s0002-9440(10)64463-x

Thomas, B., and Beal, M. F. (2007). Parkinson's disease. *Hum. Mol. Genet.* 16, R183–R194. doi: 10.1093/hmg/ddm159

Thompson, A. G., Gray, E., Heman-Ackah, S. M., Mäger, I., Talbot, K., El Andaloussi, S., et al. (2016). Extracellular vesicles in neurodegenerative disease-pathogenesis to biomarkers. *Nat. Rev. Neurol.* 12, 346–357. doi: 10.1038/nrneurol.2016.68

Tsunemi, T., Hamada, K., and Krainc, D. (2014). ATP13A2/PARK9 regulates secretion of exosomes and α-synuclein. *J. Neurosci.* 34, 15281–15287. doi: 10.1523/jneurosci.1629-14.2014

Urbanelli, L., Buratta, S., Sagini, K., Tancini, B., and Emiliani, C. (2016). Extracellular vesicles as new players in cellular senescence. *Int. J. Mol. Sci.* 17:E1408. doi: 10.3390/ijms17091408

Valadi, H., Ekström, K., Bossios, A., Sjöstrand, M., Lee, J. J., and Lötvall, J. O. (2007). Exosome-mediated transfer of mRNAs and microRNAs is a novel mechanism of genetic exchange between cells. *Nat. Cell Biol.* 9, 654–659. doi: 10.1038/ncb1596

van Balkom, B. W. M., de Jong, O. G., Smits, M., Brummelman, J., den Ouden, K., de Bree, P. M., et al. (2013). Endothelial cells require miR-214 to secrete exosomes that suppress senescence and induce angiogenesis in human and mouse endothelial cells. *Blood* 121, 3997–4006. doi: 10.1182/blood-2013-02-478925

Vidal, M., Sainte-Marie, J., Philippot, J. R., and Bienvenue, A. (1989). Asymmetric distribution of phospholipids in the membrane of vesicles released during *in vitro* maturation of guinea pig reticulocytes: evidence precluding a role for "aminophospholipid translocase". *J. Cell. Physiol.* 140, 455–462. doi: 10.1002/jcp.1041400308

Wei, H., Xu, Y., Xu, W., Zhou, Q., Chen, Q., Yang, M., et al. (2018). Serum exosomal miR-223 serves as a potential diagnostic and prognostic biomarker for dementia. *Neuroscience* 379, 167–176. doi: 10.1016/j.neuroscience.2018.03.016

Weilner, S., Keider, V., Winter, M., Harreither, E., Salzer, B., Weiss, F., et al. (2016). Vesicular Galectin-3 levels decrease with donor age and contribute to the reduced osteo-inductive potential of human plasma derived extracellular vesicles. *Aging* 8, 16–30. doi: 10.18632/aging.100865

Weilner, S., Schraml, E., Redl, H., Grillari-Voglauer, R., and Grillari, J. (2013). Secretion of microvesicular miRNAs in cellular andorganismal aging. *Exp. Gerontol.* 48, 626–633. doi: 10.1016/j.exger.2012.11.017

Weiner-Gorzel, K., Dempsey, E., Milewska, M., McGoldrick, A., Toh, V., Walsh, A., et al. (2015). Overexpression of the microRNA miR-433 promotes resistance to paclitaxel through the induction of cellular senescence in ovarian cancer cells. *Cancer Med.* 4, 745–758. doi: 10.1002/cam4.409

Westergard, T., Jensen, B. K., Wen, X., Cai, J., Kropf, E., Iacovitti, L., et al. (2016). Cell-to-cell transmission of dipeptide repeat proteins linked to C9orf72-ALS/FTD. *Cell Rep.* 17, 645–652. doi: 10.1016/j.celrep.2016.09.032

Willms, E., Johansson, H. J., Mäger, I., Lee, Y., Blomberg, K. E. M., Sadik, M., et al. (2016). Cells release subpopulations of exosomes with distinct molecular and biological properties. *Sci. Rep.* 6:22519. doi: 10.1038/srep22519

Winston, C. N., Goetzl, E. J., Akers, J. C., Carter, B. S., Rockenstein, E. M., Galasko, D., et al. (2016). Prediction of conversion from mild cognitive impairment to dementia with neuronally derived blood exosome protein profile. *Alzheimers Dement.* 3, 63–72. doi: 10.1016/j.dadm.2016.04.001

Xu, Y., and Sun, Z. (2015). Molecular basis of Klotho: from gene to function in aging. *Endocr. Rev.* 36, 174–193. doi: 10.1210/er.2013-1079

Yagi, Y., Ohkubo, T., Kawaji, H., Machida, A., Miyata, H., Goda, S., et al. (2016). Next-generation sequencing-based small RNA profiling of cerebrospinal fluid exosomes. *Neurosci. Lett.* 636, 48–57. doi: 10.1016/j.neulet.2016.10.042

Yamakuchi, M., and Lowenstein, C. J. (2009). MiR-34, SIRT1 and p53: the feedback loop. *Cell Cycle* 8, 712–715 doi: 10.4161/cc.8.5.7753

Yang, T. T., Liu, C. G., Gao, S. C., Zhang, Y., and Wang, P. C. (2018). The serum exosome derived MicroRNA-135a, -193b, and -384 were potential Alzheimer's disease biomarkers. *Biomed. Environ. Sci.* 31, 87–96. doi: 10.3967/bes2018.011

Yuyama, K., Sun, H., Usuki, S., Sakai, S., Hanamatsu, H., Mioka, T., et al. (2015). A potential function for neuronal exosomes: sequestering intracerebral amyloid-β peptide. *FEBS Lett.* 589, 84–88. doi: 10.1016/j.febslet.2014.11.027

Zhang, G., and Yang, P. (2018). A novel cell-cell communication mechanism in the nervous system: exosomes. *J. Neurosci. Res.* 96, 45–52. doi: 10.1002/jnr.24113

Zhang, Y., Pizzute, T., and Pei, M. (2014). A review of crosstalk between MAPK and Wnt signals and its impact on cartilage regeneration. *Cell Tissue Res.* 358, 633–649. doi: 10.1007/s00441-014-2010-x

13

On the Role of Adenosine A2A Receptor Gene Transcriptional Regulation in Parkinson's Disease

*Anastasia Falconi[1], Alessandra Bonito-Oliva[2], Martina Di Bartolomeo[1], Marcella Massimini[1], Francesco Fattapposta[3], Nicoletta Locuratolo[3], Enrico Dainese[1], Esterina Pascale[4], Gilberto Fisone[2] and Claudio D'Addario[1,5]**

[1] Faculty of Bioscience, University of Teramo, Teramo, Italy, [2] Department of Neuroscience, Karolinska Institute, Stockholm, Sweden, [3] Department of Human Neurosciences, Sapienza University, Rome, Italy, [4] Department of Medical-Surgical Sciences and Biotechnologies, Sapienza University, Rome, Italy, [5] Department of Clinical Neuroscience, Karolinska Institute, Stockholm, Sweden

***Correspondence:**
Claudio D'Addario
cdaddario@unite.it

Adenosine A2A receptors (A2ARs) have attracted considerable attention as an important molecular target for the design of Parkinson's disease (PD) therapeutic compounds. Here, we studied the transcriptional regulation of the A2AR gene in human peripheral blood mononuclear cells (PBMCs) obtained from PD patients and in the striatum of the well-validated, 6-hydroxydopamine (6-OHDA)-induced PD mouse model. We report an increase in A2AR mRNA expression and protein levels in both human cells and mice striata, and in the latter we could also observe a consistent reduction in DNA methylation at gene promoter and an increase in histone H3 acetylation at lysine 9. Of particular relevance in clinical samples, we also observed higher levels in the receptor gene expression in younger subjects, as well as in those with less years from disease onset, and less severe disease according to clinical scores. In conclusion, the present findings provide further evidence of the relevant role of A2AR in PD and, based on the clinical data, highlight its potential role as disease biomarker for PD especially at the initial stages of disease development. Furthermore, our preclinical results also suggest selective epigenetic mechanisms targeting gene promoter as tool for the development of new treatments.

Keywords: Parkinson's disease, adenosine A2A receptor, 6-hydroxydopamine, peripheral blood mononuclear cells, DNA methylation, histone modifications

INTRODUCTION

Parkinson's disease (PD), the second most common neurodegenerative disorder after Alzheimer's disease, affects approximately 1% of the population over 60 (Ozansoy and Basak, 2013). The pathological hallmark of PD is the degeneration of nigrostriatal dopaminergic neurons and the consequent loss of dopaminergic input to the basal ganglia, which gives rise to well-defined motor symptoms, including bradykinesia, rigidity, muscular stiffness, tremor, poor posture and balance, and sensory motor integration deficits (Marsden, 2000; Obeso et al., 2000). Epidemiological studies reveal that less than 10% of PD cases are familial, while most are sporadic. The etiology of the disease remains poorly understood and is likely the result of an intricate interplay between genetic, epigenetic, and environmental factors, among others. At present, there are no FDA-approved disease-modifying treatments.

Nowadays, dopamine replacement treatments represent the best therapy available to alleviate PD symptoms. The dopamine precursor L-3,4-dihydroxyphenylalanine (L-DOPA) is the most efficacious and commonly prescribed anti-parkinsonian drug. However, its prolonged use is limited by the occurrence of a number of debilitating side effects (LeWitt, 2015).

Among the different possible targets for symptomatic treatments, the adenosine A2ARs have attracted considerable interest. A2ARs are enriched in the medium spiny neurons (MSN) of the striatum, which is the main component of the basal ganglia (Jarvis and Williams, 1989; Svenningsson et al., 1997; Rosin et al., 1998). Importantly, A2ARs are selectively expressed on the MSNs of the indirect striatopallidal pathway (Schiffmann et al., 1991; Fink et al., 1992), where they antagonize dopamine D2 receptor-mediated transmission (Schiffmann et al., 2007).

In line with these findings, several preclinical and clinical studies point to A2ARs antagonists as a promising non-dopaminergic therapy for PD (Feigin, 2003; Pinna et al., 2005; Schwarzschild et al., 2006). Moreover, oral administration of the A2ARs antagonist KW-6002 showed a significant neuroprotective effect in a rat model of PD characterized by dopamine depletion achieved by administration of the toxin 6-hydroxydopamine (6-OHDA) (Ikeda et al., 2002).

Adenosine A2A receptors gene expression was found to be up-regulated in the striata of rats with a 6-OHDA lesion (Pinna et al., 2002), and in the putamen and peripheral blood mononuclear cells (PBMCs) of PD and mild cognitive impairment patients (Calon et al., 2004; Varani et al., 2010; Casetta et al., 2014). These observations were confirmed by PET studies, showing enhanced striatal A2ARs levels in PD patients (Ramlackhansingh et al., 2011). However, others have reported a reduction of A2ARs in the anterior and posterior caudate nucleus and anterior dorsal putamen of individuals with PD (Hurley et al., 2000), or no changes in the striata of rats with a 6-OHDA lesion (Kaelin-Lang et al., 2000; Tomiyama et al., 2004).

It has been suggested that DNA methylation, an epigenetic mark associated with gene repression (Jones, 2012), might have a key role in regulating A2AR gene transcription (Buira et al., 2010a,b). In line with this hypothesis, reduced DNA methylation in the 5′UTR region of A2AR gene was observed in advanced PD cases (Villar-Menéndez et al., 2014). Another well-studied mechanism of epigenetic regulation is the post-translational modification of histone tails. Increased histone acetylation has also been observed in experimental models of PD as well as in the brain of PD patients (Park et al., 2016), leading to the hypothesis that drugs that affect histone acetylation would have therapeutic effects (Song et al., 2011; Harrison and Dexter, 2013). So far, there are no studies that selectively focus on the role of histone modifications on A2AR gene transcription regulation in PD.

Based on this background, the present study deeply investigates the A2AR gene transcriptional regulation via epigenetic mechanisms in PD. To this aim, we employed a multidisciplinary approach, based on the use of clinical (PBMCs of PD patients) and preclinical samples (brain tissue of 6-OHDA-lesioned mice).

EXPERIMENTAL PROCEDURES

Subjects

For this study we enrolled 73 outpatients attending the Neurological Clinic in La Sapienza University, Rome, on stable pharmacological treatment. Diagnosis of sporadic PD was based on clinical symptoms according to the United Kingdom. Brain Bank Criteria for PD (Hughes et al., 1992). Patients showing a comorbid substance or alcohol abuse in the previous 2 months were ruled out. Exclusion criteria included signs of atypical parkinsonism, diagnosis of mental retardation or dementia (Mini-Mental State Examination score <23.8). The variables collected included: smoking habit, age at onset of PD, clinical form (Tremor-dominant TD, Non-Tremor-dominant NTD), motor disability by means of the Unified Parkinson's Disease rating Scale-subset III (UPDRS III), disease stage according to Hoehn & Yahr scale, duration of disease, levodopa equivalent daily dose (LEDD) calculated according to Tomlinson (Tomlinson et al., 2010). We also selected sex and age-matched healthy subjects as a control group. The exclusion criteria were: alcohol and substance abuse, neurological disorders, family history of movement disorders. Subjects suffering from metabolic disorders, severe hypertension or systemic autoimmune diseases were also excluded. No statistical difference between patients and control groups emerged in either hypertension or dyslipidemia cases. The study was approved by the local ethics committee. Written informed consent was obtained from all study participants. Demographic and clinical characteristics for the study samples are shown in **Table 1**.

Animals

Male C57BL/6J mice (25–30 g; Taconic, Tornbjerg, Denmark) were housed under a 12 h light/dark cycle with food and water *ad libitum*. Experiments were carried out in accordance with the guidelines of Research Ethics Committee of Karolinska Institutet,

TABLE 1 | Demographic and clinical characteristics of PD patients and controls.

Characteristic	Controls n = 32	PD n = 73
Male (%)	16 (50%)	40 (55%)
Smokers (%)	11 (34%)	23 (31%)
Age (yrs, mean ± SD)	71.5 ± 6.8	68.8 ± 7.2
Age at Onset (yrs, mean ± SD)	NA	62.3 ± 7.7
Disease duration (yrs, mean ± SD)	NA	7.6 ± 11.6
LEDD at last visit (mg/die, mean ± SD)	NA	509.5 ± 35
UPDRS III score	NA	14.1 ± 5.8
H&Y scale (mean ± SD)	NA	1.78 ± 0.5
1		21
1.5		3
2		36
2.5		12
3		1
Tremor dominant (%)	NA	30 (41%)

H&Y, Hohen &Yahr scale; UPDRS III, unified Parkinson's disease rating scale-subset III; LEDD, levodopa equivalent daily dose.

Swedish Animal Welfare Agency and European Communities Council Directive 86/609/EEC.

6-OHDA Lesion and Brain Dissection

Mice were anesthetized with a mixture of Hypnorm® (VetaPharma Ltd., Leed, United Kingdom), midazolam (5 mg/ml) (Hameln Pharmaceuticals GmbH, Hameln, Germany), and water (1:1:2 in a volume of 10 ml/kg) and mounted in a stereotaxic frame (David Kopf Instruments, Tujunga, CA, United States). 6-OHDA was dissolved in 0.02% ascorbic acid in saline at the concentration of 3.0 g of freebase 6-OHDA/l. Each mouse received two unilateral injections of vehicle (Sham, unlesioned) or 6-OHDA (2 μl/injection) into the right dorsal striatum as previously described (Santini et al., 2007), according to the following coordinates (in mm) (Franklin and Paxinos, 2008): anterior-posterior +1, medial-lateral −2.1, dorsal-ventral −3.2 and anterior-posterior +0.3, medial-lateral −2.3, and dorsal-ventral −3.2. Three weeks after surgery, the mice were killed by decapitation, their heads were cooled in liquid nitrogen for 6 s and striata were dissected out on an ice-cold surface and snap frozen in liquid nitrogen. The success of the lesion was assessed at the end of the experiments by measuring striatal levels of tyrosine hydroxylase (TH) in Sham *vs* unlesioned mice by Western Blot (see below). The success of the lesion was defined by ≥80% TH decrease and only the mice that met these criteria were included in the analysis.

Molecular Biology Studies

To evaluate regulation of A2ARs transcription, we analyzed mRNA and protein levels, as well as epigenetic modifications at A2AR gene promoter such as DNA methylation and histone modifications (**Figure 1**).

Real-Time Quantitative PCR (RT-qPCR)

Peripheral blood mononuclear cells were isolated from the peripheral blood of control subjects and PD patients by Fycoll-Paque PLUS density gradient medium according to manufacturer's instructions (GE Healthcare, Bio-Sciences AB Uppsala-Sweden). Total RNA was extracted from PBMCs and single striatum samples (Chomczynski and Sacchi, 2006) and checked for integrity by electrophoresis. RNA concentrations were then measured by spectrophotometry and just samples reporting an OD 260:280 ratio >2 were subjected to DNAse treatment and converted to cDNA with a commercially available kit (Thermo Fisher Scientific, Waltham, MA, United States). Diluted cDNAs were thus used to assess A2AR mRNA relative abundance by RT-qPCR, using SensiFast No-Rox Kit (Bioline) using the DNA Engine Opticon-2 detection system (Biorad, CA, United States). β-actin and GAPDH genes, properly validated to confirm that in our experimental conditions their expression was not affected, were used as reference genes to normalize the data.

Sequences of the primers used for PCR amplification are listed in **Table 2**. In a final volume of 15 μl, we used 2 μl of cDNA, 7,5 μl of SensiFAST SYBR, and 10 pmol of each primer. Duplicate samples were run and PCR conditions were: 95°C for 10 s, 60°C for 30 s, and 72 for 30 s. A2ARs relative expression was calculated by Delta-Delta Ct (ΔΔCT) method and converted to $2^{-\Delta\Delta Ct}$ for statistical analysis (Livak and Schmittgen, 2001).

DNA Methylation Analysis by Pyrosequencing

Genomic DNA, obtained from human PBMCs and striatum tissues, was bisulfite-treated according to manufacturer's instructions (Zymo Research, Irvine, CA, United States). Methylation status of human and mouse A2AR GENE was assessed using pyrosequencing of the bisulfite-converted DNA as previously reported (Cifani et al., 2015; Pucci et al., 2015).

Pyrosequencing primers were designed to focus on a series of CpG dinucleotides part of the CpG island located in two different regions both in clinical samples and in mice brain tissues (see **Figure 1** and **Table 2** for details). Bisulfite-treated DNA was amplified by PyroMark PCR Kit (Qiagen, Germany) under these PCR conditions: 95°C for 15 min; 45 cycles of 94°C for 30 s; 56°C for 30 s; 72°C for 30 s; and final step of 72°C for 10 min. Following PCR products verification by agarose electrophoresis, pyrosequencing methylation analysis was conducted using the PyroMark Q24 Software (Qiagen, Germany), which allows for each CpG site quantitative comparisons of the methylation percentage.

Chromatin Immunoprecipitation (ChIP)

Dahl and Collas protocol, with minor modifications, was used to prepare chromatin from mice frozen tissues as previously described (Dahl and Collas, 2007). Briefly, to cross-link proteins to DNA, formaldehyde was added at a final concentration of 1% in phosphate buffer saline containing a broad-range protease inhibitor cocktail (PIC) (Sigma, St. Louis, MO, United States) and sodium butyrate (Sigma, St. Louis, MO, United States), for 10 min at room temperature. Glycine, used to quench the reaction, was added to a final concentration of 0.125 M and incubating for 5 min at room temperature. Following washing, the samples were lysed using 120 μl of a lysis buffer (50 mM Tris–HCl, pH 8, 10 mM EDTA, 1% SDS) containing PIC and sodium butyrate (20 mM). The samples were incubated on ice and sonicated for 30 s for 6 times, with 30 s pause intervals each sonicated. The lysates were centrifuged at 12,000 *g* for 10 min at 4°C and the supernatants transferred into a chilled tube, leaving around 30 μl of buffer with the pellet. Lysis buffer (30 μl) was added. DNA fragments ranging in size from 200 to 500 bp were analyzed by agarose gel electrophoresis. 20 μl aliquot was used as "input" DNA, for each immunoprecipitation. Chromatin was diluted in 90 μl of RIPA buffer (10 mM Tris–HCl, pH 7.5, 1 mM EDTA, 0.5 mM EGTA, 1% Triton X-100, 0.1% SDS, 0.1% Na-deoxycholate, 140 mM NaCl) plus PIC and incubated overnight by rotation with either antibody previously coated with Protein A beads (Invitrogen, Carlsbad, CA, United States), Histone 3 acetylation at Lysine 9 (H3K9Ac) (PA5 17868, Thermo Fisher Scientific, Carlsbad, CA, United States), or Histone 3 trimethylation at Lysine 27 (H3K27me3) (PA5 17173, Thermo Fisher Scientific, Carlsbad, CA, United States). The beads and associated immune

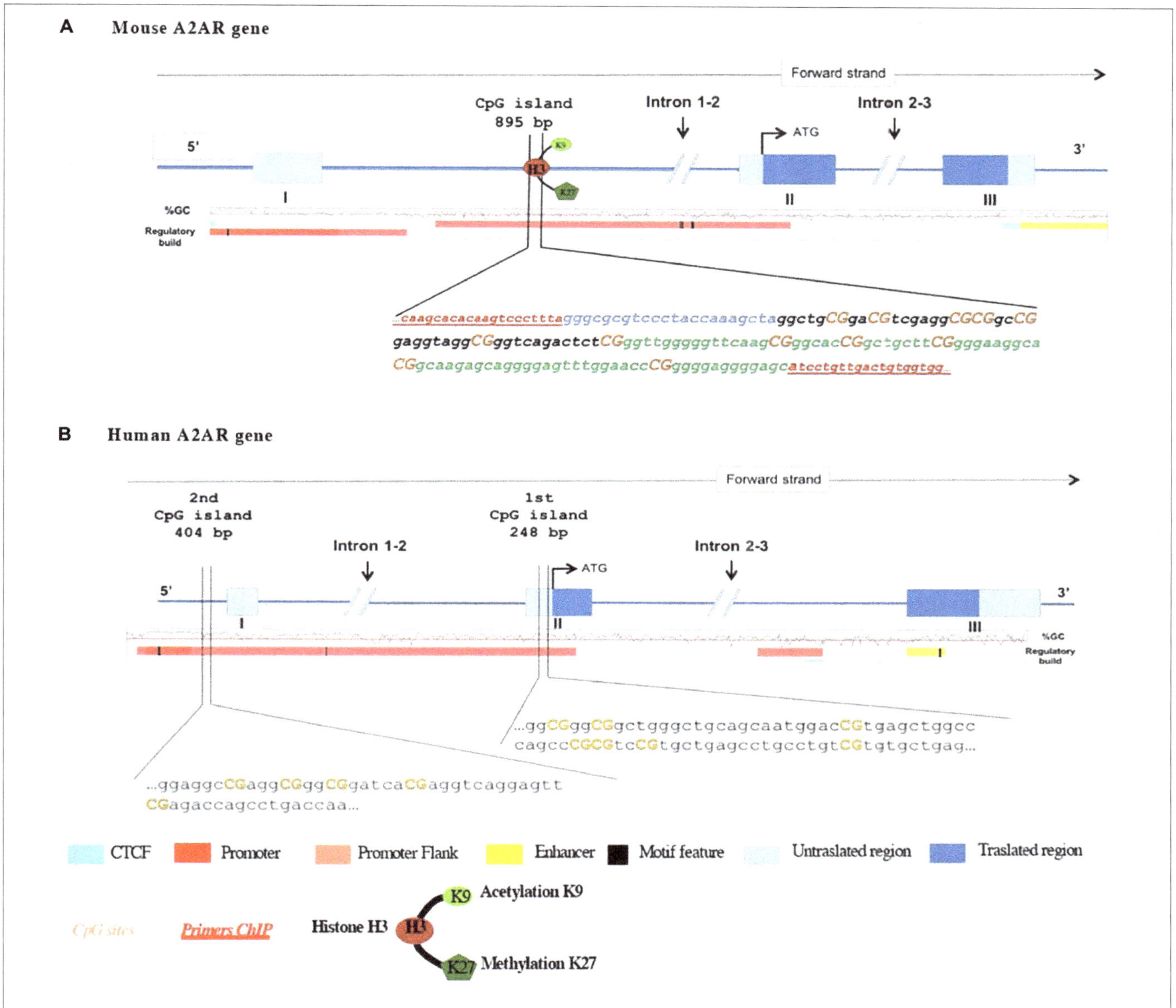

FIGURE 1 | Schematic representation of **(A)** mouse and **(B)** human A2AR gene promoters and the 5′ upstream region. Translation start code (ATG), exons and introns, CpG island, and histone modifications studied are depicted. In mouse A2AR gene promoter, two regions (region 1 in black and region 2 in green) localized in the same CpG island. Orange bold text indicates the CpG sites analyzed.

complexes were washed three times with RIPA buffer and once with Tris–EDTA buffer. The immune complexes were eluted with elution buffer (20 mM Tris-HCl, 5 mM EDTA, 50 mM NaCl) containing proteinase K (50 μg/ml) (Qiagen, Valencia, CA, United States) at 68°C for 2 h, and DNA was recovered by NucleoSpin TriPrep (Macherey-Nagel, Germany). Thereafter, to quantify A2AR gene sequences associated with the immunoprecipitated proteins, RT-qPCR was carried out using primers designed with Primer 3 software (Rozen and Skaletsky, 2000; see **Table 1**). All ChIP data were normalized to the input DNA amounts (Ct values of immunoprecipitated samples were normalized to Ct values obtained from "input"). In addition, results on DNA from lesioned animals were normalized by the DNA data obtained from control animals (control group).

Western Blot

Total cellular lysates from human PBMCs and mice tissues were prepared with different procedures. PBMCs were lysed in RIPA buffer whereas 0.3 gr of striatum tissue sample of lesioned and control animals were homogenized in T-PER lysis buffer (PIERCE, Rockford, IL, United States) containing 1% NP-40 detergent solution, 5% glycerol, 1 mM EDTA and 0.1% PIC (Sigma-Aldrich, Milan, Italy). Both human and mouse samples were sonicated and then centrifuged at 5000 *g* for 30 min at 4°C. Protein concentrations were

TABLE 2 | Primers employed during the quantitative polymerase chain reaction, chromatin immunoprecipitation, and DNA methylation assays.

		Gene expression	
Species	**Gene**	**Forward**	**Reverse**
Human	β-actin	GCACCAGATCATGTTTGAGACCT	CCATACACGATGCCAGTGGT
	GAPDH	CAGCCTCAAGATCATCAGCA	TGTGGTCATGAGTCGTTCCA
	A2AR	CATCCCGCTCCGGTACAATG	TGGTTCTTGCCCTCCTTTGG
Mouse	β-actin	AACGGGAAGCTCACTGGCAT	GTCTCAAACATGATCTGGGTC
	GAPDH	AACGGGAAGCTCACTGGCAT	AACGGGAAGCTCACTGGCAT
	A2AR	AGAGCAAGAGGCAGGTATCTC	CCCAAAGGCTTTCTCACGGA
	A2AR ChIP	CAAGCACACAAGTCCCTTTA	CAAGCACACAAGTCCCTTTA
		DNA methylation	
		Region 1	**Region 2**
Human A2AR	Forward	TTTGGGTAGGGTTGGGAGTT	AGGTGGAGGTTGTAGTGA
	Reverse	CCCAACACACCAACACATT	CCACACTCCCTCTTTTCTTT
	Sequencing	GGTAGGGTTGGGAGTTA	GGAGGTTGTAGTGAG
Mouse A2AR	Forward	PM00220542 Qiagen, Hilden, Germany	GGAGGGGATTGAATTTGTAAGTATA
	Reverse		CCAAACACCCACCCTATTATC
	Sequencing		GAGGTAGGAGGGTTAGAT

measured according to Bradford method (1976). For each sample, 50 μg of human proteins and 30 μg of mouse proteins were electrophoresed (12% acrylamide gels) and transferred to PVDF membranes (Amersham Biosciences, Piscataway, NJ, United States). Membranes, blocked with a solution of 5% non-fat dry milk for 20 min and with 5% BSA for 40 min at room temperature, were incubated with a rabbit anti-A2A polyclonal antibody (PA1-042, Thermo Fisher Scientific, Carlsbad, CA, United States, 1:5000 in blocking solution) and a rabbit anti-GAPDH monoclonal antibody (2118S, Cell Signaling, Danvers, MA, United States, 1:5000 in blocking solution) overnight in cold room. GAPDH was used to normalize samples. Antibody against TH (Chemicon, Temecula, CA, 1:1000) was used in mice samples to assess the severity of the 6-OHDA lesions. Finally, the membranes were incubated with specific horseradish peroxidase-conjugated secondary anti-rabbit antibody for 1 h at room temperature (AP307P, Millipore, Darmstadt, Germany, 1:10000 in blocking solution). The antigen-antibody complex was detected by enhanced chemiluminescence (ECL, Amersham Biosciences) and the intensities of the immunoreactive bands were quantified by densitometric analysis using the ImageJ software (NIH, Bethesda, MD, United States).

Statistical Analysis

Non-parametric statistic (Mann-Whitney *U* test) was used to compare lesioned vs. unlesioned striata, as well as the human PD and control samples. For correlation analysis, Spearman's coefficient was used. $p < 0.05$ was considered statistically significant. All the mentioned tests were performed using GraphPad Prism version 6.00 (GraphPad Software, San Diego, CA, United States).

RESULTS

Human Subjects

Patients and controls were age and gender matched to allow consistent comparisons. RT-PCR analysis revealed significantly higher A2AR mRNA levels in PD patients when compared to healthy controls (PD: 2.84 ± 0.14; Controls: 1.13 ± 0.12

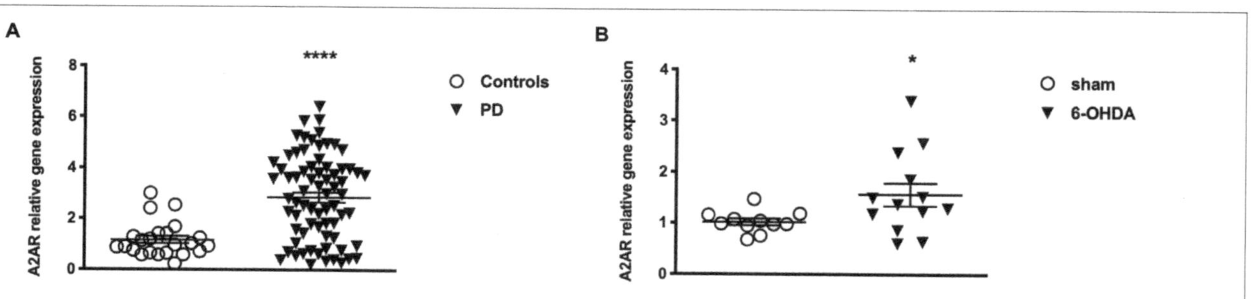

FIGURE 2 | Levels of A2AR mRNA **(A)** in PBMC from controls (n = 22) and PD patients (n = 25) and **(B)** in the striatum of Sham (n = 11) and 6-OHDA (n = 13) animals. Bars represents $2^{-\Delta\Delta Ct}$ value calculated by Delta-Delta Ct (ΔΔCt) method. *$p < 0.05$ and ****$p < 0.0001$ vs. respective control groups.

$p < 0.0001$ Mann Whitney test) (**Figure 2A**). Moreover, data stratification analysis showed a significant correlation between A2AR gene expression and age of the subjects (Spearman $r = -0.2931$; $p = 0.014$), years from disease onset (Spearman $r = -0.4046$; $p = 0.001$), as well as Hoehn & Yahr (H&Y) ($p < 0.01$ score 2 vs. score 1), UPDRS (Spearman $r = -0.2752$; $p = 0.0211$) scores, and LEDD (Spearman $r = -0.3902$; $p = 0.001$) (**Figure 3**). On the other hand, no correlation was observed between A2AR gene expression and age in controls (Spearman $r = 0.2399$; $p = 0.3226$). Correlation analysis survived Dunn's multiple comparisons test for age, UPDRS score, and LEDD. Finally, in a multiple linear regression analysis A2AR mRNA levels were found to be related to age ($p = 0.0343$) and gender ($p = 0.0335$), as well as LEDD ($p = 0.0005$).

It is interesting to note that also A2AR density, expressed as A2AR/GAPDH ratio, was significantly higher in PD patients when compared to controls (Controls: 100% ± 6.67; PD: 184.5% ± 13.07; $p = 0.0159$ Mann Whitney test) (**Figure 4A**). DNA methylation analyzed at A2AR promoter in two different CpG islands did not show any difference between PD and controls (**Table 3**).

6-OHDA Mice Model

The first result we observed in mice is the reduced TH immunoreactivity to 10.3 ± 1.22% of control Sham-lesioned animals (100.0 ± 3.39%) (see **Supplementary Figure S1**). Successively, the study of the A2AR transcriptional regulation revealed a significant up-regulation of A2AR mRNA in the striata of 6-OHDA lesioned mice, when compared to control (Sham) mice (Sham: 1.02 ± 0.06; 6-OHDA: 1.56 ± 0.22; $p = 0.0041$ Mann Whitney test) (**Figure 2B**). In agreement with these findings, we observed a parallel increase of A2AR protein levels in 6-OHDA-lesioned animals when compared to controls (Sham: 100.0 ± 7.89; 6-OHDA: 124.84 ± 7.39; $p = 0.0425$ Mann Whitney test) (**Figure 4B**). See **Supplementary Figure S2** for further details about the analysis of protein levels. We also observed a consistent reduction in DNA methylation at A2AR gene promoter selectively in one of the two regions under study, and specifically in the second CpG site (Sham: 5.06 ± 0.41; 6-OHDA: 4.45 ± 0.60; $p = 0.025$) as well as in the average of the 6 CpG sites analyzed (Sham: 3.97 ± 0.22; 6-OHDA: 3.52 ± 0.35; $p = 0.031$) (**Figure 5B**). Notably, gene expression and DNA methylation levels were inversely correlated in all samples (Spearman $r = -0.427$, $p = 0.037$) (**Figure 5C**). No changes were observed in region 1 (**Figure 5A**). Finally, we report also a significant enrichment of H3K9Ac (a histone mark exerting permissive action on gene transcription) at A2AR GENE promoter, at the level of the same region studied for DNA methylation in 6-OHDA mice (Sham: 1.06 ± 0.07; 6-OHDA: 1.52 ± 0.21; $p = 0.038$) (**Figure 6**). We also analyzed the levels of the repressive marker, H3K27me3, but we did not observe any significant change (Sham: 1.05 ± 0.07; 6-OHDA: 0.80 ± 0.11; $p = 0.075$ (**Figure 6**).

DISCUSSION

This study shows that dopamine depletion, a characteristic trait of PD experimentally induced *in vivo* by 6-OHDA, evokes in mice striata A2AR gene up-regulation as well as increase in protein receptor levels. The same alterations have also been observed in PBMCs from PD patients when compared to healthy controls.

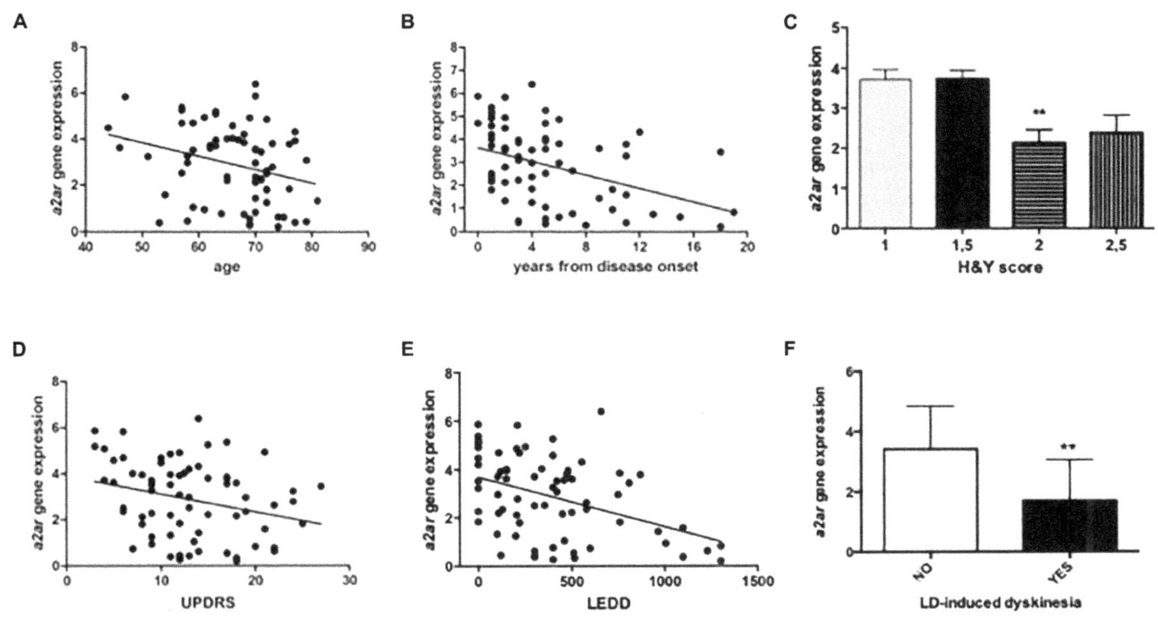

FIGURE 3 | Data stratification and correlation analysis between A2AR mRNA levels in PD human subjects and age **(A**, years from disease onset **(B)**, H&Y score **(C)**, UPDRS score **(D)**, LEDD **(E)**, and LD-induced dyskinesia **(F)**. $^{**}p < 0.01$ vs. respective control groups.

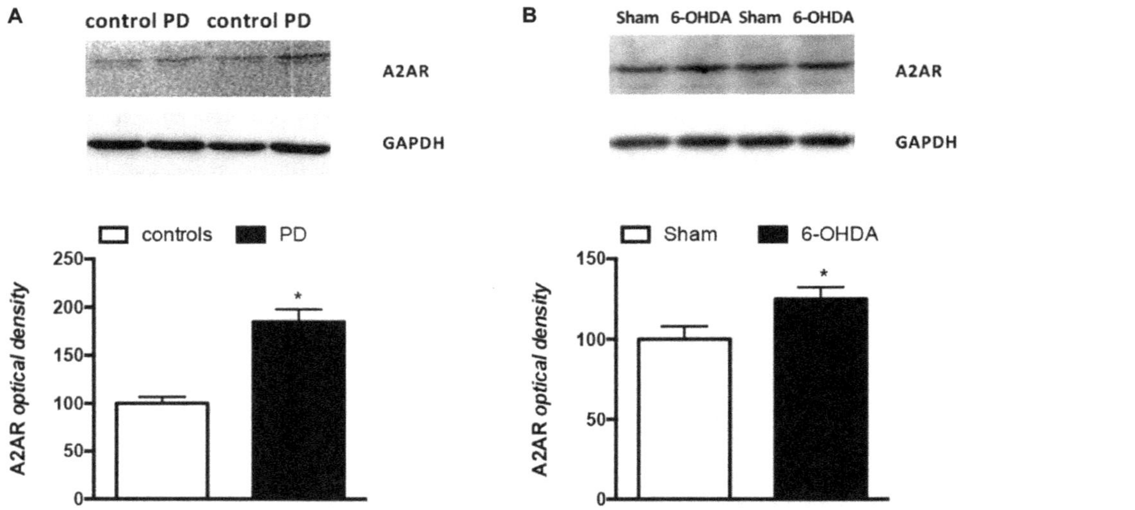

FIGURE 4 | Analysis of A2AR protein levels in PBMCs from **(A)** PD patients (n = 5) and controls (n = 4) and **(B)** Sham (n = 12) and 6-OHDA (n = 10) mice striata. Representative immunoblots of PBMCs and striata lysates reacted with specific anti-A2AR or anti-GAPDH antibodies are shown above the bars for both mice and humans. Values, expressed as means ± standard error of the mean (SEM), were normalized by GAPDH and taking the control and sham groups as 100, respectively for **(A,B)**. $^{*}p < 0.05$ vs. respective control groups.

Our data corroborate previous studies showing increased A2AR transcription in the striatum of dopamine-denervated rats (Pinna et al., 2002) and in the putamen of PD patients (Varani et al., 2010) suggesting a similar regulation in the 6-OHDA mouse model of PD as well as in PBMCs from PD subjects. In addition, we provide evidence that these changes are paralleled by a significant increase in A2AR levels, confirming the same change already observed in both 6-OHDA rat model (Bhattacharjee et al., 2011) and clinical samples (Calon et al., 2004; Varani et al., 2010; Ramlackhansingh et al., 2011; Casetta et al., 2014).

Notably, these clinical studies established a correlation between L-DOPA-induced motor complications (i.e., dyskinesia) and increased levels of A2AR. Thus, A2AR density is significantly higher in lymphocytes and neutrophils of dyskinetic than non-dyskinetic patients. Interestingly, L-DOPA-induced dyskinesia is influenced by the degree of dopamine depletion, suggesting that the increase in A2AR expression may be particularly prominent in advanced PD (Varani et al., 2010). Our findings in patients instead show different pattern of changes. In fact, data stratification based on age, as well as years from disease onset, showed higher levels in receptor gene expression in younger patients and in subjects affected for less than a few years, as well as in those with less severe disease even if it should be considered the limited range of H&Y and UPDRS scores. This is in agreement with the results from Villar-Menéndez et al. (2014) showing that the increased A2AR occurs as an early event in PD.

Importantly, these effects in mice are accompanied by consistent changes in two relevant epigenetic marks: a significant reduction in DNA methylation and a significant increase in H3K9Ac at gene promoter. DNA methylation role in A2AR gene regulation was previously reported (Buira et al., 2010a,b; Villar-Menéndez et al., 2014) and we here show in mice striata a significant and selective reduction in DNA methylation clearly correlated with the increase in gene expression.

Moreover, we observed a hitherto undiscovered increase in H3K9Ac, a permissive epigenetic mark, in line with the upregulation of gene expression. Global histone hyperacetylation represents a key epigenetic change in dopaminergic neurons and has been proposed to participate in PD pathogenesis (Villar-Menéndez et al., 2013; Kleiveland, 2015) however this is the

TABLE 3 | DNA methylation levels (mean ± SEM) at seven cytosine-guanine dinucleotide (CpG) sites (Region 1) and at five cytosine-guanine dinucleotide (CpG) sites (Region 2), within the human A2AR gene promoter, in PBMCs of control (n = 22), and PD subjects (n = 25).

Region 1	CpG site 1	CpG site 2	CpG site 3	CpG site 4	CpG site 5	CpG site 6	CpG site 7
CT	97.50 ± 0.07	95.89 ± 0.10	97.97 ± 0.16	100	81.81 ± 0.34	92.62 ± 0.21	93.07 ± 0.37
PD	97.45 ± 0.05	95.83 ± 0.10	97.31 ± 0.27	100	81.32 ± 0.20	93.03 ± 0.23	92.40 ± 0.31
Region 2	**CpG site 1**	**CpG site 2**	**CpG site 3**	**CpG site 4**	**CpG site 5**		
CT	92.02 ± 1.03	94.77 ± 0.63	85.81 ± 0.47	75.81 ± 0.47	36.49 ± 4.63		
PD	92.39 ± 0.76	95.51 ± 0.48	85.97 ± 0.75	74.93 ± 0.57	33.27 ± 0.98		

ANOVAs and subsequent post hoc tests did not indicate any significant difference in the level of methylation at CpG sites at the two regions analyzed between PD and control patients.

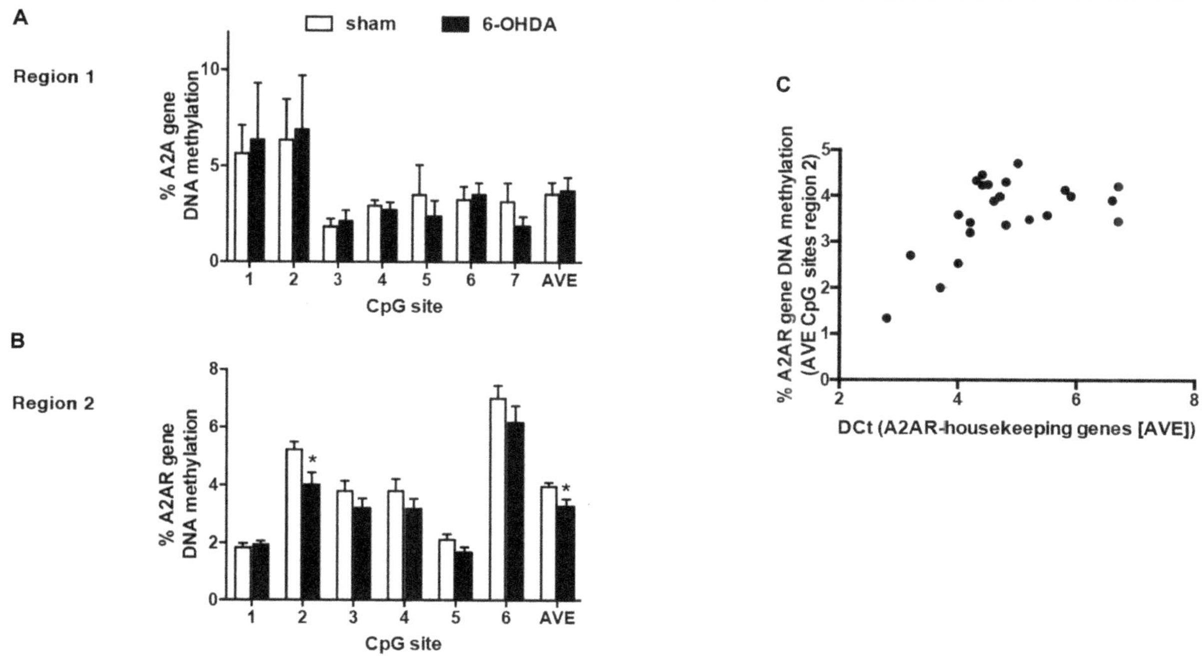

FIGURE 5 | Percentage of DNA methylation assessed with bisulfite pyrosequencing in sham (n = 12) and 6-OHDA (n = 14) mice striata at A2AR gene promoter: **(A)** Region 1 (7 CpG sites quantified). **(B)** Region 2 (6 CpG sites quantified). Values are expressed as means ± SEM. $^*p < 0.05$ vs. Sham group. **(C)** Correlation between average DNA methylation at 6 CpG sites located in Region 2 and A2AR mRNA levels in mice striata. Data were compared with non-parametric Spearman correlation analysis. $^*P = 0.0357$.

first study showing a specific change in H3 acetylation at A2AR gene in the dopamine-depleted striatum. This finding suggests that the reduction in DNA methylation of this gene might be mediated by a local state of acetylation, as previously proposed as a global effect (Cervoni and Szyf, 2001). No changes in DNA methylation levels have been observed in PBMCs from PD subjects when compared to controls. Instead, others reported a reduction of DNA methylation in two CpG sites at A2AR gene promoter in human brain samples (Villar-Menéndez et al., 2014).

In this study we used whole blood samples composed of different cell types with different DNA methylation profiles (Kleiveland, 2015). Therefore, it will be necessary to extend these findings using novel methodological approaches, such as cell-sorting, to fully elucidate the underlying epigenetic regulation of gene expression. However, it is important to underline that PBMCs share with neurons several cellular components and contain the complete epigenetic machinery present in neurons as well as in many other tissues (Joseph et al., 2018; Sen et al., 2018; Zhu et al., 2018). For this reason, their gene expression profile has been recently proposed as a substitute for cerebral markers which, on the other hand, wouldn't provide enough insight into biochemical detail in order to originate novel and more effective therapeutic intervention (Woelk et al., 2011; Arosio et al., 2014). Moreover, it would also be relevant to evaluate the molecular outcomes in mice PBMCs and compare them to the data obtained from mice brain samples as well as human PBMCs.

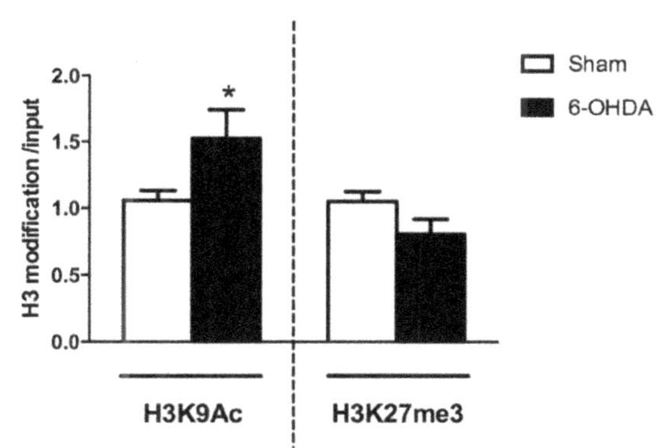

FIGURE 6 | RT-qPCR analysis of H3K9Ac and H3K27me3 immunoprecipitated fragments at A2AR gene promoter. Bars show specific histone modification levels, normalized to total input DNA in Sham (n = 11), and 6-OHDA (n = 9) animals. Values are expressed as means ± SEM. $^*p < 0.05$ vs. Sham group.

In conclusion, our results in mice indicate that loss of dopaminergic innervation to the striatum results in the upregulation of A2AR GENE expression paralleled by selective epigenetic mechanisms, thereby providing new insights into the role of this receptor in PD. Several clinical trials have shown that A2AR antagonists ameliorate the dyskinesia induced by chronic L-DOPA treatment in PD patients (Pinna et al., 2005;

Xu et al., 2005; Mizuno and Kondo, 2013) and it is possible that receptor silencing might be an alternative therapy to reduce receptors activity.

Therefore, these data may offer new vistas for therapeutic interventions in PD by targeting histone acetylation and/or DNA methylation selectively at this gene sequence. These data also suggest a possible role of A2AR transcriptional regulation as a biomarker in PD on the basis of the relevant changes occurring at early stages of disease development observed in patient samples.

AUTHOR CONTRIBUTIONS

CD'A, EP, and GF conceived and designed the experiments. AF, MD, MM, AB-O, NL, and FF conducted the experiments. CD'A, EP, and ED analyzed the data. ED, CD'A, and GF contributed to the reagents, materials, and analysis tools. CD'A, GF, and AF wrote the manuscript.

FUNDING

This study was supported by the Italian Ministry of University and Research under the grants FIRB-RBFR12DELS to CD'A and by the StratNeuro at Karolinska Institutet to AB-O.

REFERENCES

Arosio, B., D'Addario, C., Gussago, C., Casati, M., Tedone, E., Ferri, E., et al. (2014). Peripheal blood mononuclear cells as a laboratory to study dementia in the elderly. *Biomed. Res. Int.* 2014, 169203. doi: 10.1155/2014/169203

Bhattacharjee, A. K., Lang, L., Jacobson, O., Shinkre, B., Ma, Y., Niu, G., et al. (2011). Striatal adenosine A(2A) receptor-mediated positron emission tomographic imaging in 6-hydroxydopamine-lesioned rats using ((18)F)-MRS5425. *Nucl. Med. Biol.* 38, 897–906. doi: 10.1016/j.nucmedbio.2011.01.009

Buira, S. P., Albasanz, J. L., Dentesano, G., Moreno, J., Martín, M., Ferrer, I., et al. (2010a). *DNA methylation regulates adenosine A(*2A) receptor cell surface expression levels. *J. Neurochem.* 112, 1273–1285. doi: 10.1111/j.1471-4159.2009.06538.x

Buira, S. P., Dentesano, G., Albasanz, J. L., Moreno, J., Martín, M., Ferrer, I., et al. (2010b). *DNA methylation and Yin Yang*-1 repress adenosine A2A receptor levels in human brain. *J. Neurochem.* 115, 283–295. doi: 10.1111/j.1471-4159.2010.06928.x

Calon, F., Dridi, M., Hornykiewicz, O., Bédard, P. J., Rajput, A. H., and Di Paolo, T. (2004). Increased adenosine A2A receptors in the brain of Parkinson's disease patients with dyskinesias. *Brain* 127, 1075–1084. doi: 10.1093/brain/awh128

Casetta, I., Vincenzi, F., Bencivelli, D., Corciulo, C., Gentile, M., Granieri, E., et al. (2014). A(2A) adenosine receptors and Parkinson's disease severity. *Acta Neurol. Scand.* 129, 276–281. doi: 10.1111/ane.12181

Cervoni, N., and Szyf, M. (2001). Demethylase activity is directed by histone acetylation. *J. Biol. Chem.* 276, 40778–40787. doi: 10.1074/jbc.m103921200

Chomczynski, P., and Sacchi, N. (2006). The single-step method of RNA isolation by acid guanidinium thiocyanate-phenol-chloroform extraction: twenty-something years on. *Nat. Protoc.* 1, 581–585. doi: 10.1038/nprot.2006.83

Cifani, C., Micioni Di Bonaventura, M. V., Pucci, M., Giusepponi, M. E., Romano, A., Di Francesco, A., et al. (2015). Regulation of hypothalamic neuropeptides gene expression in diet induced obesity resistant rats: possible targets for obesity prediction? *Front. Neurosci.* 9:187. doi: 10.3389/fnins.2015.00187

Dahl, J. A., and Collas, P. (2007). A quick and quantitative chromatin immunoprecipitation assay for small cell samples. *Front. Biosci.* 12, 4925–4931.

Feigin, A. (2003). Nondopaminergic symptomatic therapies for Parkinson's disease: turn on or turn off? *Neurology* 61, 286–287. doi: 10.1212/wnl.61.3.286

Fink, J. S., Weaver, D. R., Rivkees, S. A., Peterfreund, R. A., Pollack, A. E., Adler, E. M., et al. (1992). Molecular cloning of the rat A2 adenosine receptor: selective co-expression with D2 dopamine receptors in rat striatum. *Brain Res. Mol. Brain Res.* 14, 186–195. doi: 10.1016/0169-328x(92)90173-9

Franklin, K. B., and Paxinos, G. (2008). *The Mouse Brain in Stereotaxic Coordinates*, 3rd Edn. San Diego, CA: Academic press.

Harrison, I. F., and Dexter, D. T. (2013). Epigenetic targeting of histone deacetylase: therapeutic potential in Parkinson's disease? *Pharmacol. Ther.* 140, 34–52. doi: 10.1016/j.pharmthera.2013.05.010

Hughes, A. J., Daniel, S. E., Kilford, L., and Lees, A. J. (1992). Accuracy of clinical diagnosis of idiopathic Parkinson's disease: a clinico-pathological study of 100 cases. *J. Neurol. Neurosurg. Psychiatry* 55, 181–184. doi: 10.1136/jnnp.55.3.181

Hurley, M. J., Mash, D. C., and Jenner, P. (2000). Adenosine A(2A) receptor mRNA expression in Parkinson's disease. *Neurosci. Lett.* 291, 54–58. doi: 10.1016/s0304-3940(00)01371-9

Ikeda, K., Kurokawa, M., Aoyama, S., and Kuwana, Y. (2002). Neuroprotection by adenosine A2A receptor blockade in experimental models of Parkinson's disease. *J. Neurochem.* 80, 262–270. doi: 10.1046/j.0022-3042.2001.00694.x

Jarvis, M. F., and Williams, M. (1989). Direct autoradiographic localization of adenosine A2 receptors in the rat brain using the A2-selective agonist, (3H)CGS 21680. *Eur. J. Pharmacol.* 168, 243–246. doi: 10.1016/0014-2999(89)90571-2

Jones, P. A. (2012). Functions of DNA methylation: islands, start sites, gene bodies and beyond. *Nat. Rev. Genet.* 13, 484–492. doi: 10.1038/nrg3230

Joseph, S., George, N. I., Green-Knox, B., Treadwell, E. L., Word, B., Yim, S., et al. (2018). Epigenome-wide association study of peripheral blood mononuclear cells in systemic lupus erythematosus: identifying DNA methylation signatures associated with interferon-related genes based on ethnicity and SLEDAI. *J. Autoimmun.* 96, 147–157. doi: 10.1016/j.jaut.2018.09.007

Kaelin-Lang, A., Liniger, P., Probst, A., Lauterburg, T., and Burgunder, J. M. (2000). Adenosine A2A receptor gene expression in the normal striatum and after 6-OH-dopamine lesion. *J. Neural. Transm.* 107, 851–859. doi: 10.1007/s007020070037

Kleiveland, C. R. (2015). "Peripheral blood mononuclear cells," in *The Impact of Food Bioactives on Health*, eds K. Verhoeckx, P. Cotter, I. López-Expósito, C. Kleiveland, T. Lea, A. Mackie, et al. (Cham: Springer).

LeWitt, P. A. (2015). Levodopa therapy for Parkinson's disease: pharmacokinetics and pharmacodynamics. *Mov. Disord.* 30, 64–72. doi: 10.1002/mds.26082

Livak, K. J., and Schmittgen, T. D. (2001). Analysis of relative gene expression data using real-time quantitative PCR and the 2(-Delta Delta C(T)) Method. *Methods.* 25, 402–408. doi: 10.1006/meth.2001.1262

Marsden, C. D. (2000). Parkinson's disease. *J. Neurol. Neurosurg. Psychiatry* 57, 672–681.

Mizuno, Y., and Kondo, T. (2013). Japanese istradefylline study group adenosine A2A receptor antagonist istradefylline reduces daily OFF time in Parkinson's disease. *Mov. Disord.* 28, 1138–1141. doi: 10.1002/mds.25418

Obeso, J. A., Rodriguez-Oroz, M. C., Chana, P., Lera, G., Rodriguez, M., and Olanow, C. W. (2000). The evolution and origin of motor complications in Parkinson's disease. *Neurology* 55, S13–S20.

Ozansoy, M., and Basak, A. N. (2013). The central theme of Parkinson's disease: alpha-synuclein. *Mol. Neurobiol.* 47, 460–465. doi: 10.1007/s12035-012-8369-3

Park, G., Tan, J., Garcia, G., Kang, Y., Salvesen, G., and Zhang, Z. (2016). Regulation of Histone Acetylation by autophagy in Parkinson disease. *J. Biol. Chem.* 291, 3531–3540. doi: 10.1074/jbc.M115.675488

Pinna, A., Corsi, C., Carta, A. R., Valentini, V., Pedata, F., and Morelli, M. (2002). Modification of adenosine extracellular levels and adenosine A(2A) receptor mRNA by dopamine denervation. *Eur. J. Pharmacol* 446, 75–82. doi: 10.1016/s0014-2999(02)01818-6

Pinna, A., Wardas, J., Simola, N., and Morelli, M. (2005). New therapies for the treatment of Parkinson's disease: adenosine A2A receptor antagonists. *Life Sci.* 77, 3259–3267. doi: 10.1016/j.lfs.2005.04.029

Pucci, M., Micioni Di Bonaventura, M. V., Giusepponi, M. E., Romano, A., Filaferro, M., Maccarrone, M., et al. (2015). Epigenetic regulation of nociceptin/orphanin FQ and corticotropin-releasing factor system genes in frustration stress-induced binge-like palatable food consumption. *Addict. Biol.* 21, 1168–1185. doi: 10.1111/adb.12303

Ramlackhansingh, A. F., Bose, S. K., Ahmed, I., Turkheimer, F. E., Pavese, N., and Brooks, D. J. (2011). Adenosine 2A receptor availability in dyskinetic and nondyskinetic patients with Parkinson disease. *Neurology* 76, 1811–1816. doi: 10.1212/WNL.0b013e31821ccce4

Rosin, D. L., Robeva, A., Woodard, R. L., Guyenet, P. G., and Linden, J. (1998). Immunohistochemical localization of adenosine A2A receptors in the rat central nervous system. *J. Comp. Neurol.* 401, 163–186. doi: 10.1002/(sici)1096-9861(19981116)401:2<163::aid-cne2>3.3.co;2-4

Rozen, S., and Skaletsky, H. (2000). Primer3 on the WWW for general users and for biologist programmers. *Methods Mol. Biol.* 132, 365–386. doi: 10.1385/1-59259-192-2:365

Santini, E., Valjent, E., Usiello, A., Carta, M., Borgkvist, A., Girault, J. A., et al. (2007). Critical involvement of cAMP/DARPP-32 and extracellular signal-regulated protein kinase signaling in L-DOPA-induced dyskinesia. *J. Neurosci.* 27, 6995–7005. doi: 10.1523/jneurosci.0852-07.2007

Schiffmann, S. N., Fisone, G., Moresco, R., Cunha, R. A., and Ferré, S. (2007). Adenosine A2A receptors and basal ganglia physiology. *Prog. Neurobiol.* 83, 277–292. doi: 10.1016/j.pneurobio.2007.05.001

Schiffmann, S. N., Libert, F., Vassart, G., and Vanderhaeghen, J. J. (1991). Distribution of adenosine A2 receptor mRNA in the human brain. *Neurosci. Lett.* 130, 177–181. doi: 10.1016/0304-3940(91)90391-6

Schwarzschild, M. A., Agnati, L., Fuxe, K., Chen, J. F., and Morelli, M. (2006). Targeting adenosine A2A receptors in Parkinson's disease. *Trends Neurosci.* 29, 647–654. doi: 10.1016/j.tins.2006.09.004

Sen, P., Kemppainen, E., and Orešič, M. (2018). Perspectives on systems modeling of human peripheral blood mononuclear cells. *Front. Mol. Biosci.* 4:96. doi: 10.3389/fmolb.2017.00096

Song, C., Kanthasamy, A., Jin, H., Anantharam, V., and Kanthasamy, A. (2011). Paraquat induces epigenetic changes by promoting histone acetylation in cell culture models of dopaminergic degeneration. *Neurotoxicology* 32, 586–595. doi: 10.1016/j.neuro.2011.05.018

Svenningsson, P., Hall, H., Sedvall, G., and Fredholm, B. B. (1997). Distribution of adenosine receptors in the postmortem human brain: an extended autoradiographic study. *Synapse* 27, 322–335. doi: 10.1002/(sici)1098-2396(199712)27:4<322::aid-syn6>3.0.co;2-e

Tomiyama, M., Mori, F., Kimura, T., Ichinohe, N., Wakabayashi, K., Matsunaga, M., et al. (2004). Hypertrophy of medial globus pallidus and substantia nigra reticulata in 6-hydroxydopamine-lesioned rats treated with L-DOPA: implication for L-DOPA-induced dyskinesia in Parkinson's disease. *Neuropathology* 24, 290–295. doi: 10.1111/j.1440-1789.2004.00559.x

Tomlinson, C. L., Stowe, R., Patel, S., Rick, C., Gray, R., and Clarke, C. E. (2010). Systematic review of levodopa dose equivalency reporting in Parkinson's disease. *Mov. Disord.* 25, 2649–2653. doi: 10.1002/mds.23429

Varani, K., Vincenzi, F., Tosi, A., Gessi, S., Casetta, I., Granieri, G., et al. (2010). A2A adenosine receptor overexpression and functionality, as well as TNF-alpha levels, correlate with motor symptoms in Parkinson's disease. *FASEB J.* 24, 587–598. doi: 10.1096/fj.09-141044

Villar-Menéndez, I., Blanch, M., Tyebji S., Pereira-Veiga, T., Albasanz, J. L., Martín, M., et al. (2013). Increased 5-methylcytosine and decreased 5-hydroxymethylcytosine levels are associated with reduced striatal A2AR levels in Huntington's disease. *Neuromolecular. Med.* 15, 295–309. doi: 10.1007/s12017-013-8219-0

Villar-Menéndez, I., Porta, S., Buira, S. P., Pereira-Veiga, T., Díaz-Sánchez, S., Albasanz, J. L., et al. (2014). Increased striatal adenosine A2A receptor levels is an early event in Parkinson's disease-related pathology and it is potentially regulated by miR-34b. *Neurobiol. Dis.* 69, 206–214. doi: 10.1016/j.nbd.2014.05.030

Woelk, C. H., Singhania, A., Pérez-Santiago, J., Glatt, S. J., and Tsuang, M. T. (2011). The utility of gene expression in blood cells for diagnosing neuropsychiatric disorders. *Int. Rev. Neurobiol.* 101, 41–63. doi: 10.1016/B978-0-12-387718-5.00003-1

Xu, K., Bastia, E., and Schwarzschild, M. (2005). Therapeutic potential of adenosine A(2A) receptor antagonists in Parkinson's disease. *Pharmacol. Ther.* 105, 267–310. doi: 10.1016/j.pharmthera.2004.10.007

Zhu, C., Mi, W., Chen, T., Zhao, H., Zuo, X., Luo, H., et al. (2018). Integration of genome-wide DNA methylation and transcription uncovered aberrant methylation-regulated genes and pathways in the peripheral blood mononuclear cells of systemic sclerosis. *Int. J. Rheumatol.* 2018:7342472. doi: 10.1155/2018/7342472

14

Introducing a Novel Approach for Evaluation and Monitoring of Brain Health Across Life Span Using Direct Non-invasive Brain Network Electrophysiology

Noa Zifman[1†], Ofri Levy-Lamdan[1†], Gil Suzin[2], Shai Efrati[2,3], David Tanne[3,4], Hilla Fogel[1] and Iftach Dolev[1]*

[1] QuantalX Neuroscience, Tel Aviv-Yafo, Israel, [2] Sagol Center for Hyperbaric Medicine and Research, Assaf Harofeh Medical Center, Ramle, Israel, [3] Sackler School of Medicine and Sagol School of Neuroscience, Tel-Aviv University, Tel Aviv-Yafo, Israel, [4] Stroke and Cognition Institute, Rambam Healthcare Campus, Haifa, Israel

***Correspondence:**
Iftach Dolev
iftach@quantalx.com;
doleviftach@gmail.com

† These authors have contributed equally to this work

Objective: Evaluation and monitoring of brain health throughout aging by direct electrophysiological imaging (DELPHI) which analyzes TMS (transcranial magnetic stimulation) evoked potentials.

Methods: Transcranial magnetic stimulation evoked potentials formation, coherence and history dependency, measured using electroencephalogram (EEG), was extracted from 80 healthy subjects in different age groups, 25–85 years old, and 20 subjects diagnosed with mild dementia (MD), over 70 years old. Subjects brain health was evaluated using MRI scans, neurocognitive evaluation, and computerized testing and compared to DELPHI analysis of brain network functionality.

Results: A significant decrease in signal coherence is observed with age in connectivity maps, mostly in inter-hemispheric temporal, and parietal areas. MD patients display a pronounced decrease in global and inter-hemispheric frontal connectivity compared to healthy controls. Early and late signal slope ratio also display a significant, age dependent, change with pronounced early slope, phase shift, between normal healthy aging, and MD. History dependent analysis demonstrates a binary step function classification of healthy brain vs. abnormal aging subjects mostly for late slope. DELPHI measures demonstrate high reproducibility with reliability coefficients of around 0.9.

Conclusion: These results indicate that features of evoked response, as charge transfer, slopes of response, and plasticity are altered during abnormal aging and that these fundamental properties of network functionality can be directly evaluated and monitored using DELPHI.

Keywords: brain, aging, DELPHI, plasticity, imaging, functional, network

INTRODUCTION

The ability to deal with the expanding risk of age associated brain disorders, such as vascular cognitive impairment, Alzheimer's disease (AD), and other neurodegenerative or psychiatric disorders, the impact of which cannot be overstated, is limited by the lack of tools which enable the evaluation and monitoring of brain functional health status. These brain disorders are mostly manifested as brain network functionality changes, particularly in the early stages changing the network function. Brain functionality refers to the network topological features of connectivity, plasticity and strength which together reflect the network hierarchy and its ability to store and process information (Greenwood, 2007; Palop et al., 2007; Berlucchi and Buchtel, 2009; Feldman, 2009; Almeida et al., 2017; Kumar et al., 2017; Schulz and Hausmann, 2017). Current clinically available brain imaging provides high resolution images of the rigid brain anatomical network. Advanced technologies such as functional MRI (fMRI), or positron emission tomography can provide functional information but use indirect measurement as blood flow in high spatial but poor temporal resolution (Gore, 2003; Cherry, 2009). Therefore, these methods are insufficient for the evaluation of brain health during normal aging or age-related pathological deterioration such as mild cognitive impairment (MCI) or mild dementia (MD).

Electrophysiology is a well-established powerful tool for evaluating brain network functionality. It is used extensively in neurophysiological research, for measuring properties of brain network functionality as network effective strength of connectivity and excitation/inhibition balance that corresponds to network short term plasticity (STP) (Markram and Tsodyks, 1996; Markram et al., 1998; Bédard et al., 2004; Covey and Carter, 2015). However, clinically, it is used mostly for epilepsy and sleep monitoring, in the form of electroencephalograph – EEG, (Niedermeyer and da Silva, 2005) measuring spontaneous activity or activity related to specific task (event related potential -ERP) but is not routinely used in the clinical environment for evaluation of brain health (Shah and Mittal, 2014). Therefore, there is a great need for an ancillary tool, which enables an objective, direct, and accessible evaluation of brain network functionality in physiological terms of network connectivity, plasticity, and strength.

Transcranial magnetic stimulation (TMS) is a non-invasive brain stimulation method that allows the study of human cortical function *in vivo* (Ilmoniemi et al., 1999; Hallett, 2007; Rossini et al., 2015). TMS enables the exploration and modulation of functional neuronal networks topology with a potential therapeutic aim (Bordet et al., 2017), both in normal brain aging and in patients with degenerative or vascular dementia (Pennisi et al., 2016). Using TMS for examining human cortical functionality is enhanced by combining it with simultaneous registration of EEG. EEG provides an opportunity to directly measure the cerebral response to TMS, measuring the cortical TMS evoked potential (TEP), and is used to assess cerebral reactivity across wide areas of neocortex (Komssi et al., 2002; Nikulin et al., 2003; Rossini et al., 2015). Studies integrating TMS with EEG (TMS-EEG) have shown that TMS produces waves of activity that reverberate throughout the cortex and that are reproducible and reliable (Komssi and Kähkönen, 2006; Lioumis et al., 2009; Casarotto et al., 2010; Farzan et al., 2010; Kerwin et al., 2018), thus providing direct information about cortical excitability and connectivity with excellent temporal resolution (Kähkönen et al., 2005; Ilmoniemi and Kicić, 2010; Chung et al., 2015; Shafi et al., 2016). By evaluating the propagation of evoked response in different behavioral states and in different tasks, TMS-EEG has been used to causally probe the dynamic effective connectivity of human brain networks (Shafi et al., 2012; Kugiumtzis and Kimiskidis, 2015; Rogasch et al., 2015; Cash et al., 2017; Ferreri et al., 2017b).

Our approach, called direct electro-physiological imaging (DELPHI), is a new methodology for evaluating brain network functionality, evaluating fundamental physiological properties of brain functionality. DELPHI is a clinically available bedside tool, combining TMS-EEG and their robust scientific infrastructure, into one complete automated acquisition, and analysis system. The DELPHI software algorithm extracts direct stimulation related properties of brain network functionality in time-frequency-location. Using DELPHI, common electro-physiological features are clustered into multi-dimensional patterns of evoked network response, characterizing a profile of brain network functional pathophysiology. This neurophysiological profile includes properties of network connectivity and plasticity measured by analyzing the evoked response to changes in magnetic stimulation to specific cortical neuronal network hubs.

Aging is a normal, yet, complex biological process associated with decline in specific brain functions (sensory, motor, and cognitive) (Mora, 2013). Brain plasticity is highly important during aging, for optimal brain health (Grady et al., 2003; Kelly et al., 2006). Evidence support the understanding that network plasticity becomes less efficient with age (Rosenzweig and Barnes, 2003; Greenwood, 2007; Sambataro et al., 2010; Wang et al., 2010). Patients with early AD, reveal an abnormally suppressed efficacy of plasticity mechanisms (Greenwood, 2007; Casarotto et al., 2011; Pascual-Leone et al., 2011; Oberman and Pascual-Leone, 2013). Although common age-related diseases, such as vascular cognitive impairment and neurodegenerative disorders, are known to share patho-physiological mechanisms of alerted cortical excitability, synaptic plasticity (Bella et al., 2013; Lanza et al., 2017), and neurotransmission pathways (Bella et al., 2016), currently, there are no available tools or methods to monitor and evaluate brain health during aging.

The purpose of this work was to evaluate age dependent brain network functional changes in healthy adults using our developed DELPHI technology, providing a potential tool, and method to distinguish between normal and abnormal aging pathophysiology.

Based on the vast published data supporting the understanding that abnormal aging processes share common measurable electrophysiological features, the experimental hypothesis of this study was that using DELPHI we can characterize normal brain network functional aging, and differentiate it from abnormal aging defined in this study as MD.

MATERIALS AND METHODS

Clinical Data Collection and Analysis

This study was carried out in accordance with the recommendation of "Assaf-Harofeh" Medical center review board. Protocol was approved by the local institutional "Ethical Committee." All subjects gave written informed consent in accordance with the Declaration of Helsinki. All participants underwent the exact same TMS-EEG stimulation and recording protocol.

Subjects

Four study groups were included in the study, defined as follows: (a) Healthy young, 25–45 years old (N = 30; mean age: 35, stdv: 6.6); (b) Healthy adults, 50–70 years old (N = 30 mean age: 61; stdv: 5.9); (c) Healthy elderly, over 70 years old; (N = 17; mean age: 75.4; stdv: 5.6); (d) MD subjects, over 70 years old (N = 20; mean age: 75.2, stdv: 4.3). Statistics of each study group is described in **Tables 1, 2**. Inclusion criteria for the healthy subject groups were as follows: (1) No neurological or psychiatric disorder documented in medical history or self-report. (2) Absence of any significant abnormal findings in MRI scan such as brain tumors, subdural hematoma, and other brain structural lesion. (3) No central nervous system (CNS) directed prescribed medication treatment. (4) A global index score and memory (verbal and non-verbal) of 95 or above (normalized to age related population) in computerized testing. MD inclusion criteria were defined as follows: (1) A clinical diagnosis of probable AD Dementia (McKhann et al., 2011). (2) Montreal cognitive assessment (MoCA) score between 11 and 22 as evaluated by neuropsychologist (Nasreddine et al., 2005; Saczynski et al., 2015). (3) Computerized testing index score of at least 1.5 standard deviations (STDV) below age related norm in verbal and non-verbal memory score and at least in one out of 3 additional computerized tests (Attention/Information Processing/Executive Function). (4) Absence of other unrelated neurological or psychiatric disorder documented in medical history or self-report. (5) Absence of any unrelated significant abnormal findings in MRI scan such as brain tumors, subdural hematoma, and other brain structural lesion. **Tables 3, 4** summarize study groups computerized cognitive score per cognitive domain. Mean MoCA score of the MD subject group was 16 ± 4.

All subjects underwent a brain MRI scan 1–2 weeks before DELPHI evaluation. Imaging was performed with a 3 Tesla system (20 channels, MAGNETOM Skyra, Siemens Medical Solutions). The MRI protocol included T2 weighted, T1 weighted, FLAIR, and susceptibility weighted imaging (SWI) sequences. All scans were evaluated at "Assaf-Harofeh" medical center by a neuro-radiologist. Assessment of cognitive functions was performed by trained neuropsychologists using the MoCA test (Nasreddine et al., 2005) and NeuroTrax *Mindstreams* Mild Impairment Battery computerized BrainCare cognitive battery tests (NeuroTrax Corp., TX, United States) (Dwolatzky et al., 2003).

TABLE 2 | Statistical differences between ages of study groups.

	p value
Mild Dementia (>70)\Healthy (>70)	ns/*p* = 0.77
Healthy (>70)\Healthy (50–70)	$p < 0.0001$
Healthy (50–70)\Healthy (25–45)	$p < 0.0001$

Each row represents two study groups, right column displays t-test p values.

TMS-EEG

Transcranial magnetic stimulation was performed with a MagPro R30 stimulator (MagVenture, Denmark) and an MCF-B65-HO figure-8 Coil (MagVenture, Denmark). 32-channel EEG data were obtained using two 32-channel TMS compatible BrainAmp DC amplifiers (5 kHz sampling rate; ±16.384 mv measurement range; analog low pass filter 1 kHz; Brain Products GmbH, Germany). These were attached to the Easy EEG cap (EasyCap GmbH, Germany) with Ag-AgCl electrodes. Electrode impedances were kept below 5 kOhm. The reference and ground electrodes were affixed to the ear lobes. EEG data were recorded using a BrainVision Recorder software (Brain Products GmbH, Germany). All data were pre-processed and analyzed using our developed fully automated DELPHI algorithm and implemented in MATLAB (R2016b, The Mathworks Inc., MA, United States).

Experimental Procedure

Transcranial magnetic stimulation coil was positioned over the left cortical motor (M1) region, at 45° toward the contralateral forehead according to guidelines (Rossini et al., 2015). Each TMS-EEG run entailed 420 pulses (biphasic pulses at 280 ms pulse width) at ranging intensities, from 25 to 60% of the maximal device intensity of stimulation varied in frequencies from 0.1 Hz up to 20 Hz. A thin (0.5 mm) foam pad was attached to the TMS coil to minimize electrode movement and bone-conducted auditory artifact. Participants were instructed to keep their eyes closed throughout the examination to reduce ocular artifacts. The operator of the system conversed with subjected between the short stimulation protocol blocks in order to avoid drowsiness.

TABLE 1 | Statistical distribution of study groups.

	Total N of subjects	N of male	N of female	N right- handed	N left- handed	Mean age (year)	Std
Mild dementia (>70)	20	11	9	19	1	75.2	4.3
Healthy (>70)	17	12	5	16	1	75.4	5.6
Healthy (50–70)	30	23	7	29	1	61	5.9
Healthy (25–45)	30	16	14	28	2	35	6.6

Each row represents different study group.

TABLE 3 | Statistical distribution of study groups computerized testing scores.

	Global score		Memory		Executive function		Attention		Information processing speed		Motor skills	
	Mean	STD	Mean	STD	Mean	STD	Mean	STD	Mean	STD	Mean	STD
Mild dementia (>70)	81	11	71	8	85	13	80	19	95	7	91	17
Healthy (>70)	108	7	109	5	113	9	103	8	108	14	110	7
Healthy (50–70)	105	6	102	9	108	9	104	8	107	11	107	5
Healthy (25–45)	103	10	103	6	104	10	101	9	101	17	107	12

Each row represents a different group in the study, each column represents a different cognitive domain that was evaluated.

TABLE 4 | Statistical differences between study groups computerized testing scores.

P values	Global score	Memory	Executive function	Attention	Information processing speed	Motor skills
Mild dementia (>70)\Healthy (>70)	0.000	0.000	0.000	0.005	0.130	0.005
Healthy (>70)\Healthy (50–70)	0.096	0. 863	0.247	0.531	0.864	0.258
Healthy (50–70) \Healthy (25–45)	0.367	0.529	0.221	0.237	0.314	0.877

Each row represents two study groups that were compared, each column represents a different cognitive domain that was evaluated and displays t-test p values.

Electrode were grouped for statistical purposes: Frontal, F3, F5 -ipsilateral and F4, F6- contralateral to stimulation. Parietal, C3, C5, CP1 -ipsilateral and C4, C6, CP2- contralateral to stimulation. Temporal CP5, CP3, CF5 -ipsilateral and CP6, CP4, FC6- contralateral to stimulation. Occipital cortex, O1, PO3 -ipsilateral and O2, PO4- contralateral to stimulation.

Sham Stimulation

For sham TMS stimulation a realistic sham was performed by spacing the TMS coil in order to maintain auditory, pressure and tactile parameters with reduced magnetic field (Veniero et al., 2009; Zanon et al., 2013; Gordon et al., 2018). The figure of 8 coil was placed over the left cortical motor (M1) region in the exact same orientation as for non-sham stimulation. After placement, the coil was moved 3 cm away from the scalp and a silicone cube (10 cm × 3 cm) filled with artificial cerebral spinal fluid (aCSF) (Dolev et al., 2013) was placed between scalp and TMS coil. Stimulation protocol (duration, intensities, and frequencies) was maintained the same as in non-sham (**Supplementary Figure 1**).

DELPHI Analysis

Direct electrophysiological imaging analyzes the regional and network TMS evoked EEG pattern of response to single and history dependent events. A single TMS pulse delivered over the primary motor cortex (M1) results in a sequence of positive and negative EEG peaks at specific latencies (i.e., N45, P60, N100, and P180; negative peaks 45 and 100 msec after stimulation, positive peaks 60 and 180 msec after stimulation, **Supplementary Figure 2**). This pattern of response indicates synaptic activity, specifically the Glutamate-excitatory and Gamma-aminobutyric acid (GABA)-inhibitory transmission balance (Du et al., 2018). It is considered that the P60 peak represents activity of α1-subunit-containing GABA-A receptors whereas the N100 represents activity of GABA-B receptors (Premoli et al., 2014a). These TMS-evoked cortical potentials last for up to 300 msec in both the vicinity of the stimulation, as well as in remote interconnected brain areas that reflect long term changes in cortical network excitation-inhibition balance, referred to as brain network plasticity (Bonato et al., 2006; Daskalakis et al., 2008; Fitzgerald et al., 2008; Casarotto et al., 2010; Premoli et al., 2014a,b). Changes in TMS evoked short term plasticity measurements provide important insights into cortical processing both in health (Massimini et al., 2005; Ferrarelli et al., 2010) and disease (Daskalakis et al., 2002; Julkunen et al., 2008; Kaster et al., 2015; Manganotti et al., 2015; Ferreri et al., 2017a). All data processing is performed automatically by the DELPHI software algorithm.

DELPHI Architecture

Direct electrophysiological imaging is composed of customized integrated hardware devices (TMS and EEG), combined with an automated acquisition and analysis software (**Figure 1**).

Direct electrophysiological imaging software algorithm architecture is divided into five layers, as outlined in **Figure 1A**. Data acquisition: automated data collection. A fixed stimulation protocol of TMS in varying intensities and frequencies, introduced to specific pre-determined locations on the skull, ensuring accuracy of the acquired TEP data. (B) Online data check: automated and continuous evaluation of the collected data quality for optimal collection at minimum acquisition time. The online data check ensures a continuous online feedback of data quality. (C) Data pre- processing: automated rapid cleaning of data following acquisition (D) Data analysis and features extraction: measured signal features are extracted and calculated for determining the relevant electrophysiological parameters of DELPHI physiological profiling. (E) Classification of population subgroups. DELPHI electrophysiological parameters constitute the subject network physiological profiling, which is displayed as numeric raw values. The reliability of DELPHI as a state and disease classification tool increases with the growth in the quantity of collected neuro-physiological biomarkers data.

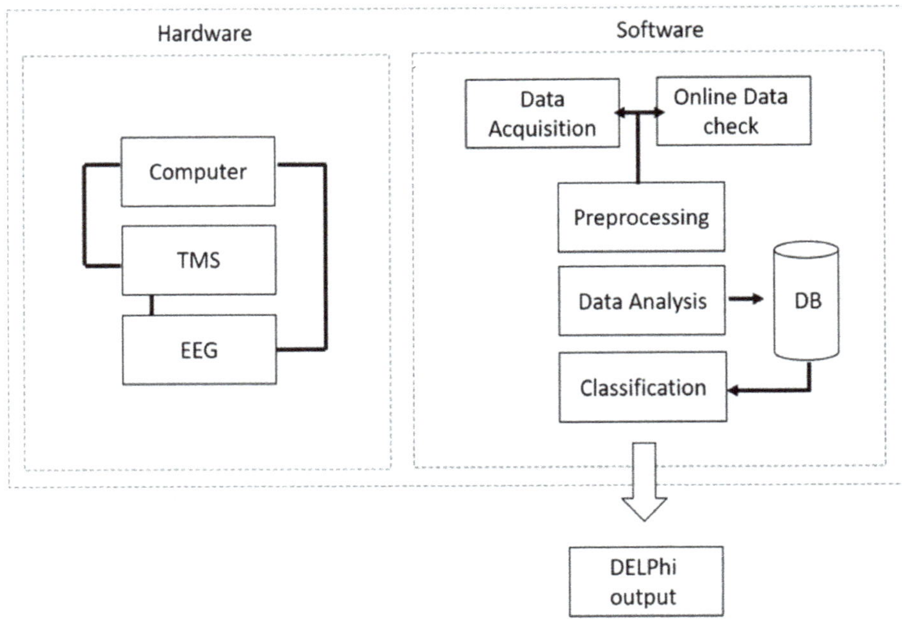

FIGURE 1 | DELPHI system hardware and software architecture: DELPHI software algorithm architecture is divided into five layers.

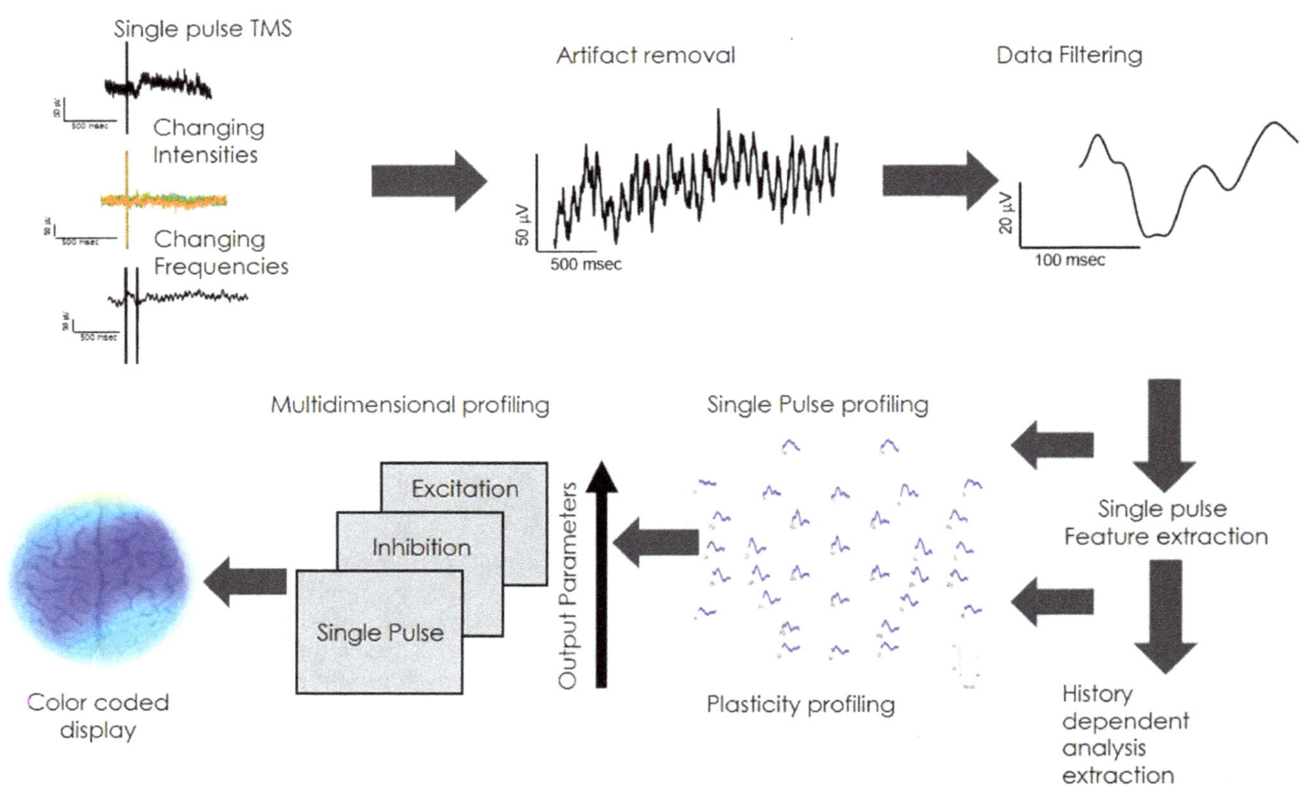

FIGURE 2 | Outline of the DELPHI functional network analysis.

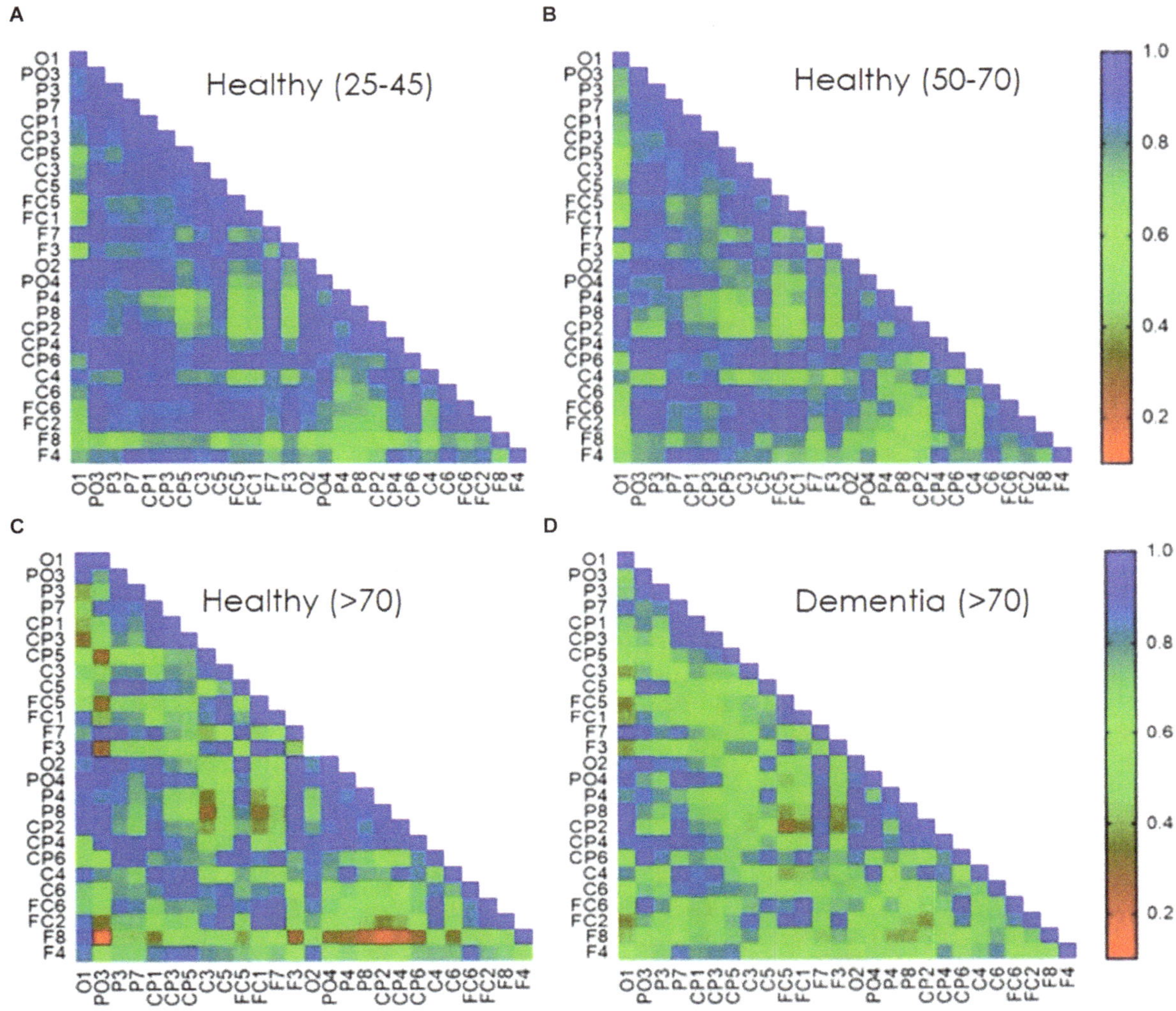

FIGURE 3 | Age dependent TEP-connectivity matrixes analysis. Pearson's correlation coefficient of bi-lateral EEG sensors single pulse evoked response. Data presents averaged population response **(A)** 25–45 years old healthy group. **(B)** 50–70 years old healthy group. **(C)** Over 70 years old healthy group. **(D)** Over 70 years old diagnosed with Mild Dementia (MD). Correlation values are presented as consecutive color-coded bar. blue, high correlation; red, low correlation.

DELPHI Physiological Network Profile Analysis

Direct electrophysiological imaging profile, characterizing brain network functionality, analyzes the physiological features of the local brain response to stimuli. The analysis regard two fundamental features of brain physiology: (1) Single pulse. This refers to the evoked response to a single TMS pulse in varying intensities, calculated as the local Input/output curve (**Supplementary Figure 2A**). Evoked response is represented as a collection of amplitudes, slopes and latencies (P60-N100 slope is referred to as the early slope and the N100-P180 slope as the late slope) (Rogasch et al., 2015; Tremblay et al., 2019). (2) Network plasticity. Refers to frequency dependent changes in evoked response, an attribute that expresses the history dependency of the network. Introducing high frequency of stimulation (>=20 Hz) evokes excitation of network response (Maeda et al., 2000; Garcia-Toro et al., 2006) while low frequency (>=5 Hz) evokes inhibition of the regional network response in a mechanism that may be similar to long term depression -LTD (Muellbacher et al., 2000; Fitzgerald et al., 2006; **Supplementary Figure 2B**). Data acquisition is performed automatically by introducing a sequence of stimuli in changing intensities and frequencies (**Figure 2A**) followed by a bilayer data cleaning step of TMS artifact removal and data filtering (**Figures 2B,C**). Average response features of charge transfer, slopes and latencies are extracted (**Figure 2D**), providing the single pulse and plasticity profile of network functionality. These physiological parameters are unified into one multidimensional neuro-physiological DELPHI profile of brain network functionality (**Figure 2E**). Cortical network values may be translated into pseudo-colored coded image describing brain network functionality (**Figure 2F**).

Reproducibility test was performed on collected and analyzed parameters. Results demonstrate high reliability and reproducibility of the DELPHI analyzed physiological parameters displaying reliability coefficient (r) of 0.87 and 0.94 (**Supplementary Figure 3**).

Statistical Analysis

Statistical data analysis was performed using GraphPad Prism 7. Reproducibility measures were compared by Pearson's correlation. Error bars shown in the figures represent standard error of the mean (SEM). The number of subjects is defined by *N*. One-way ANOVA analysis with *post hoc* Tukey was used to compare subject groups. Student's un-paired *t*-test was used to compare two groups. $^{*}p < 0.05$; $^{**}p < 0.01$; $^{***}p < 0.001$, $^{****}p < 0.0001$, ns, non-significant.

RESULTS

Evaluation of Age Dependent Changes in Network Connectivity

Brain Network Connectivity and Coherence Are Indicators of Network Health and Function. The concept of using TMS-EEG for evaluating brain neuronal network by monitoring its response has been described in numerus papers and has been shown to provide clinical evidence for functional brain network pathophysiological deterioration (Grady et al., 2003; Wang et al., 2010; Legon et al., 2016).

Direct electrophysiological imaging analysis of single pulse response is displayed as connectivity matrixes (Pearson's r) of averaged age groups (**Figure 3**). A decrease in signal coherence is observed with age, young 25–45 matrix (**Figure 3A**) display high correlation values which are slightly decreased in the healthy 50–70 group (**Figure 3B**) and decreases further in the over 70 healthy group (**Figure 3C**). A significant decrease is observed for young 25–45 and over 70 healthy group between left and right parietal and temporal areas ($p < 0.01$), but not between frontal right and left areas. A significant decrease is also displayed for frontal and parietal areas ($p < 0.01$), frontal and temporal areas ($p < 0.01$), and frontal vs. occipital areas ($p < 0.01$). There is also a significant decrease in *r* values for the 50–70 and over 70 healthy group for frontal connectivity between frontal and parietal areas ($p < 0.01$), frontal and temporal areas ($p < 0.01$), and frontal vs. occipital areas ($p < 0.01$). When comparing the MD patients, over 70 years old, with healthy over 70 controls (**Figure 3D**) a pronounced decrease in frontal inter-hemispheric connection is displayed ($p < 0.01$) as well as a decrease in connectivity values between frontal and contralateral parietal, temporal, and occipital areas ($p < 0.01$).

Direct electrophysiological imaging pinpoints two features that display a significant age dependent decrease in both early (**Figure 4A**) and late (**Figure 4B**) components of evoked response (data displayed for right hemisphere, contralateral to stimulation, parietal cortex). Moreover, comparing the two age comparable groups of healthy elderly and patients diagnosed with MD, reveals a significant difference in both components, particularly in the late slope of evoked response (**Figure 4B**). Group averaged regional ratio between these two slopes (early and late) of evoked response displays a significant, age dependent, change with pronounced differentiation between normal healthy aging, and MD, over the frontal, parietal, temporal and occipital cortical areas (**Figures 4C–F**, respectively). These extracted cortical network ratio values may be displayed as individual pseudo-color-coded images. **Figures 4G–J** presents color-coded images of subjects from the representative four study groups. 38-year-old healthy subject demonstrates high and uniform ratio between the late and early slope of evoked response reflected as a homogeneous blue colored brain (**Figure 4G**). A decline in the measured ratio is demonstrated with age, translated into light blue colored brain of a 58-year-old subject, representing the healthy 50–70 age group (**Figure 4H**), and a green-yellow colored brain presenting the over 70 years old group (**Figure 4I**). The MD group, represented by a 71 years-old subject, display a negative high ratio between late and early slopes of evoked response, reflected as orange colored cortical brain network functionality (**Figure 4J**).

Age Dependent Changes in Network Short Term Plasticity

Brain network plasticity is known to change with age (Cabeza et al., 2002; Buckner et al., 2008; Wang et al., 2010). Moreover, progression of degenerative disorders as AD, correlate with decrease in brain network plasticity (Palop et al., 2007; Kumar et al., 2017). As TMS-EEG technology has been extensively shown to enable measuring of excitability and plasticity changes in healthy and pathological condition (Tremblay et al., 2019) it provides a platform for such evaluation DELPHI Analysis of the history dependency identified two physiological parameters of network functionality that best distinguished between groups (healthy aging and MD). The ratio between the total charge transfer of response (Q) evoked to an inhibitory protocol of stimulation (STP-Q), and the ratio between the late slope component of evoked response to an inhibitory protocol of stimulation (STP-slope N100-P180) (**Figures 5A,B**). A significant age dependent increase in the charge transfer STP and a decrease in the late slope STP is observed (**Figures 5A,B** data from the right hemisphere (contralateral to stimulation) parietal cortex is displayed). Comparing the two age comparable groups of healthy elderly and patients with MD, reveals a significant difference in both parameters. Interestingly, the most significant change in STP between the two groups is observed in the STP of the late slope, in which the MD group displays positive values (**Figure 5B**) reflecting a significant change in inhibitory response ($P < 0.001$). Group averaged regional ratio between these analyzed parameters of evoked response (**Figures 5C–F**), displays a pronounced differentiation between normal, healthy aging, and early phases of dementia, over the frontal, parietal, temporal and occipital cortical areas (**Figures 5C–F**, respectively). Intriguingly, the ratio between these STP calculated parameters demonstrates lower age dependency. These extracted cortical plasticity ratio values may be displayed as individual pseudo-color-coded images. **Figures 5G–J**, displays the significant differentiation between normal, healthy aging and

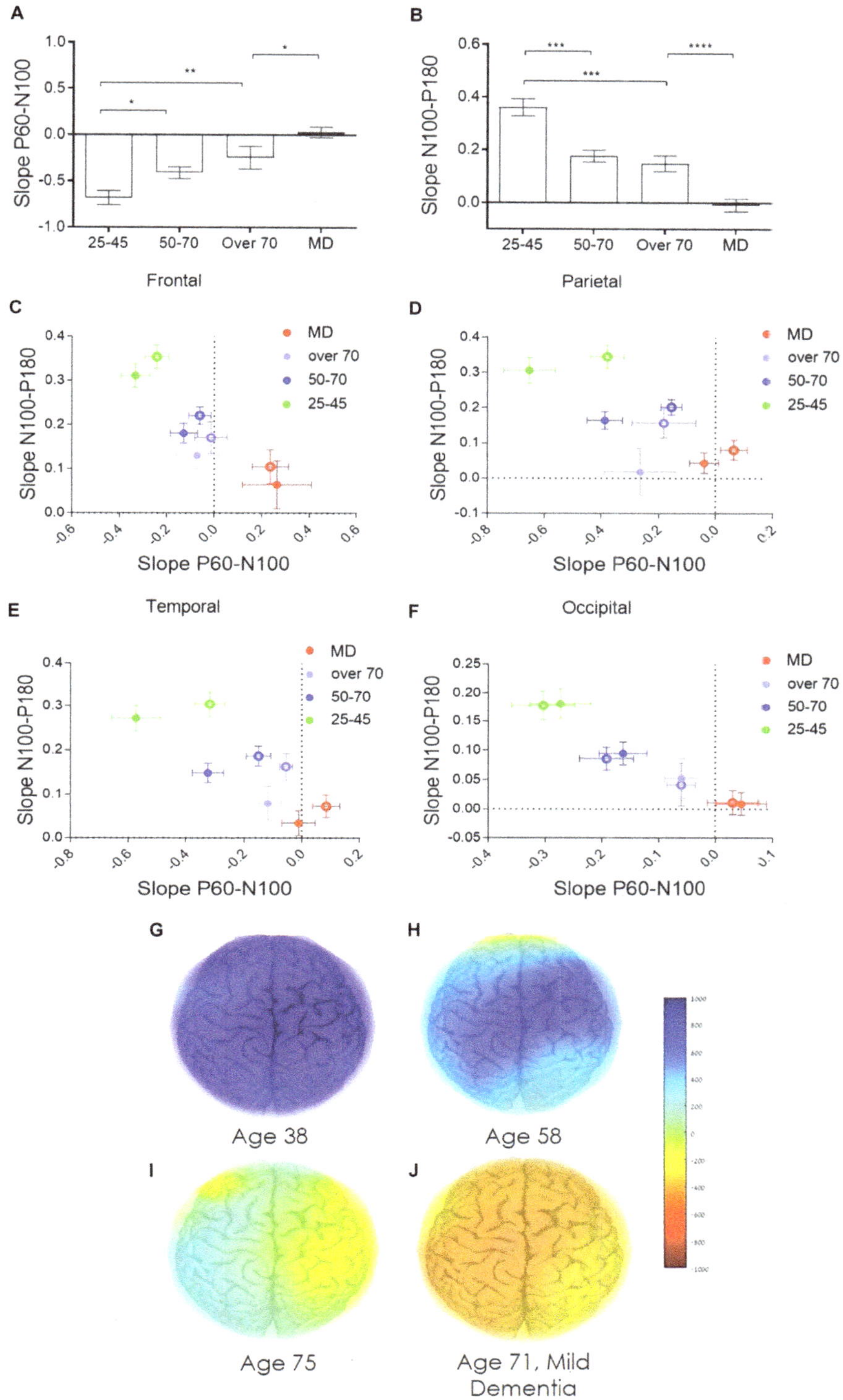

FIGURE 4 | Age dependent network strength. **(A)** Age dependent change in the early slope of evoked response (P60-N100). **(B)** Age dependent change in the late slope of evoked response (N100-P180). **(C–F)** Group average of the ratio between the early and late slopes of response measured from the frontal, parietal, temporal, and occipital cortex electrodes, respectively. **(C–F)** green dots represent the averaged young, 25–45 years old, healthy individuals. Blue dots represents the averaged healthy, 50–70 years old subjects. Purple dots represent the averaged healthy subjects, over 70 years old. Red dots represent patients diagnosed with mild dementia, over 70 years old. Full dots, left hemisphere; empty circles, right hemisphere. **(G–J)** Represent the color-coded images of representative subjects from the four study groups **(G)** 38 years old healthy subject. **(H)** 58 years old healthy subject. **(I)** 75 years old healthy subject. **(J)** 71 years old subject diagnosed with mild dementia. Color coded scale bar represent the ratio between the late slope and the early slope of evoked response.

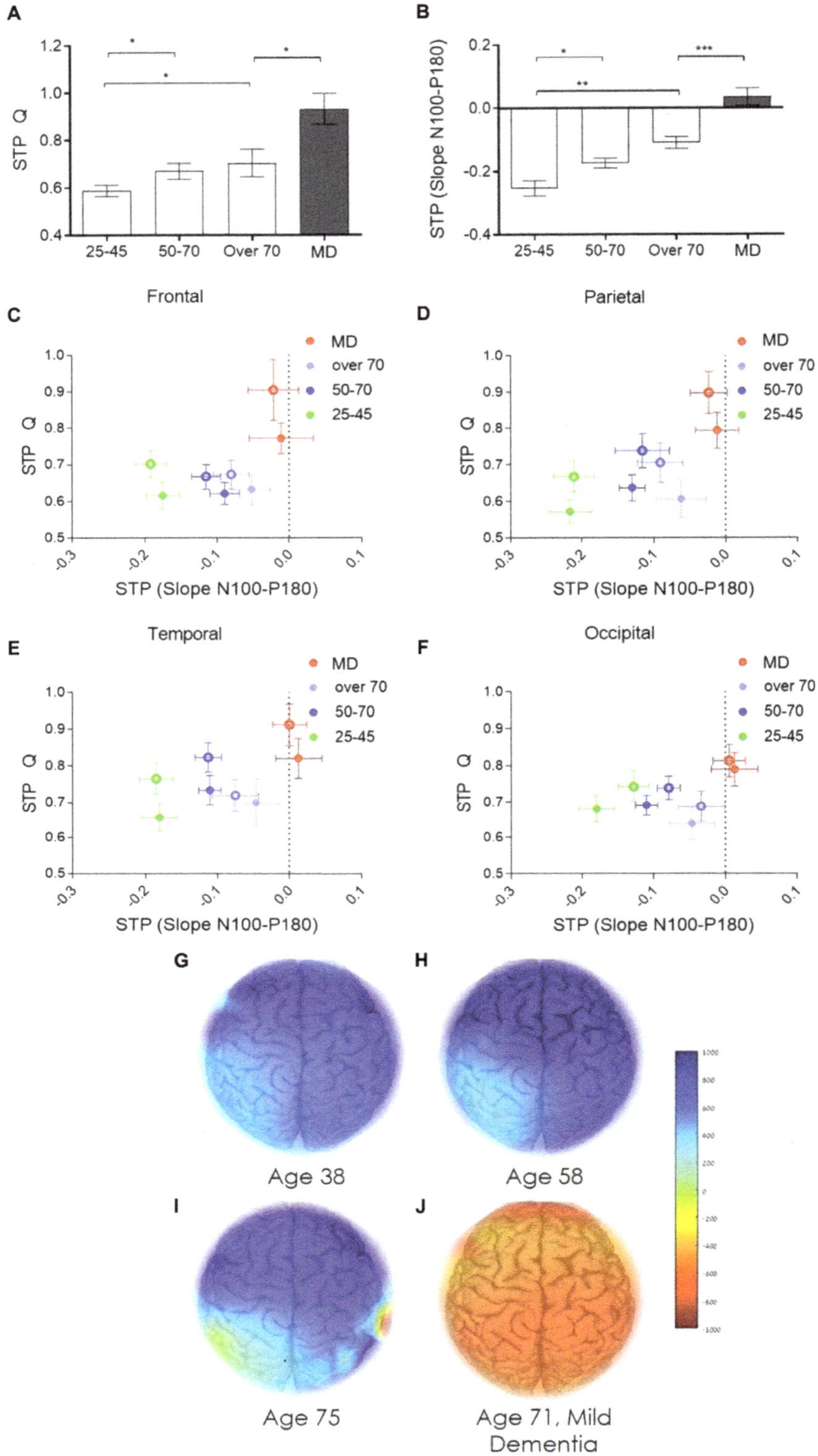

FIGURE 5 | Age dependent network short term plasticity. **(A)** Age dependent short-term plasticity of evoked response charge transfer (STP-Q). **(B)** Age dependent short-term plasticity of evoked response late slope component (STP-slope N100-P180). **(C–F)** Group average of the ratio between STP of the total charge transfer and STP of the late slope of evoked response measured from the frontal, parietal, temporal, and occipital cortex electrodes, respectively. **(C–F)** green dots represent the averaged young, 25–45 years old, healthy individuals. Blue dots represents the averaged healthy, 50–70 years old subjects. Purple dots represent the averaged *(Continued)*

FIGURE 5 | Continued
healthy subjects, over 70 years old. Red dots represent subject diagnosed with mild dementia, over 70 years old. Full dots, left hemisphere; empty circles, right hemisphere. **(G,H)** represent the color-coded images of representative subjects from the four study groups (g) 38 years old healthy subject. **(H)** 58 years old healthy subject. **(I)** 75 years old healthy subject. **(J)** 71 years old subject diagnosed with mild dementia. Color coded scale bar represent the ratio between the STP-Q and STP-slope N100-P180.

early stages of dementia, implicating that while single pulse analysis of evoked response demonstrates strong correlation with normal aging (**Figure 4**), plasticity measures seem to provide a robust parameter for separating normal from abnormal-pathological aging, as in the current case of early stages of dementia (**Figure 5**).

DISCUSSION

Current study results display the ability of DELPHI using TMS-EEG technology for measuring crucial brain network parameters of connectivity and plasticity and its relevance for monitoring brain health. Network connectivity measures displayed in this study, indicate monitorable changes that occur with age and point to the ability of this technology to monitor subtle structural and functional changes, as well as the ability to differentiate normal and abnormal aging. Connectivity maps display changes in connectivity between healthy and MD subjects mainly relating frontal areas, indicating a decrease in inter-hemispheric synchronicity, as well as decreased synchronicity between frontal and temporal or parietal areas (**Figure 3**).

These results are consistent with several structural and functional studies demonstrating intercortical disconnect such as changes in the corpus callosum (CC) in early stages of AD and MCI (Di Paola et al., 2010a,b; Frederiksen et al., 2011). Changes in transcallosal connectivity have also been displayed using TMS in a study differentiating between demented and cognitively impaired non-demented patients (Lanza et al., 2013). TEP slopes, which provide a description of TEP form and an excitation/inhibition reference (Rossi et al., 2009; Tremblay et al., 2019), display an age dependent decrease in both early and late slopes of response (**Figure 4**). This decrease may be associated with atrophy of gray and white matter or changes in excitation/inhibition balance as supported by anatomical MRI and EEG studies which indicate reduced fiber tracks in frontal and temporal areas and front-occipital reduced synchronicity (Sexton et al., 2011; Dipasquale and Cercignani, 2016; Teipel et al., 2016). In addition, TEP slopes display a clear separation of pathological MD group from healthy control which includes a phase shift represented by slope changes, these may be accounted by severe brain atrophy and/or excitation/inhibition balance shift. Short term plasticity measures (**Figure 5**), which evaluates the changes in excitation/inhibition balance, are shown to provide discrete parameter which display a sort of binary step function for differentiating the healthy and diseased brain. These results may indicate as to the nature of significant changes in pathological population that results from shifting in excitation/inhibition mechanisms as opposed to connectivity and structural changes that may account for age related changes displayed here. This study results support the significance and value of TMS in understanding and monitoring brain health and pathological aging including neurodegenerative disorders such as Alzheimer's disease (AD) and vascular dementia. Studies of connectivity, excitability and plasticity utilizing TMS have provided evidence suggesting cortical excitability changes in the early stages of the disease, as well as altered cortical inhibition and cholinergic mechanisms (Bella et al., 2013, 2016; Ni and Chen, 2015; Ferreri et al., 2017b; Lanza et al., 2017). It has also been shown that TMS-EEG evoked potentials (TEP) poses major advantages as: (A) High reproducibility of evoked response within individuals over occipital, parietal, premotor, motor and prefrontal regions (Lioumis et al., 2009; Casarotto et al., 2010; Kerwin et al., 2018). (B) Ability to measure TEP at sub MT intensities. Stimulating the M1 at intensities as low as 40% of the MEP threshold, exemplifying the sensitivity of the measure (Komssi et al., 2004; Komssi and Kähkönen, 2006). (C) Recorded both locally, and in distal electrodes, allowing for the study of the spreading of activation over cortical areas (Ilmoniemi et al., 1997; Komssi et al., 2002).

In this study, we introduce a new scientific and methodological approach, which can be used in the clinical environment, enabling healthcare providers with a bedside tool for the evaluation and monitoring of brain functional status in health and disease. Study results indicate the ability of DELPHI to clinically monitor brain structural and functional changes that may be associated with multiple pathologies, however, this study did not consider different dementia sub groups of AD and Vascular dementia or its precursor of MCI (mild cognitive impairment) and SVD (small vessel disease) this should be further explored in larger pathological populations including different dementia types and their precursor conditions, alongside longitudinal aging studies that might indicate early detection, and exploration of other pathologies.

CONCLUSION

The extent of functional changes during brain aging varies among individuals in a way that cannot be quantified using current available clinical tools. Early identification of abnormal brain aging is extensively researched, scanning genetic, biochemical, and neuropsychological aspects of the transition from normal to pathologic aging. Our findings support the notion that evaluating elecro-physiological properties of connectivity and plasticity enable the characterization of age dependent brain functional changes and the monitoring of abnormal aging processes as presented in previous studies. Data presented in this work DELPHI as clinically effective in evaluating brain functionality and may ultimately provide a clinical tool for monitoring brain network function and brain health. DELPHI automated acquisition and analysis system can be used in order to monitor brain health throughout aging and may enable early detection of abnormal pathophysiological changes leading to neurodegeneration, as for the case of MD.

AUTHOR CONTRIBUTIONS

NZ determined the study design and criteria with OL-L, HF, and ID, and conducted most of the laboratory works. OL-L and HF designed most of the DELPHI software algorithm. HF and ID contributed in designing and writing most of the manuscript and submitting the manuscript for publication. SE was principal investigator in this study. GS was responsible for the cognitive evaluation conducted in the study. DT, SE, and GS contributed in assuring the methods and the quality of the results with reviewing the manuscript, and approving for publication of the content.

REFERENCES

Almeida, S. R., Vicentini, J., Bonilha, L., De Campos, B. M., Casseb, R. F., and Min, L. L. ((2017). Brain connectivity and functional recovery in patients with ischemic stroke. *J. Neuroimaging* 27, 65–70. doi: 10.1111/jon.12362

Bédard, C., Kröger, H., and Destexhe, A. (2004). Modeling extracellular field potentials and te frequency-filtering properties of extracellular space. *Biophys. J.* 86, 1829–1842. doi: 10.1016/S0006-3495(04)74250-2

Bella, R., Cantone, M., Lanza, G., Ferri, R., Vinciguerra, L., Puglisi, V., et al. (2016). Cholinergic circuitry functioning in patients with vascular cognitive impairment-no dementia. *Brain Stimul.* 9, 225–233. doi: 10.1016/j.brs.2015.09.013

Bella, R., Ferri, R., Lanza, G., Cantone, M., Pennisi, M., Puglisi, V., et al. (2013). TMS follow-up study in patients with vascular cognitive impairment-no dementia. *Neurosci. Lett.* 534, 155–159. doi: 10.1016/j.neulet.2012.12.017

Berlucchi, G., and Buchtel, H. A. (2009). Neuronal plasticity: historical roots and evolution of meaning. *Exp. Brain. Res.* 192, 307–319. doi: 10.1007/s00221-008-1611-6

Bonato, C., Miniussi, C., and Rossini, P. M. (2006). Transcranial magnetic stimulation and cortical evoked potentials: a TMS/EEG co-registration study. *Clin. Neurophysiol.* 117, 1699–1707. doi: 10.1016/j.clinph.2006.05.006

Bordet, R., Ihl, R., Korczyn, A. D., Lanza, G., Jansa, J. R., and Hoerr, A. (2017). Towards the concept of disease-modifier in post-stroke or vascular cognitive impairment: a consensus report. *BMC Med.* 15:07. doi: 10.1186/s12916-017-0869-6

Buckner, R. L., Andrews-Hanna, J. R., and Schacter, D. L. (2008). The brain's default network: anatomy, function, and relevance to disease. *Ann. N Y Acad. Sci.* 1124, 1–38. doi: 10.1196/annals.1440.011

Cabeza, R., Anderson, N. D., Locantore, J. K., and McIntosh, A. R. (2002). Aging gracefully: compensatory brain activity in high-performing older adults. *Neuroimage* 17, 1394–1402. doi: 10.1006/nimg.2002.1280

Casarotto, S., Määttä, S., Herukka, S. K., Pigorini, A., Napolitani, M., Gosseries, O., et al. (2011). Transcranial magnetic stimulation-evoked EEG/cortical potentials in physiological and pathological aging. *Neuroreport* 22, 592–597. doi: 10.1097/WNR.0b013e328349433a

Casarotto, S., Romero Lauro, L. J., Bellina, V., Casali, A. G., Rosanova, M., Pigorini, A., et al. (2010). EEG responses to TMS are sensitive to changes in the perturbation parameters and repeatable over time. *PLoS One* 5:e10281. doi: 10.1371/journal.pone.0010281

Cash, R. F., Noda, Y., Zomorrodi, R., Radhu, N., Farzan, F., Rajji, T. K., et al. (2017). Characterization of Glutamatergic and GAB. *Neuropsychopharmacology* 42, 502–511. doi: 10.1038/npp.2016.133

Cherry, S. R. (2009). Multimodality imaging: beyond PET/CT and SPECT/CT. *Semin. Nucl. Med.* 39, 348–353. doi: 10.1053/j.semnuclmed.2009.03.001

Chung, S. W., Rogasch, N. C., Hoy, K. E., and Fitzgerald, P. B. (2015). Measuring Brain Stimulation induced changes in cortical properties using TMS-EEG. *Brain Stimul.* 8, 1010–1020. doi: 10.1016/j.brs.2015.07.029

Covey, E., and Carter, M. (2015). *Basic Electrophysiological Methods*. Oxford:Oxford University Press.

Daskalakis, Z. J., Christensen, B. K., Fitzgerald, P. B., and Chen, R. (2002). Transcranial magnetic stimulation: a new investigational and treatment tool in psychiatry. *J. Neuropsychiatry Clin. Neurosci.* 14, 406–415. doi: 10.1176/jnp.14.4.406

Daskalakis, Z. J., Farzan, F., Barr, M. S., Maller, J. J., Chen, R., and Fitzgerald, P. B. (2008). Long-interval cortical inhibition from the dorsolateral prefrontal cortex: a TMS-EEG study. *Neuropsychopharmacology* 33, 2860–2869. doi: 10.1038/npp.2008.22

Di Paola, M., Di Iulio, F., Cherubini, A., Blundo, C., Casini, A. R., Sancesario, G., et al. (2010a). When, where, and how the corpus callosum changes in MCI and AD: a multimodal MRI study. *Neurology* 74, 1136–1142. doi: 10.1212/WNL.0b013e3181d7d8cb

Di Paola, M., Luders, E., Di Iulio, F., Cherubini, A., Passafiume, D., Thompson, P. M., et al. (2010b). Callosal atrophy in mild cognitive impairment and Alzheimer's disease: different effects in different stages. *Neuroimage* 49, 141–149. doi: 10.1016/j.neuroimage.2009.07.050

Dipasquale, O., and Cercignani, M. (2016). Network functional connectivity and whole-brain functional connectomics to investigate cognitive decline in neurodegenerative conditions. *Funct. Neurol.* 31, 191–203.

Dolev, I., Fogel, H., Milshtein, H., Berdichevsky, Y., Lipstein, N., Brose, N., et al. (2013). Spike bursts increase amyloid-β 40/42 ratio by inducing a presenilin-1 conformational change. *Na.t Neurosci.* 16, 587–595. doi: 10.1038/nn.3376

Du, X., Rowland, L. M., Summerfelt, A., Wijtenburg, A., Chiappelli, J., Wisner, K., et al. (2018). TMS evoked N100 reflects local GABA and glutamate balance. *Brain Stimul.* 11, 1071–1079. doi: 10.1016/j.brs.2018.05.002

Dwolatzky, T., Whitehead, V., Doniger, G. M., Simon, E. S., Schweiger, A., Jaffe, D., et al. (2003). Validity of a novel computerized cognitive battery for mild cognitive impairment. *BMC Geriatr.* 3:4. doi: 10.1186/1471-2318-3-4

Farzan, F., Barr, M. S., Levinson, A. J., Chen, R., Wong, W., Fitzgerald, P. B., et al. (2010). Reliability of long-interval cortical inhibition in healthy human subjects: a TMS EEG study. *J. Neurophysiol.* 104, 1339–1346. doi: 10.1152/jn.00279.2010

Feldman, D. E. (2009). Synaptic mechanisms for plasticity in neocortex. *Annu. Rev. Neurosci.* 32, 33–55. doi: 10.1146/annurev.neuro.051508.135516

Ferrarelli, F., Massimini, M., Sarasso, S., Casali, A., Riedner, B. A., Angelini, G., et al. (2010). Breakdown in cortical effective connectivity during midazolam-induced loss of consciousness. *Proc. Natl. Acad. Sci. U. S. A.* 107, 2681–2686. doi: 10.1073/pnas.0913008107

Ferreri, F., Guerra, A., Vollero, L., Ponzo, D., Maatta, S., Mervaala, E., et al. (2017a). Age-related changes of cortical excitability and connectivity in healthy humans: non-invasive evaluation of sensorimotor network by means of TMS-EE. *Neuroscience* 357, 255–263. doi: 10.1016/j.neuroscience.2017.06.014

Ferreri, F., Vecchio, F., Guerra, A., Miraglia, F., Ponzo, D., Vollero, L., et al. (2017b). Age related differences in functional synchronization of EEG activity as evaluated by means of TMS-EEG coregistrations. *Neurosci. Lett.* 647, 141–146. doi: 10.1016/j.neulet.2017.03.021

Fitzgerald, P. B., Daskalakis, Z. J., Hoy, K., Farzan, F., Upton, D. J., Cooper, N. R., et al. (2008). Cortical inhibition in motor and non-motor regions: a combined TMS-EEG study. *Clin. EEG Neurosci.* 39, 112–117. doi: 10.1177/155005940803900304

Fitzgerald, P. B., Fountain, S., and Daskalakis, Z. J. (2006). A comprehensive review of the effects of rTMS on motor cortical excitability and inhibition. *Clin. Neurophysiol.* 117, 2584–1596. doi: 10.1016/j.clinph.2006.06.712

Frederiksen, K. S., Garde, E., Skimminge, A., Ryberg, C., Rostrup, E., Baaré, W. F., et al. (2011).). Corpus callosum atrophy in patients with mild Alzheimer's disease. *Neurodegener Dis.* 8, 476–482. doi: 10.1159/000327753

Garcia-Toro, M., Salva, J., Daumal, J., Andres, J., Romera, M., Lafau, O., et al. (2006). High (20-Hz) and low (1-Hz) frequency transcranial magnetic stimulation as adjuvant treatment in medication-resistant depression. *Psychiatry Res.* 146, 53–57. doi: 10.1016/j.pscychresns.2004.08.005

Gordon, P. C., Desideri, D., Belardinelli, P., Zrenner, C., and Ziemann, U. (2018). Comparison of cortical EEG responses to realistic sham versus real TMS of human motor cortex. *Brain Stimul.* 11, 1322–1330. doi: 10.1016/j.brs.2018.08.003

Gore, J. C. (2003). Principles and practice of functional MRI of the human brain. *J. Clin. Invest.* 112, 4–9. doi: 10.1172/JCI19010

Grady, C. L., McIntosh, A. R., and Craik, F. I (2003). Age-related differences in the functional connectivity of the hippocampus during memory encoding. *Hippocampus* 13, 572–586. doi: 10.1002/hipo.10114

Greenwood, P. M. (2007). Functional plasticity in cognitive aging: review and hypothesis. *Neuropsychology* 21, 657–673. doi: 10.1037/0894-4105.21.6.657

Hallett, M. (2007). Transcranial magnetic stimulation: a primer. *Neuron* 55, 187–199. doi: 10.1016/j.neuron.2007.06.026

Ilmoniemi, R. J., and Kicić, D. (2010). Methodology for combined TMS and EEG. *Brain Topogr.* 22, 233–248. doi: 10.1007/s10548-009-0123-4

Ilmoniemi, R. J., Ruohonen, J., and Karhu, J. (1999). Transcranial magnetic stimulation–a new tool for functional imaging of the brain. *Crit. Rev. Biomed Eng.* 27, 241–284.

Ilmoniemi, R. J., Virtanen, J., Ruohonen, J., Karhu, J., Aronen, H. J., Näätänen, R., et al. (1997). Neuronal responses to magnetic stimulation reveal cortical reactivity and connectivity. *Neuroreport* 8, 3537–3540. doi: 10.1097/00001756-199711100-00024

Julkunen, P., Jauhiainen, A. M., Westerén-Punnonen, S., Pirinen, E., Soininen, H., Könönen, M., et al. (2008). Navigated TMS combined with EEG in mild cognitive impairment and Alzheimer's disease: a pilot study. *J. Neurosci. Methods* 172, 270–276. doi: 10.1016/j.jneumeth.2008.04.021

Kähkönen, S., Komssi, S., Wilenius, J., and Ilmoniemi, R. J. (2005). Prefrontal transcranial magnetic stimulation produces intensity-dependent EEG responses in humans. *Neuroimage* 24, 955–960. doi: 10.1016/j.neuroimage.2004.09.048

Kaster, T. S., de Jesus, D., Radhu, N., Farzan, F., Blumberger, D. M., Rajji, T. K., et al. (2015). Clozapine potentiation of GABA mediated cortical inhibition in treatment resistant schizophrenia. *Schizophr Res.* 165, 157–162. doi: 10.1016/j.schres.2015.04.015

Kelly, K. M., Nadon, N. L., Morrison, J. H., Thibault, O., Barnes, C. A., and Blalock, E. M. (2006).). The neurobiology of aging. *Epilepsy Res.* 68(Suppl. 1), S5–S20. doi: 10.1016/j.eplepsyres.2005.07.015

Kerwin, L. J., Keller, C. J., Wu, W., Narayan, M., and Etkin, A. (2018). Test-retest reliability of transcranial magnetic stimulation EEG evoked potentials. *Brain Stimul.* 11, 536–544. doi: 10.1016/j.brs.2017.12.010

Komssi, S., Aronen, H. J., Huttunen, J., Kesäniemi, M., Soinne, L., Nikouline, V. V., et al. (2002). Ipsi- and contralateral EEG reactions to transcranial magnetic stimulation. *Clin. Neurophysiol.* 113, 175–184. doi: 10.1016/s1388-2457(01)00721-0

Komssi, S., and Kähkönen, S. (2006). The novelty value of the combined use of electroencephalography and transcranial magnetic stimulation for neuroscience research. *Brain Res. Rev.* 52, 183–192. doi: 10.1016/j.brainresrev.2006.01.008

Komssi, S., Kähkönen, S., and Ilmoniemi, R. J. (2004). The effect of stimulus intensity on brain responses evoked by transcranial magnetic stimulation. *Hum. Brain Mapp.* 21, 154–164. doi: 10.1002/hbm.10159

Kugiumtzis, D., and Kimiskidis, V. K. (2015). Direct causal networks for the study of transcranial magnetic stimulation effects on focal epileptiform discharges. *Int. J. Neural. Syst.* 25, 1550006. doi: 10.1142/S0129065715500069

Kumar, S., Zomorrodi, R., Ghazala, Z., Goodman, M. S., Blumberger, D. M., Cheam, A., et al. (2017). Extent of dorsolateral prefrontal cortex plasticity and its association with working memory in patients with Alzheimer Disease. *JAMA Psychiatry* 74, 1266–1274. doi: 10.1001/jamapsychiatry.2017.3292

Lanza, G., Bella, R., Giuffrida, S., Cantone, M., Pennisi, G., Spampinato, C., et al. (2013). Preserved transcallosal inhibition to transcranial magnetic stimulation in nondemented elderly patients with leukoaraiosis. *Biomed Res. Int.* 2013:351680. doi: 10.1155/2013/351680

Lanza, G., Bramanti, P., Cantone, M., Pennisi, M., Pennisi, G., and Bella, R. (2017). Vascular Cognitive impairment through the looking glass of transcranial magnetic stimulation. *Behav. Neurol.* 2017:1421326. doi: 10.1155/2017/1421326

Legon, W., Punzell, S., Dowlati, E., Adams, S. E., Stiles, A. B., and Moran, R. J. (2016). Altered prefrontal excitation/inhibition balance and prefrontal output: markers of aging in human memory networks. *Cereb. Cortex* 26, 4315–4326. doi: 10.1093/cercor/bhv200

Lioumis, P., Kicić, D., Savolainen, P., Mäkelä , J. P., and Kähkönen, S. (2009). Reproducibility of TMS-Evoked EEG responses. *Hum. Brain Mapp.* 30, 1387–1396. doi: 10.1002/hbm.20608

Maeda, F., Keenan, J. P., Tormos, J. M., Topka, H., and Pascual-Leone, A. (2000). Modulation of corticospinal excitability by repetitive transcranial magnetic stimulation. *Clin. Neurophysiol.* 111, 800–805. doi: 10.1016/s1388-2457(99)00323-5

Manganotti, P., Acler, M., Masiero, S., and Del Felice, A. (2015). TMS-evoked N100 responses as a prognostic factor in acute stroke. *Funct. Neurol.* 30, 125–130.

Markram, H., and Tsodyks, M. (1996). Redistribution of synaptic efficacy between neocortical pyramidal neurons. *Nature* 382, 807–810. doi: 10.1038/382807a0

Markram, H., Wang, Y., and Tsodyks, M. (1998). Differential signaling via the same axon of neocortical pyramidal neurons. *Proc. Natl. Acad. Sci. U.S.A.* 95, 5323–5328. doi: 10.1073/pnas.95.9.5323

Massimini, M., Ferrarelli, F., Huber, R., Esser, S. K., Singh, H., and Tononi, G. (2005). Breakdown of cortical effective connectivity during sleep. *Science* 309, 2228–2232. doi: 10.1126/science.1117256

McKhann, G. M., Knopman, D. S., Chertkow, H., Hyman, B. T., Jack, C. R., Kawas, C. H., et al. (2011). The diagnosis of dementia due to Alzheimer's disease: recommendations from the National Institute on Aging-Alzheimer's Association workgroups on diagnostic guidelines for Alzheimer's disease. *Alzheimers Dement.* 7, 263–269. doi: 10.1016/j.jalz.2011.03.005

Mora, F. (2013). Successful brain aging: plasticity, environmental enrichment, and lifestyle. *Dialogues Clin. Neurosci.* 15, 45–52.

Muellbacher, W., Ziemann, U., Boroojerdi, B., and Hallett, M. (2000). Effects of low-frequency transcranial magnetic stimulation on motor excitability and basic motor behavior. *Clin. Neurophysiol.* 111, 1002–1007. doi: 10.1016/s1388-2457(00)00284-4

Nasreddine, Z. S., Phillips, N. A., Bédirian, V., Charbonneau, S., Whitehead, V., Collin, I., et al. (2005). The montreal cognitive assessment, MoCA: a brief screening tool for mild cognitive impairment. *J. Am. Geriatr. Soc.* 53, 695–699. doi: 10.1111/j.1532-5415.2005.53221.x

Ni, Z., and Chen, R. (2015). Transcranial magnetic stimulation to understand pathophysiology and as potential treatment for neurodegenerative diseases. *Transl. Neurodegener* 4:22. doi: 10.1186/s40035-015-0045-x

Niedermeyer, E., and da Silva, F. H. L (2005). *Electroencephalography: Basic Principles, Clinical Applications, and Related fields.* Philadelhia: Lippincott Williams & Wilkins.

Nikulin, V. V., Kicić, D., Kähkönen, S., and Ilmoniemi, R. J. (2003). Modulation of electroencephalographic responses to transcranial magnetic stimulation: evidence for changes in cortical excitability related to movement. *Eur. J. Neurosci.* 18, 1206–1212. doi: 10.1046/j.1460-9568.2003.02858.x

Oberman, L., and Pascual-Leone, A. (2013). Changes in plasticity across the lifespan: cause of disease and target for intervention. *Prog. Brain Res.* 207, 91–120. doi: 10.1016/B978-0-444-63327-9.00016-3

Palop, J. J., Chin, J., Roberson, E. D., Wang, J., Thwin, M. T., Bien-Ly, N., et al. (2007). Aberrant excitatory neuronal activity and compensatory remodeling of inhibitory hippocampal circuits in mouse models of Alzheimer's disease. *Neuron* 55, 697–711. doi: 10.1016/j.neuron.2007.07.025

Pascual-Leone, A., Freitas, C., Oberman, L., Horvath, J. C., Halko, M., Eldaief, M., et al. (2011). Characterizing brain cortical plasticity and network dynamics across the age-span in health and disease with TMS-EEG and TMS-fMRI. *Brain Topogr.* 24, 302–315. doi: 10.1007/s10548-011-0196-8

Pennisi, M., Lanza, G., Cantone, M., Ricceri, R., Spampinato, C., Pennisi, G. V., et al. (2016). Correlation between motor cortex excitability changes and cognitive impairment in vascular depression: pathophysiological insights from a longitudinal TMS study. *Neural. Plast* 2016:8154969. doi: 10.1155/2016/8154969

Premoli, I., Castellanos, N., Rivolta, D., Belardinelli, P., Bajo, R., Zipser, C., et al. (2014a). TMS-EEG signatures of GABAergic neurotransmission in the human cortex. *J. Neurosci.* 34, 5603–5612. doi: 10.1523/JNEUROSCI.5089-13.2014

Premoli, I., Rivolta, D., Espenhahn, S., Castellanos, N., Belardinelli, P., Ziemann, U., et al. (2014b). Characterization of GABAB-receptor mediated neurotransmission in the human cortex by paired-pulse TMS-EE. *Neuroimage* 103, 152–162. doi: 10.1016/j.neuroimage.2014.09.028

Rogasch, N. C., Daskalakis, Z. J., and Fitzgerald, P. B. (2015). Cortical inhibition of distinct mechanisms in the dorsolateral prefrontal cortex is related to working memory performance: a TMS-EEG study. *Cortex* 64, 68–77. doi: 10.1016/j.cortex.2014.10.003

Rosenzweig, E. S., and Barnes, C. A. (2003). Impact of aging on hippocampal function: plasticity, network dynamics, and cognition. *Prog. Neurobiol.* 6, 143–179. doi: 10.1016/s0301-0082(02)00126-0

Rossi, S., Hallett, M., Rossini, P. M., Pascual-Leone, A., and Safety of Tms Consensus Group. (2009). Safety, ethical considerations, and application guidelines for the use of transcranial magnetic stimulation in clinical practice and research. *Clin. Neurophysiol.* 120, 2008–2039. doi: 10.1016/j.clinph.2009.08.016

Rossini, P. M., Burke, D., Chen, R., Cohen, L. G., Daskalakis, Z. R., Di Iorio, V., et al. (2015). Non-invasive electrical and magnetic stimulation of the brain, spinal cord, roots and peripheral nerves: Basic principles and procedures for routine clinical and research application. An updated report from an I.F.C.N. Committee. *Clin. Neurophysiol.* 126, 1071–1077. doi: 10.1016/j.clinph.2015.02.001

Saczynski, J. S., Inouye, S. K., Guess, J., Jones, R. N., Fong, T. G., Nemeth, E., et al. (2015). The montreal cognitive assessment: creating a crosswalk with the mini-mental state examination. *J. Am. Geriatr. Soc.* 63, 2370–2374. doi: 10.1111/jgs.13710

Sambataro, F., Murty, V. P., Callicott, J. H., Tan, H. Y., Das, S., Weinberger, R., et al. (2010). Age-related alterations in default mode network: impact on working memory performance. *Neurobiol. Aging* 31, 839–852. doi: 10.1016/j.neurobiolaging.2008.05.022

Schulz, J., and Hausmann, B. L. (2017). The malleable brain - An educational review from students to students. *J. Neurochem.* 142, 788–789. doi: 10.1111/jnc.14102

Sexton, C. E., Kalu, U. G., Filippini, N., Mackay, C. E., and Ebmeier, K. P. (2011). A meta-analysis of diffusion tensor imaging in mild cognitive impairment and Alzheimer's disease. *Neurobiol. Aging* 32, 2322.e5–2322.e18. doi: 10.1016/j.neurobiolaging.2010.05.019

Shafi, M. M., Westover, M. B., Fox, M. D., and Pascual-Leone, A. (2012). Exploration and modulation of brain network interactions with noninvasive brain stimulation in combination with neuroimaging. *Eur. J. Neurosci.* 35, 805–825. doi: 10.1111/j.1460-9568.2012.08035.x

Shafi, M. M., Whitfield-Gabrieli, S., Chu, C. J., Pascual-Leone, A., and Chang, B. S. (2016). A Multimodal imaging- and stimulation-based method of evaluating connectivity-related brain excitability in patients with epilepsy. *J. Vis Exp.* 117, 53727. doi: 10.3791/53727

Shah, A. K., and Mittal, S. (2014). Invasive electroencephalography monitoring: Indications and presurgical planning. *Ann. Indian Acad. Neurol.* 17(Suppl. 1), S89–S94. doi: 10.4103/0972-2327.128668

Teipel, S., Grothe, M. J., Zhou, J., Sepulcre, J., Dyrba, M., Sorg, C., et al. (2016). Measuring cortical connectivity in Alzheimer's Disease as a brain neural network pathology: toward clinical applications. *J. Int. Neuropsychol. Soc.* 22, 138–163. doi: 10.1017/S1355617715000995

Tremblay, S., Rogasch, N. C., Premoli, I., Blumberger, D. M., Casarotto, S., Chen, R., et al. (2019). Clinical utility and prospective of TMS-EEG. *Clin. Neurophysiol.* 130, 802–844. doi: 10.1016/j.clinph.2019.01.001

Veniero, D., Bortoletto, M., and Miniussi, C. (2009). TMS-EEG co-registration: on TMS-induced artifact. *Clin. Neurophysio.* 120, 1392–1399. doi: 10.1016/j.clinph.2009.04.023

Wang, L., Li, Y., Metzak, P., He, Y., and Woodward, T. S. (2010). Age-related changes in topological patterns of large-scale brain functional networks during memory encoding and recognition. *Neuroimage* 50, 862–872. doi: 10.1016/j.neuroimage.2010.01.044

Zanon, M., Battaglini, P. P., Jarmolowska, J., Pizzolato, G., and Busan, P. (2013). Long-range neural activity evoked by premotor cortex stimulation: a TMS/EEG co-registration study. *Front. Hum. Neurosci.* 7:803. doi: 10.3389/fnhum.2013.00803

15

Brain Structural Correlates of Odor Identification in Mild Cognitive Impairment and Alzheimer's Disease Revealed by Magnetic Resonance Imaging and a Chinese Olfactory Identification Test

Xingqi Wu[1,2], Zhi Geng[1,2], Shanshan Zhou[1,2,3], Tongjian Bai[1,2,3], Ling Wei[1,2,3], Gong-Jun Ji[2,3,4], Wanqiu Zhu[5], Yongqiang Yu[5], Yanghua Tian[1,2,3]* and Kai Wang[1,2,3,4]**

[1] Department of Neurology, The First Affiliated Hospital of Anhui Medical University, Hefei, China, [2] Anhui Province Key Laboratory of Cognition and Neuropsychiatric Disorders, Hefei, China, [3] Collaborative Innovation Center of Neuropsychiatric Disorders and Mental Health, Hefei, China, [4] Department of Medical Psychology, The First Affiliated Hospital of Anhui Medical University, Hefei, China, [5] Department of Radiology, The First Affiliated Hospital of Anhui Medical University, Hefei, China

***Correspondence:**
Kai Wang
wangkai1964@126.com
Yongqiang Yu
cjr.yuyongqiang@vip.163.com
Yanghua Tian
ayfytyh@126.com

Alzheimer's disease (AD) is a common memory-impairment disorder frequently accompanied by olfactory identification (OI) impairments. In fact, OI is a valuable marker for distinguishing AD from normal age-related cognitive impairment and may predict the risk of mild cognitive impairment (MCI)-to-AD transition. However, current olfactory tests were developed based on Western social and cultural conditions, and are not very suitable for Chinese patients. Moreover, the neural substrate of OI in AD is still unknown. The present study investigated the utility of a newly developed Chinese smell identification test (CSIT) for OI assessment in Chinese AD and MCI patients. We then performed a correlation analysis of gray matter volume (GMV) at the voxel and region-of-interest (ROI) levels to reveal the neural substrates of OI in AD. Thirty-seven AD, 27 MCI, and 30 normal controls (NCs) completed the CSIT and MRI scans. Patients (combined AD plus MCI) scored significantly lower on the CSIT compared to NCs [$F(2,91) = 62.597$, $p < 0.001$)]. Voxel-level GMV analysis revealed strong relationships between CSIT score and volumes of the left precentral gyrus and left inferior frontal gyrus (L-IFG). In addition, ROI-level GMV analysis revealed associations between CSIT score and left amygdala volumes. Our results suggest the following: (1) OI, as measured by the CSIT, is impaired in AD and MCI patients compared with healthy controls in the Chinese population; (2) the severity of OI dysfunction can distinguish patients with cognitive impairment from controls and AD from MCI patients; and (3) the left-precentral cortex and L-IFG may be involved in the processing of olfactory cues.

Keywords: Alzheimer's disease, mild cognitive impairment, olfactory disorder, Chinese smell identification test, magnetic resonance imaging, voxel-based morphometry

INTRODUCTION

Alzheimer's disease (AD) is the most common age-related neurodegenerative disorder and is characterized by progressive impairment of cognitive function, ultimately leading to incapacitation and death (McKhann et al., 2011). Thus, AD places a considerable emotional burden on families and economic burden on society (McDade and Bateman, 2017). Multiple studies have shown that neurobiological changes associated with AD are present for many years before the appearance of clinical symptoms. Many studies have focused on identifying neurological and behavioral changes that can predict AD onset and thereby allow early intervention. Mild cognitive impairment (MCI) is an intermediate state between normal age-related cognitive decline and dementia (Petersen, 2007); about 3 – 15% of MCI patients progress to AD annually (Petersen et al., 2001). Although there is still no effective treatment for AD (Miller, 2012), a previous study suggested that timely intervention can alleviate early symptoms, and delay AD progression (Baazaoui and Iqbal, 2018). Therefore, early detection of MCI is important for the short-term prognosis of AD. To this end, it is critical to identify biomarkers that can distinguish among AD, MCI, and healthy aging.

Previous studies have indicated that olfactory perception is frequently disrupted in the early stages of AD (Djordjevic et al., 2008; Silva et al., 2018), especially when preceded by MCI (Devanand, 2000; Larsson et al., 2000; Roalf et al., 2017). Impairments of olfactory perception involve deficits in several domains, including odor detection threshold, olfactory identification (OI), olfactory discrimination, and olfactory memory (Mesholam, 1998; Silva et al., 2018). Many studies have shown that olfactory dysfunction can accurately detect cognitive impairment (Graves et al., 1999; Peters, 2003; Schubert et al., 2008), differentiate AD from normal aging with high sensitivity (0.88) and specificity (0.91) (Ewers et al., 2012; Ritchie et al., 2014), and predict the potential for the progression of MCI to AD (Devanand et al., 2000, 2014; Roberts et al., 2016; Tahmasebi et al., 2019). Mounting evidence suggests that OI deficits are the predominant factor contributing to olfactory dysfunction in AD, as OI deficits occur earlier, and are more strongly correlated with memory impairments than deficits in other olfactory domains (Djordjevic et al., 2008). Moreover, impaired OI has been linked to accelerated decline in cognitive function (Dintica et al., 2019). Therefore, OI may be a valuable biomarker for preclinical AD.

There are many OI tests, such as the University of Pennsylvania Smell Identification Test (UPSIT), Connecticut Chemosensory Clinical Research Center (CCCRC) olfactory test, and "Sniffin Sticks" olfactory test. Each includes odors common in the local culture; however, performance may be affected by various semantic and cultural factors (Schab, 1991; Ayabe-Kanamura et al., 1998; Kobayashi et al., 2006). For instance, some items familiar to Western patients may not be easily recognizable by the Chinese population (and vice versa). Based on this consideration, Zhou developed the Chinese smell identification test (CSIT) (Feng et al., 2019), which adopts odor items that are familiar to and identifiable by most Chinese people. As such, the CSIT provides an effective tool (test-retest reliability of 0.92) for the assessment of olfactory function in the Chinese population. To our knowledge, however, there are few studies investigating OI dysfunction among AD and MCI patients using Chinese olfactory tests. In the present study, we examined whether CSIT can distinguish between normal aging, MCI, and AD in the Chinese population.

The neural substrates of OI dysfunction in AD and MCI patients are still unclear. Several neuroimaging studies have found associations between OI dysfunction and structural abnormities in brain regions that contribute to olfactory processing, such as the olfactory cortex (OC). The OC is the center of olfactory processing and functional and structural anomalies are strongly implicated in OI dysfunction (Thomann et al., 2009b; Servello et al., 2015; Vasavada et al., 2017). Hippocampal atrophy is a well-known pathological feature of AD and MCI (Prestia et al., 2010), and so may also contribute to OI dysfunction in AD and MCI. Indeed, several studies have reported a positive relationship between OI performance and hippocampal volume in patients with MCI or AD (Kjelvik et al., 2014). The amygdala is a key node linking the olfactory and hippocampal cortices (Price, 2003; LeDoux, 2007). Amygdala nuclei receive inputs from and send outputs to multiple brain regions subserving olfactory-associated functions, including emotional salience (Hamann, 2001). Thus, it is possible that the amygdala plays a key role in OI dysfunction among AD patients. Indeed, an vivo MRI study found that the amygdala was closely related to the olfactory loop in AD (Cavedo et al., 2011). The amygdala also has abundant neural connections with the hippocampus, and modulates both the encoding and the storage of hippocampal-dependent memories (Phelps, 2004).

Although several neuroimaging studies have implicated OC, hippocampal, and (or) amygdala abnormalities in OI dysfunction among AD and MCI patients, multiple studies have also reported contrary results. For example, Servello and colleagues (Feng et al., 2019) found no correlation between OC volume and olfactory function in AD, MCI, and NC. In contrast, several groups have found a correlation between the decline in OI and structural degeneration of the OC among AD patients (Claire Murphy, 2003; Thomann et al., 2009a; Marigliano et al., 2014; Servello et al., 2015). These discrepancies may be attributed to factors such as sample heterogeneity and differences in OI tests. In addition, neuroimaging analysis based on regions of interest (ROIs) may contribute to variability as the coordinates of specific ROIs differ markedly across studies (Ji et al., 2017). Thus, voxel-based analysis may help mitigate such inconsistencies.

In this study, we first compared OI performance among AD, MCI, and normal aging in the Chinese population using the CSIT. Subsequently, we conducted correlational analysis of CSIT scores and regional GMV at both ROI and whole-brain voxel levels to explore the neural substrates of OI.

MATERIALS AND METHODS

Study Subjects

A total of 94 right-handed participants (37 AD, 27 MCI, and 30 age-matched cognitively NCs were enrolled in this study. The AD and MCI patients were recruited from the Dysmnesia Outpatient Department at the First Affiliated Hospital of Anhui Medical University, Anhui Province, China. The NCs were recruited from the local community through advertisement or were the spouses of the study patients. The present study was approval by the Research Ethics Committee of the First Affiliated Hospital of Anhui Medical University. All subjects gave written informed consent in accordance with the Declaration of Helsinki.

Patients With AD

The AD subjects were clinically diagnosed by a specialist in accordance with NINCDS-ADRDA (McKhann et al., 1984) criteria: (a) Meeting criteria of possible or probable AD (McKhann et al., 2011), (b) mini-mental state examination (MMSE) score < 24, and (c) clinical dementia rating (CDR) score ranging from 0.5 to 2.

The exclusion criteria were as follows: (a) sudden onset, (b) early occurrence of gait disturbances, seizures, or behavioral changes, (c) focal neurological features such as hemiparesis, sensory loss, or visual field deficits, and (d) early extra-pyramidal signs or other severe disorders such as trauma, major depression, severe cerebrovascular disease, or metabolic abnormalities (Dubois et al., 2007).

Patients With MCI

Participants with MCI were clinically diagnosed by experts according to Peterson's criteria (Petersen et al., 1999) and NINCDS-ADRDA criteria as follows: (a) complaints of memory loss/other cognitive decline (including from the patient's family or doctor), (b) unexpectedly poor performance on one or more cognitive functions given the patient's age and educational background, (c) ability to maintain independence of daily living (i.e., no dementia) (Albert et al., 2011), (d) MMSE score > 24, (e) CDR score of 0.5. The exclusion criteria were the same as defined for AD patients.

Normal Controls

The NCs fulfilled the following criteria: cognitively normal, no neurological or psychiatric disorders, no psychoactive medication use, MMSE score of 28 or higher, and CDR score of 0.

Common Participant Criteria

White mater hyper-intensities (WMHs) were graded according to the Fazekas scale (Fazekas et al., 1987) based on visual assessment of both periventricular and subcortical areas (Helenius et al., 2017). However, as the presence of mild to moderate WMH frequently accompanies normal aging as well as neurodegenerative diseases (Wardlaw et al., 2013), this was not considered a criterion (Liu et al., 2011).

In order to rule out any confounds that could adversely influence the study results, we excluded subjects who engaged in long-term smoking and drinking as these behaviors have been shown to affect cognition and olfaction (Frye, 1990). We also checked for complications specific to olfactory dysfunction (e.g., nasal polyps, nasal obstruction, respiratory distress, head trauma, active sinus/upper respiratory infection, and allergies) and for contraindications to MRI (e.g., not-MRI-safe metal implants, severe claustrophobia). However, no participants were excluded from the study based upon these criteria.

Finally, 37 AD and 27 MCI patients with initial diagnosis and currently not treated with a cholinesterase inhibitor (donepezil, galantamine, or rivastigmine) were enrolled. Detailed background information on all groups is summarized in **Table 1**.

Neuropsychological Assessment

All participates underwent a clinical evaluation and neuropsychological assessment. The following neuropsychological test battery was administered to each subject for the purpose of establishing a clinical diagnosis as described previously (Lezak et al., 2004; Woodward et al., 2017). (i) General cognitive function was assessed with the Mini Mental State Examination (MMSE) (Burns, 1998) and the (global) Clinical Dementia Rating Scale (CDR) (Morris, 1993) as a proxy for disease severity. (ii) The Chinese version of the auditory verbal learning test (AVLT) was used to evaluate memory. (iii) The Hamilton Depression Rating Scale (HAMD) was used to assess depressive symptoms. (iv) Daily function was assessed using the Lawton-Brody activities of daily living (ADL) scale (Salmon and Bondi, 2009). Testing was administered by board-certified neuropsychologists and research staff under the supervision of neuropsychologists.

Olfactory Identification Assessment

The Chinese smell identification test (CSIT) developed by the Institute of Psychology, Chinese Academy of Sciences, was applied to evaluate OI performance (Feng et al., 2019). The CSIT consists of two parts. The first part is a self-assessment questionnaire (CSIT-self) that surveys medical factors that may confound olfactory function (septal deviation, difficulty breathing through one side of the nose, history of radiation or chemotherapy, history of nasal surgery) (Tabert et al., 2005). Participants were asked to rate their sense of smell relative to others on a 5-point scale as follows: 1 = poor, 2 = low, 3 = normal, 4 = good, and 5 = superior (to others).

The second part (CSIT-OI) includes olfactory tests of 40 familiar and easy to recognize odors such as strawberry, jujube, haw, and sesame oil. Subjects were required to name each odor from a list of four alternatives. The CSIT-OI test method is similar to the 40-item UPSIT (Doty et al., 1984), but CSIT is more suitable for people with a Chinese cultural background. Odorants of the CSIT were presented in felt-tip pens (Hummel et al., 1997), each filled with 1 ml of liquid. The cap of the pen was removed and the pen tip was placed approximately 2 cm in front of the subject's nostrils. Participants were requested to sniff the presented odor for 5 s then to pick the correct response. The tests were carried out in an environment with efficient air circulation and no other odors. The CSIT-IO score is the total of correct choices for the 40 odors.

Imaging Data Acquisition

Structural MRI images were acquired on a General Electric HD 750 w 3.0 T MRI scanner with an 8-channel head-coil (General Electric, Waukesha, WI, United States). Structural imaging included T1-weighted three-dimensional (3D-T1), axial

TABLE 1 | Demographics of the patients and normal controls.

	AD (mean ± SD)	MCI (mean ± SD)	NC (mean ± SD)	χ^2/F	p
Number	37	27	30		
Age (years)	66.86 ± 10.27	68.04 ± 7.58	67.23 ± 6.71	0.150	0.861
Gender (male/female)	17/20	13/14	11/19	0.896	0.639
Family history (yes/no)	3/34	2/25	1/29	0.699	0.795
Education (years)	6.78 ± 5.26	8.48 ± 5.53	12.20 ± 4.44	9.559	0.00[ab]
WMH score	1.51 ± 1.10	1.37 ± 1.15	1.30 ± 0.84	0.371	0.691

[a]p < 0.05, post-hoc when AD compared to NC, [b]p < 0.05, post-hoc when MCI compared to NC, [c]p < 0.05, post-hoc when AD compared to MCI.
Abbreviations: AD, Alzheimer's disease; MCI, mild cognitive impairment; NC, normal control; WMH, White Matter Hyper-intensities.

T2-weighted, and fluid-attenuated inversion recovery images. According to axial T2-weighted and fluid-attenuated inversion recovery images, subjects with abnormalities other than atrophy, or leukoaraiosis were excluded. The 3D-T1 images were collected using a fast-spoiled gradient recalled echo sequence [TR = 8.5 ms, TE = 3.2 ms, Inversion time (TI) = 450 ms, Matrix 256 × 256, FOV 256 mm × 256 mm, flip angle = 12°, and slice thickness of 1.0 mm without intervals]. The total scan duration for 3D-T1 image acquisition was 4 min, 30 s.

Image Processing and VBM Analyses

The VBM8 toolbox[1], a software package based on statistical parametric mapping software (SPM 8[2]) was used for VBM analyses. VBM8 was used to calculate GMV corrected for total intracranial volume, age, sex, and education level. T1-weighted images were segmented into GM, white matter, and cerebrospinal fluid using a fully automated algorithm in SPM 8. Images were normalized by diffeomorphic anatomical registration through exponentiated Lie algebra normalization, and transformed to Montreal Neurological Institute space to preserve local differences in anatomy across subjects, thereby allowing quantification. Finally, the normalized GM images were smoothed for statistical analysis (Wang et al., 2017).

For ROI-level analysis, we used SPM 8 for automatic anatomic segmentation and volumetric measurement of brain structures. We adopted the anatomical automatic labeling (AAL)-based structural ROI method for *ex vivo* measurement of each individual ROI signal (Tzourio-Mazoyer et al., 2002), and used the extracted signal for subsequent analysis. In this study, the ROIs were the hippocampus, amygdala, and OC, brain regions strongly related to olfactory processing. A voxel-based analysis was then applied over the whole brain to explore regions associated with CSIT score in AD, MCI, and NC groups.

Statistics Analysis

Statistical analyses of behavioral data were conducted using SPSS for Windows (22.0, IBM). Sex ratios were compared across diagnostic groups (AD, MCI, and NC) using the chi-square test. Demographic variables such as age, education level, neuropsychological features, and CSIT scores were compared across groups by one-way analysis of covariance (ANCOVA) (Vasavada et al., 2015) followed by a *post hoc* Bonferroni test for multiple comparisons. For non-normally distributed data [denoted by Md (p25,p75)], we used Kruskal–Wallis analysis of variance (ANOVA) to evaluate differences among groups followed by a Dunn–Bonferroni test for *post hoc* comparisons. The effectiveness of CSIT for identifying AD, MCI, and NC was assessed by receiver operating characteristic curve (ROC) analysis. The sensitivity and false positive rate (1 – specificity) of CSIT-OI, CSIT-self, and CSIT-OI + self was calculated for ROC curves, and the area under the ROC curve was used to determine classification accuracy. A $\alpha < 0.05$ (two-tailed) was considered significant for all tests.

Spearman correlation analysis was performed between CSIT scores and mean GMV of each ROI (OC, amygdala, and hippocampus). Significant correlations between CSIT and GMV of each ROI were corrected for false discovery rate. The mean GMV of each ROI was also compared between groups by ANCOVA with sex, age, and education as covariates. At the whole-brain voxel level, behavior – neuroimaging correlation analysis was conducted using SPM 8 with sex, age, and education as covariates. The statistical maps were thresholded using the Gaussian random field (GRF) correction with a voxel-level threshold of $P < 0.001$ and a cluster-level threshold of $P < 0.05$.

RESULTS

Clinical Characteristics of the Study Cohort

The demographic and baseline clinical characteristics of the study subjects are summarized in **Table 1**. There were no significant differences in age, sex ratio, family history, WMH score, and vascular risk factors among the three groups. However, there were significant differences in years of education (AD = 6.78 ± 5.26, MCI = 8.48 ± 5.53, NC = 12.20 ± 4.44; $p < 0.001$).

Neuropsychological Deficits in MCI and AD

There were significant differences in several neuropsychological test outcomes among the three groups as revealed by one-way ANOVA (**Table 2**). As expected, MMSE ($p < 0.001$) and CDR ($p < 0.001$) differed markedly, with significantly lower scores in the AD group compared to MCI and NC groups. In addition, there were significant inter-group differences in AVLT

[1]http://www.neuro.uni-jena.de/vbm/download/
[2]http://www.fil.ion.ucl.ac.uk/spm

TABLE 2 | Neuropsychological assessment of MCI, AD, and NC groups.

	AD	MCI	NC	ANOVA/Kruskal-Wallis	
	n = 37	*n* = 27	*n* = 30	χ^2/F	*p*
MMSE*	16.03 ± 4.04	26 (25, 28)	29 (28, 30)	73.253^{abc}	<0.001
CDR*	1.0 (1, 1.5)	0.5 (0.5, 0.5)	0 (0, 0)	61.189^{abc}	<0.001
AVLT (immediate)*	2.2 (1.1, 3.4)	4.64 ± 1.65	9.22 ± 1.86	72.642^{abc}	<0.001
AVLT (delay)*	0.0 (0.0, 0.5)	3.33 ± 2.51	10.57 ± 2.45	29.308^{abc}	<0.001
AVLT (recognize)*	10.0 (4.0, 13.5)	12.52 ± 2.03	14 (14, 15)	29.308^{abc}	<0.001
HAMD*	4.0 (3.0, 6.0)	5.0 (4.0, 14.0)	1.0 (0, 2.0)	31.904^{ab}	<0.001
ADL*	30.0 (26.0, 35.5)	21.0 (20.0, 22.0)	20 (20, 20)	61.443^{abc}	<0.001
CSIT score†	13.46 ± 6.09	19.11 ± 6.41	28.80 ± 3.93	62.597^{abc}	<0.001
CSIT-self*	3.0 (2.5, 4.0)	3.0 (3.0, 3.0)	3.0 (3.0, 4.0)	4.039	0.133

**Kruskal–Wallis test followed by pairwise multiple comparisons. †ANOVA with post hoc Bonferroni test. $^a p < 0.05$ (post hoc), AD vs. HC; $^b p < 0.05$ (post hoc), MCI vs. HC; $^c p < 0.05$ (post hoc), AD vs. MCI. AD, Alzheimer's disease, ADL, activities of daily living scale; AVLT, auditory verbal learning test; CDR, clinical dementia rating; CSIT-OI, Chinese smell identification test – olfactory identification; CSIT-self, Chinese smell identification test – self assessment; HAMD, hamilton depression scale; MCI, mild cognitive impairment; MMSE, mini mental state examination; NC, normal control.*

TABLE 3 | Correlations analysis of CSIT and neuro-psychological.

	All participants		AD		MCI		NC	
	R	*p*	*R*	*p*	*R*	*p*	*R*	*p*
MMSE	0.740**	0.000	0.225	0.180	0.268	0.176	0.392*	0.032
CDR	−0.775**	0.000	−0.452**	0.005	0.000	0.000	0.087	0.648
AVLT (immediate)	0.703**	0.000	0.241	0.151	0.027	0.892	0.329	0.076
AVLT (delay)	0.799**	0.000	0.417*	0.010	0.213	0.286	0.350	0.058
AVLT (recognize)	0.624**	0.000	0.459**	0.004	0.180	0.370	0.419*	0.021
HAMD	−0.46**	0.000	−0.186	0.269	0.107	0.595	−0.394*	0.031
ADL	−0.697**	0.000	−0.193	0.253	−0.246	0.216	−0.257	0.171

*R, correlation coefficient (Spearman's rho correlations). **Correlation is significant at the 0.01 level (2-tailed). *Correlation is significant at the 0.05 level (2-tailed). AD, Alzheimer's disease; MCI, mild cognitive impairment; NC, normal control; MMSE, mini mental state examination; CDR, clinical dementia rating; AVLT, auditory verbal learning test; HAMD, Hamilton depression scale, ADL, activities of daily living scale.*

(immediate, delay, or recognition; $p < 0.001$). Daily functions were significantly impaired only in AD patients; both MCI and AD groups showed a gradual decline, but a worse performance was observed in the latter patients (**Table 2**). Mean HAMD scores were higher in AD and MCI groups than in the NC group, and higher in MCI than AD (**Table 2**). The CSIT-OI score was positively correlated with AVLT [delay] and AVLT [recognize] and negatively correlated with CDR in AD patients but not in the other groups (**Table 3**).

CSIT Scores Distinguish MCI and AD From Age-Matched Controls

Group Differences in CSIT-OI and CSIT-Self Scores

There were significant differences in CSIT-OI score among groups, with significantly lower scores (indicating poorer OI) in the AD and MCI group compared to NCs ($p < 0.001$), and lower mean score in AD than MCI (**Figure 1** and **Table 2**). The CSIT-self score was also lower in AD and MCI groups compared to NCs. The CSIT-self score was positively correlated with CSIT-OI for the entire cohort ($R = 0.415$; $p < 0.001$); however, the correlation did not reach significance within individual diagnostic groups due to lack of statistical power ($p > 0.05$).

Power of Discrimination

Patients vs. normal controls

In the ROC analysis, both CSIT-OI score and combined CSIT-OI plus CSIT-self score distinguished AD from NC and MCI from NC, while CSIT-self score alone did not (note that AUC = 0.5 indicates no discriminative power) (**Figures 2A,B** and **Table 4**). Using a cut-off value of 26, CSIT-OI score distinguished MCI from NC with 80.0% sensitivity and 89.0% specificity; using a cut-off value of 22.5 distinguished AD from NC with 93% sensitivity and 95% specificity.

AD vs. MCI

According to ROC analysis, CSIT-OI score and CSIT-OI plus CSIT-self score also distinguished AD from MCI, while again CSIT-self score did not (**Figure 2C** and **Table 4**). Using a cutoff value of 18.5, CSIT-OI score distinguished AD from MCI with 70.4% sensitivity and 83.8% specificity.

Correlations Between CSIT Scores and Regional GMV Values at the ROI and Voxel Levels

At the ROI level, CSIT-OI scores of AD patients were positively correlated with left amygdala volume ($r = 0.38$, $p = 0.046$), with

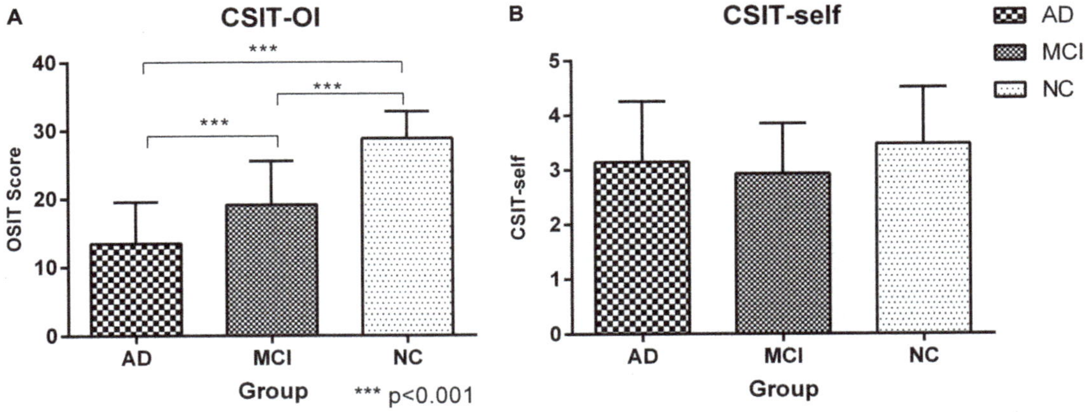

FIGURE 1 | Histogram of CSIT scores for all participants in this study. **(A)** The CSIT-OI scores of patients with AD and MCI were lower than NC, and the scores of AD were the lowest and there were significant statistical differences ($P < 0.001$); *** <0.001. **(B)** There was no difference in the CSIT-self scores of the three groups ($P > 0.05$).

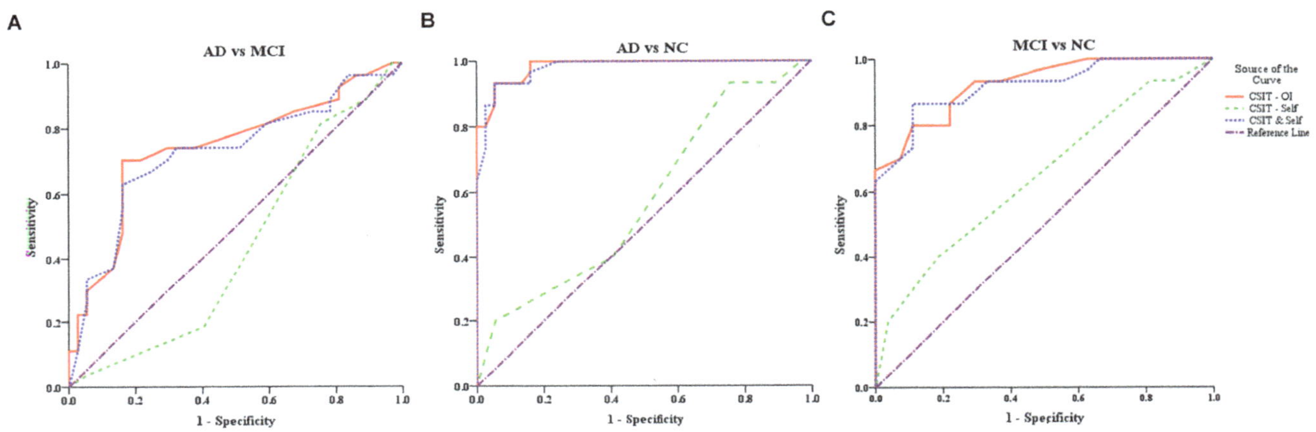

FIGURE 2 | ROC curves for the CSIT-OI, CSIT-Self and CSIT-OI + Self **(A–C)**. **(A)** ROC curves for the CSIT-OI, CSIT-self, and CSIT-OI + Self between AD and MCI. **(B)** ROC curves for the CSIT-OI, CSIT-self, and CSIT-OI + Self between AD and NC. **(C)** ROC curves for the CSIT-OI, CSIT-self, and CSIT-OI + Self between MCI and NC. The *x*-axis indicates the error of the second kind (100%-specificity). The *y*-axis indicates sensitivity. The area under the curve (AUC) shows the discriminative power between the two groups. The diagonal from (0,0) to (100,100) with AUC = 0.5 indicates a total lack of discriminative power.

TABLE 4 | Receiver operating characteristic curve analysis of CSIT in all participant.

	Variable	AUC	Cut-off value	Youden index	Sensitivity	Specificity	PPV	NPV	LR+	LR–
AD vs. MCI	CSIT-OI	0.98**	18.5	0.54	0.70	0.84	0.76	0.80	4.34	0.35
	CSIT-Self	0.58	2.5	0.06	0.81	0.24	0.44	0.64	1.08	0.76
	CSIT&Self	0.98*	22.5	0.47	0.63	0.84	0.74	0.76	3.88	0.44
AD vs. NC	CSIT-OI	0.98**	22.5	0.88	0.93	0.95	0.93	0.95	17.27	0.07
	CSIT-Self	0.58	2.5	0.18	0.93	0.24	0.92	0.88	1.23	0.27
	CSIT&Self	0.98**	25.5	0.88	0.93	0.95	0.82	0.94	17.27	0.07
MCI vs. NC	CSIT-OI	0.92**	26.0	0.69	0.80	0.89	0.89	0.80	7.20	0.23
	CSIT-Self	0.64	3.5	0.21	0.40	0.81	0.71	0.55	2.16	0.74
	CSIT&Self	0.92**	28.5	0.76	0.87	0.89	0.90	0.86	7.80	0.15

**significant at the 0.05 level (2-tailed). **significant at the 0.01 level (2-tailed).*

Abbreviations: AUC: area under the receiver operating characteristic (ROC) curve, PPV: positive prediction value, NPV: negative prediction value, LR+: positive likelihood ratio, LR–: negative likelihood ratio, CSIT-OI: Chinese smell identification test – olfactory identification, CSIT-self: Chinese smell identification test – self assessment, CSIT & self: CSIT-OI + CSIT-self.

TABLE 5 | Correlations analysis of CSIT and the GMV of ROI.

	Total participants		AD		MCI		NC	
	R	*FDR-p*	*R*	*FDR-p*	*R*	*FDR-p*	*R*	*FDR-p*
OFC-L	0.452**	0.000	0.248	0.139	0.156	0.438	0.012	0.95
OFC-R	0.487**	0.000	0.213	0.247	0.382	0.294	0.144	0.674
Amygdala-L	0.466**	0.000	0.331*	0.046	0.035	0.863	0.191	0.312
Amygdala-R	0.457**	0.000	0.192	0.255	0.144	0.71	0.02	0.918
Hippocampus-L	0.520**	0.000	0.323	0.051	0.088	0.797	0.326	0.47
Hippocampus-R	0.512**	0.000	0.242	0.224	0.231	0.737	0.167	0.757
Precentral cortex-L	0.469**	0.000	0.577**	0.000	0.283	0.152	0.172	0.363
IFG-L	0.416**	0.000	0.430**	0.008	0.174	0.769	−0.2	0.29

*R, correlation coefficient (Spearman's rho correlations); FDR-p, the p value after false discovery rate (FDR) correction. *Correlation is significant at the 0.05 level (2-tailed). **Correlation is significant at the 0.01 level (2-tailed). ROI, region of interesting; GMV, gray matter volume; L, left; R, right; OFC, olfactory cortex; IFG, inferior frontal gyrus.*

a trend observed for the left hippocampus ($r = 0.35$, $p = 0.051$) (**Table 5**). At the voxel level, CSIT-OI score was associated with volumes of the left inferior frontal gyrus (IFG, peak location $x = -33$, $y = 20$, $z = -18$, peak intensity = 0.612) and left precentral gyrus (peak location: $x = -42$, $y = -5$, $z = 33$, peak intensity = 0.707) ($p < 0.05$; **Figure 3** and **Table 5**). There was a significant relationship between CSIT-OI score and GMV in the all participants at the ROI or voxel level, but no significant relationships were found between CSIT-OI score and GMV in the MCI and NC groups at either the ROI or voxel level (**Table 5**).

DISCUSSION

We demonstrate that OI as measured by the CSIT is impaired in AD and MCI patients compared to age-matched healthy controls in the Chinese population, and that the severity of OI dysfunction can distinguish AD and MCI patients from controls and AD from MCI with high sensitivity and specificity. In addition, CSIT scores were significantly associated with specific memory assessment outcomes but not with measures of general cognitive function such as MMSE score. Based on ROI-level GMV analysis, the OI of AD patients was significantly correlated with left amygdala volume, with a similar trend observed for the left hippocampus (but not bilateral OC, right amygdala, or hippocampus); meanwhile, a voxel-level analysis revealed that the OI of AD patients was also associated with the volumes of precentral gyrus-L and IFG-L. In contrast, no such CSIT-GMV associations were found in the MCI and NC groups. Therefore, OI dysfunction as assessed by a culturally appropriate test (the CSIT) may be a convenient AD screening tool.

This study confirmed that OI is impaired in ethnic Chinese AD and MCI patients, consistent with previous studies in Western populations. In all three diagnostic groups (MCI, AD, and NC), OI decreased progressively with age (Larsson et al., 2000; Devanand et al., 2014; Roalf et al., 2017; Silva et al., 2018). There was also a disconnect between objective and subjective OI capacity, as AD patients did not rate their sense of smell as inferior despite lower CSIT-OI scores. In line with our findings (Doty et al., 1984; Burns, 1998) reported that only 6% of AD patients complained of olfactory dysfunction, while 90% had actual olfactory deficits as demonstrated by olfactory tests. Alternatively, MCI patients did provide relatively low self-assessments (Yu et al., 2018). This may result from impaired self-concept in AD but not in MCI. Further, average score among AD patients (13/40 = 32.5%) was near the chance level of 25%, indicating that sense of smell was substantially degraded. Therefore, it is necessary to measure olfactory function using sensitive and objective olfactory tests. Thus, OI may not be suitable for gauging AD progression but could be useful for measuring MCI progression and deficits during normal aging.

Although CSIT is based on UPSIT, group differences in scores were greater than in past studies using the UPSIT, suggesting better discriminative efficacy. Our ROC analysis suggests that the CSIT can distinguish MCI and AD patients from normal elderly individuals and accurately distinguish AD from MCI. This level of discrimination is similar to cerebral spinal fluid (CSF) biomarkers, only slightly inferior to amyloid imaging and structural MRI, and significantly greater than UPSIT (sensitivity: 0.88, specificity: 0.91) (Devanand, 2016; Hagemeier et al., 2016). The OI test classifies individuals showing cognitive decline correctly at a higher rate than a global cognitive test (Graves et al., 1999). Consistent with these findings, CSIT-OI score was positively correlated with memory function (AVLT-delay and -recognition), and negatively correlated with the severity of cognitive impairment (CDR score) in AD patients. This demonstrates that the OI deficit in AD is mainly related to impairment of semantic (cognitive) rather than perceptual processing (Lehrner et al., 1999) However, the CSIT-OI score was not associated with MMSE scores in AD patients, consistent with previous studies (Roalf et al., 2017; Silva et al., 2018), possibly because the MMSE is a general test of cognition that does not provide information on specific cognitive dysfunctions in AD. Therefore, we conclude that CSIT is more suitable for use in the Chinese Han population than the UPSIT, and is a useful biomarker for cognitive deficit.

Volumes of left IFG and precentral cortex were significantly associated with OI performance in AD patients, a finding that to the best of our knowledge has not been reported previously. While previous reports have indicated that OI is related to the olfactory bulb, OC, hippocampus, and parahippocampus, few have found associated changes in motor-related areas. The

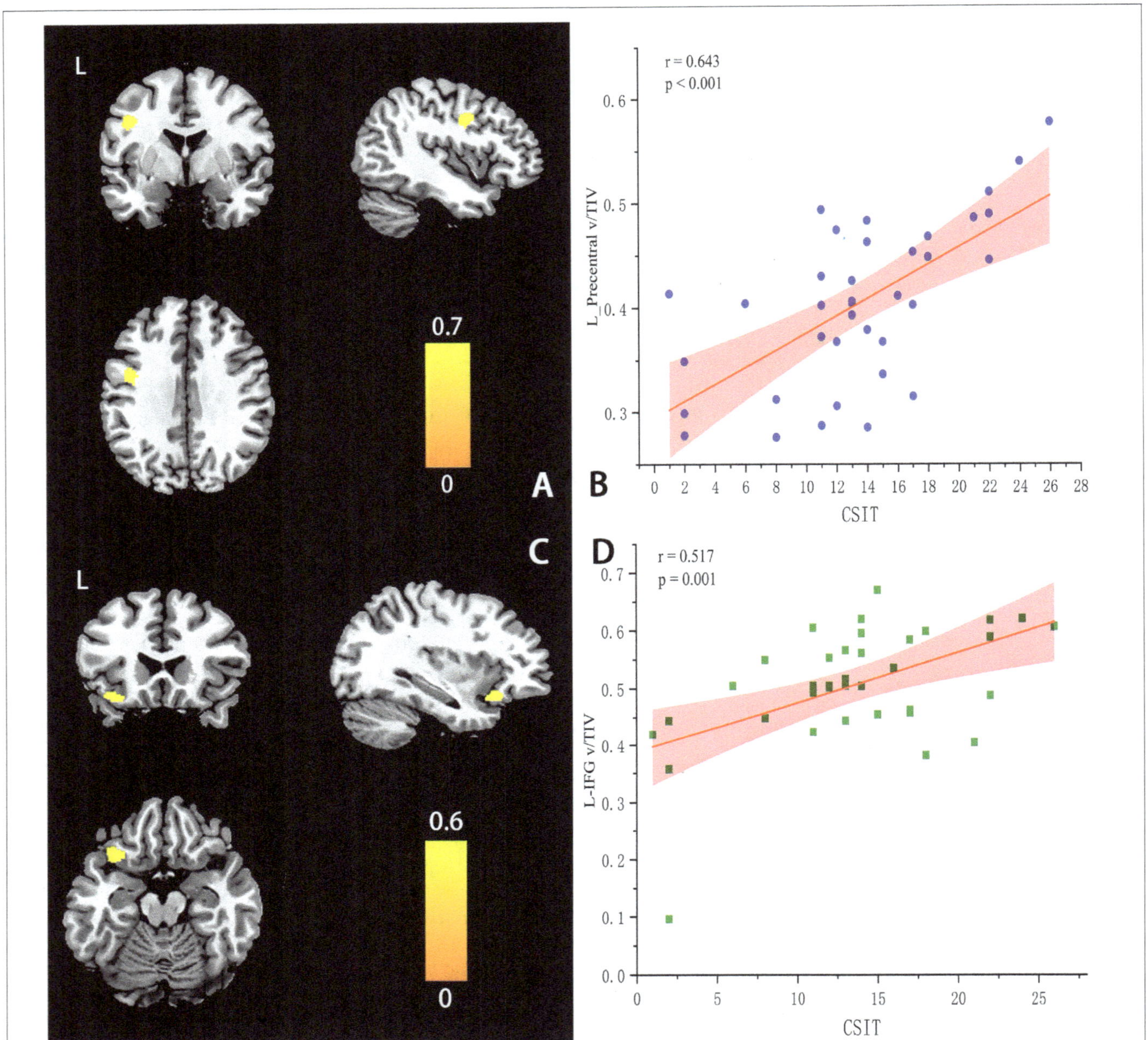

FIGURE 3 | Correlations between CSIT scores and regional GMV values at the voxel levels **(A–D)**. **(A)** The location of left-Precentral Gyrus (L-PG) (peak MINI: $x = -42$, $y = -5$, $z = 33$, Peak intensity: 0.707). **(C)** The location of left-Inferior Frontal Gyrus (L-IFG) (peak MINI $x = -33$, $y = 20$, $z = -18$, Peak intensity = 0.612). **(B,D)** The scatter plot and linear fit show the relationship between the GMV of L-PG & L-IFG and CSIT score in AD. The results suggested that the GMV of L-PG ($r = 0.643$, $p < 0.001$) & L – IFG ($r = 0.517$, $p = 0.001$) were significantly correlated with the CSIT scores in AD.

precentral cortex is an important component of the motor network (Yousry et al., 1997; Hopkins et al., 2017). In addition, however, recent reports have found that the precentral cortex participates in a variety of perceptual and integrative processes (Chen et al., 2008), including contributions to cognitive functions such as language and executive control (Ferreira et al., 2017; Mugler et al., 2018). Bi et al. (2018) found significant changes in the precentral cortex volume of AD patients compared to NCs. In addition, Rizzo et al. (2018) found that the fiber bundle connection between the amygdala and precentral gyrus is abnormal in AD. Furthermore, the strength of functional connections between posteromedial and precentral cortices was reduced, which is significantly correlated with cognitive function in AD (Wu et al., 2016). The IFG is part of Broca's area, which is involved in semantic processing and phoneme production (Mugler et al., 2018), and some studies have also reported a relationship with memory function (Smith and Jonides, 1999). The IFG does not contribute to the processing of single syllables, but rather acts in combination with the precentral gyrus for responding to understood speech, including the ordering of multiple syllables. A number of functional imaging studies have demonstrated that L-IFG and L-precentral gyrus regions are active during speech perception and comprehension (Wilson et al., 2004; Pulvermuller et al., 2006), particularly when participants listen attentively to speech signals that are noisy or degraded (Hervais-Adelman et al., 2012; Wild et al., 2012). On the ROI level, the volume of the left amygdala was significantly associated with OI performance in AD patients, suggesting that structural changes in the left amygdala are due to involvement of the olfactory network. Based on previous reports and our findings, we speculate that functional anomalies in the precentral gyrus, IFG, amygdala, and hippocampus lead to defective OI in AD patients, and that the amygdala–precentral gyrus pathway plays a predominant role in OI. Unraveling the specific contributions of this precentral gyrus shrinkage to OI deficits requires further research.

This study has several limitations. First, our AD patient group included both early-onset and late-onset patients, which may introduce heterogeneity to morphometric changes. A previous study found that patients with early-onset AD showed bilateral reductions in the medial temporal lobes, inferior parietal lobules, precuneus and perisylvian cortices, and cingulate cortices, as well as in the right inferior frontal gyrus, whereas late-onset patients with AD showed atrophy only in bilateral medial temporal cortices. Second, we did not compare differences between AD patients with and without olfactory dysfunction, and such a comparison could also reveal mechanisms underlying OI disorders. Third, this is a cross-sectional rather than a longitudinal study, so we do not know if these differences were caused by the progression of AD. Fourth, we excluded subjects who engaged in long-term smoking and drinking, as these behaviors affect cognition and olfaction (Frye, 1990). This could result in selection bias but better reflects central mechanisms of olfactory recognition (Vasavada et al., 2017). Lastly, the sample was small; therefore, studies in a larger population are needed in order to confirm whether this measure can consistently distinguish controls from AD patients.

CONCLUSION

Our study confirms that the CSIT is a culturally appropriate olfactory recognition test for the Chinese Han population that can effectively distinguish among AD, MCI, and healthy aging. Gray matter voxel-based MRI analysis demonstrated that OI is more strongly related to the left cerebral hemisphere (left hippocampus, left amygdala, left-precentral gyrus, left-IFG, and bilateral olfactory cortex) than to the right hemisphere (right hippocampus and right amygdala). We also found that the left-precentral gyrus and left-IFG may be involved in OI. We therefore speculate that language processing may contribute to the expression of olfactory recognition, and that AD patients are impaired in this domain. However, further research is needed to elucidate the precise mechanisms for OI dysfunction and relationships to other aspects of MCI and AD pathology.

AUTHOR CONTRIBUTIONS

XW performed the analysis and wrote the manuscript. ZG, SZ, LW, WZ, and YY helped to collect the behavioral and imaging data. TB and G-JJ helped in MRI data analysis. YT and KW designed and supervised the study.

FUNDING

This work was supported by the National Key R&D Program of China (Grant Nos. 2016YFC1306400, 2016YFC1305904, 2018YFC1314504, and 2018YFC1314200), the National Natural Science Foundation of China (Grant Nos. 91432301, 91732303, and 81771817), and the Provincial Natural Science Foundation Project of Anhui (Grant No. 1608085MH169).

ACKNOWLEDGMENTS

We thank the participants for their cooperation during this study and WZ for providing the CSIT Kit.

REFERENCES

Albert, M. S., DeKosky, S. T., Dickson, D., Dubois, B., Feldman, H. H., Fox, N. C., et al. (2011). The diagnosis of mild cognitive impairment due to Alzheimer's disease: recommendations from the National Institute on Aging-Alzheimer's association workgroups on diagnostic guidelines for Alzheimer's disease. *Alzheimers Dement* 7, 270–279. doi: 10.1016/j.jalz.2011.03.008

Ayabe-Kanamura, S., Schicker, I., Laska, M., Hudson, R., Distel, H., Kobayakawa, T., et al. (1998). Differences in perception of everyday odors: a Japanese-German cross-cultural study. *Chem. Senses* 23, 31–38. doi: 10.1093/chemse/23.1.31

Baazaoui, N., and Iqbal, K. (2018). A novel therapeutic approach to treat Alzheimer's disease by neurotrophic support during the period of synaptic compensation. *J. Alzheimers Dis.* 62, 1211–1218. doi: 10.3233/JAD-170839

Bi, X. A., Jiang, Q., Sun, Q., Shu, Q., and Liu, Y. (2018). Analysis of alzheimer's disease based on the random neural network cluster in fMRI. *Front. Neuroinform.* 12:60. doi: 10.3389/fninf.2018.00060

Burns, A. (1998). Key papers in geriatric psychiatry: mini-mental state: a practical method for grading the cognitive state of patients for the clinician. M. Folstein, S. Folstein and P. McHugh, journal of psychiatric research (1975) 12, 189-198. *Int. J. Geriatr. Psych.* 13, 285–285.

Cavedo, E., Boccardi, M., Ganzola, R., Canu, E., Beltramello, A., Caltagirone, C., et al. (2011). Local amygdala structural differences with 3T MRI in patients with Alzheimer disease. *Neurology* 2011:8.

Chen, J. L., Penhune, V. B., and Zatorre, R. J. (2008). Listening to musical rhythms recruits motor regions of the brain. *Cereb. Cortex* 18, 2844–2854. doi: 10.1093/cercor/bhn042

Claire Murphy, T. L. (2003). Jernigan,christine fennema, left hippocampal volume loss in Alzheimer's disease is reflected in performance on odor identification: a structural MRI study. *J. Int. Neuropsychol. Soc.* 2003:13.

Devanand, D., Lee, S., Manly, J., Andrews, H., Schupf, N., Brickman, A. M., et al. (2014). Olfactory identification deficits predict the transition from MCI to Ad in a multi-ethnic community sample. *Alzheimer Dement.* 10:803.

Devanand, D. P. (2000). Olfactory deficits in patients with mild cognitive impairment predict Alzheimer's disease at follow-up. *Am. J. Psychiatry* 2000:7.

Devanand, D. P. (2016). Olfactory identification deficits, cognitive decline, and dementia in older adults. *Am. J. Geriatr. Psychiatry* 24, 1151–1157. doi: 10.1016/j.jagp.2016.08.010

Devanand, D. P., Michaels-Marston, K. S., Liu, X. H., Pelton, G. H., Padilla, M., Marder, K., et al. (2000). Olfactory deficits in patients with mild cognitive impairment predict Alzheimer's disease at follow-up. *Am. J. Psychiat.* 157, 1399–1405. doi: 10.1176/appi.ajp.157.9.1399

Dintica, C. S., Marseglia, A., Rizzuto, D., Wang, R., Seubert, J., Arfanakis, K., et al. (2019). Impaired olfaction is associated with cognitive decline and neurodegeneration in the brain. *Neurology* 92, e700–e709. doi: 10.1212/WNL.0000000000006919

Djordjevic, J., Jones-Gotman, M., De Sousa, K., and Chertkow, H. (2008). Olfaction in patients with mild cognitive impairment and Alzheimer's disease. *Neurobiol. Aging* 29, 693–706.

Doty, R. L., Shaman, P., and Dann, M. (1984). Development of the university of pennsylvania smell identification smell identification test - a standardized microencapsulated test of olfactory function. *Physiol. Behav.* 32, 489–502. doi: 10.1016/0031-9384(84)90269-5

Dubois, B., Feldman, H. H., Jacova, C., DeKosky, S. T., Barberger-Gateau, P., Cummings, J., et al. (2007). Research criteria for the diagnosis of Alzheimer's disease: revising the NINCDS–ADRDA criteria. *Lancet Neurol.* 6, 734–746. doi: 10.1016/s1474-4422(07)70178-3

Ewers, M., Walsh, C., Trojanowski, J. Q., Shaw, L. M., Petersen, R. C., Jack, C. R., et al. (2012). Prediction of conversion from mild cognitive impairment to Alzheimer's disease dementia based upon biomarkers and neuropsychological test performance. *Neurobiol. Aging* 33, 1203–1214. doi: 10.1016/j.neurobiolaging.2010.10.019

Fazekas, F., Chawluk, J. B., Alavi, A., Hurtig, H. I., and Zimmerman, R. A. (1987). MR signal abnormalities at 1.5-T in Alzheimer dementia and normal aging. *Am. J. Roentgenol.* 149, 351–356. doi: 10.2214/ajr.149.2.351

Feng, G., Zhuang, Y., Yao, F., Ye, Y., Wan, Q., and Zhou, W. (2019). Development of the Chinese smell identification test. *Chem. Senses* 44, 189–195. doi: 10.1093/chemse/bjz006

Ferreira, D., Machado, A., Molina, Y., Nieto, A., Correia, R., Westman, E., et al. (2017). Cognitive variability during middle-age: possible association with neurodegeneration and cognitive reserve. *Front. Aging Neurosci.* 9:188. doi: 10.3389/fnagi.2017.00188

Frye, R. E. (1990). Dose-related effects of cigarette smoking on olfactory function. *JAMA* 1990:4.

Graves, A. B., Bowen, J. D., Rajaram, L., McCormick, W. C., McCurry, S. M., Schellenberg, G. D., et al. (1999). Impaired olfaction as a marker for cognitive decline - interaction with apolipoprotein E epsilon 4 status. *Neurology* 53, 1480–1487.

Hagemeier, J., Woodward, M. R., Rafique, U. A., Amrutkar, C. V., Bergsland, N. Dwyer, M. G., et al. (2016). Odor identification deficit in mild cognitive impairment and Alzheimer's disease is associated with hippocampal and deep gray matter atrophy. *Psychiatry Res. Neuroimaging* 255, 87–93. doi: 10.1016/j.pscychresns.2016.08.003

Hamann, S. (2001). Cognitive and neural mechanisms of emotional memory. *Trends Cogn. Sci.* 5, 394–400. doi: 10.1016/s1364-6613(00)01707-1

Helenius, J., Mayasi, Y., and Henninger, N. (2017). White matter hyperintensity lesion burden is associated with the infarct volume and 90-day outcome in small subcortical infarcts. *Acta Neurol. Scand.* 135, 585–592. doi: 10.1111/ane.12670

Hervais-Adelman, A. G., Carlyon, R. P., Johnsrude, I. S., and Davis, M. H. (2012). Brain regions recruited for the effortful comprehension of noise-vocoded words. *Lang. Cogn. Process.* 27, 1145–1166. doi: 10.1080/01690965.2012.662280

Hopkins, W. D., Meguerditchian, A., Coulon, O., Misiura, M., Pope, S., Mareno, M. C., et al. (2017). Motor skill for tool-use is associated with asymmetries in Broca's area and the motor hand area of the precentral gyrus in chimpanzees (Pan troglodytes). *Behav. Brain Res.* 318, 71–81. doi: 10.1016/j.bbr.2016.10.048

Hummel, T., Sekinger, B., Wolf, S. R., Pauli, E., and Kobal, G. (1997). 'Sniffin' Sticks': olfactory performance assessed by the combined testing of odor identification, odor discrimination and olfactory threshold. *Chem. Senses* 22, 39–52. doi: 10.1093/chemse/22.1.39

Ji, G.-J., Liao, W., Chen, F.-F., Zhang, L., and Wang, K. (2017). Low-frequency blood oxygen level-dependent fluctuations in the brain white matter: more than just noise. *Sci. Bull.* 62, 656–657. doi: 10.1016/j.scib.2017.03.021

Kjelvik, G., Saltvedt, I., White, L. R., Stenumgård, P., Sletvold, O., Engedal, K., et al. (2014). The brain structural and cognitive basis of odor identification deficits in mild cognitive impairment and Alzheimer's disease. *BMC Neurol.* 2014:10.

Kobayashi, M., Saito, S., Kobayakawa, T., Deguchi, Y., and Costanzo, R. M. (2006). Cross-cultural comparison of data using the odor stick identification test for Japanese (OSIT-J). *Chem. Senses* 31, 335–342. doi: 10.1093/chemse/bjj037

Larsson, M., Finkel, D., and Pedersen, N. L. (2000). Odor identification: influences of age, gender, cognition, and personality. *J. Gerontol. B.Psychol.* 55, 304–310.

LeDoux, J. (2007). The amygdala. *Curr. Biol.* 17, R868–R874.

Lehrner, J. P., Walla, P., Laska, M., and Deecke, L. (1999). Different forms of human odor memory: a developmental study. *Neurosci. Lett.* 272, 17–20. doi: 10.1016/s0304-3940(99)00566-2

Lezak, M. D., Howieson, D. B., Loring, D. W., and Fischer, J. S. (2004). *Neuropsychological Assessment.* New York, NY: Oxford University Press.

Liu, Y. W., Spulber, G., Lehtimaki, K. K., Kononen, M., Hallikainen, I., Grohn, H., et al. (2011). Diffusion tensor imaging and tract-based spatial statistics in Alzheimer's disease and mild cognitive impairment. *Neurobiol. Aging* 32, 1558–1571. doi: 10.1016/j.neurobiolaging.2009.10.006

Marigliano, V., Gualdi, G., Servello, A., Marigliano, B., Volpe, L. D., Fioretti, A., et al. (2014). Olfactory deficit and hippocampal volume loss for early diagnosis of Alzheimer Disease a pilot study. *Alzheimer Dis. Assoc. Disord.* 28:4. doi: 10.1097/WAD.0b013e31827bdb9f

McDade, E., and Bateman, R. J. (2017). Stop Alzheimer's before it starts. *Nature* 547, 153–155.

McKhann, G., Drachman, D., Folstein, M., Katzman, R., Price, D., and Stadlan, E. M. (1984). Clinical-diagnosis of Alzheimers disease report of the NINCADS-ADRDA work group under the auspices of department of health and human services task foecr on Alzheimers disease. *Neurology* 34, 939–944.

McKhann, G. M., Knopman, D. S., Chertkow, H., Hyman, B. T., Jack, C. R., Kawas, C. H., et al. (2011). The diagnosis of dementia due to Alzheimer's disease: recommendations from the national institute on Aging-Alzheimer's association workgroups on diagnostic guidelines for Alzheimer's disease. *Alzheimers Dement.* 7, 263–269.

Mesholam, R. I. (1998). Olfaction in neurodegenerative disease a meta-analysis of olfactory functioning in Alzheimer's and Parkinson's diseases. *Arch. Neurol.* 1998:7.

Miller, G. (2012). Stopping Alzheimer's before it starts. *Science* 337, 790–792. doi: 10.1126/science.337.6096.790

Morris, J. C. (1993). The clinical dementia rating (CDR) - current version and scoring rules. *Neurology* 43, 2412–2414.

Mugler, E. M., Tate, M. C., Livescu, K., Templer, J. W., Goldrick, M. A., and Slutzky, M. W. (2018). Differential representation of articulatory gestures and phonemes in precentral and inferior frontal gyri. *J. Neurosci.* 38, 9803–9813. doi: 10.1523/JNEUROSCI.1206-18.2018

Peters, J. M. (2003). Olfactory function in mild cognitive impairment and Alzheimer's disease: an investigation using psychophysical and electrophysiological techniques. *Am. J. Psychiatry* 2003:8.

Petersen, R. C. (2007). Mild cognitive impairment: current research and clinical implications. *Semin. Neurol.* 27, 22–31.

Petersen, R. C., Doody, R., Kurz, A., Mohs, R. C., Morris, J. C., Rabins, P. V., et al. (2001). Current concepts in mild cognitive impairment. *Arch. Neurol.* 58, 1985–1992.

Petersen, R. C., Smith, G. E., Waring, S. C., Ivnik, R. J., Tangalos, E. G., and Kokmen, E. (1999). Mild cognitive impairment: clinical characterization and outcome. *Arch. Neurol.* 56, 303–308.

Phelps, E. A. (2004). Human emotion and memory: interactions of the amygdala and hippocampal complex. *Curr. Opin. Neurobiol.* 14, 198–202. doi: 10.1016/j.conb.2004.03.015

Prestia, A., Drago, V., Rasser, P. E., Bonetti, M., Thompson, P. M., and Frisoni, G. B. (2010). Cortical changes in incipient Alzheimer's disease. *J. Alzheimers. Dis.* 22, 1339–1349. doi: 10.3233/jad-2010-101191

Price, J. L. (2003). "Comparative aspects of amygdala connectivity," in *Amygdala in Brain Function: Bacic and Clinical Approaches*, eds P. ShinnickGallagher, A. Pitkanen, A. Shekhar, and L. Cahill, (New York: New York Acadmic Sciences), 50–58. doi: 10.1111/j.1749-6632.2003.tb07070.x

Pulvermuller, F., Huss, M., Kherif, F., Martin, F., Hauk, O., and Shtyrov, Y. (2006). Motor cortex maps articulatory features of speech sounds. *Proc. Natl. Acad. Sci. U.S.A.* 103, 7865–7870. doi: 10.1073/pnas.0509989103

Ritchie, C., Smailagic, N., Noel-Storr, A. H., Takwoingi, Y., Flicker, L., Mason, S. E., et al. (2014). Plasma and cerebrospinal fluid amyloid beta for the diagnosis of Alzheimer's disease dementia and other dementias in people with mild cognitive impairment (MCI)*. *Cochrane Database Syst. Rev.* CD008782. doi: 10.1002/14651858.CD008782.pub4

Rizzo, G., Milardi, D., Bertino, S., Basile, G. A., Di Mauro, D., Calamuneri, A., et al. (2018). The limbic and sensorimotor pathways of the human amygdala: a structural connectivity study. *Neuroscience* 385, 166–180. doi: 10.1016/j.neuroscience.2018.05.051

Roalf, D. R., Moberg, M. J., Turetsky, B. I., Brennan, L., Kabadi, S., Wolk, D. A., et al. (2017). A quantitative meta-analysis of olfactory dysfunction in mild cognitive impairment. *J. Neurol. Neurosurg. Psychiatry* 88, 226–232. doi: 10.1136/jnnp-2016-314638

Roberts, R. O., Christianson, T. J., Kremers, W. K., Mielke, M. M., Machulda, M. M., Vassilaki, M., et al. (2016). Association between olfactory dysfunction and amnestic mild cognitive impairment and Alzheimer Disease Dementia. *JAMA Neurol.* 73, 93–101. doi: 10.1001/jamaneurol.2015.2952

Salmon, D. P., and Bondi, M. W. (2009). Neuropsychological assessment of dementia. *Annu. Rev. Psychol.* 60, 257–282. doi: 10.1146/annurev.psych.57.102904.190024

Schab, F. R. (1991). Odor memory - taking stock. *Psychol. Bull.* 109, 242–251. doi: 10.1037//0033-2909.109.2.242

Schubert, C. R., Carmichael, L. L., Murphy, C., Klein, B. E. K., Klein, R., and Cruickshanks, K. J. (2008). Olfaction and the 5-year incidence of cognitive impairment in an epidemiological study of older adults. *J. Am. Geriatr. Soc.* 56, 1517–1521. doi: 10.1111/j.1532-5415.2008.01826.x

Servello, A., Fioretti, A., Gualdi, G., Di Biasi, C., Pittalis, A., Sollaku, S., et al. (2015). Olfactory dysfunction, olfactory bulb volume and Alzheimer's disease: is there a correlation? a pilot study1. *J. Alzheimers Dis.* 48, 395–402. doi: 10.3233/JAD-150232

Silva, M. M. E., Mercer, P. B. S., Witt, M. C. Z., and Pessoa, R. R. (2018). Olfactory dysfunction in Alzheimer's disease systematic review and meta-analysis. *Dement Neuropsychol.* 12, 123–132. doi: 10.1590/1980-57642018dn12-020004

Smith, E. E., and Jonides, J. (1999). Neuroscience - storage and executive processes in the frontal lobes. *Science* 283, 1657–1661. doi: 10.1126/science.283.5408.1657

Tabert, M. H., Liu, X., Doty, R. L., Serby, M., Zamora, D., Pelton, G. H., et al. (2005). A 10-item smell identification scale related to risk for Alzheimer's disease. *Ann. Neurol.* 58, 155–160. doi: 10.1002/ana.20533

Tahmasebi, R., Zehetmayer, S., Pusswald, G., Kovacs, G., Stogmann, E., and Lehrner, J. (2019). Identification of odors, faces, cities and naming of objects in patients with subjective cognitive decline, mild cognitive impairment and Alzheimer s disease: a longitudinal study. *Int. Psychogeriatr.* 31, 537–549. doi: 10.1017/S1041610218001114

Thomann, P. A., Dos Santos, V., Seidl, U., Toro, P., Essig, M., and Schroder, J. (2009a). MRI-derived atrophy of the olfactory bulb and tract in mild cognitive impairment and Alzheimer's disease. *J. Alzheimers Dis.* 17, 213–221. doi: 10.3233/JAD-2009-1036

Thomann, P. A., Dos Santos, V., Toro, P., Schonknecht, P., Essig, M., and Schroder, J. (2009b). Reduced olfactory bulb and tract volume in early Alzheimer's disease–a MRI study. *Neurobiol. Aging* 30, 838–841. doi: 10.1016/j.neurobiolaging.2007.08.001

Tzourio-Mazoyer, N., Landeau, B., Papathanassiou, D., Crivello, F., Etard, O., Delcroix, N., et al. (2002). Automated anatomical labeling of activations in SPM using a macroscopic anatomical parcellation of the MNI MRI single-subject brain. *Neuroimage* 15, 273–289. doi: 10.1006/nimg.2001.0978

Vasavada, M. M., Martinez, B., Wang, J., Eslinger, P. J., Gill, D. J., Sun, X., et al. (2017). Central olfactory dysfunction in Alzheimer's disease and mild cognitive impairment: a functional MRI study *J. Alzheimers Dis.* 59, 359–368. doi: 10.3233/JAD-170310

Vasavada, M. M., Wang, J. L., Eslinger, F. J., Gill, D. J., Sun, X. Y., Karunanayaka, P., et al. (2015). Olfactory cortex degeneration in Alzheimer's disease and mild cognitive impairment. *J. Alzheimers Dis.* 45, 947–958. doi: 10.3233/JAD-141947

Wang, J. J., Wei, Q., Bai, T. J., Zhou, X. Q., Sun, H., Becker, B., et al. (2017). Electroconvulsive therapy selectively enhanced feedforward connectivity from fusiform face area to amygdala in major depressive disorder. *Soc. Cogn. Affect. Neur.* 12, 1983–1992. doi: 10.1093/scan/nsx100

Wardlaw, J. M., Smith, E. E., Biessels, G. J., Cordonnier, C., Fazekas, F., Frayne, R., et al. (2013). Neuroimaging standards for research into small vessel disease and its contribution to ageing and neurodegeneration. *Lancet Neurol.* 12, 822–838. doi: 10.1016/S1474-4422(13)70124-8

Wild, C. J., Yusuf, A., Wilson, D. E., Peelle, J. E., Davis, M. H., and Johnsrude, I. S. (2012). Effortful listening: the processing of degraded speech depends critically on attention. *J. Neurosci.* 32, 14010–14021. doi: 10.1523/JNEUROSCI.1528-12.2012

Wilson, S. M., Saygin, A. P., Sereno, M. I., and Iacoboni, M. (2004). Listening to speech activates motor areas involved in speech production. *Nat. Neurosci.* 7, 701–702. doi: 10.1038/nn1263

Woodward, M. R., Amrutkar, C. V., Shah, H. C., Benedict, R. H. B., Rajakrishnan, S., Doody, R. S., et al. (2017). Validation of olfactory deficit as a biomarker of Alzheimer disease. *Neurol.Clin. Pract.* 7, 5–14. doi: 10.1212/CPJ.0000000000000293

Wu, Y., Zhang, Y., Liu, Y., Liu, J., Duan, Y., Wei, X., et al. (2016). Distinct changes in functional connectivity in posteromedial cortex subregions during the progress of Alzheimer's disease. *Front. Neuroanat.* 10:41. doi: 10.3389/fnana.2016.00041

Yousry, T. A., Schmid, U. D., Alkadhi, H., Schmidt, D., Peraud, A., Buettner, A., et al. (1997). Localization of the motor hand area to a knob on the precentral gyrus - A new landmark. *Brain* 120, 141–157. doi: 10.1093/brain/120.1.141

Yu, Q., Guo, P., Li, D., Zuo, L., Lian, T., Yu, S., et al. (2018). Olfactory dysfunction and its relationship with clinical symptoms of Alzheimer disease. *Aging Dis.* 9, 1084–1095. doi: 10.14336/AD.2018.0819

16

Elevations in Serum Dickkopf-1 and Disease Progression in Community-Dwelling Older Adults with Mild Cognitive Impairment and Mild-to-Moderate Alzheimer's Disease

Laura Tay[1], Bernard Leung[2,3], Audrey Yeo[4], Mark Chan[4,5] and Wee Shiong Lim[4,5]*

[1] Department of General Medicine, Sengkang General Hospital, Singapore, Singapore, [2] Department of Rheumatology, Allergy and Immunology, Tan Tock Seng Hospital, Singapore, Singapore, [3] Health and Social Sciences, Singapore Institute of Technology, Singapore, Singapore, [4] Institute of Geriatrics and Active Ageing, Tan Tock Seng Hospital, Singapore, Singapore, [5] Department of Geriatric Medicine, Tan Tock Seng Hospital, Singapore, Singapore

***Correspondence:**
Laura Tay
laura.tay.b.g@singhealth.com.sg

Background: Disruption of Wnt signaling has been implicated in dysfunctional synaptic plasticity, the degree of which correlates with Alzheimer's disease severity. We sought to examine whether serum levels of Dickkopf-1 (Dkk-1), a Wnt antagonist, are associated with global disease progression in older adults with mild cognitive impairment (MCI) and mild-to-moderate AD.

Methods: We prospectively followed 88 older adults with MCI and mild-to-moderate AD attending a Memory Clinic. Cognitive performance, functional performance and neuropsychological symptoms were assessed at baseline and after 1 year. We reviewed neuroimaging for white matter changes and medial temporal atrophy, and performed ApoE genotyping at baseline. Serum Dkk-1 was assayed at baseline and 1 year, along with blood biomarkers of inflammation and endocrine dysfunction. We defined global disease progression ("progressors") as an increase in Clinical Dementia Rating Sum-of-Boxes (CDR-SB) score by $\geq$2 points at 1 year.

Results: Fifteen (17.0%) participants had global disease progression. At baseline, there was no difference in cognitive performance and neuropsychiatric symptoms between groups, although progressors were more impaired in instrumental activities of daily living ($p = 0.008$). Progressors had significantly greater deterioration in cognitive performance ($p = 0.002$), with significantly worse functional performance and more severe neuropsychiatric symptoms ($p = 0.042$) at follow-up. Serum inflammatory and endocrine biomarkers at baseline and 1 year were similar between progressors and non-progressors. Serum Dkk-1 had increased significantly from baseline amongst progressors, while non-progressors exhibited decremental Dkk-1 over time (Dkk-1_{change}: 354.304 ± 670.467 vs. −173.582 ± 535.676 ng/ml, p = 0.001). Adjusting for age, gender and baseline cognitive performance, incremental Dkk-1 independently predicted global cognitive decline (p = 0.012).

Conclusion: Our results suggest progressively dysfunctional Wnt signaling through Dkk-1 antagonism contributes to disease progression amongst older adults with MCI and mild-moderate AD.

Keywords: Dickkopf-1, mild cognitive impairment, Alzheimer's disease, disease progression, inflammation

INTRODUCTION

Alzheimer's disease (AD) is the most common form of dementia, with significant impact on the individual, caregiver, health systems and society. Current treatment strategies remain only symptomatic, with no known cure or disease-modifying therapy. While a natural trajectory of decline is anticipated, disease progression in AD is significantly heterogeneous with high variability in the rate of cognitive decline amongst afflicted persons (Lam et al., 2013). Risk factors for dementia have been widely reported in the literature, and a recent study suggested that rapid progression may be influenced by demographic and clinical factors as well as genetic interactions (Ferrari et al., 2018).

Synaptic dysfunction occurs early in the course of AD, before evidence of neuronal cell death, and the loss of synapses correlates best with cognitive decline (Terry et al., 1991; Palop and Mucke, 2010). Extracellular plaques of amyloid β (Aβ) and neurofibrillary tangles of hyperphosphorylated tau are the neuropathological hallmarks of AD and contribute to synaptic toxicity and neuronal loss. Wnt signaling has a key role in synaptic plasticity and memory, being neuroprotective against Aβ-induced toxicity, tau phosphorylation, neuroinflammation and apoptosis (Vallee and Lecarpentier, 2016; Tapia-Rojas and Inestrosa, 2018a). Dickkopf-1 protein (Dkk-1) is a secreted Wnt antagonist and found to be elevated in post-mortem brain samples from AD patients (Caricasole et al., 2004). Mouse models have demonstrated Dkk-1 as a critical participant in synaptic disassembly induced by Aβ, with short-term exposure to Aβ yielding increasing expression of Dkk-1 with consequent rapid synaptic loss (Purro et al., 2012). The observed enhanced working memory and memory consolidation in old mice deficient in Dkk-1 suggests that neutralization of Dkk-1 may be beneficial in counteracting age-related cognitive decline (Seib et al., 2013). There has been only one prior study that examined the relationship between circulating Dkk-1 levels and cognition in older adults, in which baseline Dkk-1 predicted decline in cognitive performance during follow-up (Ross et al., 2018). However, the study specifically recruited participants with subjective memory concerns and excluded those with confirmed clinical diagnoses of mild cognitive impairment (MCI) and dementia.

Dkk-1 appears to play a role in chronic inflammation (Diarra et al., 2007; Sato et al., 2010; Chae et al., 2016), which has been implicated in the neuropathological profile of AD (Uchihara et al., 1997; Vehmas et al., 2003). Plasma levels of inflammatory cytokines had also been associated with pathological severity, with significant elevations in peripheral inflammatory signals over time amongst AD patients who exhibited rapid cognitive decline (Leung et al., 2013).

The objective of this exploratory study was to investigate whether circulating Dkk-1 is associated with disease progression in older adults with MCI and mild-to-moderate Alzheimer's dementia. In addition, we measured serum markers representing inflammation and the endocrine axes due to reported associations with AD. If established, the study findings would support the potential role of Dkk-1 antagonist molecules to ameliorate AD progression.

MATERIALS AND METHODS

Study Population

This is a prospective study of community-dwelling older adults from a tertiary Memory Clinic in Singapore. We recruited 96 subjects with a diagnosis of MCI or mild-moderate Alzheimer's dementia (AD) between December 2012 and November 2013. 88 participants completed a 1-year follow up.

Informed written consent was obtained from the patient or legally acceptable representative where appropriate. Ethics approval was obtained from the Domain Specific Review Board (DSRB) of the National Healthcare Group (NHG).

Diagnostic Categories

MCI was operationalized as follows: (1) global Clinical Dementia Rating (CDR) (Morris, 1993) score of 0.5; (2) presence of subjective memory complaint with corroboration by a reliable informant; (3) delayed recall > 1 SD below the age and education-adjusted means of healthy community-dwelling subjects based on an earlier normative study (Sahadevan et al., 2002); (4) relatively normal general cognitive function, defined as Chinese Mini Mental State Examination (CMMSE) (Sahadevan et al., 2000) score ≥21 for subjects with ≤6 years education and ≥24 for those with >6 years of education; (5) largely intact activities of daily living; and (6) no clinical dementia.

Mild-moderate AD subjects were diagnosed according to National Institute of Neurological and Communicative Disorders and Stroke and the Alzheimer's Disease and Related Disorders Association (NINCDS-ADRDA) criteria for *probable AD* (McKhann et al., 1984), with global CDR of 0.5, 1 or 2, for very mild, mild or moderate dementia, respectively. We excluded subjects with a diagnosis of *possible AD* in view of the confounding co-morbid diagnoses and differing clinical course in these individuals.

Eligibility Criteria

Potentially eligible subjects must have been aged $\geq$55 years, with a diagnosis of MCI or mild to moderate AD at baseline, community-dwelling, and accompanied by a reliable caregiver informant.

Subjects with presence of other central nervous conditions (stroke disease, Parkinson's disease, subdural hematoma, normal pressure hydrocephalus, and brain tumor); presence of systemic conditions that can contribute to cognitive impairment (hypothyroidism, B12 deficiency, and hypercalcaemia); and presence of any active neuropsychiatric conditions producing disability were excluded. Residents of sheltered or nursing homes were also excluded.

The validity of the overall cognitive evaluation process and CDR scoring has been previously established (Chong and Sahadevan, 2003; Lim et al., 2005). All patients had undergone laboratory investigations and neuroimaging to exclude potentially reversible causes of dementia. All cases were discussed in a multidisciplinary consensus meeting in which all relevant results were reviewed for accurate clinical phenotyping. Patients meeting study eligibility criteria were then recruited.

Measures

Cognitive Assessment

We used the CDR (Morris, 1993), a structured clinician rating, to assess cognitive change and determine dementia severity. The CDR is a global dementia rating scale encompassing assessment across six domains – memory, orientation, judgment-problem solving, community affairs, home hobbies, and personal care – providing both a global and sum-of-boxes (CDR-SB) score (range 0 to 18). Global CDR 0 indicates no dementia, and CDR 1, 2 and 3 correspond to mild, moderate, and severe dementia, respectively. A global CDR stage of 0.5 can be representative of either very mild dementia or MCI, with the latter diagnosis being assigned when the cognitive impairment does not fulfill dementia criteria. CDR-SB provides a finer gradation of impairment and has demonstrated sensitivity to progression in dementia (Williams et al., 2013). The attending geriatrician, trained in administration of the CDR, rated each patient's CDR at baseline and 1-year follow-up. We defined disease progression as an increase $\geq$2 points from baseline on the CDR-SB, based on an observed annual rate of change in CDR-SB score of 1.91 $\pm$ 0.07 amongst participants with mild AD (Williams et al., 2013).

Cognitive performance was assessed using the Chinese Mini-Mental State Examination (CMMSE). MCI subjects also underwent a neuropsychological assessment, which was modeled after the Consortium to Establish a Registry for Alzheimer's Disease (CERAD) psychometric instrument, with local validation and education adjustment (Sahadevan et al., 2002). The battery of tests provides for assessment across multiple cognitive domains – memory (word list for immediate and delayed recall, and recognition memory), language (category fluency and modified Boston Naming Test), executive function (category fluency and Color Trail 2), and visuo-spatial ability (Block Design subtest of the Weschler Adult Intelligence Scale-revised).

Blood Biomarkers

All subjects underwent blood biomarker measurements at baseline and 1 year. Participants fasted for 8 h before the blood draw, and the aliquoted serum was frozen and stored at $-80°$C until the tests were performed. Inflammatory status was assessed by serum levels of Dkk-1, soluble tumor necrosis factor-α receptor-1 (TNF-R1, both R&D Systems, Minneapolis, MN, United States), and interleukin-6 (high sensitive IL-6, eBioscience, San Diego, CA, United States) via ELISA. The endocrine markers insulin-like growth factor-1 (IGF-1) and dehydroepiandrosterone sulfate (DHEA-S) were quantified using commercial ELISA assays (BioVendor, Brno, Czech Republic and Abcam, Cambridge, United Kingdom, respectively). All biomarkers were measured in duplicates according to manufacturers' recommendations, and the average value was reported for all assays. Detection limits were as follows: DHEAS, 0.2 μmol/L; Dkk-1, 30 pg/ml; IGF-1, 2 ng/ml; IL-6, 0.1 pg/ml; TNF-R1, 30 pg/ml.

Other Co-variates

Demographic data and co-morbid vascular risk factors - hypertension, hyperlipidemia, diabetes mellitus, atrial fibrillation, peripheral vascular disease, smoking history, and ischemic heart disease – were documented at baseline. We reviewed participants' medical records for the presence of chronic inflammatory disease and any active treatment with steroids or immunosuppressant medication.

At both baseline and 1-year follow-up, functional performance was evaluated using Barthel's basic activities of daily living (ADL) index (Mahoney and Barthel, 1965) and Lawton and Brody's instrumental ADL (iADL) index (Barberger-Gateau et al., 1992), while severity of neuropsychological symptoms was assessed using the Neuropsychiatric Inventory Questionnaire (Cummings, 1997).

We reviewed each subject's neuroimaging scan - brain computed tomography (CT) scan (27 subjects) or magnetic resonance imaging (MRI) (68 subjects). White matter lesion (WML) severity was graded using the Age-Related White Matter Changes (ARWMC) scale applicable to both CT and MRI (using T2-weighted axial slices), in five different regions and separately for the right and left hemispheres – frontal area, parieto-occipital area, temporal area, infra-tentorial area, and basal ganglia. Each region was graded on a 4-point scale, and the global white matter score derived from summation of the individual scores (range 0–30), with higher ARWMC score reflecting a greater burden of white matter lesions (Wahlund et al., 2001). Medial temporal atrophy (MTA) score reflecting neurodegeneration was scored on T1-weighted coronal slices for MRI or non-enhanced CT, parallel to the brainstem axis and perpendicular to the hippocampal axis, by a consensus method where the scores range from 0 (no atrophy) to 4 (severe atrophy) (Wahlund et al., 2000). Visual ratings for ARWMC and MTA were performed by a blinded rater.

APOE genotyping into *APOEε2,3,4* isoforms was performed via restriction enzyme analysis using the Applied Biosystems platform ABI Prism 310 Genetic Analyzer.

Statistical Analyses

Descriptive data are presented as means (± SD) or median (interquartile range, IQR) for quantitative variables and as absolute and relative frequencies for categorical variables. We performed univariate analyses comparing progressors and non-progressors in baseline demographics, co-morbidities and neuroimaging markers, along with changes in cognitive, functional performance and blood biomarker measures, using independent-sample *t*-test and Wilcoxon Rank-Sum test for parametric and non-parametric continuous variables, respectively, and Chi-square test for categorical variables. Pearson's correlation was performed to examine the relationship between changes in individual blood biomarkers and cognition as measured on both CMMSE and CDR-SB, for the overall cohort as well as subgroup analyses by baseline diagnosis (MCI or AD).

Multiple logistic regression, with disease progression (CDR-SB increase ≥ 2 points) as the outcome variable, was performed to examine the independent role of blood biomarkers. The full model included *a priori* age, gender, and baseline cognitive performance, in addition to each predictor biomarker showing significant univariate association with the outcome of interest. The chosen variables were guided by our sample size and prior literature on factors potentially influencing disease progression in AD, while ensuring no multi-collinearity.

Statistical analyses were performed using SPSS version 24. All statistical tests were two-tailed, with p-value ≤ 0.05 considered statistically significant. Owing to the number of blood biomarkers examined in our correlation analyses, we applied Bonferroni correction (0.05 divided by 5 blood biomarkers) to control for family wise error rate, such that only a p-value ≤ 0.01 would be considered significant for blood biomarker changes.

RESULTS

Clinical Characteristics (Table 1)

The mean age of our cohort was 77.0 ± 6.8 years, with 15 (15.6%) having a diagnosis of MCI, 69 (71.9%) mild AD, and 12 (12.5%) moderate AD. Eighty-eight (91.7%) of the 96 participants completed 1-year follow-up, of whom 14 had MCI and 74 had mild-moderate AD at baseline. There was no significant difference in age, gender, and baseline cognitive performance between participants who completed vs. those who were lost to follow-up.

Fifteen (17.0%) of 88 participants who completed 1-year follow-up exhibited global disease progression. Fourteen (18.9%) of participants with mild-moderate AD at diagnosis fulfilled CDR-SB cut-off for progression, while only 1 participant (7.1%) in the MCI group had progressed.

Baseline cognitive diagnosis (MCI, mild or moderate AD), cognitive performance and severity of neuropsychiatric symptoms were similar between participants with and without disease progression. However, progressors had significantly greater functional impairment in instrumental ADLs at baseline (15.6 ± 5.4 vs. 12.5 ± 3.4, $p = 0.008$) and follow-up. At 1-year follow-up, there was significantly greater decline in cognitive performance and increased severity of neuropsychiatric symptoms amongst progressors compared with non-progressors.

TABLE 1 | Clinical characteristics and disease progression.

	Progressors *N* = 15	Non-progressors *N* = 73	*p*-value
Demographics			
Age	76.2 (6.2)	76.9 (6.7)	0.726
Gender (Female)	11 (73.3%)	47 (64.4%)	0.505
Ethnicity (Chinese)	14 (93.3%)	68 (93.2%)	0.745
Education (years)	5.8 (5.1)	5.9 (4.5)	0.949
Comorbidities			
Hypertension	11 (73.3%)	47 (64.4%)	0.505
Diabetes mellitus	3 (20%)	24 (32.9%)	0.325
Hyperlipidemia	7 (46.7%)	47 (64.4%)	0.199
Ischemic heart disease	1 (6.7%)	14 (19.2%)	0.451
Atrial fibrillation	0	2 (2.7%)	1.00
Stroke/TIA	0	3 (4.1%)	1.00
Baseline diagnosis			0.540
MCI	1 (6.7%)	13 (17.8%)	
Mild AD	12 (80%)	53 (72.6%)	
Moderate AD	2 (13.3%)	7 (9.6%)	
Cognitive performance			
$CMMSE_{baseline}$	16.5 (4.7)	18.7 (4.9)	0.116
$CMMSE_{1-yr}$	13.0 (6.4)	18.2 (5.7)	0.003**
$CMMSE_{change}$	−3.6 (3.2)	−0.6 (3.1)	0.002**
Mood			
$Depression_{baseline}$	0	2 (2.7%)	1.00
$Depression_{1-yr}$	0	0	
Behavioral			
$NPI\text{-}sev_{baseline}$	5.3 (5.1)	3.4 (3.3)	0.198
$NPI\text{-}sev_{1-yr}$	7.0 (6.8)	3.0 (4.0)	0.042*
$NPI\text{-}sev_{change}$	1.7 (4.7)	−0.4 (3.2)	0.033*
Functional			
$MBI_{baseline}$	100 (90–100)	100 (95–100)	0.092
MBI_{1-yr}	95 (90–100)	100 (95–100)	0.019*
MBI_{change}	0 (−5–0)	0 (−2.5–0)	0.234
$iADL_{baseline}$	12.5 (3.4)	15.6 (5.4)	0.008**
$iADL_{1-yr}$	9.1 (4.3)	14.5 (5.5)	0.001**
$iADL_{change}$	−3.4 (4.3)	−8.2 (1.1)	0.059
Neuroimaging			
ARWMC total (*n* = 86)	5.31 (5.98)	5.71 (4.03)	0.405
MTA (*n* = 83)	1.46 (1.13)	1.51 (1.03)	0.868
ApoE4 positive	6 (40%)	25 (34.7%)	0.654
Use of cognitive enhancer	13 (86.7%)	55 (76.4%)	0.506

*AD, Alzheimer's disease; ARWMC, age-related white matter changes; CMMSE, Chinese Mini Mental State Examination; iADL, Lawton and Brody's instrumental activities of daily living; MBI, Modified Barthel Index; MCI, mild cognitive impairment; MTA, medial temporal atrophy; NPI, neuropsychiatric inventory questionnaire. Mean (SD) or median (IQR), unless otherwise indicated. *P < 0.05; **P < 0.01.*

Vascular burden, as reflected by comorbidities and extent of white matter lesions on neuroimaging, was similar between progressors and non-progressors. There was no difference in severity of hippocampal atrophy at baseline, and ApoE-4 status was similar, between progressors and non-progressors.

Blood Biomarkers

Association of Disease Progression With Blood Biomarkers at Baseline and 1 Year (Table 2)

While there was no significant difference in baseline Dkk-1, serum Dkk-1 at 1 year was significantly higher in progressors compared with non-progressors (1045.762 ± 553.839 vs. 714.429 ± 366.852, p = 0.005). Contrary to the observed decremental Dkk-1 at 1 year relative to baseline amongst non-progressors, Dkk-1 had increased significantly from baseline amongst progressors ($DKK\text{-}1_{change}$: 354.304 ± 670.467 vs. -173.582 ± 535.676, p = 0.001).

Other serum inflammatory and endocrine biomarkers - both at baseline and 1 year - were similar between progressors and non-progressors. There was also no difference in magnitude of individual inflammatory (IL-6 and TNF-R1) and endocrine biomarker change from baseline to 1 year between progressors and non-progressors.

Correlation Between Changes in Blood Biomarkers and Cognitive Performance (Table 3)

In analysis for the overall cohort of 88 participants, we observed no significant correlation between decline in CMMSE score and magnitude of change in individual biomarkers over time. Amongst the individual blood biomarkers, only incremental serum Dkk-1 over time correlated significantly with change in CDR sum-of-boxes score (r = 0.275, p = 0.010).

In subgroup analysis amongst MCI participants, there was no correlation between any blood biomarker with either CMMSE or CDR-SB score change. However, we observed significant moderate correlation between incremental serum Dkk-1 and progressively higher CDR-SB scores over time in participants with mild-moderate AD at diagnosis (r = 0.346, p = 0.003).

Multiple Logistic Regression Model for Global Cognitive Decline (Table 4)

In multiple logistic regression, adjusting for age, gender, and baseline cognitive performance, incremental Dkk-1 over time independently predicted global disease progression. Incremental Dkk-1 within the upper quartile conferred 4.91-fold higher odds (95% confidence interval: 1.43–16.93, p = 0.012) for global cognitive decline.

We repeated the multiple logistic regression model for the subgroup with diagnosis of mild-moderate AD at baseline. Incremental Dkk-1 in the upper quartile significantly increased the odds for disease progression (Odds ratio = 3.96, 95% confidence interval: 1.07–14.39, p = 0.039). As only 1 MCI participant exhibited CDR-SB cut-off for progression, subgroup analysis was not performed for MCI.

DISCUSSION

This is the first study to demonstrate an association between circulating Dkk-1 and progressive decline in a cohort of older adults with MCI and mild-moderate AD. Deterioration in cognitive performance was paralleled by greater dependence in functional performance and increased neuropsychological symptoms, supporting the role of Dkk-1 in overall disease progression, particularly with established Alzheimer's dementia. Notably, there was no difference in baseline vascular burden, hippocampal atrophy, and ApoE-4 status, nor was there a difference in other inflammatory and endocrine blood biomarkers.

TABLE 2 | Blood biomarkers and disease progression.

	Progressors N = 15	Non-progressors N = 73	p-value
$IL6_{baseline}$ (pg/ml)	0.170 (0.060 – 0.262)	0.227 (0.105 – 0.506)	0.190
$IL6_{1-yr}$ (pg/ml)	0.420 (0.290 – 0.668)	0.500 (0.300 – 1.582)	0.424
$IL6_{change}$ (pg/ml)	0.308 (0.140 – 0.450)	0.251 (0.058 – 0.564)	0.786
$TNFR1_{baseline}$ (pg/ml)	6858.91 (4791.03 – 9214.85)	6929.04 (5248.25 – 8648.16)	0.837
$TNFR1_{1-yr}$ (pg/ml)	2497.58 (1713.54 – 3483.35)	3465.24 (1978.96 – 4638.76)	0.146
$TNFR1_{change}$ (pg/ml)	−4689.65 (− 7501.31 – 490.83)	−4429.02 (− 6298.33 – 329.34)	0.606
$IGF1_{baseline}$ (ng/ml)	129.25 (72.43 – 136.84)	110.74 (72.38 – 167.58)	0.960
$IGF1_{1\ year}$ (ng/ml)	87.118 (75.787 – 134.751)	102.235 (75.091 – 152.205)	0.706
$IGF1_{change}$ (ng/ml)	−12.33 (− 53.745 – 5.504)	−3.281 (− 27.381 – 18.614)	0.434
$DHEAS_{baseline}$ µmol/L	1.387 (0.700 – 2.193)	1.865 (1.056 – 2.979)	0.310
$DHEAS_{1-yr}$ µmol/L	1.552 (0.773 – 2.122)	1.943 (1.176 – 3.100)	0.136
$DHEAS_{change}$ µmol/L	0.025 (− 0.830 – 0.502)	0.187 (− 0.621 – 0.721)	0.534
$Dkk\text{-}1_{baseline}$ (pg/ml)	611.270 (493.09 – 855.650)	824.790 (687.335 – 1057.795)	0.064
$Dkk\text{-}1_{1-yr}$ (pg/ml)	1021.120 (863.560 – 1317.650)	731.180 (419.931 – 1047.955)	0.024*
$Dkk\text{-}1_{change}$ (pg/ml)	487.610 (24.046 – 899.060)	−142.910 (− 605.305 – 179.605)	0.003**

*DHEAS, dehydroepiandrosterone sulfate; Dkk-1, Dickkopf-1; IGF1, insulin-like growth factor-1; IL6, interleukin-6; TNFR1, tumor necrosis factor-α receptor-1. *P < 0.05; **P < 0.01.*

TABLE 3 | Correlation between changes in blood biomarkers and cognitive performance.

	Overall cohort (N = 88)		MCI (N = 14)		AD (N = 74)	
	CMMSE change (r, p value)	**CDR-SB change (r, p value)**	**CMMSE change (r, p value)**	**CDR-SB change (r, p value)**	**CMMSE change (r, p value)**	**CDR-SB change (r, p value)**
$IL6_{change}$	−0.130 (0.233)	0.002 (0.983)	0.093 (0.751)	0.110 (0.709)	−0.232 (0.050)	0.023 (0.899)
$TNFR1_{change}$	−0.093 (0.395)	−0.012 (0.915)	−0.199 (0.494)	0.284 (0.325)	−0.077 (0.521)	−0.054 (0.647)
$IGF\text{-}1_{change}$	−0.017 (0.879)	−0.055 (0.609)	−0.056 (0.849)	0.141 (0.630)	−0.018 (0.884)	−0.068 (0.567)
$DHEAS_{change}$	0.102 (0.352)	−0.072 (0.506)	−0.059 (0.841)	−0.300 (0.298)	0.089 (0.457)	−0.032 (0.785)
$Dkk\text{-}1_{change}$	−0.137 (0.208)	0.275 (0.010)*	−0.357 (0.210)	−0.125 (0.295)	−0.125 (0.295)	0.346 (0.003)**

*DHEAS, dehydroepiandrosterone sulfate; Dkk-1, Dickkopf-1; IGF1, insulin-like growth factor-1; IL6, interleukin-6; TNFR1, tumor necrosis factor-α receptor-1. *P < 0.05; **p < 0.01.*

TABLE 4 | Multiple logistic regression for global cognitive decline.

	Overall cohort (N = 88)		AD (N = 74)	
	OR (95% CI)	***p*-value**	**OR (95% CI)**	***p*-value**
Age	1.002 (0.917–1.093)	0.972	0.968 (0.883–1.062)	0.489
Female	1.015 (0.258–3.989)	0.983	1.448 (0.323–6.499)	0.629
Baseline CMMSE	0.906 (0.793–1.036)	0.149	0.929 (0.801–1.077)	0.527
$Dkk\text{-}1_{change(topquartile)}$	4.913 (1.426–16.929)	0.012*	3.960 (1.074–14.593)	0.039*

*Overall cohort: R^2 = 0.169; AD: R^2 = 0.142. *P < 0.05.*

The Wnt signaling pathway is fundamental to the development of the central nervous system and also plays critical roles in the adult brain, having been implicated in synaptic plasticity and cognition (Ortiz-Matamoros et al., 2013; Inestrosa and Varela-Nallar, 2014). Inhibition of Wnt signaling in mouse models of AD has been associated with accelerated onset and progression of AD neuropathology and memory loss (Tapia-Rojas and Inestrosa, 2018b). As a negative modulator of Wnt signaling, Dkk-1 has been demonstrated to trigger synaptic loss mediated by amyloid-β (Purro et al., 2012). Mouse models suggest that Dkk-1 increases with age and its deletion attenuates age-related cognitive decline (Seib et al., 2013). To date, there is only one other study which examined serological Dkk-1 in a cohort of older adults with subjective cognitive concerns but in the absence of clinically diagnosed dementia (Ross et al., 2018). Although baseline Dkk-1 was negatively related to the annual rate of change in global cognition, this association between Dkk-1 and cognition was however lost following exclusion of participants who developed dementia during follow-up, suggesting that Dkk-1 may be more predictive of dementia than mere cognitive change. Our results complement this earlier study by examining a cohort of older adults across the spectrum of cognitive impairment ranging from MCI to mild-moderate AD. Increased Dkk-1 over time correlated with progressive disease severity as indicated by the change in CDR-SB scores. Specifically, our subgroup analysis also showed incremental Dkk-1 was significantly associated with progressively higher CDR-SB scores amongst participants with mild-moderate dementia, but not at the MCI stage. The apparent lack of correlation between changes in Dkk-1 and disease progression in MCI may be attributable to the slower natural progression in MCI compared with dementia given the relatively short duration of follow-up in our study (Storandt et al., 2002), as well as the etiological heterogeneity of MCI, although patients with non-amnestic presentations as well as central nervous or systemic conditions that could potentially contribute to cognitive impairment were excluded. In line with the present findings, Dkk-3 - a related Dkk-1 protein - was also noted to be elevated in both plasma and cerebrospinal fluid of patients with AD (Zenzaimer et al., 2009), although its action on the Wnt-pathway is context-dependent and its induction of vascular endothelial growth factor with dual effects in the central nervous system may occur independently of the Wnt signaling pathway (Busceti et al., 2018). Interestingly, we observed decremental Dkk-1 over time amongst non-progressors, which could not be accounted for by cognitive enhancer use or clinical comorbidities, although our data limits further exploration for possible mechanisms for restoration of Wnt-activity. With synaptic failure underlying the cognitive manifestations of AD, our data suggests that Dkk-1 may contribute to AD progression through synaptic dysfunction consequent to Wnt antagonism.

Contrary to the established role of inflammation in pathogenesis of AD (Perry et al., 2001; Heppner et al., 2015; Bagyinszky et al., 2017), we found no association between blood biomarkers of inflammation and global cognitive decline in our cohort of cognitively impaired older adults. Despite elevated concentrations of inflammatory markers within senile plaques and neurofibrillary tangles (Hosfield and Humpel, 2015), studies examining circulating levels of inflammatory markers and cognitive decline or clinical AD have had conflicting results (Tan et al., 2007; Sundelof et al., 2009). Furthermore, clinical trials of non-steroidal anti-inflammatory drugs have failed to demonstrate benefit on both risk and progression of AD (Aisen et al., 2003; Szekely et al., 2008). In the current study, the lack of relationship between peripheral inflammatory markers and disease progression may be attributed to the effect of the blood-brain barrier such that circulating inflammatory biomarkers may have limited utility in reflecting the changes occurring within the brain.

Disease progression in MCI and mild-moderate AD was also not associated with baseline or changes in serum concentrations of IGF-1 and DHEA-S. Beyond its role on somatic growth and development, IGF-1 has a neurotrophic role and is involved in the regulation of synaptic plasticity (Nieto-Estevez et al., 2016). While the liver is the primary site of IGF-1 production and systemic IGF-1 readily permeates the blood-brain barrier, there is also small local production in brain regions, including the hippocampus (Nieto-Estevez et al., 2016). Earlier studies on the relationship between serum IGF-1 and cognition in older adults have yielded mixed evidence, including the interesting observation of a possible U-shaped relationship where both high and low serum concentrations of IGF-1 were associated with poorer cognitive function (Frater et al., 2018). Most of the earlier studies involved healthy older adults, although in a small cohort of older persons with MCI, higher serum IGF-1 was associated with better cognitive performance, while lower IGF-1 concentration was also found to be associated with MCI (Calvo et al., 2013; Doi et al., 2015). However, with the earlier analyses being cross-sectional, it remains uncertain whether individual changes may potentially affect the rate of cognitive decline over time. Our results suggest that disease progression following established clinical manifestation of AD is independent of circulating IGF-1 changes.

Despite biologic evidence for the neuroprotective effects of androgens against amyloid-β induced apoptosis and tau hyperphosphorylation, we found no association between DHEA-S and disease progression. Our findings are consistent with an earlier study in which plasma DHEA-S was not associated with presence of AD, impairment in cognitive domains, or cumulative mortality (Bo et al., 2006), albeit in contradiction to a subsequent study reporting lower plasma DHEA in AD patients respective to age-matched controls (Aldred and Mecocci, 2010). Further, DHEA levels within cerebrospinal fluid were significantly higher in AD patients compared with cognitively normal controls and correlated with Braak neuropathological disease stage. Postulated reasons for the observed elevation include compensatory mechanisms in AD, heightened stress in more severely ill patients with AD, as well as induction by amyloid-β, indicating an adaptive response (Naylor et al., 2008). However, while CSF DHEA levels were similarly elevated in AD relative to controls in a separate study, CSF DHEA-S levels were notably significantly lower, suggesting that DHEA elevation may be consequent to its accumulation from reduced downstream transformation, rather than being a neuroprotective mechanism (Kim et al., 2003). On the contrary, DHEA positively modulates excitatory *N*-methyl-D-aspartate receptors while it negatively modulates inhibitory γ-aminobutyric receptors, potentially driving the excitotoxicity in AD and thus representing a non-adaptive response that may be driving AD pathophysiology (Naylor et al., 2008).

The strength of this study lies in our careful phenotyping and exclusion of participants with other central nervous conditions, such that the findings may be more specific to AD pathology, particularly for MCI which is etiologically heterogeneous. With regards to study limitations, we acknowledge that the relatively small sample size of only 15 progressors in our exploratory study may have contributed to the failure to demonstrate an association between disease progression and inflammatory as well as endocrine biomarkers. However, even with the whole cohort pooled, there was no correlation between serial change in inflammatory-endocrine biomarkers and change in cognitive performance or global disease severity. It also remains to be ascertained whether serum levels of biomarkers may reflect their concentrations in the brain. For instance, while circulating IGF-1 readily crosses the blood-brain barrier, local paracrine production has been postulated to be the major source of IGF-1 within the brain. The possibility of circulating biomarker levels being downstream of ongoing pathological changes in the brain cannot be definitively excluded, particularly with the absence of a normal control group. Further, the lack of cognitively healthy elderly precludes inference on the diagnostic or predictive utility of the examined biomarkers and the pathophysiology driving the initial symptomatic manifestations of AD.

In conclusion, our study provides preliminary clinical evidence for progressively dysfunctional Wnt signaling through DKK-1 antagonism in contributing to disease progression amongst cognitively impaired older adults with MCI and mild-moderate AD. The findings offer a platform to encourage further search for Dkk-1 antagonist molecules as potential therapeutic agents to ameliorate AD progression.

AUTHOR CONTRIBUTIONS

LT, MC, and WL contributed to the conception and design of the study. BL performed the blood biomarker analysis. AY contributed to data collection. LT wrote the first draft of the manuscript. BL and WL wrote sections of the manuscript. All authors contributed to manuscript revision, and read and approved the submitted version.

FUNDING

This study was funded by NHG Clinician Scientist Career Scheme CSCS 12002 and NHG CSCS 13001.

REFERENCES

Aisen, P. S., Schafer, K. A., Grundman, M., Pfeiffer, E., Sano, M., Davis, K. L., et al. (2003). Effects of rofecoxib or naproxen vs placebo on Alzheimer disease progression: a randomized controlled trial. *JAMA* 289, 2819–2826. doi: 10.1001/jama.289.21.2819

Aldred, S., and Mecocci, P. (2010). Decreased dehydroepiandrosterone (DHEA) and dehydroepiandrosterone sulphate (DHEAS) concentrations in plasma of Alzheimer's disease (AD) patients. *Arch. Gerontol. Geriatr.* 51, e16–e18. doi: 10.1016/j.archger.2009.07.001

Bagyinszky, E., Giau, V. V., Shim, K., Suk, K., An, S. S. A., and Kim, S. (2017). Role of inflammatory molecules in the Alzheimer's disease progression and diagnosis. *J. Neurol. Sci.* 376, 242–254. doi: 10.1016/j.jns.2017.03.031

Barberger-Gateau, P., Commenges, D., Gagnon, M., Letenneur, L., Sauvel, C., and Dartigues, J. F. (1992). Instrumental activities of daily living as a screening tool for cognitive impairment and dementia in elderly community dwellers. *J. Am. Geriatr. Soc.* 40, 1129–1134. doi: 10.1111/j.1532-5415.1992.tb01802.x

Bo, M., Massaia, M., Zannella, P., Cappa, G., Ferrario, E., Rainero, I., et al. (2006). Dehydroepiandrosterone sulphate (DHEA-S) and Alzheimer's dementia in older subjects. *Int. J. Geriatr. Psychiatry* 21, 1065–1070. doi: 10.1002/gps.1608

Busceti, C. L., Di Menna, L., Bianchi, F., Mastroiacovo, F., Di Petro, P., Traficante, A., et al. (2018). Dickkopf-3 causes neuroprotection by inducing vascular endothelial growth factor. *Front. Cell Neurosci.* 12:292. doi: 10.3389/fncel.2018.00292

Calvo, D., Gunstad, J., Miller, L. A., Glickman, E., and Spitznagel, M. B. (2013). Higher serum insulin-like growth factor-1 is associated with better cognitive performance in persons with mild cognitive impairment. *Psychogeriatrics* 13, 170–174. doi: 10.1111/psyg.12023

Caricasole, A., Copani, A., Caraci, F., Aronica, E., Rozemuller, A. J., Caruso, A., et al. (2004). Induction of Dickkopf-1, a negative modulator of the Wnt pathway, is associated with neuronal degeneration in Alzheimer's brain. *J. Neurosci.* 24, 6021–6027. doi: 10.1523/JNEUROSCI.1381-04.2004

Chae, W. J., Ehrlick, A. K., Chan, P. Y., Teixeira, A. M., Henegariu, O., Hao, H., et al. (2016). The Wnt antagonist dicckopf-1 promotes pathological type 2 cell-mediated inflammation. *Immunity* 44, 246–258. doi: 10.1016/j.immuni.2016.01.008

Chong, M. S., and Sahadevan, S. (2003). An evidence-based clinical approach to the diagnosis of dementia. *Ann. Acad. Med. Singapore* 23, 740–749.

Cummings, J. L. (1997). The neuropsychiatric inventory: assessing psychopathology in dementia patients. *Neurology* 48(Suppl. 6), S10–S16.

Diarra, D., Stolina, M., Polzer, K., Zwerina, J., Ominsky, M. S., Dwyer, D., et al. (2007). Dickkopf-1 is a master regulator of joint remodeling. *Nat. Med.* 13, 156–163. doi: 10.1038/nm1538

Doi, T., Shimada, H., Makizako, H., Tsutsumimoto, K., Hotta, R., Nakakubo, S., et al. (2015). Association of insulin-like growth factor-1 with mild cognitive impairment and slow gait speed. *Neurobiol. Aging* 36, 942–947. doi: 10.1016/j.neurobiolaging.2014.10.035

Ferrari, C., Lombardi, G., Polito, C., Lucidi, G., Bagnoli, S., Piaceri, I., et al. (2018). Alzheimer's disease progression: factors influencing cognitive decline. *J. Alzheimers Dis.* 61, 785–791. doi: 10.3233/JAD-170665

Frater, J., Lie, D., Bartlett, P., and McGrath, J. J. (2018). Insulin-like growth factor 1 (IGF-1) as a marker of cognitive decline in normal ageing: a review. *Ageing Res. Rev.* 42, 14–27. doi: 10.1016/j.arr.2017.12.002

Heppner, F. L., Ransohoff, R. M., and Becher, B. (2015). Immune attack: the role of inflammation in Alzheimer disease. *Nat. Rev. Neurosci.* 16, 358–372. doi: 10.1038/nrn3880

Hosfield, L. A., and Humpel, C. (2015). Migration of blood cells to β-amyloid plaques in Alzheimer's disease. *Exp. Gerontol.* 65, 8–15. doi: 10.1016/j.exger.2015.03.002

Inestrosa, N. C., and Varela-Nallar, L. (2014). Wnt signaling in the nervous system and in Alzheimer's disease. *J. Mol. Cell Biol.* 6, 64–74. doi: 10.1093/jmcb/mjt051

Kim, S. B., Hill, M., Kwak, Y. T., Hampl, R., Jo, D. H., and Morfin, R. (2003). Neurosteroids: cerebrospinal fluid levels for Alzheimer's disease and vascular dementia diagnostics. *J. Clin. Endocrinol. Metab.* 88, 5199–5206. doi: 10.1210/jc.2003-030646

Lam, B., Masellis, M., Freedman, M., Stuss, D. T., and Black, S. E. (2013). Clinical, imaging and pathological heterogeneity of the Alzheimer's disease syndrome. *Alzheimers Res. Ther.* 5:1. doi: 10.1186/alzrt155

Leung, R., Proitsi, P., Simmons, A., Lunnon, K., Guntert, A., Kronenberg, D., et al. (2013). Inflammatory proteins in plasma are associated with severity of Alzheimer's disease. *PLoS One* 8:e64971. doi: 10.1371/journal.pone.0064971

Lim, W. S., Chin, J. J., Lam, C. K., Lim, P. P., and Sahadevan, S. (2005). Clinical dementia rating: experience of a multi-racial Asian population. *Alzheimer Dis. Assoc. Disord.* 19, 135–142. doi: 10.1097/01.wad.0000174991.60709.36

Mahoney, F. I., and Barthel, D. (1965). Functional evaluation: the barthel index. *Md. State Med. J.* 14, 56–61.

McKhann, G., Drachmann, D. A., Folstein, M., Katzman, R., Price, D., Stadlan, E. M., et al. (1984). Clinical diagnosis of Alzheimer's disease – report to the NINCDS-ADRDA workgroup under the auspices of department of health and human services task force on alzheimer's disease. *Neurology* 34, 939–944.

Morris, J. C. (1993). The Clinical Dementia Rating (CDR): current version and scoring rules. *Neurology* 43, 2412–2414.

Naylor, J. C., Hulette, C. M., Steffens, D. C., Shampine, L. J., Ervin, J. F., Payne, V. M., et al. (2008). Cerebrospinal fluid dehydroepiandrosterone levels are correlated with brain dehydroepiandrosterone levels, elevated in Alzheimer's disease and related to neuropathological disease stage. *J. Clin. Endocrinol. Metab.* 93, 3173–3178. doi: 10.1210/jc.2007-1229

Nieto-Estevez, V., Defterali, C., and Vicario-Abejon, C. (2016). IGF-1: a key growth factor that regulates neurogenesis and synaptogenesis from embryonic to adult stages of the brain. *Front. Neurosci.* 10 52. doi: 10.3389/fnins.2016.00052

Ortiz-Matamoros, A., Salcedo-Tello, P., Avila-Munoz, E., Zepeda, A., and Arias, C. (2013). Role of Wnt signaling in the control of adult hippocampal functioning in health and disease: therapeutic implications. *Curr. Neuropharmacol.* 11, 465–476. doi: 10.2174/1570159X11311050001

Palop, J. J., and Mucke, L. (2010). Amyloid-β-induced neuronal dysfunction in Alzheimer's disease: from synapses toward neural networks. *Nat. Neurosci.* 13, 812–818. doi: 10.1038/nn.2583

Perry, R. T., Collins, J. S., Wiener, H., Acton, R., and Go, R. C. (2001). The role of TNF and its receptors in Alzheimer disease. *Neurobiol. Aging* 22, 873–883. doi: 10.1016/s0197-4580(01)00291-3

Purro, S. A., Dickins, E. M., and Salinas, P. C. (2012). The secreted wnt antagonist dickkopf-1 is required for amyloid β-mediated synaptic loss. *J. Neurosci.* 32, 3492–3498. doi: 10.1523/JNEUROSCI 4562-11.2012

Ross, R. D., Shah, R. C., Leurgans, S., Bottiglieri, T., Wilson, R. S., and Sumner, D. R. (2018). Circulating Dkk1 and TRAIL are associated with cognitive decline in community-dwelling older adults with cognitive concerns. *J. Gerontol. A Biol. Sci. Med. Sci.* 73, 1688–1694. doi: 10.1093/gerona/glx252

Sahadevan, S., Lim, J. P., Tan, N. J., and Chan, S. P. (2002). Psychometric identification of early Alzheimer disease in an elderly Chinese population with differing educational levels. *Alzheimer Dis. Assoc. Disord.* 16, 65–72. doi: 10.1097/00002093-200204000-00003

Sahadevan, S., Lim, P. P., Tan, N. J., and Chan, S. P. (2000). Diagnostic performance of two mental status tests in the older Chinese: influence of education and age on cut-off values. *Int. J. Geriatr. Psychiatry* 15, 234–241. doi: 10.1002/(sici)1099-1166(200003)15:3<234::aid-gps99>3.0.co;2-g

Sato, N., Yambuki, T., Takano, A., Koinuma, J., Aragaki, M., Masuda, K., et al. (2010). Wnt-inhibitor dicckopf-1 as a target for passive cancer immunotherapy. *Cancer Res.* 70, 5326–5336. doi: 10.1158/0008-5472.CAN-09-3879

Seib, D. R. M., Corsini, N. S., Ellwanger, K., Plaas, C., Mateos, A., Pitzer, C., et al. (2013). Loss of Diskkopf-1 restores neurogenesis in old age, and counteracts cognitive decline. *Cell Stem Cell* 12, 204–214. doi: 10.1016/j.stem.2012.11.010

Storandt, M., Grant, E. A., Miller, P., and Morris, J. C. (2002). Rates of progression in mild cognitive impairment, and early Alzheimer's disease. *Neurology* 59, 1034–1041.

Sundelof, J., Kilander, L., Helmersson, J., Larsson, A., Ronnemma, E., Degerman-Gunnarson, A., et al. (2009). Systemic inflammation and the risk of Alzheimer's disease and dementia: a prospective population-based study. *J. Alzheimers Dis.* 18, 79–87. doi: 10.3233/JAD-2009-1126

Szekely, C. A., Green, R. C., Bretiner, J. C., Ostybye, T., Beiser, A. S., Corrada, M. M., et al. (2008). No advantage of A beta-42 lowering NSAIDs for prevention of Alzheimer dementia in six pooled cohort studies. *Neurology* 70, 2291–2298. doi: 10.1212/01.wnl.0000313933.17796.f6

Tan, Z. S., Beiser, A. S., Vasan, R. S., Roubenoff, R., Dinarello, C. A., Harris, T. B., et al. (2007). Inflammatory markers and the risk of Alzheimer disease: the framingham study. *Neurology* 68, 1902–1908. doi: 10.1212/01.wnl.0000263217.36439.da

Tapia-Rojas, C., and Inestrosa, N. C. (2018a). Loss of canonical Wnt signaling is involved in the pathogenesis of Alzheimer's disease. *Neural Regen. Res.* 13, 1705–1710. doi: 10.4103/1673-5374.238606

Tapia-Rojas, C., and Inestrosa, N. C. (2018b). Wnt signaling loss accelerates the appearance of neuropathological hallmarks of Alzheimer's disease in J20-APP transgenic and wild type mice. *J. Neurochem.* 144, 443–465. doi: 10.1111/jnc.14278

Terry, R. D., Masliah, E., Salmon, D. P., Butters, N., DeTeresa, R., Hill, R., et al. (1991). Physical basis of cognitive alterations in Alzheimer's disease: synapse loss is the major correlate of cognitive impairment. *Ann. Neurol.* 30, 572–580. doi: 10.1002/ana.410300410

Uchihara, T., Akiyama, H., Kondo, H., and Ikeda, K. (1997). Activated microglial cells are colocalized with perivascular deposits of amyloid-(protein in Alzheimer's disease brain. *Stroke* 28, 1948–1950. doi: 10.1161/01.str.28.10.1948

Vallee, A., and Lecarpentier, Y. (2016). Alzheimer disease: crosstalk between the canonical Wnt/Beta-catenin pathway and PPARs alpha and gamma. *Front. Neurosci.* 10:459. doi: 10.3389/fnins.2016.00459

Vehmas, A. K., Kawas, C. H., Stewart, W. F., and Troncoso, J. C. (2003). Immune reactive cells in senile plaques and cognitive decline in Alzheimer's disease. *Neurobiol. Aging* 24, 321–331. doi: 10.1016/s0197-4580(02)00090-8

Wahlund, L. O., Barkhof, F., Fazekas, F., Bronge, L., Augustin, M., Sjögren, M., et al. (2001). A new rating scale for age-related white matter changes applicable to MRI and CT. *Stroke* 32, 1318–1322. doi: 10.1161/01.str.32.6.1318

Wahlund, L. O., Julin, P., Johansson, S. E., and Scheltens, P. (2000). Visual rating and volumetry of the medial temporal lobe on magnetic resonance imaging in dementia: a comparative study. *J. Neurol. Neurosurg. Psychiatry* 69, 630–635. doi: 10.1136/jnnp.69.5.630

Williams, M. M., Storandt, M., Roe, C. M., and Morris, J. C. (2013). Progression of Alzheimer's disease as measured by clinical dementia rating sum-of-boxes scores. *Alzheimer Dement.* 9(1 Suppl.), S39–S44. doi: 10.1016/j.jalz.2012.01.005

Zenzaimer, C., Marksteiner, J., Kiefer, A., Berger, P., and Humpel, C. (2009). Dkk-3 is elevated in CSF and plasma of Alzheimer's disease patients. *J. Neurochem.* 110, 653–661. doi: 10.1111/j.1471-4159.2009.06158

17

Brain Amide Proton Transfer Imaging of Rat with Alzheimer's Disease Using Saturation with Frequency Alternating RF Irradiation Method

Runrun Wang[1†], Peidong Chen[1†], Zhiwei Shen[1,2], Guisen Lin[1], Gang Xiao[3], Zhuozhi Dai[1], Bingna Zhang[4], Yuanfeng Chen[1], Lihua Lai[1], Xiaodan Zong[1], Yan Li[1], Yanyan Tang[1] and Renhua Wu[1]*

[1] Department of Medical Imaging, The Second Affiliated Hospital, Shantou University Medical College, Shantou, China, [2] Philips Healthcare, Shantou, China, [3] Department of Mathematics and Statistics, Hanshan Normal University, Chaozhou, China, [4] Translational Medicine, The Second Affiliated Hospital, Shantou University Medical College, Shantou, China

***Correspondence:**
Renhua Wu
cjr.wurenhua@vip.163.com

† These authors have contributed equally to this work

Amyloid-β (Aβ) deposits and some proteins play essential roles in the pathogenesis of Alzheimer's disease (AD). Amide proton transfer (APT) imaging, as an imaging modality to detect tissue protein, has shown promising features for the diagnosis of AD disease. In this study, we chose 10 AD model rats as the experimental group and 10 sham-operated rats as the control group. All the rats underwent a Y-maze test before APT image acquisition, using saturation with frequency alternating RF irradiation (APT_{SAFARI}) method on a 7.0 T animal MRI scanner. Compared with the control group, APT (3.5 ppm) values of brain were significantly reduced in AD models ($p < 0.002$). The APT_{SAFARI} imaging is more significant than APT imaging ($p < 0.0001$). AD mode mice showed spatial learning and memory loss in the Y-maze experiment. In addition, there was significant neuronal loss in the hippocampal CA1 region and cortex compared with sham-operated rats. In conclusion, we demonstrated that APT imaging could potentially provide molecular biomarkers for the non-invasive diagnosis of AD. APT_{SAFARI} MRI could be used as an effective tool to improve the accuracy of diagnosis of AD compared with conventional APT imaging.

Keywords: Alzheimer's disease, amide proton transfer, saturation with alternating frequency RF irradiation, chemical exchange saturation transfer, magnetic resonance imaging

INTRODUCTION

Alzheimer's disease (AD) is the most prevalent neurodegenerative disease in the world, which is characterized with progressive memory decline (Chen et al., 2018). Currently there is no definitive diagnosis or effective treatment for AD (Goozee et al., 2017). Many pathogenic mechanisms have been reported, including the accumulation of amyloid plaques, neuronal loss, neurofibrillary tangles (NFTs), excessive acetylcholinesterase activity and neurovascular dysfunction (Vanderstichele et al., 2006). Biomarkers based on protein aggregation play important roles in evaluating AD. The reliable AD model rat can be made by intracerebroventricular (icv) injection of well-characterized toxic soluble Aβ species into rat brain (Kasza et al., 2017). The injection of Aβ species in rat induced loss of learning and memory behavior, which could be detected using the Y-maze (Hwang et al., 2017). The rat model of AD was used to observe the effect of drug therapy (Fahanik-Babaei et al., 2018) and was often used to establish and validate biomarkers as a surrogate for patients (Prestia et al., 2018) as well.

Magnetic resonance imaging (MRI) is essential for early diagnosis of AD (Matsuda, 2017), including conventional MRI, diffusion tension imaging (DTI) (Promteangtrong et al., 2015), proton magnetic resonance spectroscopy (MRS) (Zhang N. et al., 2014). The accuracy of AD diagnosis may be increased using advanced MRI techniques. Up to now, further reliable imaging technique for early AD diagnosis is still desired. Amide proton transfer (APT) imaging based on chemical exchange saturation transfer (CEST) is a novel molecular MRI technique (Kamimura et al., 2018), by which low-concentration endogenous mobile proteins and peptides in tissue could be detected non-invasively (Xu et al., 2014). Furthermore, multiple sources of exchanging magnetization, like amide (Lin et al., 2018), amine (Zhang et al., 2018) and hydroxyl protons from macromolecules and various protons (Kanazawa et al., 2018), could also be detected. AD is associated with the accumulation of abnormal proteins in the central nervous system (Li et al., 2017). However, the quantitative method to detect protein *in vivo* is limited. To our knowledge, few studies have been reported to diagnose AD by APT method.

Zaiss and Bachert (2013) proved from algorithms and theoretical formulas that chemical exchange observed by NMR saturation transfer (CEST) and spin-lock (SL) experiments provided a MRI contrast by indirect detection of exchanging protons. A comprehensive signature of protein unfolding detectable by CEST was observed in a set of model solutions containing BSA and in yeast cells (Goerke et al., 2015). Zollner et al. (2018) demonstrated that APT-weighted CEST imaging is sensitive to ammonia introduced protein denaturation. Using APT to detect tau-pathology in regions of low NFT density is also a method to study AD in mouse model of tauopathy (rTg4510) (Wells et al., 2015). In Chen et al. (2019) study, a new sequence (radial-sampling steady-state sequence based ultrashort echo time readout) was used to image the contributions from mobile proteins at the frequency offsets for both aliphatic proton (–3.6 ppm) and protein amide proton (+3.6 ppm) signals. Their results showed significantly reduced ΔST (–3.6) signal in AD mouse, which was more sensitive. In this study, we use the AD model (based on intracerebrovascular injection of the beta amyloid 1-40). Target APT imaging could potentially provide molecular biomarkers for diagnosis of AD. These results suggested that APT_{SAFARI} MRI could be used as an effective tool to improve the accuracy for the diagnosis of AD.

In this study, we hypothesized that the accumulation of abnormal cytoplasmic proteins in some specific cerebral areas was associated with low APT signal. Meanwhile, saturation with frequency alternating radiofrequency irradiation (SAFARI) method was used to improve accuracy of APT signal by removing the direct water saturation (DS) effect, magnetization transfer (MT) effect and MT asymmetry (Scheidegger et al., 2011).

MATERIALS AND METHODS

Alzheimer Disease Model Preparation

Sprague-Dawley (SD) male rats weighting 275 ± 25 g (aged 10–12 weeks) were purchased from the Animal Center of Shantou University Medical College (Guangdong, China). All animal experiments were performed according to the guidelines of the National Institutes of Health guide and approved by the Ethics Committee of Shantou University Medical College. The rats were randomly divided into two groups: sham-operated control group rats (n = 10) and AD model group rats (n = 10). Both groups were placed in a geomagnetic environment. The rats were housed in an air-conditioned room with a constant temperature (22 ± 1°C), humidity (50 ± 10%), and were kept under reversed light/dark (12 h each) cycle.

At Sigma-Aldrich (St. Louis, MO, United States), we purchased Aβ1–40. To obtain aggregated Aβ1-40, Aβ1-40 was dissolved at the concentration of 1 g/L in distilled water and was incubated for 48 h at 37°C. Then it was diluted to the final concentration with saline just before the experiments (Guerra de Souza et al., 2018). After aggregation, the sample was stored at 4°C. The SD rats received icv injection of Aβ1-40 as described before (Rasool et al., 2018). Briefly, the rats were anesthetized with 3 mg/ml sodium pentobarbital (1 ml/100 g, i.p. body weight). Then they were placed in stereotaxic apparatus. For a single icv injection of aggregated Aβ1-40, a 28-G needle (stainless-steel) was inserted into lateral ventricular (1.0 mm lateral, 3.6 mm central to bregma and 0.8 mm posterior). And then AD model group rats were administered with Aβ1-40 10 μg per rat (1 mg/ml) using Hamilton microsyringe at a speed of 0.6 μl/min. Sham-operated control group rats were given the same volume of normal saline. The cannula was left for 2–3 min after the injection to facilitate drug diffusion. The wound as an additional antiseptic measure was then sealed with sterile wax.

Behavioral Testing

All rats underwent Y-maze testing 14 days after the model was built. The Y-maze test was used to assess the spatial learning and memory of the rats (Zhang L. et al., 2014). The spontaneous alternation behavior, the time spent in the new arm, total distance and the total new arm distance were measured to assess the learning ability of the rats (Conrad et al., 2003). Behavioral studies were carried out 2 h after last work between 9 am and 5 pm in a quiet room. Before testing the next rat, the device was cleaned with 10% ethanol. The tests were recorded using a video camera and later scored by a trained observer who was blind to the grouping of the rats. Each rat was placed at the start arm and moved freely through the maze for 10 min. An alternation was defined as successive entries into all three arms on consecutive choices (i.e., BCA, ABC, or CAB but not ABA). Spontaneous alternation, as a measure of cognitive functions, assesses short-term spatial memory. The percentage of spontaneous alternation was calculated as alternation rate (%) = 100 × [1 – mistake number/(total number – 2)] (Bak et al., 2017). The second test aimed to test spatial learning. The three arms were set as the starting arm (animal entry), the common arm and the new arm. In the first step, which was the acquisition period, the new arm was closed, and the rats were free to explore to the other two arms for 3 min. Two hours later, the second step (recall phase) began. All the arms were opened, the animals were free to move for 3 min in the three arms. The time and distance of exploration in each arm were recorded.

MRI Experiments

After behavioral testing, all AD model rats were scanned 15 days after model was built. All images were acquired on a 7.0T horizontal bore small animal MR scanner (Agilent Technologies, Santa Clara, CA, United States) with a standard 9563 volume coil for transmission and reception. Parameters of T2WI MRI were as follows. TR = 3,140 ms, TE = 37 ms, FOV = 40 mm × 40 mm, matrix = 240 × 320, and slice thickness = 1 mm. We scanned 6 slices for T2w images and selected the largest slice of the hippocampus for shimming.

The main magnetic field (B_0) was shimmed. The axial APT images were acquired using a single slice echo planar imaging (EPI) sequence with continuous wave (CW) pre-saturating RF irradiation. FOV = 35 × 35 mm, slice thickness = 3.5 mm, matrix size = 128 × 128, repetition time (TR) = 5,000 ms, echo time (TE) = 20 ms, and bandwidth = 267,000 Hz. The APT imaging and Z-spectra were acquired, which ranged from 5 to −5 ppm, with the use of a B1 of 1.3 μT (56 Hz) and a saturation time of 4 s. A saturation pulse was applied at 101 frequency offsets that cover the range of ±5 ppm and step of 0.1 ppm to contain around ±3.5 ppm of APT saturation peaks. The APT imaging was 8 min and 40 s. S_0 was acquired at saturation frequency offset of 33.33 ppm as a reference image. Saturation with frequency alternating RF irradiation (SAFARI) was achieved by setting a dual frequency preparation of a gauss pulse saturation at ±3.5 ppm (Scheidegger et al., 2011). Then 101 frequency offsets images were detected using a gauss pulse saturation with the same range and step as CW pulse sequence. The total time of SAFARI imaging was 8 min and 45 s. The B_0 and B1 fields were also measured, as well as T1 and T2 maps. T1 maps were acquired using the same geometry and spatial resolution as CEST MRI. An IR-FSEMS sequence with Inversion recovery time = 0.010, 0.023, 0.051, 0.115, 0.260, 0.588, 1.328, 3 s was used for T1 maps. While the T2 map was obtained by a multi-slice multi-echo (MSME) MRI with echo number = 16. Echo time = 8.2, 16.3, 24.5, 32.7, 40.8, 49.0, 57.2, 65.3, 73.5, 81.7, 89.8, 98.0, 106.2, 114.4, 122.5, 130.7 ms was used for T2 maps.

Image Analysis

Images were analyzed in MATLAB (MathWorks, R2012b). For APT acquisition, we normalized voxels of images by the corresponding unsaturated reference image S_0. Then B_0 correction was performed for the z-spectrum scans according the water saturation shift referencing (WASSR) method (Kim et al., 2009). Evaluation of the APT effect by conventional MT ratio asymmetry analysis after B_0 correction (Wada et al., 2016):

$$MTR_{asym} = \frac{S_{sat}(-3.5ppm) - S_{sat}(+3.5ppm)}{S_0}$$

For the APT_{SAFARI} scans, calculated the quantitative maps of MTR_{SAFARI} as described previously (Scheidegger et al., 2011):

$$MTR_{SAFARI} = \frac{S_{sat}(+3.5ppm) + S_{sat}(-3.5ppm)}{S_0} - \frac{S_{sat}(SAFARI) + S_{sat}(SAFARI')}{S_0}$$

where S_{sat} (SAFARI) is the signal after alternating frequency irradiation and S_{sat} (SAFARI′) is a similar image but with the order of positive and negative frequencies reversed to minimize any system error related timing (Scheidegger et al., 2011).

The hippocampus is the primary structure affected in the early AD pathology which control the learning and cognitive function (Zhang et al., 2017). Therefore, we selected the largest slice of hippocampus on EPI-based image according to the high spatial resolution atlases exist for MRI (Johnson et al., 2010) as our APT slice. ROIs across all slices containing cortex, hippocampus and thalamus were manually drawn by the same expert with visual reference to a rat brain atlas. The T2w image demonstrates the ROIs in the coronal brain slices for the cortex (CX), hippocampus (HI), and thalamus (TH). The red dotted lines indicate the ROI tissues (**Figure 3A**). ROIs for the APT image were manually drawn on the EPI-based image (**Figure 3B**).

Histology and Histomorphometry

After imaging scanning, rats were anesthetized and perfused *via* the left ventricle with 100 mL of 4% paraformaldehyde followed by 100 mL of normal saline at a flow rate of 3 mL/min. After perfusion, the brains were obtained and kept in 4% para formaldehyde (24 h) and embedded in paraffin before being dispatched for histology (Wang et al., 2018).

Axial slices (5 μm) were incubated at 55°C for 45 min. Hematoxylin-eosin (HE) staining was used to assesse neuropathology. Finally, the slices were examined under a Zeiss microscope (Zeiss Instruments Inc.).

The process of double-labeling immunofluorescence was as follows. Staining coverslips with 70 nm serial sections were done as previously described (Kay et al., 2013). Paraffin-embedded sections were rehydrated with reduced concentrations of ethanol and subjected to a standard antigen- retrieval procedure consisting of being microwaved in 5% goat serum for 20 min (ZLI-9056, China). The sections were cooled for about 40 min at 4°C. They were then blocked with 5% normal goat serum for 1 h at room temperature. Finally, they were incubated with the primary antibody overnight at 4°C. After 24 h, the sections were deparaffinized and washed through a series of xylene and ethanol to rehydrate. With anti-GFAP to label astrocytes, all primary antibodies were diluted in PBS. Slides were incubated for the secondary antibody and fluorescently labeled for 1 h. Finally, the coverslips were mounted on glass slides and then observed using the Zeiss laser confocal microscope.

Statistical Analysis

All data were analyzed using the SPSS22.0. Imaging data of AD models and control subjects were compared using *t*-test for

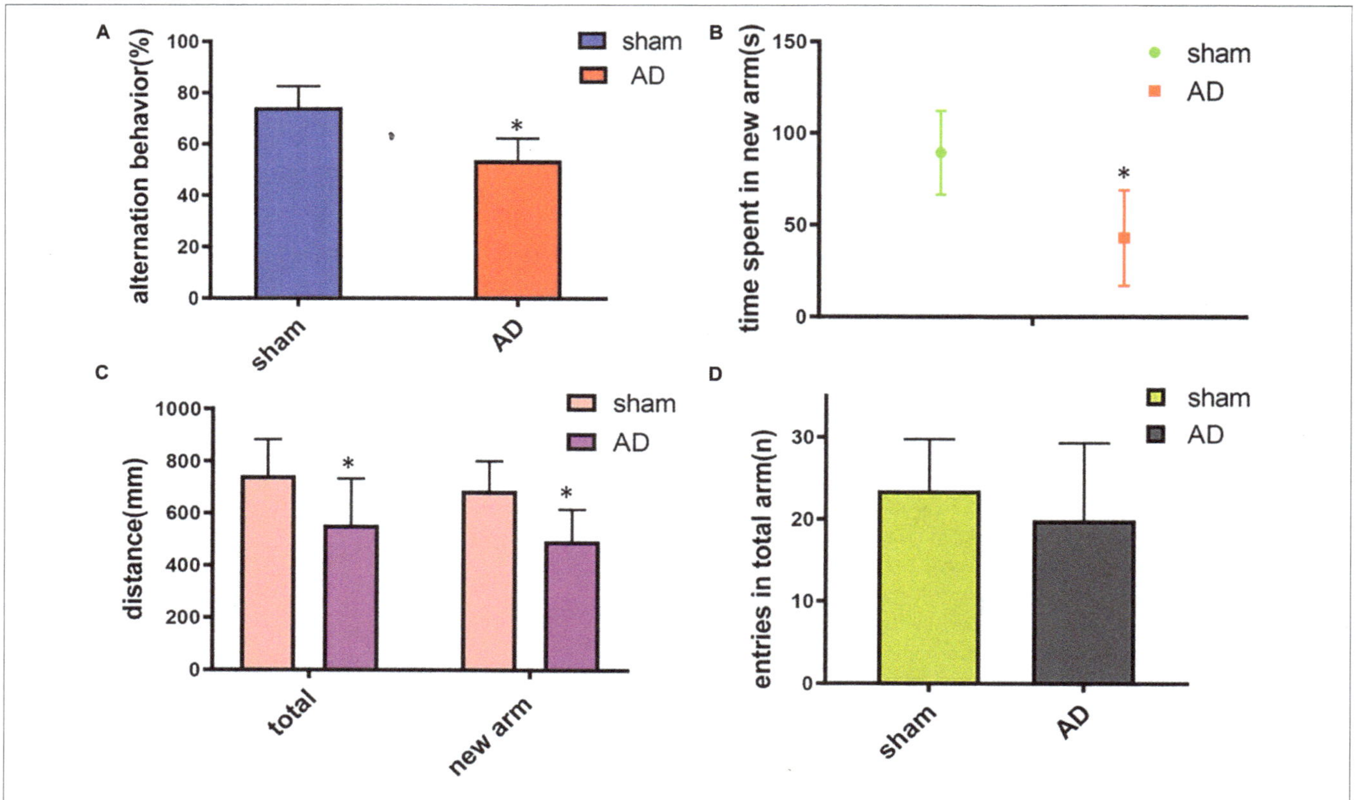

FIGURE 1 | Learning and memory assessment of AD model group and sham operated control group measured by Y-maze. **(A)** Alternation behavior: AD model group had significantly decreased the spontaneous alternation behavior compared with the sham operated control group. **(B)** Time spent in the new arm: The time spent in the new arm of AD model group decreased significantly compared with the sham operated control group. **(C)** Total distance and the total new arm distance: AD model group had significant decrease of the total distance and the total new arm distance compared with the sham operated control group. **(D)** There was no significant difference between two groups on the numbers of arm entries. *$p < 0.05$.

pairwise comparison. One-way analysis of variance (ANOVA) followed by multiple comparisons were used to investigate the associations between Y-maze. A level of $p < 0.05$ was considered as statistically significant for all tests.

RESULTS

Y-Maze Test Results of AD Model Rat

In the Y-maze test, significant decrease of the spontaneous alternation was found in AD model group compared with the sham operated control group ($p < 0.05$, **Figure 1A**). Meanwhile, a significant decrease of the time, total distance and the total distance in the new arm were also found in AD model group compared with the sham-operated control group ($p < 0.05$, **Figures 1B,C**). There was no significant difference between the two groups in the numbers of arm entries (**Figure 1D**). These results demonstrated the AD model had loss spatial learning and memory.

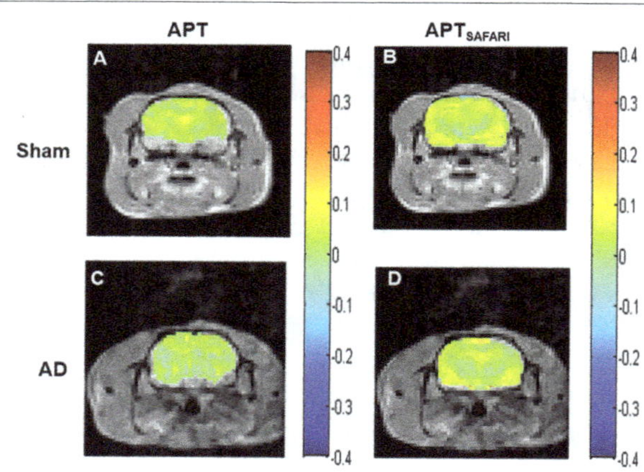

FIGURE 2 | **(A)** APT imaging of sham operated control, **(B)** APT_{SAFARI} imaging of sham operated control, **(C)** APT imaging of AD model, **(D)** APT_{SAFARI} imaging of AD model.

Results of APT Imaging and SAFARI Imaging

The Z-spectra and MTR_{asym} curves showed that there were significant differences between AD models and sham operated controls in the whole brain (**Figure 4A**), there are more significant reductions when hippocampus regions are compared (**Figure 4B**). ΔMTR_{asym} was maximal with a 1.3 μT B_1 power and the peak of MTR_{asym} curve was at 3.5 ppm. The APT

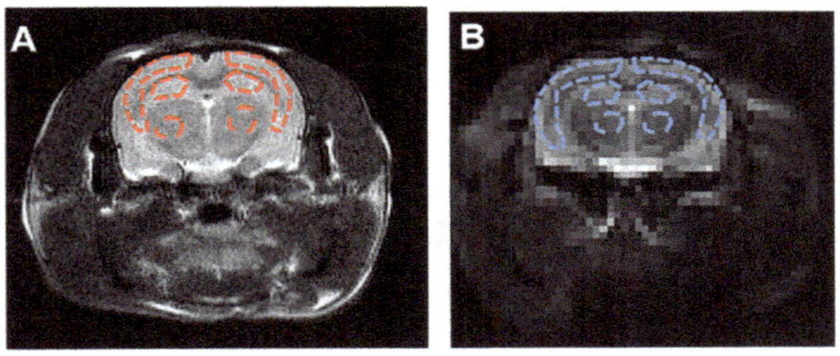

FIGURE 3 | (A) The T2w image demonstrates the ROIs in the coronal brain slices for the cortex (CX), hippocampus (HI) and thalamus (TH). The red dotted lines indicate the ROI tissues. **(B)** ROIs for the APT image were manually drawn on the EPI-based image. The blue dotted lines indicate the ROI tissues.

maps of AD model and sham control were showed in the **Figures 2A,C**. The APT_{SAFARI} maps of AD model and sham control were showed in the **Figures 2B,D**. Image uniformity and image contrast of the SAFARI method were all better than that acquired from APT imaging. T2w anatomical only-image is added for the readers to understand the exact geometrical position of the selected slice (**Figure 3A**). ROIs for the APT image were manually drawn on the EPI-based image (**Figure 3B**). AD model rats (n = 10) had reduced APT effect compared to the sham groups. The APT effects of AD model rats were 4.7 ± 1.2, 5.9 ± 1.4, 2.78 ± 0.9, and 3.3 ± 1.1% at CX, HI, TH and whole brain (WB), respectively APT effects at CX, HI and WB were lower than that in sham controls (7.5 ± 1.3%, 9.6 ± 1.5%, 5.2 ± 0.9%, $p < 0.05$). At TH, no significant differences in APT effect were observed between two groups ($p > 0.05$) (**Figure 4C**). The APT_{SAFARI} effects of AD model in above four regions were 8.5 ± 1.2, 9.6 ± 1.3, 7.7 ± 1.3, and 8.2 ± 1.2%, respectively. APT_{SAFARI} effects at CX, HI and WB, were lower than that in sham controls (16.8 ± 1.4%, 18.7 ± 1.1%, 13.5 ± 1.3%, $p < 0.01$). At TH, no significant differences in APT effect were observed at two groups ($p > 0.05$) (**Figure 4D**).

Results of T1 and T2 Maps

In our study, in order to examine the possible difference of T1 and T2 maps between two groups (**Figure 5**), we scanned T1 and T2 maps. The T1 map values were found to be 1.43 ± 0.07 and 1.51 ± 0.12 s for the cortex of the AD rats and sham rats, respectively; while the T2 map values were 0.047 ± 0.003 s (AD rats) and 0.051 ± 0.002 s (sham rats). No significant difference was observed between AD and sham rats (p = 0.29 and 0.21 for the

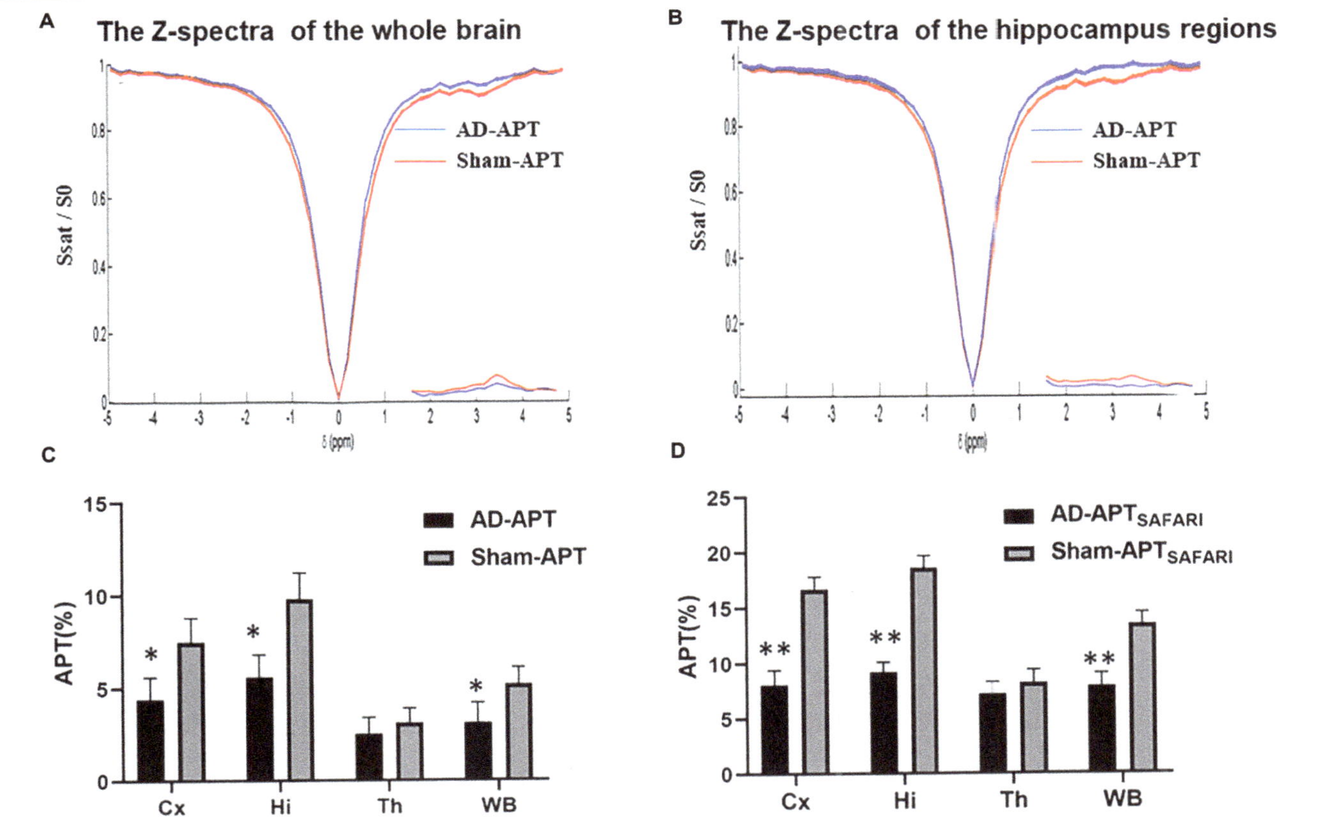

FIGURE 4 | (A) The Z-spectra and MTR_{asym} curve between AD model and sham controls in the whole brain, **(B)** The Z-spectra and MTR_{asym} curve between AD model and sham controls in hippocampus regions, **(C)** The plot for the different region APT effect in AD model and sham groups, **(D)** The plot for the different region APT_{SAFARI} effect in AD model and sham groups. *$p < 0.05$, **$p < 0.01$.

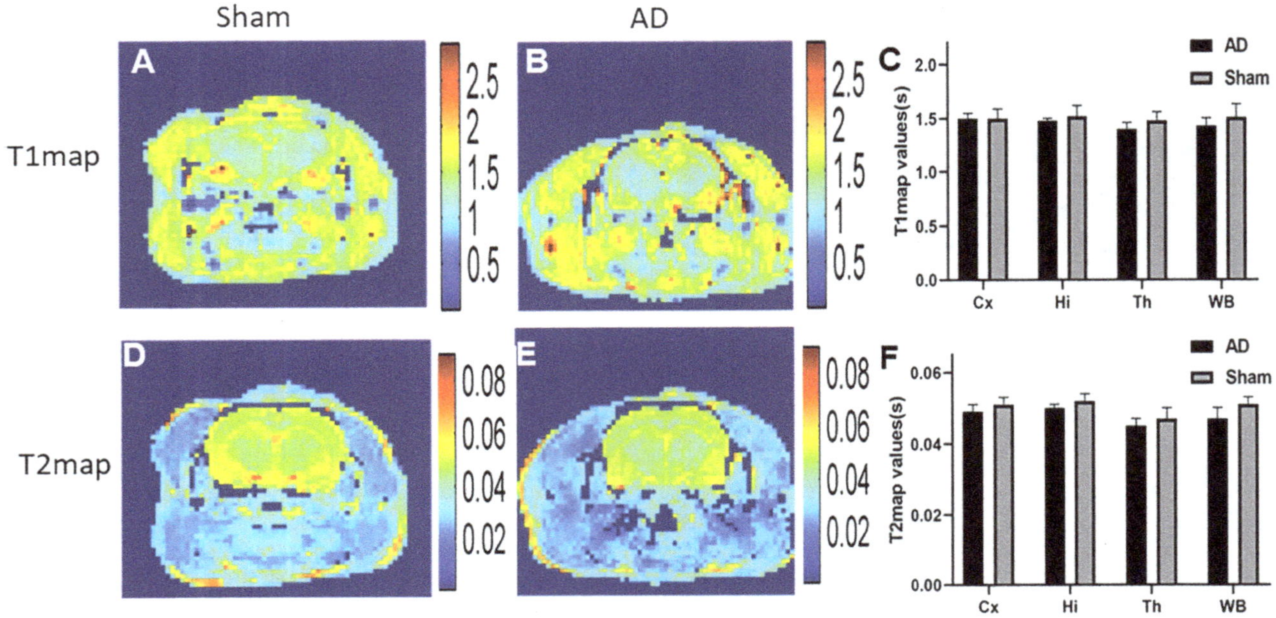

FIGURE 5 | (A) T1 map of sham operated control, **(B)** T1 map of AD model, **(C)** The plot for the different region T1 map values in AD model and sham groups, **(D)** T2 map of sham operated control, **(E)** T2 map of AD model, **(F)** The plot for the different region T2 map values in AD model and sham groups.

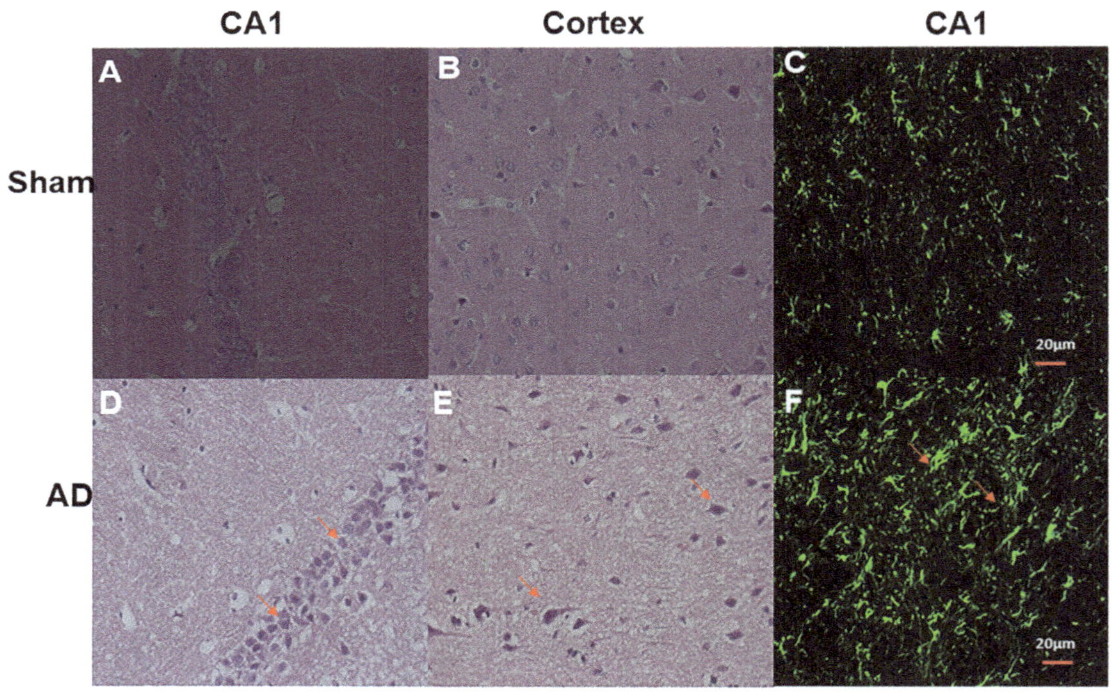

FIGURE 6 | HE staining and double-labeling immunofluorescence and confocal microscopy of GFAP (green) of Hippocampal CA1 and cortex. HE staining **(A)** CA1 region of sham operated control, **(B)** Cortex of sham operated control, **(D)** CA1 region of AD model, **(E)** Cortex of AD model (above all original magnification × 40). AD model group showed significant neuronal loss in the hippocampus CA1 region and cortex (red arrows); Double-labeling immunofluorescence **(C)** Hippocampal CA1 region of sham operated control, **(F)** Hippocampal CA1 region of AD model; GFAP staining is strongly enhanced in reactive astrocytes identified by double-labeling immunofluorescence (red arrows) in AD model, Scale bars = 20 μm.

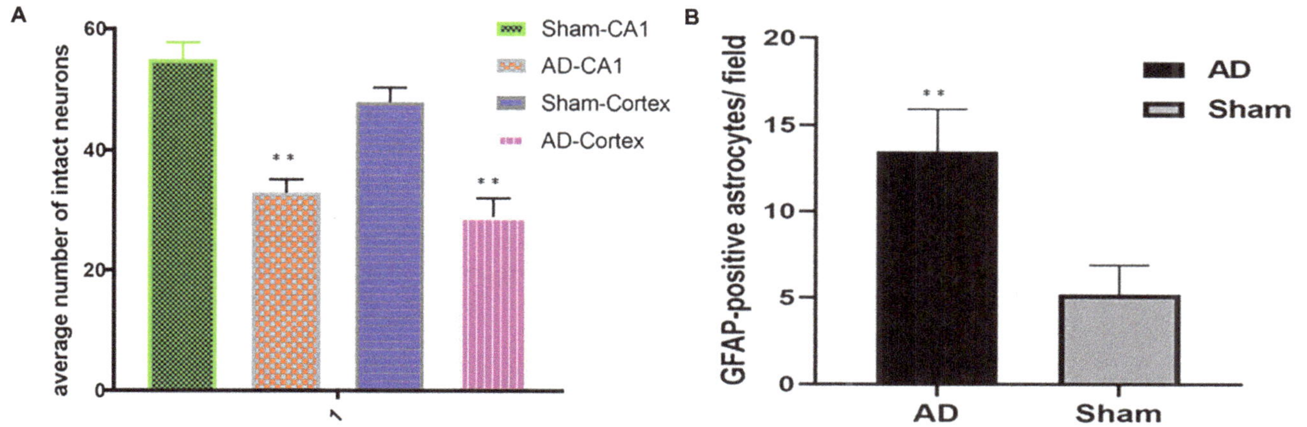

FIGURE 7 | (A) HE staining, AD model group showed significant neuronal loss in the hippocampus CA1 region and cortex compared sham operated control, **(B)** Bar graphs of mean densities of GFAP-positive reactive astrocytes of AD model and sham group. $^{**}p < 0.01$.

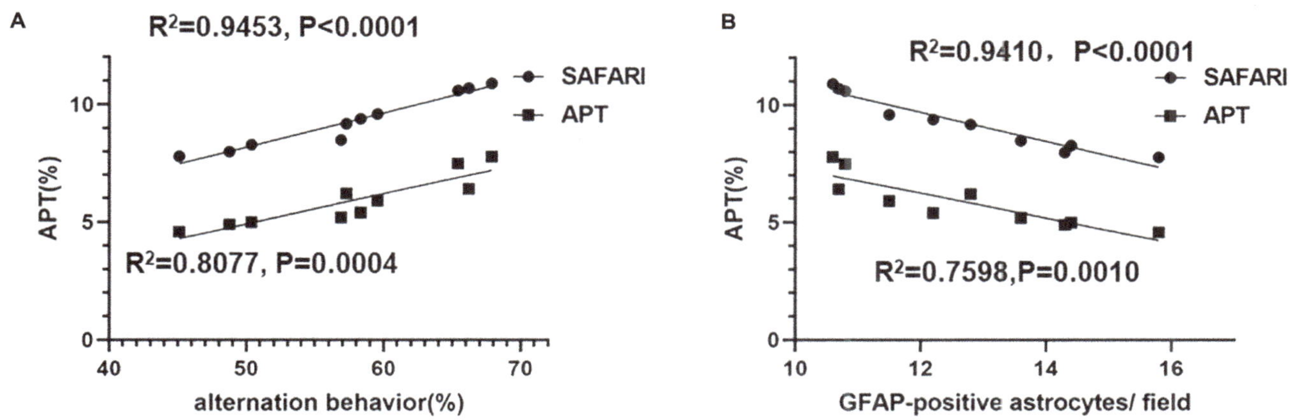

FIGURE 8 | (A) The linear regression analysis of the correlation between alternation behavior (%) and the APT (%) of the hippocampus in AD model rats (R^2 = 0.9453, $p < 0.0001$ and R^2 = 0.8077, p = 0.0004 for the APT_{SAFARI} and APT values, respectively). **(B)** The linear correlation between the APT (%) and GFAP-positive astrocytes/field of the hippocampus in AD model rats (R^2 = 0.9410, $p < 0.0001$ and R^2 = 0.7598, p = 0.0010 for the APT_{SAFARI} and APT values, respectively).

T1 and T2 map values, respectively). No significant differences in different regions of T1 and T2 map values were observed either between two groups ($p > 0.05$) (**Figures 5C,F**).

Results of Histological Examinations

Significant changes in neuron morphology in each group were revealed in histological studies. For HE staining, the number of intact neurons in the hippocampal CA1 was markedly decreased in the AD model group compared with those in the sham operated control group (**Figure 7A**). The AD model group showed significant neuronal loss in the hippocampus CA1 region and cortex (**Figures 6D,E**, red arrows). GFAP staining was strongly enhanced in reactive astrocytes identified by double-labeling immunofluorescence in the AD model (**Figure 6F**, red arrows). **Figures 6A–C** are the pathological results of the corresponding region of sham operated controls. The total number of GFAP-positive astrocytes was expressed as the mean number per field of view. A significant increase in the number of GFAP-positive astrocytes was observed in the hippocampus CA1 region of the AD model, as compared to sham rats (**Figure 7B**).

Correlation Analysis

The linear regression analysis revealed a positive correlation between alternation behavior (%) and the APT (%) of the hippocampus in AD model rats (R^2 = 0.9453, $p < 0.0001$ and R^2 = 0.8077, p = 0.0004 for the APT_{SAFARI} and APT values, respectively) (**Figure 8A**). A negative correlation between the APT (%) and GFAP-positive astrocytes/field of the hippocampus was found in AD model rats (R^2 = 0.9410, $p < 0.0001$ and R^2 = 0.7598, p = 0.0010 for the APT_{SAFARI} and APT values, respectively) (**Figure 8B**). In terms of goodness of fit. APT_{SAFARI} was better than APT for both behavior and pathology correlation. These results demonstrated that APT_{SAFARI} was a more sensitive method to detect CEST signal change compared with that using APT method.

DISCUSSION

In this study, we used both APT and APT_{SAFARI} (Scheidegger et al., 2011) methods to assess the APT value in AD models at 7.0T. These results indicate the APT is a potential method that can non-invasively visualize the protein concentration of AD *in vivo*. APT imaging is a novel molecular MRI technique for detecting endogenous mobile proteins. APT could be affected by many other factors, including tissue water content, pH, temperature, and the background MT effect (Togao et al., 2014). In our study, the results showed significantly reduced signal for the AD model compared to the control group, which is due to the effect of protein aggregation involved in AD (Chen et al., 2019). Several studies of APT have shown that the protein concentration is homogenous throughout the brain (Xu et al., 2016). APT is highly sensitive to changes of pH in tissue, although it is designed to provide a direct measurement of proton exchange. The pathology of AD also includes vascular compromise that can result in hypoperfusion, local tissue hypoxia, and acidosis (Eugenin et al., 2016). Brain acidification in AD patients has already been observed (Fang et al., 2010). This reduced pH results in a reduced rate of exchange of amide protons because the chemical exchange of the amide in the protein is base catalyzed (Zhang et al., 1995). Exchange of these amide protons with water results in a reduction in MR imaging signal that is highly pH-sensitive (Jin et al., 2017). In particular, it may serve as an important biomarker when evaluating the efficacy of novel therapeutics that target pH-sensitive pathways (Anand et al., 2014). Because of the reduced mobile protein content and decrease of pH, AD should have lower APT value than normal control. Our study also demonstrated this viewpoint.

The key to the SAFARI technology is the simultaneous application of RF radiation to acquire images at both the amide proton ($\omega s = +3.5$ ppm) and control ($-\omega s$) frequencies. There is a range of RF acquisition which the amide proton saturation is independent of power. SAFARI only needs to acquire three MR images, and the sum of these images can eliminate the symmetrical MT effects (Scheidegger et al., 2011). A series of SAFARI acquisitions may be used to more selectively detect specific endogenous biomolecules with a unique chemical exchange rate (Bateman et al., 2012). Compared with a conventional MTRasym measurement, the SAFARI method has the advantage of reducing the effect of MT, direct water saturation, and field inhomogeneity and measurement times.

T1 and T2 maps have emerged to be able to adequately identify the biochemical composition and changes of the cartilaginous tissue (Ying et al., 2019). These sequences also enable the direct quantification of T1, T2 values of the myocardium (Kim et al., 2017). In our study, no clear differences were observed between AD and sham rats. Chen et al. (2019) study showed similar finding to our analysis.

The animal behavioral test is essential to understand the bases of neurologic and psychological disorders (Bello-Arroyo et al., 2018). The Y-maze test was implemented to assess immediate spatial working memory of animals (Xu et al., 2018). Because of the simple structure and convenient operation of automated Y-maze applications, more and more animal experiments have adopted the Y-maze to explore the learning and memory of animals (Ru and Liu, 2018). The numbers of arm entries and time spent in the new arm have been identified as well indices of short-term spatial memory (Lewis et al., 2017). The spontaneous alternation behavior, the time spent in the new arm, total distance and the total new arm distance were measured to assess the learning ability of the rats (Conrad et al., 2003).

Crescenzi et al. (2017) revealed that a reduced glutamate chemical exchange saturation transfer (GluCEST) in 3.0 ppm occurred in the subhippocampal fields of AD. Our previous study had found the best parameters for scanning APT (Shen et al., 2017). So, in this study, the APT signals most of the contribution comes from the mobile protein with amide proton, rather than glutamate and glutamine. The increased GFAP in pathology and the loss of neurons in HE staining indicated that amyloid protein toxicity led to glial cell proliferation and neuronal loss (Trias et al., 2017), indicating that the modeling was successful and abnormal protein deposition was the cause of APT signal change.

Limitations

The calculation of APT CEST metric in this study was conventional MTRasym. More specific analysis using the fitting algorithm, which we are currently still working on, would reduce the impact of several unwanted contributors of the APT contrast and make the result more accurate.

CONCLUSION

This report demonstrated the value of APT_{SAFARI} as a non-invasive MRI technique for assessment of AD rat model. The non-invasive nature of APT data collection may allow for a relatively easy translation into the clinical setting. However, further standardization and improvement are required to provide useful diagnostic data within clinically feasible imaging times. We demonstrated abnormality in AD models compared to the sham operated controls, as confirmed by subsequent analysis of histological examinations. In summary, this is the first report of using APT technique with SAFARI method to detect AD. Our study provides evidence of the feasibility of APT imaging in the detection of cerebral abnormality in AD model and it has great potential for clinical application.

AUTHOR CONTRIBUTIONS

RRW and PC were responsible for the study design, acquisition and drafting the manuscript. ZS and ZD was responsible for interpretation of data. BZ undertook the immunohistochemistry analyses. GX and GL performed the CEST data analysis and CEST imaging processing. RRW, YT, and YL built the AD model. YC, XZ, and LL assisted in Y-maze test. RHW was responsible for the study concept and design, study supervision, obtaining funding.

FUNDING

This work was supported by the National Key Research and Development Program of China (Grant No: 2016YFC1305900), the National Natural Science Foundation of China (Grant Nos: 31870981 and 81471730), and the Natural Science Foundation of Guangdong Province (Grant Nos: 2017A030307020 and 2018A030307057).

REFERENCES

Anand, R., Gill, K. D., and Mahdi, A. A. (2014). Therapeutics of Alzheimer's disease: past, present and future. *Neuropharmacology* 76(Pt A), 27–50. doi: 10.1016/j.neuropharm.2013.07.004

Bak, J., Pyeon, H. I., Seok, J. I., and Choi, Y. S. (2017). Effect of rotation preference on spontaneous alternation behavior on Y maze and introduction of a new analytical method, entropy of spontaneous alternation. *Behav. Brain Res.* 320, 219–224. doi: 10.1016/j.bbr.2016.12.011

Bateman, R. J., Xiong, C., Benzinger, T. L. S., Fagan, A. M., Goate, A., Fox, N. C., et al. (2012). Clinical and biomarker changes in dominantly inherited Alzheimer's disease. *N. Engl. J. Med.* 367, 795–804. doi: 10.1056/NEJMoa1202753

Bello-Arroyo, E., Roque, H., Marcos, A., Orihuel, J., Higuera-Matas, A., Desco, M., et al. (2018). MouBeAT: a new and open toolbox for guided analysis of behavioral tests in mice. *Front. Behav. Neurosci.* 12:201. doi: 10.3389/fnbeh.2018.00201

Chen, L., Wei, Z., Chan, K. W. Y., Cai, S., Liu, G., Lu, H., et al. (2019). Protein aggregation linked to Alzheimer's disease revealed by saturation transfer MRI. *Neuroimage* 188, 380–390. doi: 10.1016/j.neuroimage.2018.12.018

Chen, Y., Fu, A. K. Y., and Ip, N. Y. (2018). Synaptic dysfunction in Alzheimer's disease: mechanisms and therapeutic strategies. *Pharmacol. Ther.* 195, 186–198. doi: 10.1016/j.pharmthera.2018.11.006

Conrad, C. D., Grote, K. A., Hobbs, R. J., and Ferayorni, A. (2003). Sex differences in spatial and non-spatial Y-maze performance after chronic stress. *Neurobiol. Learn. Mem.* 79, 32–40. doi: 10.1016/s1074-7427(02)00018-7

Crescenzi, R., DeBrosse, C., Nanga, R. P. R., Byrne, M. D., Krishnamoorthy, G., D'Aquilla, K., et al. (2017). Longitudinal imaging reveals subhippocampal dynamics in glutamate levels associated with histopathologic events in a mouse model of tauopathy and healthy mice. *Hippocampus* 27, 285–302. doi: 10.1002/hipo.22693

Eugenin, J., Vecchiola, A., Murgas, P., Arroyo, P., Cornejo, F., and von Bernhardi, R. (2016). Expression pattern of scavenger receptors and amyloid-beta phagocytosis of astrocytes and microglia in culture are modified by acidosis: implications for Alzheimer's Disease. *J. Alzheimers. Dis.* 53, 857–873. doi: 10.3233/JAD-160083

Fahanik-Babaei, J., Baluchnejadmojarad, T., Nikbakht, F., and Roghani, M. (2018). Trigonelline protects hippocampus against intracerebral Abeta(1-40) as a model of Alzheimer's disease in the rat: insights into underlying mechanisms. *Metab. Brain Dis.* 34, 191–201. doi: 10.1007/s11011-018-0338-8

Fang, B., Wang, D., Huang, M., Yu, G., and Li, H. (2010). Hypothesis on the relationship between the change in intracellular pH and incidence of sporadic Alzheimer's disease or vascular dementia. *Int. J. Neurosci.* 120, 591–595. doi: 10.3109/00207454.2010.505353

Goerke, S., Zaiss, M., Kunz, P., Klika, K. D., Windschuh, J. D., Mogk, A., et al. (2015). Signature of protein unfolding in chemical exchange saturation transfer imaging. *NMR Biomed.* 28, 906–913. doi: 10.1002/nbm.3317

Goozee, K., Chatterjee, P., James, I., Shen, K., Sohrabi, H. R., Asih, P. R., et al. (2017). Alterations in erythrocyte fatty acid composition in preclinical Alzheimer's disease. *Sci. Rep.* 7:676. doi: 10.1038/s41598-017-00751-752

Guerra de Souza, A. C., Goncalves, C. L., de Souza, V., Hartwig, J. M., Farina, M., and Prediger, R. D. (2018). Agmatine attenuates depressive-like behavior and hippocampal oxidative stress following amyloid beta (Abeta1-40) administration in mice. *Behav. Brain Res.* 353, 51–56. doi: 10.1016/j.bbr.2018.06.032

Hwang, E.-S., Kim, H.-B., Lee, S., Kim, M.-J., Lee, S.-O., Han, S.-M., et al. (2017). Loganin enhances long-term potentiation and recovers scopolamine-induced learning and memory impairments. *Physiol. Behav.* 171, 243–248. doi: 10.1016/j.physbeh.2016.12.043

Jin, T., Wang, P., Hitchens, T. K., and Kim, S.-G. (2017). Enhancing sensitivity of pH-weighted MRI with combination of amide and guanidyl CEST. *Neuroimage* 157, 341–350. doi: 10.1016/j.neuroimage.2017.06.007

Johnson, G. A., Badea, A., Brandenburg, J., Cofer, G., Fubara, B., Liu, S., et al. (2010). Waxholm space: an image-based reference for coordinating mouse brain research. *Neuroimage* 53, 365–372. doi: 10.1016/j.neuroimage.2010.06.067

Kamimura, K., Nakajo, M., Yoneyama, T., Takumi, K., Kumagae, Y., Fukukura, Y., et al. (2018). Amide proton transfer imaging of tumors: theory, clinical applications, pitfalls, and future directions. *JPN. J. Radiol.* 37, 109–116. doi: 10.1007/s11604-018-0787-3

Kanazawa, Y., Fushimi, Y., Sakashita, N., Okada, T., Arakawa, Y., and Miyazaki, M. (2018). B1 power optimization for chemical exchange saturation transfer imaging: a phantom study using egg white for amide proton transfer imaging applications in the human brain. *Magn. Reson. Med. Sci.* 17, 86–94. doi: 10.2463/mrms.tn.2016-0069

Kasza, A., Penke, B., Frank, Z., Bozso, Z., Szegedi, V., Hunya, A., et al. (2017). Studies for improving a rat model of Alzheimer's Disease: icv administration of well-characterized beta-amyloid 1-42 oligomers induce dysfunction in spatial memory. *Molecules* 22, E2007. doi: 10.3390/molecules22112007

Kay, K. R., Smith, C., Wright, A. K., Serrano-Pozo, A., Pooler, A. M., Koffie, R., et al. (2013). Studying synapses in human brain with array tomography and electron microscopy. *Nat. Protoc.* 8, 1366–1380. doi: 10.1038/nprot.2013.078

Kim, M., Gillen, J., Landman, B. A., Zhou, J., and van Zijl, P. C. M. (2009). Water saturation shift referencing (WASSR) for chemical exchange saturation transfer (CEST) experiments. *Magn. Reson. Med.* 61, 1441–1450. doi: 10.1002/mrm.21873

Kim, P. K., Hong, Y. J., Im, D. J., Suh, Y. J., Park, C. H., Kim, J. Y., et al. (2017). Myocardial T1 and T2 mapping: techniques and clinical applications. *Korean J. Radiol.* 18, 113–131. doi: 10.3348/kjr.2017.18.1.113

Lewis, S. A., Negelspach, D. C., Kaladchibachi, S., Cowen, S. L., and Fernandez, F. (2017). Spontaneous alternation: a potential gateway to spatial working memory in *Drosophila*. *Neurobiol. Learn. Mem.* 142, 230–235. doi: 10.1016/j.nlm.2017.05.013

Li, Y., Jiao, Q., Xu, H., Du, X., Shi, L., Jia, F., et al. (2017). Biometal dyshomeostasis and toxic metal accumulations in the development of Alzheimer's Disease. *Front. Mol. Neurosci.* 10:339. doi: 10.3389/fnmol.2017.00339

Lin, G., Zhuang, C., Shen, Z., Xiao, G., Chen, Y., Shen, Y., et al. (2018). APT weighted MRI as an effective imaging protocol to predict clinical outcome after acute ischemic stroke. *Front. Neurol* 9:901. doi: 10.3389/fneur.2018.00901

Matsuda, H. (2017). [The application of magnetic resonance imaging in Alzheimer's Disease]. *Brain Nerve* 69, 799–807. doi: 10.11477/mf.1416200823

Prestia, F. A., Galeano, P., Martino Adami, P. V., Do Carmo, S., Castano, E. M., Cuello, A. C., et al. (2018).). Platelets bioenergetics screening reflects the impact of brain abeta plaque accumulation in a rat model of alzheimer. *Neurochem. Res.* 44, 1375–1386. doi: 10.1007/s11064-018-2657-x

Promteangtrong, C., Kolber, M., Ramchandra, P., Moghbel, M., Houshmand, S., Scholl, M., et al. (2015). Multimodality imaging approach in alzheimer disease. part i: structural mri, functional MRI, diffusion tensor imaging and magnetization transfer imaging. dement. *Neuropsychol* 9, 318–329. doi: 10.1590/1980-57642015DN94000318

Rasool, M., Malik, A., Waquar, S., Tul-Ain, Q., Jafar, T. H., Rasool, R., et al. (2018). In-silico characterization and in-vivo validation of albiziasaponin-A, iso-orientin, and salvadorin using a rat model of Alzheimer's Disease. *Front. Pharmacol.* 9:730. doi: 10.3389/fphar.2018.00730

Ru, M., and Liu, H. (2018). Association between Y-Maze acquisition learning and major histocompatibility complex class II polymorphisms in mice. *Biomed. Res. Int.* 2018:6381932. doi: 10.1155/2018/6381932

Scheidegger, R., Vinogradov, E., and Alsop, D. C. (2011). Amide proton transfer imaging with improved robustness to magnetic field inhomogeneity and magnetization transfer asymmetry using saturation with frequency alternating RF irradiation. *Magn. Reson. Med.* 66, 1275–1285. doi: 10.1002/mrm.22912

Shen, Y., Xiao, G., Shen, Z., Zhang, X., Tang, X., Hu, W., et al. (2017). Imaging of nuclear overhauser enhancement at 7 and 3 T. *NMR Biomed.* 30:e3735. doi: 10.1002/nbm.3735

Togao, O., Yoshiura, T., Keupp, J., Hiwatashi, A., Yamashita, K., Kikuchi, K., et al. (2014). Amide proton transfer imaging of adult diffuse gliomas: correlation with histopathological grades. *Neuro. Oncol.* 16, 441–448. doi: 10.1093/neuonc/not158

Trias, E., Ibarburu, S., Barreto-Nunez, R., and Barbeito, L. (2017). Significance of aberrant glial cell phenotypes in pathophysiology of amyotrophic lateral sclerosis. *Neurosci. Lett.* 636, 27–31. doi: 10.1016/j.neulet.2016.07.052

Vanderstichele, H., De Vreese, K., Blennow, K., Andreasen, N., Sindic, C., Ivanoiu, A., et al. (2006). Analytical performance and clinical utility of the INNOTEST PHOSPHO-TAU181P assay for discrimination between Alzheimer's disease and dementia with Lewy bodies. *Clin. Chem. Lab. Med.* 44, 1472–1480. doi: 10.1515/CCLM.2006.258

Wada, T., Togao, O., Tokunaga, C., Funatsu, R., Kobayashi, K., and Nakamura, Y. (2016). Effect of the saturation pulse duration on chemical exchange saturation transfer in amide proton transfer MR imaging: a phantom study. *Radiol. Phys. Technol.* 9, 15–21. doi: 10.1007/s12194-015-0326-1

Wang, M., Bi, W., Fan, K., Li, T., Yan, T., Xiao, F., et al. (2018). Ameliorating effect of *Alpinia oxyphylla-Schisandra chinensis* herb pair on cognitive impairment in a mouse model of Alzheimer's disease. *Biomed. Pharmacother.* 97, 128–135. doi: 10.1016/j.biopha.2017.10.088

Wells, J. A., O'Callaghan, J. M., Holmes, H. E., Powell, N. M., Johnson, R. A., Siow, B., et al. (2015). In vivo imaging of tau pathology using multi-parametric quantitative MRI. *Neuroimage* 111, 369–378. doi: 10.1016/j.neuroimage.2015.02.023

Xu, J., Yadav, N. N., Bar-Shir, A., Jones, C. K., Chan, K. W. Y., Zhang, J., et al. (2014). Variable delay multi-pulse train for fast chemical exchange saturation transfer and relayed-nuclear overhauser enhancement MRI. *Magn. Reson. Med.* 71, 1798–1812. doi: 10.1002/mrm.24850

Xu, M., Xiao, F., Wang, M., Yan, T., Yang, H., Wu, B., et al. (2018). Schisantherin B improves the pathological manifestations of mice caused by behavior desperation in different ages-depression with cognitive impairment. *Biomol. Ther.* 27, 160–167. doi: 10.4062/biomolther.2018.074

Xu, X., Yadav, N. N., Zeng, H., Jones, C. K., Zhou, J., van Zijl, P. C. M., et al. (2016). Magnetization transfer contrast-suppressed imaging of amide proton transfer and relayed nuclear overhauser enhancement chemical exchange saturation transfer effects in the human brain at 7T. *Magn. Reson. Med.* 75, 88–96. doi: 10.1002/mrm.25990

Ying, J., Han, Z., Zeng, Y., Du, Y., Pei, S., Su, L., et al. (2019). Evaluation of intervertebral disc regeneration with injection of mesenchymal stem cells encapsulated in PEGDA-microcryogel delivery system using quantitative T2 mapping: a study in canines. *Am. J. Transl. Res.* 11, 2028–2041.

Zaiss, M., and Bachert, P. (2013). Exchange-dependent relaxation in the rotating frame for slow and intermediate exchange – modeling off-resonant spin-lock and chemical exchange saturation transfer. *NMR Biomed.* 26, 507–518. doi: 10.1002/nbm.2887

Zhang, L., Li, K., Sun, R., Zhang, Y., Ji, J., Huang, P., et al. (2014). Minocycline ameliorates cognitive impairment induced by whole-brain irradiation: an animal study. *Radiat. Oncol.* 9, 281. doi: 10.1186/s13014-014-0281-8

Zhang, N., Song, X., Bartha, R., Beyea, S., D'Arcy, R., Zhang, Y., et al. (2014). Advances in high-field magnetic resonance spectroscopy in Alzheimer's disease. *Curr. Alzheimer Res.* 11, 367–388. doi: 10.2174/15672050116661403022 00312

Zhang, N., Gordon, M. L., and Goldberg, T. E. (2017). Cerebral blood flow measured by arterial spin labeling MRI at resting state in normal aging and Alzheimer's disease. *Neurosci. Biobehav. Rev.* 72, 168–175. doi: 10.1016/j.neubiorev.2016.11.023

Zhang, X.-Y., Wang, F., Xu, J., Gochberg, D. F., Gore, J. C., and Zu, Z. (2018). Increased CEST specificity for amide and fast-exchanging amine protons using exchange-dependent relaxation rate. *NMR Biomed.* 31, e3863. doi: 10.1002/nbm.3863

Zhang, Y. Z., Paterson, Y., and Roder, H. (1995). Rapid amide proton exchange rates in peptides and proteins measured by solvent quenching and two-dimensional NMR. *Protein Sci.* 4, 804–814. doi: 10.1002/pro.5560040420

Zollner, H. J., Butz, M., Kircheis, G., Klinker, S., Haussinger, D., Schmitt, B., et al. (2018). Ammonia-weighted imaging by chemical exchange saturation transfer MRI at 3 T. *NMR Biomed.* 31:e3947. doi: 10.1002/nbm.3947

18

Age-Dependent Relationship Between Plasma Aβ40 and Aβ42 and Total Tau Levels in Cognitively Normal Subjects

*Lih-Fen Lue[1], Ming-Chyi Pai[2], Ta-Fu Chen[3], Chaur-Jong Hu[4,5], Li-Kai Huang[4,5], Wei-Che Lin[6], Chau-Chung Wu[7], Jian-Shing Jeng[3], Kaj Blennow[8,9], Marwan N. Sabbagh[10], Sui-Hing Yan[11], Pei-Ning Wang[12,13], Shieh-Yueh Yang[14,15], Hiroyuki Hatsuta[16,17], Satoru Morimoto[16,18], Akitoshi Takeda[17], Yoshiaki Itoh[17], Jun Liu[19], Haiqun Xie[20] and Ming-Jang Chiu[3]**

[1]Civin Neuropathology Laboratory, Banner Sun Health Research Institute, Sun City, AZ, United States, [2]Division of Behavioral Neurology, Department of Neurology, National Cheng Kung University Hospital, College of Medicine, National Cheng Kung University, Tainan, Taiwan, [3]Department of Neurology, National Taiwan University Hospital, College of Medicine, National Taiwan University, Taipei, Taiwan, [4]Department of Neurology, Taipei Medical University, Taipei, Taiwan, [5]Department of Neurology, Shuang Ho Hospital, Taipei Medical University, New Taipei City, Taiwan, [6]Department of Neurology, Kaohsiung Chang Gung Memorial Hospital, Kaohsiung, Taiwan, [7]Department of Internal Medicine, National Taiwan University Hospital, College of Medicine, National Taiwan University, Taipei, Taiwan, [8]Clinical Neurochemistry Laboratory, Sahlgrenska University Hospital, Mölndal, Sweden, [9]Department of Psychiatry and Neurochemistry, Institute of Neuroscience and Physiology, University of Gothenburg, Mölndal, Sweden, [10]Lou Ruvo Center for Brain Health, Cleveland Clinic Nevada, Las Vegas, NV, United States, [11]Department of Neurology, Renai Branch, Taipei City Hospital, Taipei, Taiwan, [12]Department of Neurology, National Yang-Ming University, Taipei, Taiwan, [13]Department of Neurology, Taipei Veterans General Hospital, Taipei, Taiwan, [14]MagQu Company Limited, New Taipei City, Taiwan, [15]MagQu LLC, Surprise, AZ, United States, [16]Hatsuta Neurology Clinic, Osaka, Japan, [17]Department of Neurology, Osaka City University Graduate School of Medicine, Osaka, Japan, [18]Department of Physiology, School of Medicine, Keio University, Tokyo, Japan, [19]Departemnt of Neurology, Sun Yat-Sen Memorial Hospital, Sun Yat-Sen University, Guangzhou, China, [20]Department of Neurology, Foshan Hospital of Sun Yat-Sen University, Foshan, China

***Correspondence:**
Ming-Jang Chiu
mjchiu@ntu.edu.tw

Both amyloid plaques and neurofibrillary tangles are pathological hallmarks in the brains of patients with Alzheimer's disease (AD). However, the constituents of these hallmarks, amyloid beta (Aβ) 40, Aβ42, and total Tau (t-Tau), have been detected in the blood of cognitively normal subjects by using an immunomagnetic reduction (IMR) assay. Whether these levels are age-dependent is not known, and their interrelation remains undefined. We determined the levels of these biomarkers in cognitively normal subjects of different age groups. A total of 391 cognitively normal subjects aged 23–91 were enrolled from hospitals in Asia, Europe, and North America. Healthy cognition was evaluated by NIA-AA guidelines to exclude subjects with mild cognitive impairment (MCI) and AD and by cognitive assessment using the Mini Mental State Examination and Clinical Dementia Rating (CDR). We examined the effect of age on plasma levels of Aβ40, Aβ42, and t-Tau and the relationship between these biomarkers during aging. Additionally, we explored age-related reference intervals for each biomarker. Plasma t-Tau and Aβ42 levels had modest but significant correlations with chronological age (r = 0.127, p = 0.0120 for t-Tau; r = −0.126, p = 0.0128 for Aβ42), ranging from ages 23 to 91. Significant positive correlations were detected between Aβ42 and t-Tau in the groups aged 50 years and older, with Rho values ranging from 0.249 to 0.474. Significant negative correlations were detected between Aβ40 and t-Tau from age 40 to 91 (r ranged from −0.293 to −0.582) and between Aβ40 and Aβ42 in the age groups of 30–39 (r = −0.562, p = 0.0235), 50–59 (r = −0.261, p = 0.0142), 60–69 (r = −0.303, p = 0.0004), and 80–91 (r = 0.459, p = 0.0083). We also provided age-related reference intervals for each biomarker. In this multicenter study, age had weak but significant effects on the levels of Aβ42 and t-Tau in plasma. However, the age group defined by decade revealed the emergence of a relationship between Aβ40, Aβ42, and t-Tau in the 6th and 7th decades. Validation of our findings in a large-scale and longitudinal study is warranted.

Keywords: Alzheimer, plasma, amyloid, tau, immunomagnetic reduction, cognitively normal subjects

INTRODUCTION

The greatest risk factor for developing late-onset Alzheimer's disease (AD) is age. At age 65, the incidence of AD is 3%, and every 5–6 years, the incidence rate doubles (Kukull et al., 2002; Ziegler-Graham et al., 2008). As the population of the world is living longer, it is estimated that there will be over 100 million people with AD by 2050 (Alzheimer's Association, 2013). To meet the challenges ahead, the development of effective disease-modifying therapeutics and preventative strategies is being accelerated. In the meantime, there is also a pressing need for developing biomarkers whose intended use is for identifying preclinical AD or subjects at risk of AD for clinical trials. Studies have shown that by combining various biomarkers, such as amyloid positron emission tomography (PET), fluorodeoxyglucose (FDG)-PET, magnetic resonance imaging (MRI), and cerebral spinal fluid (CSF) measures of amyloid beta (Aβ), total Tau (t-Tau), and phosphorylated Tau (p-Tau), the accuracy for identifying preclinical AD could be improved (Dubois et al., 2014, 2016; Jack et al., 2016, 2018).

Currently, there are no blood-based biomarkers for identifying the preclinical stage of AD. The progress in developing blood-based biomarkers has been hampered previously by the lack of sensitivity and other technical limitations (Blennow, 2017; Lue et al., 2017a). The most widely used immunoassays for measuring AD biomarkers in CSF produced discordant findings when used in blood (Fei et al., 2011; Olsson et al., 2016; Lövheim et al., 2017; Hanon et al., 2018). Recently, several new technologies have offered superior detection sensitivity and accuracy in measuring blood-based biomarkers (Andreasson et al., 2016; Zetterberg and Blennow, 2018). These innovative technologies include immunomagnetic reduction (IMR) assay (Chiu et al., 2012), single-molecule assay (SIMOA; Janelidze et al., 2016), immuno-infrared-sensor assay (Nabers et al., 2018), and immunoprecipitation-mass spectrophotometry (Nakamura et al., 2018).

Some of these technologies are being validated for classifying mild cognitive impairment (MCI) and AD and for prescreening for PET scans (Chiu et al., 2012, 2013; Tzen et al., 2014; Lue et al., 2017b; Verberk et al., 2018). AD pathological formation precedes the clinical symptoms by one to two decades (Jack et al., 2013). To identify the earliest changes in the blood to reflect the brain pathological state, it is necessary to first establish the normal ranges of the biomarkers Aβ40, Aβ42, and t-Tau. Therefore, in this study, we characterized the age-associated levels of these biomarkers and their relationship within different age groups and finally provided age-related reference intervals for each biomarker. To generalize our research results, this study was conducted in young, middle-aged and older adults with normal cognition across various countries. It is worth noting that this study is cross-sectional, not longitudinal.

MATERIALS AND METHODS

Participating Sites

A total of 391 cognitively normal subjects aged 23–91 were enrolled from 2010 to 2018 from the following six hospitals in Taiwan: National Taiwan University Hospital (NTUH), Taipei Medical University Shuang-Ho Hospital (SHH), Renai Branch of Taipei City Hospital (RAH), Taipei Veterans General Hospital (TVGH), National Cheng Kung University Hospital (NCKUH), and Kaohsiung Chang Gung Memorial Hospital (KCGMH); Sahlgrenska University Hospital (SUH) in Guttenberg, Sweden; Banner Sun Health Research Institute (BSHRI) in Sun City, AZ, USA; two hospitals in the cities of Foshan, Foshan Hospital (FH) and Guangzhou, Sun Yat-Sen Memorial Hospital (SYSMH), Guangdong, China; and finally two hospitals in Japan: Hatsuta Neurology Clinic (HNC) in Osaka, and Osaka City University Hospital (OCUH) in Osaka. All participants were older than 21 years of age and gave their own written informed consent. The study was approved by the Institutional Review Board (IRB) or Research Ethics Committee (REC) of each participating hospital in the respective countries, namely, NTUH REC, Taipei Medical University-Joint IRB for SHH, Taipei City Hospital REC for RAH, TVGH IRB, NCKUH IRB, KCGMH IRB, Central Ethical Review Board-University of Gothenburg for SUH, Banner Health IRB for BSHRI, Sun Yat-Sen University Hospital (SYSUH) Cancer Center IRB, Asai Dermatology Clinic IRB and Osaka City University IRB.

Cognition Assessment and Criteria for Recruitment

The purpose of the recruitment criteria was to exclude subjects with diagnoses of MCI and dementia. All study sites followed the NIA-AA criteria for the diagnosis of dementia and MCI due to AD (Albert et al., 2011; McKhann et al., 2011).

TABLE 1 | The means and standard deviations (SD) of age (years) of the normal-cognition subjects in each participating site*

Site No.	Name of Sites	Subject No.	Median (years)	Minimum (years)	Maximum (years)	Age, years Mean ± SD
1	NTUH-1	90	57	23	81	53.60 ± 17.91
2	NTUH-2	79	69	56	89	70.35 ± 8.12
3	NTUH-3	24	46	26	89	49.54 ± 18.41
4	NCKUH	48	54	33	70	54.15 ± 7.49
5	SHH	38	65	56	76	64.97 ± 5.63
6	KCGMH	27	60	50	72	61.15 ± 4.93
7	SU	18	71	53	89	70.50 ± 9.60
8	BSHRI	16	82	71	91	81.94 ± 5.99
9	RAH	11	64	58	74	64.91 ± 5.05
10	TVGH	17	60	54	88	64.06 ± 10.23
11	SYSH	9	66	45	79	62.67 ± 10.25
12	HNC/OCUH	14	65	53	83	64.93 ± 7.21

**Normal cognition: CDR = 0, MMSE: 28-30, and meet NIA-AA guidelines published in 2011. Name of sites: NTUH, National Taiwan University Hospital; NCKUH, National Cheng Kung University Hospital; SHH, Shuang Ho Hospital; KCGMH, Kaohsiung Chang Gung Memorial Hospital; SUH, Sahlgrenska University Hospital; BSHRI, Banner Sun Health Research Institute; RAH, Renai Branch Taipei City Hospital; TVGHL, Taipei Veterans General Hospital; SYSMH, Sun Yet-Sen Memory Hospital; FH, Foshan Hospital; HNC, Hatsuta Neurology Clinic; OCUH, Osaka City University; SD, standard deviation.*

In addition to clinical criteria, basic cognitive assessment tools [Mini-Mental State Examination (MMSE) and Clinical Dementia Rating (CDR)] were also used. The criteria for normal cognition were MMSE $\geq$ 28 and CDR = 0. Brain imaging and CSF biomarkers were used as supplementary tools. Brain (FDG)-PET were used by HNC/OCUH, Japan, and Subjects from SUH, Sweden had CSF Aβ > 530 pg/ml and t-Tau < 350 pg/ml (Sutphen et al., 2015; Teunissen et al., 2018). Subjects who had acute or chronic systemic diseases or neuropsychiatric disorders, visual or auditory dysfunction severe enough to interfere with cognitive assessments were all excluded.

Numbers of subjects and age profiles of participating hospitals are shown in **Table 1**.

Preparation of Plasma Samples

Nonfasting plasma samples were collected in EDTA-coated vacutainers (Becton Dickinson, New Jersey, NJ, USA) followed by centrifugation at speeds ranging from 1,500 g to 2,500 g for 15 min at room temperature. The upper layer (plasma) was transferred to a new 15-ml tube, aliquoted into 1.5 ml tubes, and stored at −70°C or lower. Sample aliquots were shipped on dry ice to MagQu Company Limited for IMR assays of Aβ1–40, Aβ1–42 and t-Tau. Assays were performed without knowing the demographic features of the subjects.

Assays of Aβ40, Aβ42 and t-Tau in Human Plasma

Before the assays, frozen aliquoted samples were thawed on ice. Sample preparation and assays were performed at room temperature. Assays were performed in duplicate for each sample for Aβ40, Aβ42 and t-Tau. The volumes of the reagents and plasma samples were 80 μl reagent (MF-AB0–0060, MagQu) and 40 μl plasma for the Aβ40 assay, 60 μl reagent (MF-AB2–0060, MagQu) and 60 μl plasma for the Aβ42 assay, and 80 μl reagent (MF-TAU-0060, MagQu) and 40 μl plasma for the t-Tau assay. Samples and reagents were mixed briefly in special-sized glass tubes and sealed. The tubes were then placed inside the sample channels of the IMR analyzer (XacPro-S, MagQu) for assay. The concentrations of Aβ40, Aβ42, and t-Tau were calculated according to the standard curves respective to each biomarker. The means of the values obtained from duplicate measurements were calculated for each biomarker and each sample.

Statistical Analysis

Statistical analysis was performed with MedCalc statistical software version 17.4.4[1]. The statistical significance was defined as $p < 0.05$. Continuous variables according to age groups were analyzed by one-way analysis of variance followed by pairwise differences using the *Student-Newman-Keuls test*. Spearman's correlations were performed to determine the correlation between the levels of each plasma biomarker and demographic features such as age, sex, and the presence of the ApoEε4 allele. The relationship between different biomarkers was also analyzed according to the age groups defined by the intervals of 10 years starting from 20 years of age. Three participants aged 91 were combined into a group of ages 80–89. Multiple stepwise regression analysis was used to determine whether age, ApoE ε4 allele, and biomarkers (Aβ40, Aβ42, and t-Tau) had a significant contribution to the levels of a particular biomarker. MedCalc software was used for the construction of age-related reference intervals, and the values of the biomarkers at the 2.5th and 97.5th percentiles were tabulated.

RESULTS

Cohort Characteristics

This study included a total of 391 cognitively normal subjects aged 23–91 years from 12 participating hospitals. The relative frequency of age distribution is shown in **Figure 1**. The ApoE genotype information is shown in **Table 2**. We then determined whether carrying one or two ApoE ε4 alleles had effects on any of the biomarker levels. The results in **Table 3** show that the only genotype effect was on Aβ40. The Apo-ε4 carriers had significantly lower levels of Aβ40.

[1] www.medcalc.org

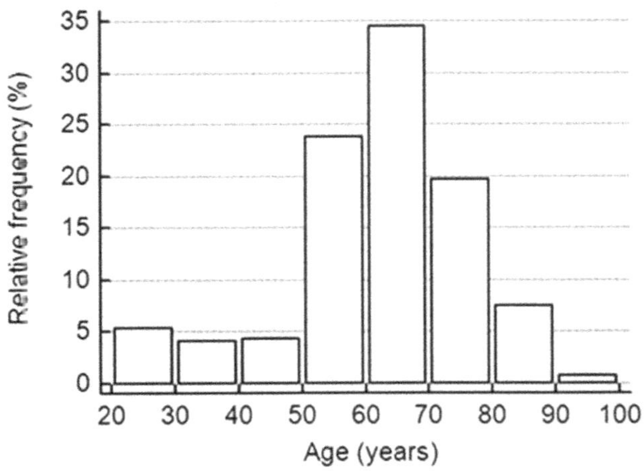

FIGURE 1 | The vertical bar on the y-axis shows the frequency as the percentage in the number of all participants in the cohort, and the x-axis indicates the age groups in 10-year intervals.

TABLE 2 | The numbers of subjects according to ApoE genotypes.

ApoE genotypes	Number (%)
2/3	19 (11.9)
2/4	3 (1.9)
3/3	110 (68.8)
3/4	27 (16.9)
4/4	1 (0.6)

TABLE 3 | The levels of Aβ40, Aβ42, and t-Tau in pg/ml grouped by ApoE ε4 carrier status.

ApoE ε4	Aβ40 mean ± SD (*n*)	Aβ42 mean ± SD (*n*)	t-Tau mean ± SD (*n*)
Non-carriers	58.59 ± 15.61* (125)	15.20 ± 2.17 (129)	18.90 ± 8.24 (129)
Carriers	52.36 ± 10.25* (31)	15.13 ± 2.02 (31)	20.83 ± 8.64 (31)

**Denotes statistical significance p < 0.05.*

TABLE 4 | Plasma AD bioboconcentrations (pg/ml) by age groups.

Age groups	Aβ40 mean ± SD (*n*)	Aβ42 mean ± SD (*n*)	t-Tau mean ± SD (*n*)
20–29	62.21 ± 5.19 (21)	15.71 ± 0.41 (21)	16.51 ± 5.91 (21)
30–39	61.23 ± 9.14 (16)	15.57 ± 2.28 (16)	17.18 ± 6.12 (16)
40–49	56.48 ± 8.60 (15)	16.47 ± 3.73 (17)	18.83 ± 10.54 (16)
50–59	57.95 ± 11.30 (88)	15.42 ± 1.78 (93)	16.07 ± 7.92 (93)
60–69	59.58 ± 13.99 (132)	15.40 ± 2.52 (135)	17.85 ± 8.92 (135)
70–79	60.72 ± 15.02 (74)	15.13 ± 2.35 (77)	17.98 ± 9.21 (77)
80–91	58.61 ± 17.84 (32)	15.60 ± 2.23 (32)	22.37 ± 5.48 (32)

SD, standard deviation; n, number of subjects.

TABLE 5 | Relationship between Aβ40, Aβ42, and t-Tau within each age group.

Age group	Aβ40 vs. t-Tau	Aβ42 vs. t-Tau	Aβ40 vs. Aβ42
20–29	$\rho = -0.087$ $p = 0.7074$ $n = 21$	$\rho = -0.308$ $p = 0.07074$ $n = 21$	$\rho = -0.126$ $p = 0.5875$ $n = 21$
30–39	$\rho = 0.076$ $p = 0.7783$ $n = 16$	$\rho = 0.282$ $p = 0.2893$ $n = 16$	$\rho = -0.562$ $p = 0.0235$ $n = 16$
40–49	$\rho = -0.582$ $p = 0.0228$ $n = 15$	$\rho = 0.444$ $p = 0.0745$ $n = 17$	$\rho = -0.321$ $p = 0.2427$ $n = 15$
50–59	$\rho = -0.445$ $p < 0.0001$ $n = 88$	$\rho = 0.474$ $p < 0.0001$ $n = 93$	$\rho = -0.261$ $p = 0.0142$ $n = 88$
60–69	$\rho = -0.458$ $p < 0.0001$ $n = 132$	$\rho = 0.341$ $p < 0.0001$ $n = 135$	$\rho = -0.303$ $p = 0.0004$ $n = 132$
70–79	$\rho = -0.293$ $p = 0.0113$ $n = 74$	$\rho = 0.249$ $p = 0.0292$ $n = 77$	$\rho = -0.116$ $p = 0.3235$ $n = 74$
80–91	$\rho = -0.252$ $p = 0.1634$ $n = 32$	$\rho = 0.459$ $p = 0.0083$ $n = 32$	$\rho = -0.120$ $p = 0.5147$ $n = 32$

Correlations of Age With the Concentrations and Ratios of Aβ40, Aβ42, and t-Tau

To determine the relationship between age and plasma concentrations and the ratios of Aβ40, Aβ42, and t-Tau, Spearman's rank correlation analyses were performed. A significant positive correlation was detected between age and t-Tau concentrations ($r = 0.127$, $p = 0.0120$), and a negative correlation was detected between age and Aβ42 concentrations ($r = -0.126$, $p = 0.0128$). There was also a significant correlation with the ratio of Aβ42 to t-Tau ($r = -0.155$, $p = 0.0022$). These correlation coefficients were modest. No correlation was detected between age and Aβ40 concentrations or ratios.

Relationship Between Core AD Bioarkers Within Age Groups

To further examine the age effect, we grouped all participants by 10-years intervals starting from age 20 to 29 years, the third decade. Aβ40, Aβ42, and t-Tau levels for these age groups are shown in **Table 4**. None of these biomarkers had age-group differences. To determine how age affected the relationship between the AD biomarkers in plasma, Spearman's rank correlation analyses between the biomarkers within each age group were performed (**Table 5**).

We observed an increasing presence of the relationship between AD biomarkers as age advances. A negative correlation was found between Aβ40 and Aβ42 in the age group ranging from 30 to 69 with the exception of the people in the 5th decade (age 40–49). Plasma t-Tau and Aβ40 concentrations were negatively correlated in age groups starting at age 40 and up to age 79. The t-Tau and Aβ42 concentrations correlated positively in age groups starting from age 50 to 59 to the oldest age group. These findings demonstrated that the levels of all three AD biomarkers in plasma became associated with each other in the 6th and 7th decades of life.

We also assessed whether the age group, ApoE ε4 carrier status, and plasma AD biomarkers could be useful for predicting the concentration of a specific AD biomarker (**Table 6**). Stepwise multiple regression analyses were performed for each biomarker by entering data in the order of age group, ApoE ε4 allele status, and the other two biomarkers. The results showed that ApoE ε4 allele status was not a significant contributor to the prediction of any biomarker levels. By contrast, age

TABLE 6 | Multiple regression of age group, ApoE ε4 allele, and plasma biomarkers.

	Variables in regression equation	F-ratios	p	Co-efficient of determination	Variables excluded from equation
Aβ40	Age group, t-Tau	7.13	= 0.0001	0.1538	ApoEε4, Aβ42
Aβ42	Age group, t-Tau	21.35	<0.0001	0.3612	ApoEε4, Aβ40
t-Tau	Age group, Aβ40, Aβ42	23.05	<0.0001	0.3702	ApoEε4

group contributed to the prediction of the AD biomarker concentrations. Plasma t-Tau concentrations could be predicted by a combination of age group and plasma concentrations of Aβ42 and Aβ40 with a coefficient of determination of 0.3701 ($p < 0.0001$). The coefficient of determination for predicting Aβ42 concentrations was 0.3433 ($p < 0.0001$) when age group and t-Tau concentrations were included in the model. The coefficient of determination for Aβ40 concentration prediction was 0.1205 ($p = 0.0001$) with age group and t-Tau in the model.

Age-Related Reference Intervals of Plasma AD Biomarkers

As blood-based biomarkers have the potential to be used for screening subjects at the preclinical stage or those with MCI or early AD in the clinic or for clinical trials, we performed an analysis of the age-related reference intervals of Aβ40, Aβ42, and t-Tau concentrations from 391 subjects. The temporal concentration range of each biomarker is shown by age group at the 2.5th and 97.5th centiles in **Table 7**. Additional 10th and 90th centiles for each biomarker are illustrated in **Figures 2A–C**.

DISCUSSION

In this cross-sectional study, we characterized the relationship between age and three plasma AD core biomarkers and the relationship between these biomarkers within a given age group. The 391cognitively normal subjects spanning 23–91 years of age were enrolled from 12 participating hospitals located in Asia, the USA, and Europe. The statistical analyses were performed in all participants as one large multicenter cohort. Our study detected weak but significant correlations between chronological years of age and plasma Aβ42 and t-Tau. Plasma Aβ42 decreased as age increased, in contrast to t-Tau, which increased with age. As the age span of the cohort was quite large, we grouped ages into 10-years intervals to assess whether the changes in plasma biomarker levels were more prominent in certain decades. By grouping ages into 10-years intervals, we did not detect age-group-associated differences in all three biomarkers. However, our important finding came from an analysis of the relationship between biomarkers within a given decade of life. There was an emerging prevalence of relationships between AD biomarkers during ages 50–70. Although no significant relationship between any two AD biomarkers was detected in the middle-aged groups, e.g., the 3rd and 4th decades of life, positive correlations between Aβ42 and t-Tau were detected from the 6th to 9th decades; negative correlations were detected between Aβ40 and Aβ42 in age groups from the 4th, 6th, and 7th decades and between Aβ40 and t-Tau during the 5th to 8th decades. During the 6th and 7th decade of life, all three biomarkers showed a significant relationship, positively correlated between Aβ42 and t-Tau and negatively correlated between Aβ40 and Aβ42 and Aβ40 and t-Tau. These relationships provided significant insights into the aging-associated patterns of changes in AD plasma biomarkers. Previous IMR studies reported AD-associated increases in Aβ42 and t-Tau (Chiu et al., 2013). This supports that during the 6th to 8th decades of life, the expression patterns of plasma biomarkers coincided with the pattern observed in MCI and early AD.

TABLE 7 | Age-related plasma biomarker reference intervals (pg/ml).

Age (years)	Aβ40		Aβ42		t-Tau	
	0.025	0.975	0.025	0.975	0.025	0.975
30	47.87	72.98	14.35	17.18	5.18	28.33
40	41.37	74.42	13.19	18.26	3.23	30.56
50	37.73	77.74	12.27	18.90	1.83	32.06
60	35.80	81.82	11.65	19.18	1.24	33.11
70	34.48	85.52	11.42	19.20	1.77	34.01
80	32.62	87.71	11.65	19.02	3.69	35.02
90	29.0	87.28	12.43	18.72	7.29	36.45

There have been only a few studies analyzing the effect of age on the levels of Aβ and t-Tau in incognitively normal subjects. One study reported a decrease in plasma Aβ40 levels with age (Kleinschmidt et al., 2016). Another study, dividing 245 subjects into age groups of young (≤34), adult (35≤ age ≤64), and old (>64), showed the lowest plasma Aβ42 concentration in the youngest group but no differences between the two older groups. The assay used in this study was Innogenetics ELISA (Belgium; Zecca et al., 2018). A study in Korean healthy adults aged 40–69 reported the effects of age and sex on the plasma levels and ratios of Aβ42 and Aβ40 (Kim et al., 2016). The assays of the study were also performed in ELISA format (Immuno-Biological Laboratories, Japan). A previous study on the plasma of healthy controls using IMR assays detected significantly higher tau levels in subjects aged 65–95 years than in the group aged 45–64 years (Chiu et al., 2017). If the participants in the present study were divided into only two groups, younger than 65 and older than 65, similar results were found (higher tau in the older group, $P = 0.0378$). The differences in findings between the reports could be due to the types of assays used for obtaining data, the age ranges, the age grouping, and the number of subjects in age groups.

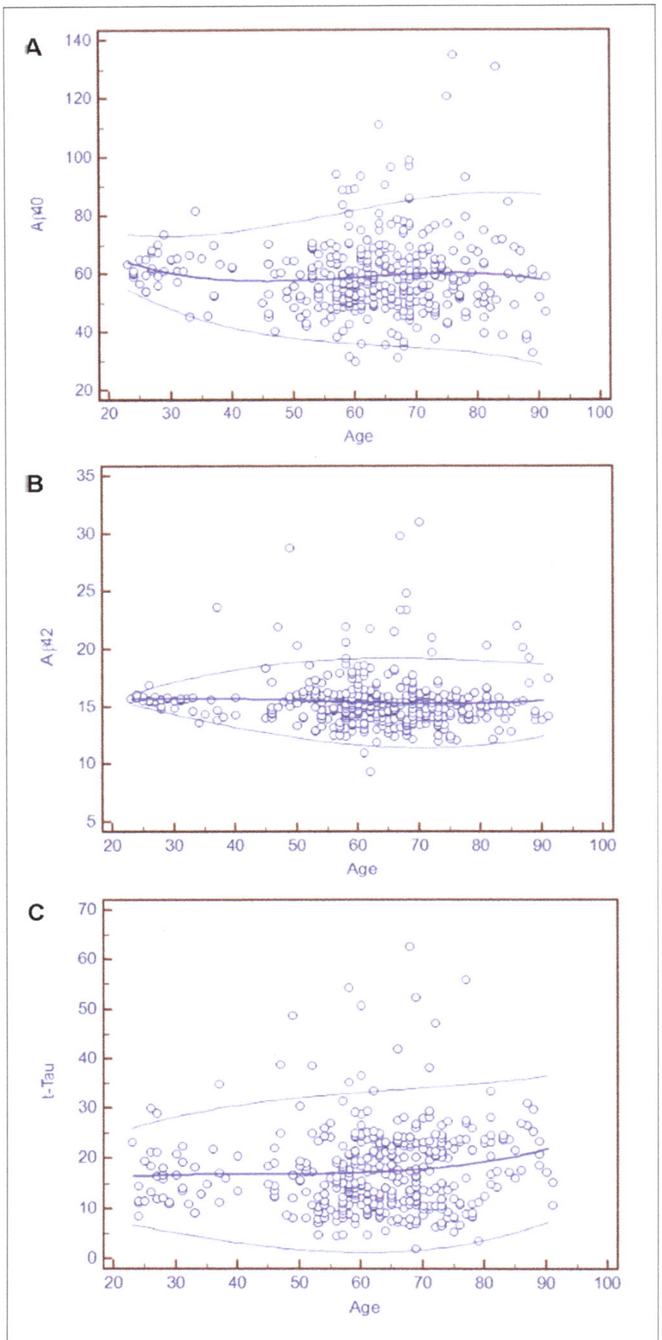

FIGURE 2 | Age-related plasma biomarker reference intervals: means and centiles. The scatter plots illustrate the reference intervals for Aβ40 **(A)**, Aβ42 **(B)**, and t-Tau **(C)**. The age range in years is indicated on the x-axis, and the reference intervals of each marker are shown in circles in the figure. The units of the reference intervals are pg/ml. The central lines are the calculated means, and the top and bottom lines are the 90th and 10th centile curves.

The physiological significance of these relationships found in this study is not readily understood. It is possible that as age advances, various upstream/downstream molecular mechanisms in the brain (production, accumulation) and/or periphery (excretion, destruction) that affect circulating levels of Aβ40, Aβ42, and t-Tau could converge or interact, resulting in the formation of a relationship. Evidence has supported that amyloid pathological events in the brain precede and trigger Tau pathology and even synergize with each other (Small and Duff, 2008; Han and Shi, 2016). Notably, the relationships between these AD biomarkers were most prominently detected during the 6th and 7th decades of life, the time when AD pathology had increasingly accumulated in the brain and CSF Aβ42 changes were already detectable (Buchhave et al., 2012).

It has been demonstrated with different preclinical AD classification systems that in cognitively normal subjects in their 70s and older, AD pathology is prevalent (Dubois et al., 2016; Jack et al., 2016; Kern et al., 2018). Our finding that the relationship between plasma AD biomarkers was most prominently present in the age group of 60–69 suggested that age-related changes in the brain might be captured in plasma, as observed in the relationship between AD biomarkers during aging.

It has been well established that the decreases in CSF Aβ42 coincide with increased brain amyloid plaque pathology (Seeburger et al., 2015; Doecke et al., 2018). In CSF, Aβ changes were detected before the changes in t-Tau in cognitively normal adults (Buchhave et al., 2012), and the change could be observed as early as middle-age (Sutphen et al., 2015). It is important to establish the relationship of core AD biomarkers between CSF and plasma. A recent study reported a significant but small positive correlation between IMR-assayed plasma Aβ42 levels and ELISA-assayed CSF Aβ42 levels in incognitively normal subjects (Teunissen et al., 2018). Further studies using the same assay platforms are needed to understand this relationship.

The mechanisms by which the ApoE ε4 genotype increases the risk of developing AD have been an important topic of research. Much evidence has indicated that ApoE ε4 forms less stable complexes with Aβ (Chiu et al., 2013). How this might affect soluble Aβ levels in the circulation has not been understood because of the complexity of the potential mechanisms involved in brain and peripheral clearance as well as the degradation of the complexes. In this study, we detected higher plasma Aβ40 levels in ApoE ε4 noncarriers than in ApoE ε4 carriers. Nevertheless, a cross-sectional cognitively normal population-based study that determined how ApoE ε4 status affected the relationship between plasma levels of Aβ species and soluble receptors for Aβ, the soluble low-density lipoprotein receptor-related protein-1 (sLRP1) and soluble receptor for advanced glycation end products (sRAGE), found positive correlations of the receptors with Aβ40 but not with Aβ42 in ApoE ε4 noncarriers (Tai et al., 2014). This finding led to speculation that part of the reason why the noncarriers had higher levels of Aβ40 in plasma than the carriers could be because more clearance receptors were available in the noncarriers. This possibility will require further studies in different cohorts to validate the findings by Gao et al. (2018) and us as well as research to delineate the genotype-specific mechanisms in the brain-periphery clearance associated with these two Aβ receptors (Deane et al., 2009; Zlokovic et al., 2010).

CONCLUSION

Previously, plasma levels of Aβ or t-Tau were considered to have limited value as biomarkers for disease classification. However, new technologies with superior technical sensitivity bring hope to the potential of using blood-based biomarkers in identifying preclinical, MCI, and early AD subjects. In this study, we provided the normal ranges of Aβ species and t-Tau in plasma as well as the development of a dynamic relationship between the biomarkers from middle to old age. Future studies will move towards a better understanding of the biology and dynamics of plasma Aβ and Tau in health and disease, as well as vigorous assessment of the clinical utility of IMR-assayed plasma Aβ and Tau in identifying preclinical AD, MCI, and early AD, and the study findings should be comparable with those from CSF biomarker and imaging studies.

AUTHOR CONTRIBUTIONS

M-CP, T-FC, C-JH, L-KH, W-CL, C-CW, J-SJ, KB, MS, S-HY, P-NW, HH, SM, AT, YI, JL, HX, and M-JC enrolled subjects and performed clinical diagnosis for all participants. S-YY was responsible for IMR measurements. L-FL conducted the statistical analysis and prepared the manuscript. M-JC critically reviewed and revised the manuscript.

FUNDING

We acknowledge the funding support of the Arizona Alzheimer Consortium for the study conducted in the United States, Ulvac Inc., for the study conducted in Osaka and Innovative Biotechnology Limited for the study conducted in Foshan and Guangzhou. The study conducted in National Taiwan University Hospital was supported in part by National Health Research Institutes, Taiwan (05A1-PHSP03-028) and in part by Ministry of Science and Technology Taiwan (106~108-2321-B-002-018,075,002).

REFERENCES

Albert, M. S., DeKosky, S. T., Dickson, D., Dubois, B., Feldman, H. H., Fox, N. C., et al. (2011). The diagnosis of mild cognitive impairment due to Alzheimer's disease: recommendations from the National Institute on Aging-Alzheimer's Association workgroups on diagnostic guidelines for Alzheimer's disease. *Alzheimers Dement.* 7, 270–279. doi: 10.1016/j.jalz.2011.03.008

Alzheimer's Association. (2013). Alzheimer's disease facts and figures. *Alzheimers Dement.* 9, 208–245. doi: 10.1016/j.jalz.2013.02.003

Andreasson, U., Blennow, K., and Zetterberg, H. (2016). Update on ultrasensitive technologies to facilitate research on blood biomarkers for central nervous system disorders. *Alzheimers Dement.* 3, 98–102. doi: 10.1016/j.dadm.2016.05.005

Blennow, K. (2017). A review of fluid biomarkers for Alzheimer's disease: moving from CSF to blood. *Neurol. Ther.* 6, 15–24. doi: 10.1007/s40120-017-0073-9

Buchhave, P., Minthon, L., Zetterberg, H., Wallin, A. K., Blennow, K., and Hansson, O. (2012). Cerebrospinal fluid levels of β-amyloid 1-42, but not of tau, are fully changed already 5 to 10 years before the onset of Alzheimer dementia. *Arch. Gen. Psychiatry* 69, 98–106. doi: 10.1001/archgenpsychiatry.2011.155

Chiu, M. J., Fan, L. Y., Chen, T. F., Chen, Y. F., Chieh, J. J., and Horng, H. E. (2017). Plasma tau levels in cognitively normal middle-aged and older adults. *Front. Aging Neurosci.* 9:51. doi: 10.3389/fnagi.2017.00051

Chiu, M. J., Yang, S. Y., Chen, T. F., Chieh, J. J., Huang, T. Z., Yip, P. K., et al. (2012). New assay for old markers-plasma β amyloid of mild cognitive impairment and Alzheimer's disease. *Curr. Alzheimer Res.* 9, 1142–1148. doi: 10.2174/156720512804142967

Chiu, M. J., Yang, S. Y., Horng, H. E., Yang, C. C., Chen, T. F., Chieh, J. J., et al. (2013). Combined plasma biomarkers for diagnosing mild cognition impairment and Alzheimer's disease. *ACS Chem. Neurosci.* 4, 1530–1536. doi: 10.1021/cn400129p

Deane, R., Bell, R. D., Sagare, A., and Zlokovic, B. V. (2009). Clearance of amyloid-beta peptide across the blood-brain barrier: implication for therapies in Alzheimer's disease. *CNS Neurol. Disord. Drug Targets* 8, 16–30. doi: 10.2174/187152709787601867

Doecke, J. D., Rembach, A., Villemagne, V. L., Varghese, S., Rainey-Smith, S., Sarros, S., et al. (2018). Concordance between cerebrospinal fluid biomarkers with Alzheimer's disease pathology between three independent assay platforms. *J. Alzheimers Dis.* 61, 169–183. doi: 10.3233/jad-170128

Dubois, B., Feldman, H. H., Jacova, C., Hampel, H., Molinuevo, J. L., Blennow, K., et al. (2014). Advancing research diagnostic criteria for Alzheimer's disease: the IWG-2 criteria. *Lancet Neurol.* 13, 614–629. doi: 10.1016/S1474-4422(14)70090-0

Dubois, B., Hampel, H., Feldman, H. H., Scheltens, P., Aisen, P., Andrieu, S., et al. (2016). Preclinical Alzheimer's disease: definition, natural history, and diagnostic criteria. *Alzheimers Dement.* 12, 292–323. doi: 10.1016/j.jalz.2016.02.002

Fei, M., Jianghua, W., Rujuan, M., Wei, Z., and Qian, W. (2011). The relationship of plasma Aβ levels to dementia in aging individuals with mild cognitive impairment. *J. Neurol. Sci.* 305, 92–96. doi: 10.1016/j.jns.2011.03.005

Gao, L., Jiang, Y., Wei, S., Shang, S., Li, P., Chen, C., et al. (2018). The level of plasma amyloid-β40 is correlated with peripheral transport proteins in cognitively normal adults: A population-based cross-sectional study. *J. Alzheimers Dis.* 65, 951–961. doi: 10.3233/JAD-180399

Han, P., and Shi, J. (2016). A theoretical analysis of the synergy of amyloid and tau in Alzheimer's disease. *J. Alzheimers Dis.* 52, 1461–1470. doi: 10.3233/jad-151206

Hanon, O., Vidal, J. S., Lehmann, S., Bombois, S., Allinquant, B., Treluyer, J. M., et al. (2018). Plasma amyloid levels within the Alzheimer's process and correlations with central biomarkers. *Alzheimers Dement.* 14, 858–868. doi: 10.1016/j.jalz.2018.01.004

Jack, C. R. Jr., Bennett, D. A., Blennow, K., Carrillo, M. C., Dunn, B., Haeberlein, S. B., et al. (2018). NIA-AA research framework: toward a biological definition of Alzheimer's disease. *Alzheimers Dement.* 14, 535–562. doi: 10.1016/j.jalz.2018.02.018

Jack, C. R. Jr., Bennett, D. A., Blennow, K., Carrillo, M. C., Feldman, H. H., Frisoni, G. B., et al. (2016). A/T/N: an unbiased descriptive classification scheme for Alzheimer disease biomarkers. *Neurology* 87, 539–547. doi: 10.1212/wnl.0000000000002923

Jack, C. R. Jr., Knopman, D. S., Jagust, W. J., Petersen, R. C., Weiner, M. W., Aisen, P. S., et al. (2013). Tracking pathophysiological processes in Alzheimer's disease: an updated hypothetical model of dynamic biomarkers. *Lancet Neurol.* 12, 207–216. doi: 10.1016/s1474-4422(12)70291-0

Janelidze, S., Stomrud, E., Palmqvist, S., Zetterberg, H., van Westen, D., Jeromin, A., et al. (2016). Plasma β-amyloid in Alzheimer's disease and vascular disease. *Sci. Rep.* 6:26801. doi: 10.1038/srep26801

Kern, S., Zetterberg, H., Kern, J., Zettergren, A., Waern, M., Hoglund, K., et al. (2018). Prevalence of preclinical Alzheimer disease: comparison of current classification systems. *Neurology* 90, e1682–e1691. doi: 10.1212/wnl.0000000000005476

Kim, M. Y., Kim, K. N., Cho, H. M., Lee, D. J., and Cho, D. Y. (2016). Reference intervals for plasma amyloid β in Korean adults without cognitive impairment. *Ann. Lab. Med.* 36, 595–598. doi: 10.3343/alm.2016.36.6.595

Kleinschmidt, M., Schoenfeld, R., Gottlich, C., Bittner, D., Metzner, J. E., Leplow, B., et al. (2016). Characterizing aging, mild cognitive impairment, and dementia with blood-based biomarkers and neuropsychology. *J. Alzheimers Dis.* 50, 111–126. doi: 10.3233/jad-143189

Kukull, W. A., Higdon, R., Bowen, J. D., McCormick, W. C., Teri, L., Schellenberg, G. D., et al. (2002). Dementia and Alzheimer disease incidence: a prospective cohort study. *Arch. Neurol.* 59, 1737–1746. doi: 10.1001/archneur.59.11.1737

Lövheim, H., Elgh, F., Johansson, A., Zetterberg, H., Blennow, K., Hallmans, G., et al. (2017). Plasma concentrations of free amyloidβ cannot predict the development of Alzheimer's disease. *Alzheimers Dement.* 13, 778–782. doi: 10.1016/j.jalz.2016.12.004

Lue, L. F., Guerra, A., and Walker, D. G. (2017a). Amyloid *β* and tau as Alzheimer's disease blood biomarkers: promise from new technologies. *Neurol. Ther.* 6, 25–36. doi: 10.1007/s40120-017-0074-8

Lue, L. F., Sabbagh, M. N., Chiu, M. J., Jing, N., Snyder, N. L., Schmitz, C., et al. (2017b). Plasma levels of Aβ42 and tau identified probable Alzheimer's dementia: findings in two cohorts. *Front. Aging Neurosci.* 9:226. doi: 10.3389/fnagi.2017.00226

McKhann, G. M., Knopman, D. S., Chertkow, H., Hyman, B. T., Jack, C. R. Jr., Kawas, C. H., et al. (2011). The diagnosis of dementia due to Alzheimer's disease: recommendations from the National Institute on Aging-Alzheimer's Association workgroups on diagnostic guidelines for Alzheimer's disease. *Alzheimers Dement.* 7, 263–269. doi: 10.1016/j.jalz.2011.03.005

Nabers, A., Perna, L., Lange, J., Mons, U., Schartner, J., Güldenhaupt, J., et al. (2018). Amyloid blood biomarker detects Alzheimer's disease. *EMBO Mol. Med.* 10:e8763. doi: 10.15252/emmm.201708763

Nakamura, A., Kaneko, N., Villemagne, V. L., Kato, T., Doecke, J., Dore, V., et al. (2018). High performance plasma amyloid-β biomarkers for Alzheimer's disease. *Nature* 554, 249–254. doi: 10.1038/nature25456

Olsson, B., Lautner, R., Andreasson, U., Öhrfelt, A., Portelius, E., Bjerke, M., et al. (2016). CSF and blood biomarkers for the diagnosis of Alzheimer's disease: a systematic review and meta-analysis. *Lancet Neurol.* 15, 673–684. doi: 10.1016/S1474-4422(16)00070-3

Seeburger, J. L., Holder, D. J., Combrinck, M., Joachim, C., Laterza, O., Tanen, M., et al. (2015). Cerebrospinal fluid biomarkers distinguish postmortem-confirmed Alzheimer's disease from other dementias and healthy controls in the OPTIMA cohort. *J. Alzheimers Dis.* 44, 525–539. doi: 10.3233/JAD-141725

Small, S. A., and Duff, K. (2008). Linking Aβ and tau in late-onset Alzheimer's disease: a dual pathway hypothesis. *Neuron* 60, 534–542. doi: 10.1016/j.neuron.2008.11.007

Sutphen, C. L., Jasielec, M. S., Shah, A. R., Macy, E. M., Xiong, C., Vlassenko, A. G., et al. (2015). Longitudinal cerebrospinal fluid biomarker changes in preclinical Alzheimer disease during middle age. *JAMA Neurol.* 72, 1029–1042. doi: 10.1001/jamaneurol.2015.1285

Tai, L. M., Mehra, S., Shete, V., Estus, S., Rebeck, G. W., and Bu, G. (2014). LaDu MJ: Soluble apoE/Aβ complex: mechanism and therapeutic target for *APOE4*-induced AD risk. *Mol. Neurodegener.* 9:2. doi: 10.1186/1750-1326-9-2

Teunissen, C. E., Chiu, M. J., Yang, C. C., Yang, S. Y., Scheltens, P., Zetterberg, H., et al. (2018). Plasma Amyloid-β (Aβ42) correlates with cerebrospinal fluid Aβ42 in Alzheimer's disease. *J. Alzheimers Dis.* 62, 1857–1863. doi: 10.3233/JAD-170784

Tzen, K. Y., Yang, S. Y., Chen, T. F., Cheng, T. W., Horng, H. E., Wen, H. P., et al. (2014). Plasma Aβ but not tau is related to brain PiB retention in early Alzheimer's disease. *ACS Chem. Neurosci.* 5, 830–836. doi: 10.1021/cn500101j

Verberk, I. M. W., Slot, R. E., Verfaillie, S. C. J., Heijst, H., Prins, N. D., van Berckel, B. N. M., et al. (2018). Plasma amyloid as prescreener for the earliest Alzheimer pathological changes. *Ann. Neurol.* 84, 648–658. doi: 10.1002/ana.25334

Zecca, C., Tortelli, R., Panza, F., Arcuti, S., Piccininni, M., Capozzo, R., et al. (2018). Plasma β-amyloid1–42 reference values in cognitively normal subjects. *J. Neurol. Sci.* 391, 120–126. doi: 10.1016/j.jns.2018.06.006

Zetterberg, H., and Blennow, K. (2018). From cerebrospinal fluid to blood: the third wave of fluid biomarkers for Alzheimer's disease. *J. Alzheimers Dis.* 64, S271–S279. doi: 10.3233/JAD-179926

Ziegler-Graham, K., Brookmeyer, R., Johnson, E., and Arrighi, H. M. (2008). Worldwide variation in the doubling time of Alzheimer's disease incidence rates. *Alzheimers Dement.* 4, 316–323. doi: 10.1016/j.jalz.2008.05.2479

Zlokovic, B. V., Deane, R., Sagare, A. P., and Bell, R. D. (2010). Winkler EA: Low-density lipoprotein receptor-related protein-1: a serial clearance homeostatic mechanism controlling Alzheimer's amyloid beta-peptide elimination from the brain. *J. Neurochem* 115, 1077–1089. doi: 10.1111/j.1471-4159.2010.07002.x

19

Biological Sex: A Potential Moderator of Physical Activity Efficacy on Brain Health

Cindy K. Barha[1,2,3]*, *Chun-Liang Hsu*[1,2,3], *Lisanne ten Brinke*[1,2,3] and *Teresa Liu-Ambrose*[1,2,3]

[1]*Department of Physical Therapy, University of British Columbia, Vancouver, BC, Canada,* [2]*Djavad Mowafaghian Centre for Brain Health, University of British Columbia, Vancouver, BC, Canada,* [3]*Centre for Hip Health and Mobility, Vancouver Coastal Health Research Institute, Vancouver, BC, Canada*

Correspondence:
Cindy K. Barha
cindy.barha@ubc.ca

The number of older people worldwide living with cognitive impairment and neurodegenerative diseases is growing at an unprecedented rate. Despite accumulating evidence that engaging in physical activity is a promising primary behavioral strategy to delay or avert the deleterious effects of aging on brain health, a large degree of variation exists in study findings. Thus, before physical activity and exercise can be prescribed as "medicine" for promoting brain health, it is imperative to understand how different biological factors can attenuate or amplify the effects of physical activity on cognition at the individual level. In this review article, we briefly discuss the current state of the literature, examining the relationship between physical activity and brain health in older adults and we present the argument that biological sex is a potent moderator of this relationship. Additionally, we highlight some of the potential neurobiological mechanisms underlying this sex difference for this relatively new and rapidly expanding line of research.

Keywords: sex differences, exercise, physical activity, cognition, hippocampus, prefrontal cortex, aging, dementia

INTRODUCTION

The worldwide population is aging at an unprecedented rate, with the proportion of people aged over 60 years projected to increase from 12% in 2015 to 22% in 2050, resulting in over 2 billion people aged 60 and over (WHO, 2018). Normative aging is characterized by multifaceted changes in cognitive function and brain structure. In particular, the domains of memory and executive functions show declines in performance, which is further reflected in atrophy in the brain regions that subserve these cognitive domains, namely the hippocampus and the prefrontal cortex (PFC; Salthouse, 2011). In non-normative cognitive aging, decline is much more dramatic and is associated with increased dementia risk.

Dementia is one of the major causes of disability in older adults (ASC, 2010). Worldwide, over 47 million people have dementia and current projections estimate that this number will reach 74.7 million by the 2030 and 131.5 million by 2050 (Prince et al., 2015). Within this context, these demographic changes in the population will lead to increasing challenges for healthcare systems. Therefore, identifying strategies that bolster healthy cognitive aging is of upmost importance globally.

As there is no effective pharmaceutical treatment currently available for cognitive impairment and dementia, there is great interest in the utility of lifestyle approaches. Physical activity (PA) is a promising primary behavioral non-pharmacological strategy to delay or avert the deleterious effects of aging on brain health (Phillips, 2017; Petersen et al., 2018). However, before

PA can be prescribed as "medicine" for promoting brain health in the diseased and non-diseased brain, it is imperative to understand how different biological factors can attenuate or amplify the effects of PA on cognition at the individual level.

One such endogenous factor that appears to moderate PA efficacy is biological sex (Barha et al., 2017a,c; Loprinzi and Frith, 2018). The need to assess potential sex differences in this context is further highlighted by the greater prevalence of mild cognitive impairment (MCI) in males (Petersen et al., 2010), but faster rates of progression from MCI to Alzheimer's disease (AD) in females (Li et al., 2016; Podcasy and Epperson, 2016). Here, we briefly review the current evidence that PA and exercise promote cognitive health in older adults with and without cognitive impairment. We present supporting evidence that biological sex is an important moderator of the relationship between PA and cognition and highlight some of the potential underlying mechanisms for this relatively new and rapidly expanding line of inquiry. We have limited our review mainly to studies in humans. We refer readers to several excellent review articles of exercise studies conducted in rodents (Cotman et al., 2007; Voss et al., 2013; Patten et al., 2015; Triviño-Paredes et al., 2016; Barha et al., 2017b; Cooper et al., 2018).

THE HIPPOCAMPUS AND PREFRONTAL CORTEX: BRAIN STRUCTURES IMPLICATED IN BRAIN AGING

The process of aging is accompanied by declines in memory and executive functions which is further reflected in atrophy in the brain regions that subserve these cognitive domains, namely the hippocampus and the PFC (Salthouse, 2011). Episodic memory, memory for events that occur in a specific place and time, shows age-associated decline (Rönnlund et al., 2005) and relies on the integrity of the hippocampus, a medial temporal lobe brain structure. Executive functions refer to the higher-level mental processes required to control, plan and coordinate other cognitive abilities and behaviors (Espy, 2004); typically executive functions are divided into three general abilities, inhibition, working memory, and cognitive flexibility (Diamond, 2013), and rely on the PFC. Gray matter volume declines with increasing age are most prominent in the PFC, with more moderate declines in the hippocampus (Terry and Katzman, 2001; Raz et al., 2004). Interestingly, 82.5% of the longitudinal age-associated reduction in the executive function of inhibition was explained by changes in structural and functional connectivity (Fjell et al., 2017). Sex differences in the rate of regional volume loss, including the frontal lobe and hippocampus, in older adults have been found, with females faring better (Armstrong et al., 2019), though not all studies find this (Raz et al., 2010; Persson et al., 2016).

PHYSICAL ACTIVITY AND BRAIN HEALTH

PA, any bodily movement produced by skeletal muscles, can be categorized into occupational, sports, conditioning, household, or other types of activities requiring energy expenditure (Caspersen et al., 1985). Exercise is a subtype of PA that must be planned, structured and be repetitive with the goal of improving or maintaining physical fitness (Caspersen et al., 1985). Generally, there are two main types of exercise: (1) aerobic training (AT; e.g., walking, running) which aims to improve cardiovascular fitness; and (2) resistance training (RT; e.g., weightlifting) which aims to improve muscle mass and strength. The vast majority of the literature has focused on the effects of AT on cognitive health in older adults, although in more recent years the efficacy of RT has been shown (for examples see Cassilhas et al., 2007; Liu-Ambrose et al., 2010, 2012; Nagamatsu et al., 2012; Best et al., 2015; Bolandzadeh et al., 2015). Evidence from epidemiological and randomized controlled trials (RCTs) supports the notion that engaging in PA and exercise are promising strategies for dementia prevention and disease modification. In a meta-analysis, Northey et al. (2018) found that to maximize the effectiveness to improve cognition in older adults, exercise bouts should be 45–60 min in duration and at least done at a moderate intensity.

Prospective, epidemiological studies historically observe the association between the amount of PA engaged in and changes in cognitive performance or dementia risk. Overall, the evidence from these studies supports the relationship between higher levels of PA and better cognitive outcomes, reduced dementia risk, and longevity. A meta-analysis of 21 cohort studies found that in older, community-dwelling individuals, higher levels of PA were associated with a 35% reduction in the risk for cognitive decline compared to lower levels of PA (Blondell et al., 2014). These findings built upon an earlier meta-analysis of 15 prospective studies among participants without dementia that found higher levels of PA were associated with a 38% lower risk of cognitive decline, and low to moderate levels of PA were associated with a 35% reduction (Sofi et al., 2011). Higher levels of PA are also associated with a reduction in risk for dementia (~14%) as seen in a meta-analysis of 26 cohort studies (Blondell et al., 2014). The protective effects of high levels of PA may be more pronounced for those with AD compared to all-cause dementia and vascular dementia (Guure et al., 2017). Importantly, using data from the Netherlands Cohort Study, a higher total daily non-occupational PA was associated with greater odds of surviving to 90 years of age in men, and in women engaging in 60 min/day of non-occupational PA was associated with the greatest odds of surviving (Brandts and van den Brandt, 2019). Additionally, greater functional fitness is associated with better general cognition; however, the specific aspects of functional fitness that correlate with cognition differ between males and females (Guo et al., 2018).

Some epidemiological studies have also employed neuroimaging techniques to better understand the neural correlates underlying the relationship between PA and cognitive function in older age. For example, in adults 65 years and older at baseline, greater amounts of PA quantified as the number of blocks walked in 1 week at baseline, predicted greater gray matter volumes of the prefrontal, occipital, entorhinal, and hippocampal regions 9 years later, and this greater volume was related to a two-fold reduction in the risk for cognitive impairment at year 13 (Erickson et al., 2010). Further, engaging in PA in midlife was associated with larger total brain volume and gray matter volume of the frontal cortex 21 years later (Rovio et al., 2010). Importantly, better maintenance of PA levels over 10 years in older age is associated with less reductions in hippocampal volume, smaller increases in global gray matter mean diffusivity and white matter axial diffusivity, and maintenance of global cognitive function, independent of baseline levels of PA, demographics, and APOE4 status (Best et al., 2017). In individuals at risk for AD who experience greater rates of brain atrophy, engaging in PA levels that meet or exceed the current PA recommendations is associated with greater volumes of the inferior and anterior temporal lobes compared to those not meeting the PA recommendations (Dougherty et al., 2016). Thus, the association between how much PA is engaged in, and maintenance of cognition in older age appears related to sparing of gray matter volume of brain regions susceptible to age-related atrophy, including the frontal and prefrontal lobes and the hippocampus (Gordon et al., 2008).

Although prospective cohort studies typically include large samples of individuals, causality cannot be established and the potential for unmeasured confounding variables is often present. Thus, stronger evidence for the importance of PA and exercise in brain health has come from RCTs. The vast majority of RCTs of exercise have focused on AT, which we will focus on in this review. However it is worth noting that RT has been shown to significantly improve cognition and brain function (for a recent review see Landrigan et al., 2019). Several meta-analyses of RCTs in older adults suggest that cognitive processes that are highly susceptible to age-related declines are amendable to AT benefits (Heyn et al., 2004; Etnier et al., 2006; Barha et al., 2017a; Northey et al., 2018), particularly the domain of executive functions (Colcombe and Kramer, 2003), an umbrella term for a suite of higher order cognitive processes required for goal-directed behavior. A seminal study in the field of exercise neuroscience conducted by Kramer et al. (1999) found that older adults randomized to a 6 month AT intervention (i.e., brisk walking) showed significant improvements in executive functions compared to participants randomized to a stretching and toning control group. In a follow-up study, the AT group showed increased gray and white matter volumes in the temporal and prefrontal regions of the brain compared to the control group (Colcombe et al., 2006). In addition to improvements in executive functions, a 12-month RCT found that AT increased hippocampal volume by 2%, coinciding with improvements in spatial memory performance compared to the stretching and toning control group that showed a 1.4% decline in volume (Erickson et al., 2011), which is comparable to the 1–2% annual hippocampal shrinkage typically seen in older adults (Raz et al., 2005). More recently, several meta-analyses of RCTs have provided further support for the protective effects of AT on cognition in older adults (Colcombe and Kramer, 2003; Heyn et al., 2004; Etnier et al., 2006; Barha et al., 2017a; Northey et al., 2018). Notably, AT benefits for cognition are seen in cognitively healthy older adults as well as across different clinical populations, including MCI, vascular dementia, and AD (Lautenschlager et al., 2008; Baker et al., 2010; Erickson et al., 2011; Nagamatsu et al., 2013; Liu-Ambrose et al., 2016; Morris et al., 2017). RCTs with neuroimaging outcomes indicate that AT interventions also lead to enhanced functional brain plasticity as indexed by changes in brain structure, activation, and connectivity variables (Voss et al., 2010; Erickson et al., 2011; Nishiguchi et al., 2015; ten Brinke et al., 2015; Gajewski and Falkenstein, 2016; Hsu et al., 2017, 2018). Specifically for gray matter changes, RCTs of AT consistently show increases in the volume of the hippocampus (Colcombe et al., 2006; Erickson et al., 2011; Niemann et al., 2014; Maass et al., 2015; Kleemeyer et al., 2016; Rosano et al., 2017), which subserves memory, and the PFC (Colcombe et al., 2006; Erickson et al., 2010; Ruscheweyh et al., 2011; Tamura et al., 2015; Jonasson et al., 2017), which subserves executive functions.

Despite the large body of evidence supporting the therapeutic potential of AT, variation exists in the ability of exercise to prevent and alleviate declines in cognition and brain health. Some meta-analyses of RCTs do not conclude that AT exerts a significant positive effect on cognition in older adults (Smith et al., 2010; Gates et al., 2013; Kelly et al., 2014; Öhman et al., 2014; Young et al., 2015). Notably, one of the largest RCTs of exercise conducted to date, did not find a significant effect of 24-months of exercise on cognitive performance in 1,635 older adults compared to a health education program (Sink et al., 2015). More recently, Lamb et al. (2018) found that a 4 month program consisting of supervised moderate to high intensity AT and RT in combination with unsupervised home-based exercises was associated with slight declines in global cognition several months after the supervised training ended in older adults with moderate dementia. Thus, to better understand the variation seen in study outcomes, it is imperative to identify biological moderators that either attenuate or amplify the effects of exercise on brain health. This knowledge will allow for more efficient and targeted deployment of current PA interventions and potentially spur development of alternative strategies. We argue here that biological sex is a key moderator of aerobic exercise efficacy, such that females show greater cognitive benefits than males.

SEX DIFFERENCES, PHYSICAL ACTIVITY AND BRAIN HEALTH

Sex differences exist in the magnitude of beneficial effects seen in cognitive function from engaging in aerobic exercise (see **Table 1**). Meta-analytical evidence from Colcombe and Kramer (2003) first suggested that older females showed greater cognitive gains from AT than older males. Our recent meta-analysis of RCTs conducted with cognitively healthy older adults confirmed this, as AT was associated with larger effect sizes in studies that included a higher percentage of female participants compared to studies with a lower percentage of female participants for the cognitive domain of executive functions (Barha et al., 2017a). Sex differences were not seen for other domains, including episodic memory and visuospatial function. Interestingly, AT enhanced word fluency to a greater extent in studies with a lower percentage of female participants. Thus, for tasks associated with verbal learning and memory, AT may be more advantageous for males than females. Moreover, our meta-analysis of studies

TABLE 1 | Evidence for sex differences in the effect of physical activity on cognition and the brain in older humans.

Study	Population	Study type and Physical activity	Results and conclusions
Baker et al. (2010)	- 15 older females with MCI - 14 older males with MCI	RCT - 6 months of high intensity AT - Stretching control	In females, AT improved performance in 4/5 tests of executive function (Symbol-Digit, Verbal Fluency, Stroop, Trails B). In males, AT only improved performance in 1/5 tests (Trails B).
Barha et al. (2017d)	- 29 older females with SIVCI - 29 older males with SIVCI	RCT - 6 months of moderate intensity AT - Usual care plus education control	In females, AT improved executive functioning on the Trail Making Test. In males, AT did not improve executive functioning.
Barha et al. (2019)	- 1,497 older females cognitively healthy (177 females with MRI) - 1,376 older males cognitively healthy (126 males with MRI)	Epidemiological cohort study - Self-reported time spent walking (mins/week) each year for 10 years	In females, maintaining PA over 10 years predicted less declines in executive functioning on the Digit Symbol Substitution Test and was associated with greater volume of the left dorsolateral prefrontal cortex. In males, maintaining PA did not predict executive functioning.
van Uffelen et al. (2008)	- 67 older females with MCI - 85 older males with MCI	RCT - 12 months of moderate intensity AT - Low intensity, non-aerobic balance and flexibility exercise control	In females, increased adherence to the AT program was associated with improved executive functioning on the Stroop test and on an auditory verbal memory test. In males, attendance in at least 75% of AT classes was required before improvements in only auditory verbal memory were seen.
Varma et al. (2015)	- 64 older females cognitively healthy - 28 older males cognitively healthy	Sub study of an RCT - Daily walking activity measuring using a step activity monitor worn on the dominant ankle for 3–7 days	In females, greater amount, duration, and frequency of total daily walking were all associated with larger hippocampal volume. In males, associations were not significant.

in middle-aged and aged rodents found a female-advantage in gains for hippocampus-dependent spatial learning and memory in studies that utilized forced AT paradigms (Barha et al., 2017b). Unfortunately, we could not examine potential sex differences in AT efficacy for executive functions as there was a lack of such studies conducted with rodents. Regardless, altogether, the meta-analytic evidence available thus far indirectly supports the notion that biological sex is an important moderator of the relationship between AT and cognition in older age.

To date, a small number of human studies have attempted to directly compare males and females to determine whether AT effects on cognition are sex-dependent. In a study sample of 29 older adults (15 women) with MCI, Baker et al. (2010) showed that 6-months of high intensity AT increased performance on four of five tests of cognition in females and only on one test in males compared to the controls. Further, in a 12-month study of moderate intensity AT, sex stratified analyses indicated that increased adherence to the AT program was associated with improved attention and memory in older females with MCI but only with memory in older males (van Uffelen et al., 2008). More recently, we provided further support for a female advantage in AT-induced gains in executive functions with a secondary analysis of a 6-month RCT in participants with mild subcortical ischemic vascular cognitive impairment (Barha et al., 2017d). The progressive, moderate intensity AT program improved the executive function of set-shifting by 36% in females compared to the controls, whereas in males AT reduced performance by 31% compared to the controls. Interestingly, the beneficial effect of AT was retained 6 months after trial completion. Epidemiological evidence for this sex difference in AT efficacy was recently provided in our study that examined whether longitudinal changes in PA over 10 years predicted changes in global cognition, executive functions and processing speed differently in males and females using data from the Health, Aging, and Body Composition Study (HABC; Barha et al., 2019). Participants were 2,873 community-dwelling older adults aged 70–79 years at year 1 and PA was assessed annually from years 1–10 through self-reported time spent walking. Independent of demographics and disease-related variables, initial time spent walking and maintenance of PA over the 10 years predicted less declines in executive functions and processing speed as assessed by the Digit Symbol Substitution Test (DSST) in females but not males. Maintenance of PA over time predicted better global cognitive function on the Modified Mini-Mental Status Examination (3MS) in both males and females. Thus, accumulating evidence from intervention and epidemiological studies suggest that engaging in targeted exercise training of sufficient duration and intensity, as well as how PA levels change over time, protect different domains of cognition in females compared to males.

Investigations into the neural underpinnings of AT-induced enhancements have also shown potential sex differences. Varma et al. (2015) showed that greater amount, duration, and frequency of objectively measured daily walking over the span of 3–7 days were associated with larger hippocampal volume among older females but not males. In a follow-up study that explored hippocampal sub-regions, increased daily walking in females only was associated specifically with a larger subiculum which is part of the posterior hippocampus (Varma et al., 2016). We have recently expanded upon these findings showing that subjective assessment of time spent walking in year 1 of a 10 year study was associated with a larger left hippocampus in older males and a smaller hippocampus in older females (Barha et al., 2019). This discrepancy in the direction of the relationship between PA and hippocampal volume in females between studies may be related to differences in how walking behaviors were measured (i.e., objective vs. subjective) and the duration of measurement (i.e., 7 days vs. 10 years). Additionally, it may be the case that connectivity of the hippocampus to other brain regions may be a better indicator of functional performance than mere hippocampal volume (Burdette et al., 2010). Indeed, there is some evidence in the literature to support this as an AT intervention-induced increase in hippocampal volume in older females was associated with lower performance on an episodic memory task (ten Brinke et al., 2015). Thus, in addition to volumetric imaging, future studies should use multimodal techniques to delve further into this intriguing sex difference to focus on changes in functional connectivity of the hippocampus and its relationship to cognition and exercise.

In addition to the hippocampus, we have recently shown that greater maintenance of PA over 10 years is associated with a greater volume of the left dorsolateral PFC (DL-PFC) among older females, but not males (Barha et al., 2019). The DL-PFC subserves executive functions (Wagner et al., 2001), one of the domains in which PA improves performance in females (Baker et al., 2010; Barha et al., 2017d), and shows extensive volume loss in older age (Jernigan et al., 2001). Previous work also shows that AT is associated with a larger volume of this brain region (Erickson et al., 2010; Best et al., 2017) and the volume mediates the relationship between cardiovascular fitness level and performance on executive functioning tasks (Weinstein et al., 2012), though, vitally, sex differences were not assessed in these studies.

Notwithstanding the lack of understanding in the effects of PA on sex differences associated with the functional architecture of the brain, evidence suggests the presence of sex differences in the patterns of neural network coupling. For instance, compared to men, women seemed to exhibit stronger connectivity between amygdala and middle temporal gyrus, inferior frontal gyrus, postcentral gyrus and hippocampus (Kogler et al., 2016). Moreover, one cross-sectional study investigated whether difference in sex and hormonal fluctuations across menstrual cycle would impact functional connectivity patterns of the frontoparietal network (Hjelmervik et al., 2014). From examining 16 healthy younger women and 15 younger men, the study showed women typically displayed higher frontoparietal connectivity compared to men, irrespective of the influences exerted by fluctuating sex hormones through various phases in the menstrual cycle. Aligning with this finding, the UK Biobank study reported that across 2,750 female and 2,466 male participants between the age of 44–77 years, a significantly stronger connectivity in the default mode network was observed in females compared to males (Ritchie et al., 2018), for which the same findings were reported in a separate, multi-site community-based study conducted previously with 1,093 participants between 18–60 years old (Biswal et al., 2010). In 559 cognitively healthy adults 70 years and older, Jamadar et al. (2019) confirmed the finding of greater connectivity within the default mode network in females and further showed greater connectivity within the salience network in males, two important resting-state networks that consistently show age-associated connectivity declines (Geerligs et al., 2015). Further, examining time-varying properties of connectivity patterns, de Lacy et al. (2019) demonstrated that dynamic connectivity of neural networks is significantly different between males and females, which complements observations made by classic methods of quantifying functional connectivity. These results, in conjunction, offer insights into sex differences in the functional organization of the brain such that women may be more proficient in social, self-referential and memory processes, in line with conclusions derived from brain structural connectomics (Ingalhalikar et al., 2014).

POTENTIAL MECHANISMS UNDERLYING THE SEX DIFFERENCE

The mechanisms underlying the sex difference in the relationship between PA and cognitive and brain health have only recently been speculated upon in the literature (Barha et al., 2017c; Barha and Liu-Ambrose, 2018; Loprinzi and Frith, 2018). A large body of evidence, stemming mainly from animal studies, highlights the importance of neurotrophic factors, in particular brain derived neurotrophic factor (BDNF), in the AT-induced enhancements in cognition, brain function and neuroplasticity (Cotman et al., 2007). BDNF supports neuroplasticity, synaptic plasticity and the cellular mechanisms involved in learning and memory (Leal et al., 2015) and has been the focus of several AT studies. Several rodent studies indicate that central BDNF levels, particularly within the hippocampus, mediate the beneficial effects of AT on the brain (Voss et al., 2011, 2013; Triviño-Paredes et al., 2016). Additionally, an acute bout of running increases BDNF within the PFC of male mice (Baranowski et al., 2017). In contrast, evidence linking AT and increases in circulating BDNF levels is less clear in humans, although the majority of studies do support the role of BDNF in mediating AT efficacy (Knaepen et al., 2010; Szuhany et al., 2015). Several potential reasons for this lack of consistency in the literature have been proposed, including: (i) length of time between AT and BDNF assessment; (ii) intensity of AT; (iii) duration of AT; (iv) BDNF Val66Met genotype; and (v) sex of participants (Coelho et al., 2013; Szuhany et al., 2015; Maass et al., 2016; Barha et al., 2017c). Sex differences do exist in some of the functions attributed to BDNF (Phillips et al., 2014; Leal et al., 2015; Atwi et al., 2016; Chan and Ye, 2017; Scharfman and MacLusky, 2017). Indeed, a meta-analysis of 29 AT studies of different exercise paradigms (AT and RT, different durations and lengths) in humans of any age showed that sex was a significant moderator such that studies with more males showed greater BDNF changes from exercise (Szuhany et al., 2015). In contrast to these findings, a meta-analysis of studies of AT in older rodents showed that BDNF gains were greater in studies utilizing female rodents compared to male rodents (Barha et al., 2017b). Further, we recently showed in older humans with SIVCI, that 6-months of moderate intensity AT increased circulating BDNF levels in females but not males (Barha et al., 2017d). Altogether, these findings highlight the need for further studies of biological sex differences in the contributions of neurotrophic factors to AT benefits for brain health.

In addition to neurotrophic factors, the sex difference in the PA-induced cognitive and brain region volume response, may be related to several other factors, including alterations in neuroplastic processes, hormones, neurotransmitter systems, and physiological adaptations to exercise. For example, AT induces changes in neurogenesis, synaptogenesis, and angiogenesis in key brain regions involved in learning and memory (Voss et al., 2013; Prakash et al., 2015; Duzel et al., 2016; Triviño-Paredes et al., 2016). Many of these neuroplastic processes show sex differences (Barha and Liu-Ambrose, 2018); thus, it is possible that AT effects on these outcomes may be sex-dependent.

There have been relatively few studies that examine sex steroid hormone responses to long term PA within the context of aging. In older sedentary men, a 6-week intervention of moderate intensity aerobic exercise alone (Hayes et al., 2015) and when followed by 6-weeks of high intensity interval training (Hayes et al., 2017) was associated with increased circulating levels of total testosterone, although not all studies have found this association (for a review of the literature, see Hayes and Elliott, 2019). In older healthy women, a meta-analysis of 18 RCTs found that PA, particularly of high intensity, was associated with a small but statistically significant decrease in circulating total estradiol, as well as reductions in free testosterone (Ennour-Idrissi et al., 2015). In contrast to circulating levels of sex hormones, local, tissue-specific synthesis of testosterone and estradiol may be of more importance for brain health. For example, an acute bout of running in young rodents led to increased levels of testosterone in skeletal muscles in both males and females, whereas levels of estradiol only increased in males (Aizawa et al., 2008). On the other hand, using a rodent model of surgical menopause, Shi et al. (2019) recently found that longer-term running led to increased levels of estradiol in skeletal muscle in females. Studies looking at the effects of PA on local synthesis of sex steroids within the brain are scarce. In young male rodents, low intensity running led to increased *de novo* synthesis of dihydrotestosterone, a non-aromatizable androgen, in the hippocampus (Okamoto et al., 2012). Significantly, in the same study, depletion of circulating levels of androgens *via* castration did not abolish the beneficial effect of running on the hippocampus, supporting the importance of locally synthesized sex steroids in PA-effects in brain function. In addition to sex steroid hormones, other hormones may be involved in the sex difference in PA effects on the brain. For example, recently Yüksel et al. (2019) showed that 6 weeks of voluntary running increased oxytocin levels in the brain and periphery in female mice, which correlated with increased empathy-like behavior. In male mice, oxytocin was only increased in the brain, and levels did not correlate with empathy-like behavior. Further, PA may be exerting its influence on the brain through alterations in the hypothalamic-pituitary-adrenal axis (for a review, see Chen et al., 2017), and there are well established sex differences within this axis (for a recent review, see Rincón-Cortés et al., 2019).

PA also influences different neurotransmitter systems (Vecchio et al., 2018), including the dopaminergic system. PA in the form of aerobic exercise has been shown to increase dopamine levels and dopamine transmission within the brain of rodents and humans, including the hippocampus and PFC (Fisher et al., 2013; Robertson et al., 2016; Ko et al., 2019). Further support for the link between PA and dopamine comes from studying common polymorphisms within dopamine-related genes that alter dopamine signaling in humans. For example, carriers of the catechol-O-methyltransferase (COMT) Val158Met polymorphism, which is associated with dysregulated levels of dopamine in the brain, showed less cognitive improvements in response to 17 weeks of exercise (Stroth et al., 2010). Importantly, there are known sex differences in the effect of the COMT Val158Met polymorphism on the brain (Gurvich and Rossell, 2015) as well as in dopaminergic neurotransmission (Riccardi et al., 2011).

Sex differences exist within the respiratory, musculoskeletal and cardiovascular systems, leading to sex differences in the physiological responses of these systems to PA (Deschenes and Kraemer, 2002; Sheel et al., 2004; Green et al., 2016), with females typically at a disadvantage (Sheel et al., 2004; Harms and Rosenkranz, 2008). Potentially compounding this is the fact that older females engage in less PA and are more sedentary than older males (Kaplan et al., 2001; Lee, 2005), which has greater consequences for processing speed in females (Fagot et al., 2019). Therefore, increasing engagement in PA may lead to more appreciable effects on cognition and brain health in older females than older males. For a more comprehensive review of potential sex differences in mechanisms underlying AT effects on the brain, please see Barha and Liu-Ambrose (2018).

CONCLUDING REMARKS

Engaging in PA is a relatively simple, highly implementable, and cost-effective lifestyle intervention with great promise in affording neuroprotection against cognitive decline in both normative and non-normative aging. Despite many studies supporting the utility of PA in preserving brain health in older age, a large degree of variation in PA efficacy exists (Smith et al., 2010; Gates et al., 2013; Kelly et al., 2014; Öhman et al., 2014; Young et al., 2015). Garnering a greater understanding of the sources of this variation will be a fundamental step towards the ultimate goal of prescribing PA as "medicine" for brain health. In this review article, we argued that biological sex is a potent moderator of the effectiveness of PA for both cognitive and neural outcomes. Future studies that aim to understand the mechanisms underlying PAs effects on the brain should take these profound sex differences into consideration.

AUTHOR CONTRIBUTIONS

CB wrote the first draft of the manuscript. C-LH, LB, and TL-A wrote sections of the manuscript. All authors read and approved the submitted version.

FUNDING

This work was supported by a Canadian Institutes of Health Research grant to TL-A (MOP-142206). TL-A is a Canada Research Chair (Tier 2) in Physical Activity, Mobility and Cognitive Neuroscience. CB is an Alzheimer's Association USA and Brain Canada Research Fellow. Funding sources were not involved in the writing of this review or in the decision to submit this review for publication.

REFERENCES

Aizawa, K., Iemitsu, M., Otsuki, T., Maeda, S., Miyauchi, T., and Mesaki, N. (2008). Sex differences in steroidogenesis in skeletal muscle following a single bout of exercise in rats. *J. Appl. Physiol.* 104, 67–74. doi: 10.1152/japplphysiol.00558.2007

Armstrong, N. M., An, Y., Beason-Held, L., Doshi, J., Erus, G., Ferrucci, L., et al. (2019). Sex differences in brain aging and predictors of neurodegeneration in cognitively healthy older adults. *Neurobiol. Aging* 81, 146–156. doi: 10.1016/j.neurobiolaging.2019.05.020

ASC. (2010). *Rising Tide: The Impact of Dementia on Canadian Society.* Toronto, ON: Alzheimer Society of Canada.

Atwi, S., McMahon, D., Scharfman, H., and MacLusky, N. J. (2016). Androgen modulation of hippocampal structure and function. *Neuroscientist* 22, 46–60. doi: 10.1177/1073858414558065

Baker, L. D., Frank, L. L., Foster-Schubert, K., Green, P. S., Wilkinson, C. W., Mctiernan, A., et al. (2010). Effects of aerobic exercise on mild cognitive impairment: a controlled trial. *Arch. Neurol.* 67, 71–79. doi: 10.1001/archneurol.2009.307

Baranowski, B. P., Peppler, W. T., and MacPherson, E. K. (2017). Acute exercise rescues cortex BDNF signaling in high fat fed male mice. *FASEB J.* 31:lb707.

Barha, C. K., Best, J. R., Rosano, C., Yaffe, K., Catov, J. M., Liu-Ambrose, T., et al. (2019). Sex-specific relationship between long-term maintenance of physical activity and cognition in the health ABC study: potential role of hippocampal and dorsolateral prefrontal cortex volume. *J. Gerontol. A Biol. Sci. Med. Sci.* doi: 10.1093/gerona/glz093 [Epub ahead of print].

Barha, C. K., Davis, J. C., Falck, R. S., Nagamatsu, L. S., and Liu-Ambrose, T. (2017a). Sex differences in exercise efficacy to improve cognition: a systematic review and meta-analysis of randomized controlled trials in older humans. *Front. Neuroendocrinol.* 46, 71–85. doi: 10.1016/j.yfrne.2017.04.002

Barha, C. K., Falck, R. S., Davis, J. C., Nagamatsu, L. S., and Liu-Ambrose, T. (2017b). Sex differences in aerobic exercise efficacy to improve cognition: a systematic review and meta-analysis of studies in older rodents. *Front. Neuroendocrinol.* 46, 86–105. doi: 10.1016/j.yfrne.2017.06.001

Barha, C. K., Galea, L. A., Nagamatsu, L. S., Erickson, K. I., and Liu-Ambrose, T. (2017c). Personalising exercise recommendations for brain health: considerations and future directions. *Br. J. Sports Med.* 51, 636–639. doi: 10.1136/bjsports-2016-096710

Barha, C. K., Hsiung, G. R., Best, J. R., Davis, J. C., Eng, J. J., Jacova, C., et al. (2017d). Sex difference in aerobic exercise efficacy to improve cognition in older adults with vascular cognitive impairment: secondary analysis of a randomized controlled trial. *J. Alzheimers Dis.* 60, 1397–1410. doi: 10.3233/JAD-170221

Barha, C. K., and Liu-Ambrose, T. (2018). Exercise and the aging brain: considerations for sex differences. *Brain Plast.* 4, 53–63. doi: 10.3233/BPL-180067

Best, J. R., Chiu, B. K., Liang Hsu, C., Nagamatsu, L. S., and Liu-Ambrose, T. (2015). Long-term effects of resistance exercise training on cognition and brain volume in older women: results from a randomized controlled trial. *J. Int. Neuropsychol. Soc.* 21, 745–756. doi: 10.1017/s1355617715000673

Best, J. R., Rosano, C., Aizenstein, H. J., Tian, Q., Boudreau, R. M., Ayonayon, H. N., et al. (2017). Long-term changes in time spent walking and subsequent cognitive and structural brain changes in older adults. *Neurobiol. Aging* 57, 153–161. doi: 10.1016/j.neurobiolaging.2017.05.023

Biswal, B. B., Mennes, M., Zuo, X. N., Gohel, S., Kelly, C., Smith, S. M., et al. (2010). Toward discovery science of human brain function. *Proc. Natl. Acad. Sci. U S A* 107, 4734–4739. doi: 10.1073/pnas.0911855107

Blondell, S. J., Hammersley-Mather, R., and Veerman, J. L. (2014). Does physical activity prevent cognitive decline and dementia? a systematic review and meta-analysis of longitudinal studies. *BMC Public Health* 14:510. doi: 10.1186/1471-2458-14-510

Bolandzadeh, N., Tam, R., Handy, T. C., Nagamatsu, L. S., Hsu, C. L., Davis, J. C., et al. (2015). Resistance training and white matter lesion progression in older women: exploratory analysis of a 12-month randomized controlled trial. *J. Am. Geriatr. Soc.* 63, 2052–2060. doi: 10.1111/jgs.13644

Brandts, L., and van den Brandt, P. A. (2019). Body size, non-occupational physical activity and the chance of reaching longevity in men and women: findings from the Netherlands Cohort Study. *J Epidemiol. Community Health* 73, 239–249. doi: 10.1136/jech-2018-211410

Burdette, J. H., Laurienti, P. J., Espeland, M. A., Morgan, A., Telesford, Q., Vechlekar, C. D., et al. (2010). Using network science to evaluate exercise-associated brain changes in older adults. *Front. Aging Neurosci.* 2:23. doi: 10.3389/fnagi.2010.00023

Caspersen, C. J., Powell, K. E., and Christenson, G. M. (1985). Physical activity, exercise, and physical fitness: definitions and distinctions for health-related research. *Public Health Rep.* 100, 125–131.

Cassilhas, R. C., Viana, V. A., Grassmann, V., Santos, R. T., Santos, R. F., Tufik, S., et al. (2007). The impact of resistance exercise on the cognitive function of the elderly. *Med. Sci. Sports Exerc.* 39, 1401–1407. doi: 10.1249/mss.0b013e318060111f

Chan, C. B., and Ye, K. (2017). Sex differences in brain-derived neurotrophic factor signaling and functions. *J. Neurosci. Res.* 95, 328–335. doi: 10.1002/jnr.23863

Chen, C., Nakagawa, S., An, Y., Ito, K., Kitaichi, Y., and Kusumi, I. (2017). The exercise-glucocorticoid paradox: How exercise is beneficial to cognition, mood, and the brain while increasing glucocorticoid levels. *Front. Neuroendocrinol.* 44, 83–102. doi: 10.1016/j.yfrne.2016.12.001

Coelho, F. G., Gobbi, S., Andreatto, C. A., Corazza, D. I., Pedroso, R. V., and Santos-Galduroz, R. F. (2013). Physical exercise modulates peripheral levels of brain-derived neurotrophic factor (BDNF): a systematic review of experimental studies in the elderly. *Arch. Gerontol. Geriatr.* 56, 10–15. doi: 10.1016/j.archger.2012.06.003

Colcombe, S. J., Erickson, K. I., Scalf, P. E., Kim, J. S., Prakash, R., Mcauley, E., et al. (2006). Aerobic exercise training increases brain volume in aging humans. *J. Gerontol. A Biol. Sci. Med. Sci.* 61, 1166–1170. doi: 10.1093/gerona/61.11.1166

Colcombe, S., and Kramer, A. F. (2003). Fitness effects on the cognitive function of older adults: a meta-analytic study. *Psychol. Sci.* 14, 125–130. doi: 10.1111/1467-9280.t01-1-01430

Cooper, C., Moon, H. Y., and van Praag, H. (2018). On the run for hippocampal plasticity. *Cold Spring Harb. Perspect. Med.* 8:a029736. doi: 10.1101/cshperspect.a029736

Cotman, C. W., Berchtold, N. C., and Christie, L. A. (2007). Exercise builds brain health: key roles of growth factor cascades and inflammation. *Trends Neurosci.* 30, 464–472. doi: 10.1016/j.tins.2007.06.011

de Lacy, N., McCauley, E., Kutz, J. N., and Calhoun, V. D. (2019). Sex-related differences in intrinsic brain dynamism and their neurocognitive correlates. *Neuroimage* 202:116116. doi: 10.1016/j.neuroimage.2019.116116

Deschenes, M. R., and Kraemer, W. J. (2002). Performance and physiologic adaptations to resistance training. *Am. J. Phys. Med. Rehabil.* 81, S3–S16. doi: 10.1097/00002060-200211001-00003

Diamond, A. (2013). Executive functions. *Annu. Rev. Psychol.* 64, 135–168. doi: 10.1146/annurev-psych-113011-143750

Dougherty, R. J., Ellingson, L. D., Schultz, S. A., Boots, E. A., Meyer, J. D., Lindheimer, J. B., et al. (2016). Meeting physical activity recommendations may be protective against temporal lobe atrophy in older adults at risk for Alzheimer's disease. *Alzheimers Dement. Amst.* 4, 14–17. doi: 10.1016/j.dadm.2016.03.005

Duzel, E., van Praag, H., and Sendtner, M. (2016). Can physical exercise in old age improve memory and hippocampal function? *Brain* 139, 662–673. doi: 10.1093/brain/awv407

Ennour-Idrissi, K., Maunsell, E., and Diorio, C. (2015). Effect of physical activity on sex hormones in women: a systematic review and meta-analysis of randomized controlled trials. *Breast Cancer Res.* 17:139. doi: 10.1186/s13058-015-0647-3

Erickson, K. I., Raji, C. A., Lopez, O. L., Becker, J. T., Rosano, C., Newman, A. B., et al. (2010). Physical activity predicts gray matter volume in late adulthood: the Cardiovascular Health Study. *Neurology* 75, 1415–1422. doi: 10.1212/WNL.0b013e3181f88359

Erickson, K. I., Voss, M. W., Prakash, R. S., Basak, C., Szabo, A., Chaddock, L., et al. (2011). Exercise training increases size of hippocampus and improves memory. *Proc. Natl. Acad. Sci. U S A* 108, 3017–3022. doi: 10.1073/pnas.1015950108

Espy K. A. (2004). Using developmental, cognitive and neuroscience approaches to understand executive control in young children. *Dev. Neuropsychol.* 26, 379–384. doi: 10.4324/9780203764428-1

Etnier, J. L., Nowell, P. M., Landers, D. M., and Sibley, B. A. (2006). A meta-regression to examine the relationship between aerobic fitness and cognitive performance. *Brain Res. Rev.* 52, 119–130. doi: 10.1016/j.brainresrev.2006.01.002

Fagot, D., Chicherio, C., Albinet, C. T., Andre, N., and Audiffren, M. (2019). The impact of physical activity and sex differences on intraindividual variability in inhibitory performance in older adults. *Neuropsychol. Dev. Cogn. B Aging Neuropsychol. Cogn.* 26, 1–23. doi: 10.1080/13825585.2017.1372357

Fisher, B. E., Li, Q., Nacca, A., Salem, G. J., Song, J., Yip, J., et al. (2013). Treadmill exercise elevates striatal dopamine D2 receptor binding potential in patients with early Parkinson's disease. *Neuroreport* 24, 509–514. doi: 10.1097/wnr.0b013e328361dc13

Fjell, A. M., Sneve, M. H., Grydeland, H., Storsve, A. B., and Walhovd, K. B. (2017). The disconnected brain and executive function decline in aging. *Cereb. Cortex* 27, 2303–2317. doi: 10.1093/cercor/bhw082

Gajewski, P. D., and Falkenstein, M. (2016). Physical activity and neurocognitive functioning in aging - a condensed updated review. *Eur. Rev. Aging Phys. Act.* 13:1. doi: 10.1186/s11556-016-0161-3

Gates, N., Fiatarone Singh, M. A., Sachdev, P. S., and Valenzuela, M. (2013). The effect of exercise training on cognitive function in older adults with mild cognitive impairment: a meta-analysis of randomized controlled trials. *Am. J. Geriatr. Psychiatry* 21, 1086–1097. doi: 10.1016/j.jagp.2013.02.018

Geerligs, L., Renken, R. J., Saliasi, E., Maurits, N. M., and Lorist, M. M. (2015). A brain-wide study of age-related changes in functional connectivity. *Cereb. Cortex* 25, 1987–1999. doi: 10.1093/cercor/bhu012

Gordon, B. A., Rykhlevskaia, E. I., Brumback, C. R., Lee, Y., Elavsky, S., Konopack, J. F., et al. (2008). Neuroanatomical correlates of aging, cardiopulmonary fitness level and education. *Psychophysiology* 45, 825–838. doi: 10.1111/j.1469-8986.2008.00676.x

Green, D. J., Hopkins, N. D., Jones, H., Thijssen, D. H., Eijsvogels, T. M., and Yeap, B. B. (2016). Sex differences in vascular endothelial function and health in humans: impacts of exercise. *Exp. Physiol.* 101, 230–242. doi: 10.1113/ep085367

Guo, Y., Yang, M., Yan, Y., Wang, L., and Gong, J. (2018). Sex differentials in relationships between functional fitness and cognitive performance in older adults: a canonical correlation analysis. *Sci. Rep.* 8:4146. doi: 10.1038/s41598-018-22475-7

Gurvich, C., and Rossell, S. L. (2015). Dopamine and cognitive control: sex-by-genotype interactions influence the capacity to switch attention. *Behav. Brain Res.* 281, 96–101. doi: 10.1016/j.bbr.2014.11.045

Guure, C. B., Ibrahim, N. A., Adam, M. B., and Said, S. M. (2017). Impact of physical activity on cognitive decline, dementia and its subtypes: meta-analysis of prospective studies. *Biomed. Res. Int.* 2017:9016924. doi: 10.1155/2017/9016924

Harms, C. A., and Rosenkranz, S. (2008). Sex differences in pulmonary function during exercise. *Med. Sci. Sports Exerc.* 40, 664–668. doi: 10.1249/mss.0b013e3181621325

Hayes, L. D., and Elliott, B. T. (2019). Short-term exercise training inconsistently influences basal testosterone in older men: a systematic review and meta-analysis. *Front. Physiol.* 9:1878. doi: 10.3389/fphys.2018.01878

Hayes, L. D., Herbert, P., Sculthorpe, N. F., and Grace, F. M. (2017). Exercise training improves free testosterone in lifelong sedentary aging men. *Endocr. Connect.* 6, 306–310. doi: 10.1530/ec-17-0082

Hayes, L. D., Sculthorpe, N., Herbert, P., Baker, J. S., Spagna, R., and Grace, F. M. (2015). Six weeks of conditioning exercise increases total, but not free testosterone in lifelong sedentary aging men. *Aging Male* 18, 195–200. doi: 10.3109/13685538.2015.1046123

Heyn, P., Abreu, B. C., and Ottenbacher, K. J. (2004). The effects of exercise training on elderly persons with cognitive impairment and dementia: a meta-analysis. *Arch. Phys. Med. Rehabil.* 85, 1694–1704. doi: 10.1016/j.apmr.2004.03.019

Hjelmervik, H., Hausmann, M., Osnes, B., Westerhausen, R., and Specht, K. (2014). Resting states are resting traits—an FMRI study of sex differences and menstrual cycle effects in resting state cognitive control networks. *PLoS One* 9:e103492. doi: 10.1371/journal.pone.0103492

Hsu, C. L., Best, J. R., Davis, J. C., Nagamatsu, L. S., Wang, S., Boyd, L. A., et al. (2018). Aerobic exercise promotes executive functions and impacts functional neural activity among older adults with vascular cognitive impairment. *Br. J. Sports Med.* 52, 184–191. doi: 10.1136/bjsports-2016-096846

Hsu, C. L., Best, J. R., Wang, S., Voss, M. W., Hsiung, R. G. Y., Munkacsy, M., et al. (2017). The impact of aerobic exercise on fronto-parietal network connectivity and its relation to mobility: an exploratory analysis of a 6-month randomized controlled trial. *Front. Hum. Neurosci.* 11:449. doi: 10.3389/fnhum.2017.00449

Ingalhalikar, M., Smith, A., Parker, D., Satterthwaite, T. D., Elliott, M. A., Ruparel, K., et al. (2014). Sex differences in the structural connectome of the human brain. *Proc. Natl. Acad. Sci. U S A* 111, 823–828. doi: 10.1073/pnas.1316909110

Jamadar, S. D., Sforazzini, F., Raniga, P., Ferris, N. J., Paton, B., Bailey, M. J., et al. (2019). Sexual dimorphism of resting-state network connectivity in healthy ageing. *J. Gerontol. B Psychol. Sci. Soc. Sci.* 74, 1121–1131. doi: 10.1093/geronb/gby004

Jernigan, T. L., Archibald, S. L., Fennema-Notestine, C., Gamst, A. C., Stout, J. C., Bonner, J., et al. (2001). Effects of age on tissues and regions of the cerebrum and cerebellum. *Neurobiol. Aging* 22, 581–594. doi: 10.1016/s0197-4580(01)00217-2

Jonasson, L. S., Nyberg, L., Kramer, A. F., Lundquist, A., Riklund, K., and Boraxbekk, C. J. (2017). Aerobic exercise intervention, cognitive performance and brain structure: results from the physical influences on brain in aging (PHIBRA) study. *Front. Aging Neurosci.* 8:336. doi: 10.3389/fnagi.2016.00336

Kaplan, M. S., Newsom, J. T., Mcfarland, B. H., and Lu, L. (2001). Demographic and psychosocial correlates of physical activity in late life. *Am. J. Prev. Med.* 21, 306–312. doi: 10.1016/s0749-3797(01)00364-6

Kelly, M. E., Loughrey, D., Lawlor, B. A., Robertson, I. H., Walsh, C., and Brennan, S. (2014). The impact of exercise on the cognitive functioning of healthy older adults: a systematic review and meta-analysis. *Ageing Res. Rev.* 16, 12–31. doi: 10.1016/j.arr.2014.05.002

Kleemeyer, M. M., Kuhn, S., Prindle, J., Bodammer, N. C., Brechtel, L., Garthe, A., et al. (2016). Changes in fitness are associated with changes in hippocampal microstructure and hippocampal volume among older adults. *Neuroimage* 131, 155–161. doi: 10.1016/j.neuroimage.2015.11.026

Knaepen, K., Goekint, M., Heyman, E. M., and Meeusen, R. (2010). Neuroplasticity—exercise-induced response of peripheral brain-derived neurotrophic factor: a systematic review of experimental studies in human subjects. *Sports Med.* 40, 765–801. doi: 10.2165/11534530-000000000-00000

Ko, I. G., Kim, C. J., and Kim, H. (2019). Treadmill exercise improves memory by up-regulating dopamine and down-regulating D2 dopamine receptor in traumatic brain injury rats. *J. Exerc. Rehabil.* 15, 504–511. doi: 10.12965/jer.1938316.158

Kogler, L., Muller, V. I., Seidel, E. M., Boubela, R., Kalcher, K., Moser, E., et al. (2016). Sex differences in the functional connectivity of the amygdalae in association with cortisol. *Neuroimage* 134, 410–423. doi: 10.1016/j.neuroimage.2016.03.064

Kramer, A. F., Hahn, S., Cohen, N. J., Banich, M. T., Mcauley, E., Harrison, C. R., et al. (1999). Ageing, fitness and neurocognitive function. *Nature* 400, 418–419. doi: 10.1038/22682

Lamb, S. E., Sheehan, B., Atherton, N., Nichols, V., Collins, H., Mistry, D., et al. (2018). Dementia and Physical Activity (DAPA) trial of moderate to high intensity exercise training for people with dementia: randomised controlled trial. *BMJ* 361:k1675. doi: 10.1136/bmj.k1675

Landrigan, J. F., Bell, T., Crowe, M., Clay, O. J., and Mirman, D. (2019). Lifting cognition: a meta-analysis of effects of resistance exercise on cognition. *Psychol. Res.* doi: 10.1007/s00426-019-01145-x [Epub ahead of print].

Lautenschlager, N. T., Cox, K. L., Flicker, L., Foster, J. K., Van Bockxmeer, F. M., Xiao, J., et al. (2008). Effect of physical activity on cognitive function in older adults at risk for Alzheimer disease: a randomized trial. *JAMA* 300, 1027–1037. doi: 10.1001/jama.300.9.1027

Leal, G., Afonso, P. M., Salazar, I. L., and Duarte, C. B. (2015). Regulation of hippocampal synaptic plasticity by BDNF. *Brain Res.* 1621, 82–101. doi: 10.1016/j.brainres.2014.10.019

Lee, Y. S. (2005). Gender differences in physical activity and walking among older adults. *J. Women Aging* 17, 55–70. doi: 10.1300/j074v17n01_05

Li, J. Q., Tan, L., Wang, H. F., Tan, M. S., Tan, L., Xu, W., et al. (2016). Risk factors for predicting progression from mild cognitive impairment to Alzheimer's disease: a systematic review and meta-analysis of cohort studies. *J. Neurol. Neurosurg. Psychiatry* 87, 476–484. doi: 10.1136/jnnp-2014-310095

Liu-Ambrose, T., Best, J. R., Davis, J. C., Eng, J. J., Lee, P. E., Jacova, C., et al. (2016). Aerobic exercise and vascular cognitive impairment: a randomized controlled trial. *Neurology* 87, 2082–2090. doi: 10.1212/WNL.0000000000003332

Liu-Ambrose, T., Nagamatsu, L. S., Graf, P., Beattie, B. L., Ashe, M. C., and Handy, T. C. (2010). Resistance training and executive functions: a 12-month randomized controlled trial. *Arch. Intern. Med.* 170, 170–178. doi: 10.1001/archinternmed.2009.494

Liu-Ambrose, T., Nagamatsu, L. S., Voss, M. W., Khan, K. M., and Handy, T. C. (2012). Resistance training and functional plasticity of the aging brain: a 12-month randomized controlled trial. *Neurobiol. Aging* 33, 1690–1698. doi: 10.1016/j.neurobiolaging.2011.05.010

Loprinzi, P. D., and Frith, E. (2018). The role of sex in memory function: considerations and recommendations in the context of exercise. *J. Clin. Med.* 7:E132. doi: 10.3390/jcm7060132

Maass, A., Duzel, S., Brigadski, T., Goerke, M., Becke, A., Sobieray, U., et al. (2016). Relationships of peripheral IGF-1, VEGF and BDNF levels to exercise-related changes in memory, hippocampal perfusion and volumes in older adults. *Neuroimage* 131, 142–154. doi: 10.1016/j.neuroimage.2015.10.084

Maass, A., Duzel, S., Goerke, M., Becke, A., Sobieray, U., Neumann, K., et al. (2015). Vascular hippocampal plasticity after aerobic exercise in older adults. *Mol. Psychiatry* 20, 585–593. doi: 10.1038/mp.2014.114

Morris, J. K., Vidoni, E. D., Johnson, D. K., Van Sciver, A., Mahnken, J. D., Honea, R. A., et al. (2017). Aerobic exercise for Alzheimer's disease: a randomized controlled pilot trial. *PLoS One* 12:e0170547. doi: 10.1371/journal.pone.0170547

Nagamatsu, L. S., Chan, A., Davis, J. C., Beattie, B. L., Graf, P., Voss, M. W., et al. (2013). Physical activity improves verbal and spatial memory in older adults with probable mild cognitive impairment: a 6-month randomized controlled trial. *J. Aging Res.* 2013:861893. doi: 10.1155/2013/861893

Nagamatsu, L. S., Handy, T. C., Hsu, C. L., Voss, M., and Liu-Ambrose, T. (2012). Resistance training promotes cognitive and functional brain plasticity in seniors with probable mild cognitive impairment. *Arch. Intern. Med.* 172, 666–668. doi: 10.1001/archinternmed.2012.379

Niemann, C., Godde, B., and Voelcker-Rehage, C. (2014). Not only cardiovascular, but also coordinative exercise increases hippocampal volume in older adults. *Front. Aging Neurosci.* 6:170. doi: 10.3389/fnagi.2014.00170

Nishiguchi, S., Yamada, M., Tanigawa, T., Sekiyama, K., Kawagoe, T., Suzuki, M., et al. (2015). A 12-week physical and cognitive exercise program can improve cognitive function and neural efficiency in community-dwelling older adults: a randomized controlled trial. *J. Am. Geriatr. Soc.* 63, 1355–1363. doi: 10.1111/jgs.13481

Northey, J. M., Cherbuin, N., Pumpa, K. L., Smee, D. J., and Rattray, B. (2018). Exercise interventions for cognitive function in adults older than 50: a systematic review with meta-analysis. *Br. J. Sports Med.* 52, 154–160. doi: 10.1136/bjsports-2016-096587

Öhman, H., Savikko, N., Strandberg, T. E., and Pitkälä, K. H. (2014). Effect of physical exercise on cognitive performance in older adults with mild cognitive impairment or dementia: a systematic review. *Dement. Geriatr. Cogn. Disord.* 38, 347–365. doi: 10.1159/000365388

Okamoto, M., Hojo, Y., Inoue, K., Matsui, T., Kawato, S., Mcewen, B. S., et al. (2012). Mild exercise increases dihydrotestosterone in hippocampus providing evidence for androgenic mediation of neurogenesis. *Proc. Natl. Acad. Sci. U S A* 109, 13100–13105. doi: 10.1073/pnas.1210023109

Patten, A. R., Yau, S. Y., Fontaine, C J., Meconi, A., Wortman, R. C., and Christie, B. R. (2015). The benefits of exercise on structural and functional plasticity in the rodent hippocampus of different disease models. *Brain Plast.* 1, 97–127. doi: 10.3233/bpl-150016

Persson, N., Ghisletta, P., Dahle, C. L., Bender, A. R., Yang, Y., Yuan, P., et al. (2016). Regional brain shrinkage and change in cognitive performance over two years: the bidirectional influences of the brain and cognitive reserve factors. *Neuroimage* 126, 15–26. doi: 10.1016/j.neuroimage.2015.11.028

Petersen, R. C., Lopez, O., Armstrong, M. J., Getchius, T. S. D., Ganguli, M., Gloss, D., et al. (2018). Practice guideline update summary: mild cognitive impairment: report of the guideline development, dissemination and implementation subcommittee of the American academy of neurology. *Neurology* 90, 126–135. doi: 10.1212/wnl.0000000000006040

Petersen, R. C., Roberts, R. O., Knopman, D. S., Geda, Y. E., Cha, R. H., Pankratz, V. S., et al. (2010). Prevalence of mild cognitive impairment is higher in men. The Mayo Clinic Study of Aging. *Neurology* 75, 889–897. doi: 10.1212/WNL.0b013e3181f11d85

Phillips, C. (2017). Lifestyle modulators of neuroplasticity: how physical activity, mental engagement, and diet promote cognitive health during aging. *Neural Plast.* 2017:3589271. doi: 10.1155/2017/3589271

Phillips, C., Baktir, M. A., Srivatsan, M., and Salehi, A. (2014). Neuroprotective effects of physical activity on the brain: a closer look at trophic factor signaling. *Front. Cell. Neurosci.* 8:170. doi: 10.3389/fncel.2014.00170

Podcasy, J. L., and Epperson, C. N. (2016). Considering sex and gender in Alzheimer disease and other dementias. *Dialogues Clin. Neurosci.* 18, 437–446.

Prakash, R. S., Voss, M. W., Erickson, K. I., and Kramer, A. F. (2015). Physical activity and cognitive vitality. *Annu. Rev. Psychol.* 66, 769–797. doi: 10.1146/annurev-psych-010814-015249

Prince, M., Wimo, A., Guerchet, M., Ali, G. C., Wu, Y. T., Prina, M., et al. (2015). *World Alzheimer Report 2015.* London: Alzheimer's Disease International (ADI).

Raz, N., Ghisletta, P., Rodrigue, K. M., Kennedy, K. M., and Lindenberger, U. (2010). Trajectories of brain aging in middle-aged and older adults: regional and individual differences. *Neuroimage* 51, 501–511. doi: 10.1016/j.neuroimage.2010.03.020

Raz, N., Lindenberger, U., Rodrigue, K. M., Kennedy, K. M., Head, D., Williamson, A., et al. (2005). Regional brain changes in aging healthy adults: general trends, individual differences and modifiers. *Cereb. Cortex* 15, 1676–1689. doi: 10.1093/cercor/bhi044

Raz, N., Rodrigue, K. M., Head, D., Kennedy, K. M., and Acker, J. D. (2004). Differential aging of the medial temporal lobe: a study of a five-year change. *Neurology* 62, 433–438. doi: 10.1212/01.wnl.0000106466.09835.46

Riccardi, P., Park, S., Anderson, S., Doop, M., Ansari, M. S., Schmidt, D., et al. (2011). Sex differences in the relationship of regional dopamine release to affect and cognitive function in striatal and extrastriatal regions using positron emission tomography and $[^{18}F]$fallypride. *Synapse* 65, 99–102. doi: 10.1002/syn.20822

Rincón-Cortés, M., Herman, J. P., Lupien, S., Maguire, J., and Shansky, R. M. (2019). Stress: influence of sex, reproductive status and gender. *Neurobiol. Stress* 10:100155. doi: 10.1016/j.ynstr.2019.100155

Ritchie, S. J., Cox, S. R., Shen, X., Lombardo, M. V., Reus, L. M., Alloza, C., et al. (2018). Sex differences in the adult human brain: evidence from 5216 UK biobank participants. *Cereb. Cortex* 28, 2959–2975. doi: 10.1093/cercor/bhy109

Robertson, C. L., Ishibashi, K., Chudzynski, J., Mooney, L. J., Rawson, R. A., Dolezal, B. A., et al. (2016). Effect of exercise training on striatal dopamine D2/D3 receptors in methamphetamine users during behavioral treatment. *Neuropsychopharmacology* 41, 1629–1636. doi: 10.1038/npp.2015.331

Rönnlund, M., Nyberg, L., Backman, L., and Nilsson, L. G. (2005). Stability, growth and decline in adult life span development of declarative memory: cross-sectional and longitudinal data from a population-based study. *Psychol. Aging* 20, 3–18. doi: 10.1037/0882-7974.20.1.3

Rosano, C., Guralnik, J., Pahor, M., Glynn, N. W., Newman, A. B., Ibrahim, T. S., et al. (2017). Hippocampal response to a 24-month physical activity intervention in sedentary older adults. *Am. J. Geriatr. Psychiatry* 25, 209–217. doi: 10.1016/j.jagp.2016.11.007

Rovio, S., Spulber, G., Nieminen, L. T., Niskanen, E., Winblad, B., Tuomilehto, J., et al. (2010). The effect of midlife physical activity on structural brain changes in the elderly. *Neurobiol. Aging* 31, 1927–1936. doi: 10.1016/j.neurobiolaging.2008.10.007

Ruscheweyh, R., Willemer, C., Kruger, K., Duning, T., Warnecke, T., Sommer, J., et al. (2011). Physical activity and memory functions: an interventional study. *Neurobiol. Aging* 32, 1304–1319. doi: 10.1016/j.neurobiolaging.2009.08.001

Salthouse, T. A. (2011). Neuroanatomical substrates of age-related cognitive decline. *Psychol. Bull.* 137, 753–784. doi: 10.1037/a0023262

Scharfman, H. E., and MacLusky, N. J. (2017). Sex differences in hippocampal area CA3 pyramidal cells. *J. Neurosci. Res.* 95, 563–575. doi: 10.1002/jnr.23927

Sheel, A. W., Richards, J. C., Foster, G. E., and Guenette, J. A. (2004). Sex differences in respiratory exercise physiology. *Sports Med.* 34, 567–579. doi: 10.2165/00007256-200434090-00002

Shi, R., Tian, X., Feng, Y., Cheng, Z., Lu, J., Brann, D. W., et al. (2019). Expression of aromatase and synthesis of sex steroid hormones in skeletal muscle following exercise training in ovariectomized rats. *Steroids* 143, 91–96. doi: 10.1016/j.steroids.2019.01.003

Sink, K. M., Espeland, M. A., Castro, C. M., Church, T., Cohen, R., Dodson, J. A., et al. (2015). Effect of a 24-month physical activity intervention vs health education on cognitive outcomes in sedentary older adults: the LIFE randomized trial. *JAMA* 314, 781–790. doi: 10.1001/jama.2015.9617

Smith, P. J., Blumenthal, J. A., Hoffman, B. M., Cooper, H., Strauman, T. A., Welsh-Bohmer, K., et al. (2010). Aerobic exercise and neurocognitive performance: a meta-analytic review of randomized controlled trials. *Psychosom. Med.* 72, 239–252. doi: 10.1097/psy.0b013e3181d14633

Sofi, F., Valecchi, D., Bacci, D., Abbate, R., Gensini, G. F., Casini, A., et al. (2011). Physical activity and risk of cognitive decline: a meta-analysis of prospective studies. *J. Intern. Med.* 269, 107–117. doi: 10.1111/j.1365-2796.2010.02281.x

Stroth, S., Reinhardt, R. K., Thone, J., Hille, K., Schneider, M., Hartel, S., et al. (2010). Impact of aerobic exercise training on cognitive functions and affect associated to the COMT polymorphism in young adults. *Neurobiol. Learn. Mem.* 94, 364–372. doi: 10.1016/j.nlm.2010.08.003

Szuhany, K. L., Bugatti, M., and Otto, M. W. (2015). A meta-analytic review of the effects of exercise on brain-derived neurotrophic factor. *J. Psychiatr. Res.* 60, 56–64. doi: 10.1016/j.jpsychires.2014.10.003

Tamura, M., Nemoto, K., Kawaguchi, A., Kato, M., Arai, T., Kakuma, T., et al. (2015). Long-term mild-intensity exercise regimen preserves prefrontal cortical volume against aging. *Int. J. Geriatr. Psychiatry* 30, 686–694. doi: 10.1002/gps.4205

ten Brinke, L. F., Bolandzadeh, N., Nagamatsu, L. S., Hsu, C. L., Davis, J. C., Miran-Khan, K., et al. (2015). Aerobic exercise increases hippocampal volume in older women with probable mild cognitive impairment: a 6-month randomised controlled trial. *Br. J. Sports Med.* 49, 248–254. doi: 10.1136/bjsports-2013-093184

Terry, R. D., and Katzman, R. (2001). Life span and synapses: will there be a primary senile dementia? *Neurobiol. Aging* 22, 347–348; discussion 353–354. doi: 10.1016/s0197-4580(00)00250-5

Triviño-Paredes, J., Patten, A. R., Gil-Mohapel, J., and Christie, B. R. (2016). The effects of hormones and physical exercise on hippocampal structural plasticity. *Front. Neuroendocrinol.* 41, 23–43. doi: 10.1016/j.yfrne.2016.03.001

van Uffelen, J. G., Chinapaw, M. J., Van Mechelen, W., and Hopman-Rock, M. (2008). Walking or vitamin B for cognition in older adults with mild cognitive impairment? A randomised controlled trial. *Br. J. Sports Med.* 42, 344–351. doi: 10.1136/bjsm.2007.044735

Varma, V. R., Chuang, Y. F., Harris, G. C., Tan, E. J., and Carlson, M. C. (2015). Low-intensity daily walking activity is associated with hippocampal volume in older adults. *Hippocampus* 25, 605–615. doi: 10.1002/hipo.22397

Varma, V. R., Tang, X., and Carlson, M. C. (2016). Hippocampal sub-regional shape and physical activity in older adults. *Hippocampus* 26, 1051–1060. doi: 10.1002/hipo.22586

Vecchio, L. M., Meng, Y., Xhima, K., Lipsman, N., Hamani, C., and Aubert, I. (2018). The neuroprotective effects of exercise: maintaining a healthy brain throughout aging. *Brain Plast.* 4, 17–52. doi: 10.3233/bpl-180069

Voss, M. W., Nagamatsu, L. S., Liu-Ambrose, T., and Kramer, A. F. (2011). Exercise, brain, and cognition across the life span. *J. Appl. Physiol.* 111, 1505–1513. doi: 10.1152/japplphysiol.00210.2011

Voss, M. W., Prakash, R. S., Erickson, K. I., Basak, C., Chaddock, L., Kim, J. S., et al. (2010). Plasticity of brain networks in a randomized intervention trial of exercise training in older adults. *Front. Aging Neurosci.* 2:32. doi: 10.3389/fnagi.2010.00032

Voss, M. W., Vivar, C., Kramer, A. F., and Van Praag, H. (2013). Bridging animal and human models of exercise-induced brain plasticity. *Trends Cogn. Sci.* 17, 525–544. doi: 10.1016/j.tics.2013.08.001

Wagner, A. D., Maril, A., Bjork, R. A., and Schacter, D. L. (2001). Prefrontal contributions to executive control: fMRI evidence for functional distinctions within lateral prefrontal cortex. *Neuroimage* 14, 1337–1347. doi: 10.1006/nimg.2001.0936

Weinstein, A. M., Voss, M. W., Prakash, R. S., Chaddock, L., Szabo, A., White, S. M., et al. (2012). The association between aerobic fitness and executive function is mediated by prefrontal cortex volume. *Brain Behav. Immun.* 26, 811–819. doi: 10.1016/j.bbi.2011.11.008

WHO. (2018). *Ageing and Health Fact Sheet [Online].* World Health Organization. Available online at: http://www.who.int/news-room/fact-sheets/detail/ageing-and-health. Accessed February 5, 2018.

Young, J., Angevaren, M., Rusted, J., and Tabet, N. (2015). Aerobic exercise to improve cognitive function in older people without known cognitive impairment. *Cochrane Database Syst. Rev.* 4:CD005381. doi: 10.1002/14651858.cd005381.pub4

Yüksel, O., Ateş, M., Kızıldağ, S., Yüce, Z., Koç, B., Kandiş, S., et al. (2019). Regular aerobic voluntary exercise increased oxytocin in female mice: the cause of decreased anxiety and increased empathy-like behaviors. *Balkan Med. J.* 36, 257–262. doi: 10.4274/balkanmedj.galenos.2019.2018.12.87

20

Longitudinal Assessment of Amyloid-β Deposition by [18F]-Flutemetamol PET Imaging Compared with [11C]-PIB Across the Spectrum of Alzheimer's Disease

Shizuo Hatashita [1], Daichi Wakebe [2], Yuki Kikuchi [3] and Atsushi Ichijo [3]*

[1]Department of Neurology, Shonan-Atsugi Hospital, Atsugi, Japan, [2]Department of Radiology, Shonan-Atsugi Hospital, Atsugi, Japan, [3]Department of Radiopharmacology, Shonan-Atsugi Hospital, Atsugi, Japan

***Correspondence:**
Shizuo Hatashita
shizu@olive.ocn.ne.jp

This study evaluates the longitudinal changes in the amyloid-β (Aβ) deposition with [18F]-flutemetamol (FMM) PET imaging across the spectrum of Alzheimer's disease (AD), compared with [11C]-Pittsburgh Compound-B (PIB) PET. Eleven AD, 17 mild cognitive impairment (MCI) and 13 cognitively normal (CN) subjects underwent neuropsychological assessment and amyloid PET imaging using [18F]-FMM and [11C]-PIB during a follow-up period. Regions of interest were defined on co-registered MRI, and the FMM and PIB standardized uptake value ratio (SUVR) was used in the same cortical regions. The annual rate of change in FMM and PIB SUVRs was calculated. Cortical FMM SUVR in amyloid-positive subjects increased over a follow-up of 3.1 ± 0.5 years. An individual FMM SUVR was significantly correlated with PIB SUVR at baseline and at follow-up in the same AD, MCI, and CN subjects. The annual rate of increase in FMM SUVR was significantly greater in typical amyloid-positive (0.033 ± 0.023, n = 7), focal positive MCI (0.076 ± 0.034, n = 4) and positive CN (0.039 ± 0.027, n = 4) while that in AD (0.020 ± 0.018, n = 11) was smaller. Among amyloid-positive patients, the baseline FMM SUVR was inversely related with the increased rate in FMM SUVR ($r=-0.44$, $n = 26$, $p < 0.05$). An individual annual rate in change of cortical FMM SUVR was significantly correlated with that in cortical PIB SUVR. Our results suggest that the [18F]-FMM PET imaging can clarify the longitudinal assessment of Aβ deposition across the AD spectrum, similarly to [11C]-PIB PET. The Increase in Aβ deposition is faster in the predementia stage but not at a constant rate across the clinical stages of the AD spectrum.

Keywords: Alzheimer's disease, amyloid imaging, PET, amyloid beta, flutemetamol

INTRODUCTION

The National Institute on Aging Alzheimer's Association (NIA-AA) workgroup has proposed diagnostic criteria for the spectrum of Alzheimer's disease (AD) supported by biomarkers of the underlying pathophysiological process (Jack et al., 2011). This disease framework for AD with biomarkers is an important advance in clinical and pathophysiological progression. Among the biomarkers, amyloid PET imaging is the biomarker of the amyloid-β (Aβ) plaques which represents the earliest evidence of AD neuropathological change currently detectable in living persons and determines whether individuals are on the AD spectrum. Amyloid PET imaging is a key approach for the AD spectrum in general clinical practice.

Amyloid PET imaging with [11C]-labeled Pittsburgh Compound-B (PIB), which has a high affinity for fibrillar Aβ, detects Aβ deposition in the brain and is a distinctive and reliable Aβ biomarker. The [11C]-PIB PET imaging has demonstrated the usefulness of assessing the Aβ plaque status of subjects and has been well established (Klunk et al., 2004; Hatashita and Yamasaki, 2010). [11C]-PIB PET imaging has been extensively used in clinical research, trial and practice for AD. However, [11C]-PIB PET tracer can only be used in large PET centers with their own on-site cyclotron and radiopharmacy facilities due to the 20 min half-life of [11C]. Following the success of [11C]-PIB, several fluorine-18 [18F]-labeled Aβ-selective radiopharmaceuticals have been developed for clinical purposes. They are more suitable radioisotopes for more routine clinical usefulness because the 110 min half-life of [18F] allows distribution from a production site to multiple PET centers. [18F]-labeled amyloid PET imaging has been recently approved and has replaced [11C]-PIB PET imaging (Morris et al., 2016). In particular, [18F]-flutemetamol (FMM) is a fluorinated derivative of [11C]-PIB and is structurally identical to [11C]-PIB. [18F]-FMM PET imaging has been demonstrated to reliably detect Aβ deposition in the brain with imaging-to autopsy comparison, and distinguish AD patients from healthy controls (HC) subjects with both visual reads and quantification in the cortical regions, similar to [11C]-PIB PET imaging (Ikonomovic et al., 2008; Hatashita et al., 2014).

The longitudinal assessment of the increasing amyloid accumulation during the AD process is an important aspect of the clinical progression of the disease across the AD spectrum. Some longitudinal studies with [11C]-PIB PET imaging have shown that Aβ deposition increases continuously from levels in HC to those in AD dementia, and Aβ deposition slows in the later stages of AD (Jack et al., 2013; Villemagne et al., 2013). In contrast, using [18F]-FMM PET imaging, the longitudinal change of Aβ deposition has not yet been successfully clarified across the AD spectrum. It is still unknown whether the clinical progression of the disease across the spectrum of AD is associated with the amount in Aβ deposition and/or the rate of increase in Aβ deposition.

The aim was to evaluate the longitudinal change in the Aβ deposition across the spectrum of AD using amyloid PET imaging with [18F]-FMM and comparing this with [11C]-PIB. We sought to clarify the relationship between the amount of Aβ deposition, the annual rate of change in Aβ deposition, and the clinical progression of the disease.

MATERIALS AND METHODS

Subjects

Forty one subjects aged 60–90 years were recruited from our memory clinic and a community advertisement, and then included in a longitudinal study. Some subjects had participated in our earlier baseline study (Hatashita et al., 2014). All subjects underwent neurological and neuropsychological assessment, and amyloid PET imaging using [18F]-FMM and [11C]-PIB at baseline and one or more during the 3.1 ± 0.5 years of follow-up (range: 2.5–4.5 years). Global cognitive status was assessed with the Mini-Mental-State Examination (MMSE; Folstein et al., 1975) and the severity of dementia was rated on the Clinical Dementia Rating (CDR) scale and CDR sum of boxes (CDR SB; Morris, 1998). Memory measurement of immediate and delayed recall of a paragraph from the Wechsler Memory Scale-Revised (WMS-R) Logical Memory II was performed as a simple episodic memory test (Wechsler, 1987). The apolipoprotein E (APOE) genotype was determined at baseline.

Of these participants, 11 patients with AD dementia met the core clinical criteria of the NIA-AA for probable AD (McKham et al., 2011). The MMSE score was less than or equal to 23 and a CDR score was greater than 0.5. Seventeen patients with mild cognitive impairment (MCI) met the core clinical criteria for MCI by the NIA-AA (Albert et al., 2011), including an MMSE score greater than or equal to 24 and a global CDR score of at least 0.5 in the memory domain. Thirteen cognitively normal (CN) subjects had normal cognitive function with a MMSE score of 28 or greater and a global CDR score of 0. Participants were excluded if they had other systemic or brain diseases, including degenerative, vascular, depressive, traumatic, medical comorbidities, mixed disease, or traumatic brain injury.

The study was approved by the Ethics Committee of the Mirai Iryo Research Center Incorporation (Tokyo, Japan). All subjects or their caregivers provided written informed consent for participation.

PET Imaging

The [18F]-FMM and [11C]-PIB were produced in our PET center with good manufacturing practice guidelines (PIC/S GMP Guide Annex 3) according to standard procedures, as previously described (Hatashita et al., 2014).

All subjects underwent a [11C]-PIB PET scan on the same day as the cognitive testing, and a [18F]-FMM PET scan on the next day. PET imaging was conducted using a Siemens ECAT ACCEL scanner with an axial field of view of 155 mm, providing 63 contiguous 2.4 mm slices with a 5.6mm transaxial and a 5.4 mm axial resolution. Images were reconstructed with an iterative reconstruction algorithm, using a Gaussian filter of 3.5 mm full-width at half-maximum. The subject's head was immobilized to minimize motion during the scan. In each case, 10 min of transmission data were acquired for attenuation and scatter correction before the emission scan.

The [11C]-PIB was injected intravenously as a bolus with a mean dose of 550 ± 10% MBq. Dynamic PET scanning in the three-dimensional mode was performed for 60 min using a predetermined protocol. A single dose of [18F]-FMM of 190 ± 10% MBq was injected as a bolus. The image acquisition window of the [18F]-FMM extended from 85 to 115 min. All subjects underwent T1-weighed MRI (1.5 Tesla) for screening and subsequent co-registration with the PET images.

Image Analysis

A region of interest (ROI) analysis was performed on individual PET images. MRI-based correction of the PET data for partial volume effects was carried out using the PMOD software (PMOD Technologies Limited, Adliswil, Switzerland). The ROIs were manually drawn on the co-registered MRI in each subject and included the following 20 bilateral cortical regions: lateral temporal cortex (LTC), medial temporal cortex (MTC), frontal cortex (FC), occipital cortex (OC), parietal cortex (PC), sensory motor cortex (MC), anterior cingulate gyrus (ACG), posterior cingulate gyrus (PCG), precuneus cortex (Pre) and cerebellar cortex. The cerebellar gray matter was used as a reference region. The ROIs of the follow-up PET images were co-registered with the initial PET images, and the same ROIs were applied to both the baseline and follow-up images.

The retention of [18F]-FMM was calculated as the regional-to-cerebellum standardized uptake value ratios (SUVR). The regional FMM SUVR in each cortical region and cortical FMM SUVR for the mean of the regional SUVR over the nine cortical regions, including LTC, MTC, FC, OC, PC, MC, ACG, PCG, and Pre, were defined. The retention of [11C]-PIB was calculated as SUVR for 35–60 min. Regional and cortical PIB SUVR values were defined in the same regions as the FMM SUVR.

The cut-off values of FMM SUVR and PIB SUVR for amyloid positivity were based on the bimodal distribution in 56 CN controls and 32 AD patients. The cut-off value of FMM SUVR was 1.36 in cortical region while that of PIB SUVR was 1.39, as previously described (Hatashita et al., 2014). A typical amyloid-positive scan had more than cut-off values of cortical FMM and PIB SUVRs, and of regional FMM and PIB SUVRs in at least four cortical regions of LTC, FC, PC and Pre. The focal amyloid-positive scan had more than the cut-off value of regional FMM and PIB SUVRs in at least one or two regional cortical regions. An amyloid-negative scan had less than the cut-off value of regional FMM and PIB SUVRs in all of the cortical regions.

Data Management

The subjects underwent clinical assessments and [18F]-FMM PET and [11C]-PIB PET imaging approximately 12 months apart during the follow-up period. Annual changes in the [18F]-FMM and [11C]-PIB SUVRs of each cortical region were calculated for each subject at the last follow-up visit using the following equation: annual change = [(SUVR at last follow-up − SUVR at baseline)/follow-up period (year)].

Statistical Analysis

Data were analyzed with Statcel 3 software (OMS Inc., Tokyo, Japan). Paired *t*-tests were used to study changes between baseline and follow-up data. Clinical group differences were evaluated with two-sample Student's *t*-tests. Multiple comparisons of the difference in cortical regions were performed using Bonferroni *post hoc* test. Pearson's correlation analyses were conducted among the FMM SUVR, PIB SUVR, and clinical features. Categorical variables were examined with Fisher's exact test. Results were considered significant at $p < 0.05$. Data were presented as means ± standard deviations (SD).

RESULTS

Amyloid Positivity

All the 11 subjects with AD dementia had typical amyloid-positive scans. Eleven of the 17 MCI patients were amyloid-positive while six patients were amyloid-negative. Seven of the 11 amyloid-positive MCI patients had typical positive scans and four patients had focal positive scans. Two of four focal positive MCI patients were amyloid-positive in both precuneus and parietal or frontal cortical regions while two were only in precuneus. Four of the 13 CN subjects had typical amyloid-positive scans, and nine subjects were amyloid-negative.

Clinical Data and Cognitive Function

The demographic characteristics of the AD, MCI and CN subjects at baseline and follow-up are shown in **Table 1**. There was no difference in a mean age, education level, and sex among these groups. An APOEε4 allele was present in 6 (54%) of 11 AD patients, 6 (54%) of 11 amyloid-positive MCI patients and two (50%) of four amyloid-positive CN subjects. The proportion of APOEε4 carriers in these amyloid-positive subjects was larger than that in the amyloid-negative MCI or CN subjects.

The 11 AD patients had a mean MMSE score of 21.0 ± 2.1, a global CDR score of 0.8 ± 0.2 and a CDR SB score of 2.8 ± 1.1 at baseline, having significantly greater cognitive impairment compared with the amyloid-positive MCI and CN subjects. At follow-up of 3.3 ± 0.3 years, the mean MMSE score significantly decreased to 16.1 ± 3.2 ($n = 11, p < 0.05$), and global CDR and CDR SB deteriorated to 1.3 ± 0.4 ($n = 11, p < 0.05$) and 5.5 ± 2.5 ($n = 11$, $p < 0.05$), respectively. In contrast, the four amyloid-positive and nine negative CN subjects had no cognitive impairment on MMSE, global CDR or WMS-R Immediate and Delayed Recall scores at baseline and follow-up. None of the CN subjects progressed to MCI or AD during the follow-up period.

The seven typical positive MCI patients had a mean MMSE score of 26.1 ± 1.4 and a CDR SB of 0.7 ± 0.2 at baseline, similarly to the focal positive and amyloid-negative MCI patients. A mean WMS-R Delayed Recall score in typical positive MCI patients was 1.4 ± 2.6, which was smaller than that in the amyloid-negative MCI patients. Five (71%) of the seven typical positive MCI patients progressed to AD during the follow-up of 3.0 ± 0.2 years (range: 2.5–3.5 years). At follow-up, MMSE scores in typical positive MCI patients decreased to 22.0 ± 0.8 ($n = 7$, $p < 0.05$) and CDR SB scores increased to 2.1 ± 0.9 ($n = 7$, $p < 0.05$). In contrast, none of the four focal positive MCI patients progressed to AD during a follow-up of 3.0 ± 0.1 years. The MMSE and CDR SB scores at follow-up did not significantly differ from those at baseline. None of the six amyloid-negative MCI patients progressed to any dementia. There were no significant differences in MMSE and CDR SB scores between at baseline and follow-up.

Aβ Deposition

Mean cortical FMM SUVR values at baseline and follow-up in AD, MCI, and CN subjects are presented in **Figure 1**. The cortical FMM SUVR in AD patients was 1.87 ± 0.29 ($n = 11$, $p < 0.01$) at baseline, which was higher than that in amyloid-negative

TABLE 1 | Demographic characteristics of Alzheimer's disease (AD), mild cognitive impairment (MCI) and cognitively normal (CN) subjects at baseline and follow-up.

	AD	MCI typ	MCI foc	MCI−	CN+	CN−
n	11	7	4	6	4	9
Female	8 (73%)	4 (57%)	3 (75%)	2 (33%)	3 (75%)	6 (66%)
Age (years)	71.1 ± 8.3	76.2 ± 3.1	67.4 ± 4.9	75.0 ± 6.0	69.2 ± 2.3	66.5 ± 4.4
Education (years)	11.2 ± 2.0	11.7 ± 2.1	11.2 ± 1.3	12.3 ± 2.8	12.5 ± 0.8	13.7 ± 1.7
APOEε4 car	6 (54%)	3 (43%)	3 (75%)	1 (16%)	2 (50%)	2 (22%)
at baseline						
MMSE	21.0 ± 2.1	26.1 ± 1.4	27.5 ± 1.5	27.5 ± 1.6	29.2 ± 0.8	29.6 ± 0.6
CDR	0.8 ± 0.2	0.5	0.5	0.5	0	0
CDR SB	2.8 ± 1.1	0.7 ± 0.2	0.6 ± 0.2	0.5 ± 0.1	0	0
Imm rec	2.4 ± 2.1	5.5 ± 3.8	7.2 ± 2.0	7.8 ± 4.1	13.0 ± 1.8	15.1 ± 2.8
Del rec	0.1 ± 0.2	1.4 ± 2.6	3.5 ± 2.5	5.3 ± 3.9	11.5 ± 2.1	13.4 ± 2.8
at last follow-up						
MMSE	16.1 ± 3.2*	22.0 ± 0.8*	26.5 ± 2.0	26.1 ± 1.7	29.5 ± 0.8	29.6 ± 0.6
CDR	1.3 ± 0.4*	0.7 ± 0.2	0.5	0.5	0	0
CDR SB	5.5 ± 2.5*	2.1 ± 0.9*	0.6 ± 0.2	0.7 ± 0.3	0	0
Imm rec	0.8 ± 0.9	2.2 ± 1.7	6.5 ± 4.5	6.6 ± 4.6	12.0 ± 1.0	15.2 ± 3.5
Del rec	0.1 ± 0.3	0	4.7 ± 3.5	5.0 ± 4.4	9.7 ± 2.0	13.6 ± 4.0
Foll-up (years)	3.3 ± 0.3	3.0 ± 0.2	3.0 ± 0.1	3.0 ± 0.5	3.0 ± 0.3	3.5 ± 0.4

*typ, typical amyloid-positive; foc, focal amyloid-positive; +, amyloid-positive; −, amyloid-negative; n, number of patients; APOEε4 car, apolipoprotein Eε4 carriers; MMSE, Mini-Mental State Examination; CDR, Clinical Dementia Rating; Imm rec, WMS-R Immediate recall score; Del rec, WMS-R Delayed recall score; Foll-up, follow-up; data are presented as means ± SD. *Statistically significant difference from baseline by paired t-test (p < 0.05).*

CN (1.19 ± 0.09, $n = 9$) or amyloid-negative MCI patients (1.25 ± 0.06, $n = 6$). The typical positive MCI patients had high cortical FMM SUVR of 1.86 ± 0.14 ($n = 7$), being the same high level as AD. In amyloid-positive CN subjects, cortical FMM SUVR was also high (1.62 ± 0.08, $n = 4$), which was slightly lower than AD patient. At follow-up, AD and amyloid-positive MCI and CN subjects had significantly higher cortical FMM SUVR than that at baseline. The cortical FMM SUVR in AD patients increased to 1.94 ± 0.29, which was not different from that in typical positive MCI (1.95 ± 0.13) or CN subjects (1.73 ± 0.09). In focal positive MCI patients, the cortical FMM SUVR increased significantly from 1.32 ± 0.02 at baseline to 1.50 ± 0.05 ($n = 4$, $P < 0.05$). The amyloid-negative MCI and CN subjects had no significant change in cortical FMM SUVR at follow-up.

The individual cortical FMM SUVR values at baseline in the AD patients, the typical and focal positive MCI patients, the amyloid-negative MCI patients and the amyloid-positive and negative CN subjects are shown in **Figure 2**. All 22 subjects with typical amyloid-positive scans had high cortical FMM SUVR of above 1.50. Five of seven typical positive MCI patients had a higher FMM SUVR of above 1.81, all of whom progressed to AD. Although four focal positive MCI patients had a cortical FMM SUVR of below 1.36, all of them had high regional FMM SUVR of above 1.50 in precuneus; two of them had high regional FMM SUVR in another cortical regions, and one had a regional FMM SUVR of 1.40 in the parietal cortical region while the other had 1.37 in the frontal cortical region. Four amyloid-positive CN subjects had a high cortical FMM SUVR of 1.55–1.74.

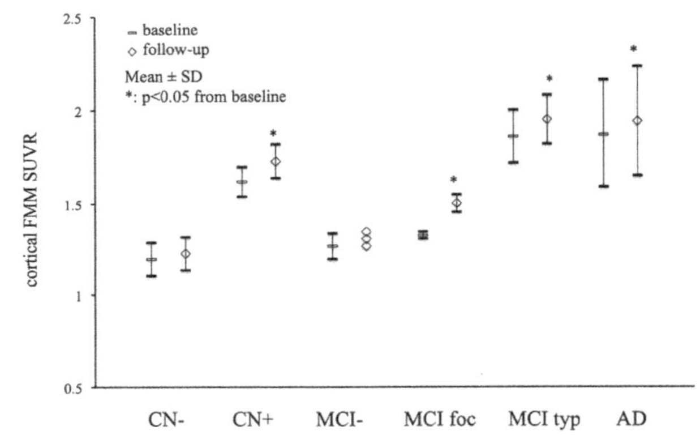

FIGURE 1 | Mean cortical [18F]-flutemetamol (FMM) standardized uptake value ratio (SUVR) at baseline and follow-up in Alzheimer's disease (AD) patients, typical positive mild cognitive impairment (MCI typ) and focal positive MCI patients (MCI foc), amyloid-negative MCI patients (MCI−), amyloid-positive cognitively normal (CN) subjects (CN+), and amyloid-negative CN subjects (CN−). Data are presented as mean ± standard deviations (SD). *Statistically significant difference from baseline by paired *t*-test ($p < 0.05$).

Changes in Aβ Deposition

The mean annual rates of change in the cortical FMM SUVR in the AD, MCI and CN subjects are shown in **Figure 3**. The annual rates of increase in cortical FMM SUVR in typical positive MCI patients (0.033 ± 0.024, $n = 7$, $p < 0.05$) and amyloid-positive CN subjects (0.039 ± 0.023, $n = 4$, $p < 0.05$) were significantly greater than those in amyloid-negative CN subjects (0.007 ± 0.016, $n = 9$). The annual increase rate in AD patients (0.020 ± 0.018, $n = 11$) was small, being not significantly different from the amyloid-negative CN subjects. In the focal positive MCI patients in particular, the annual rate of increase was the greatest among these groups (0.076 ± 0.034, $n = 4$, $p < 0.01$). The increase of cortical FMM SUVR was 5.8% per year.

The annual rate of change in regional FMM SUVR for four different cortical regions in AD, typical and focal positive MCI, amyloid-negative MCI and amyloid-positive and negative CN subjects are shown in **Table 2**. Among these cortical regions, the

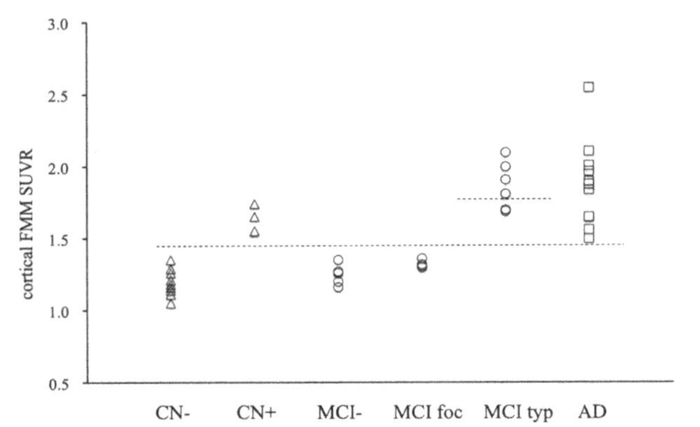

FIGURE 2 | Individual cortical FMM SUVR values at baseline in AD, typical positive MCI (MCI typ) and focal positive MCI (MCI foc), amyloid-negative MCI (MCI−), amyloid-positive CN (CN+) and negative CN subjects (CN−). The upper dotted line indicates the FMM SUVR of 1.81, while the lower line indicates the FMM SUVR of 1.50.

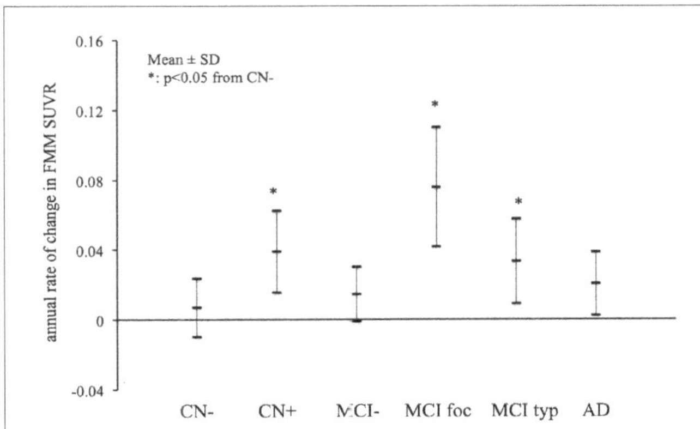

FIGURE 3 | The mean annual rate of change in the cortical FMM SUVR in AD, typical positive MCI (MCI typ) and focal positive MCI (MCI foc), amyloid-negative MCI (MCI−), amyloid-positive CN (CN+) and negative CN subjects (CN−). *Statistically significant difference from CN− by Student's *t*-test ($p < 0.05$).

annual rate of increase in regional FMM SUVR was the greatest in precuneus in focal positive MCI patients (0.097 ± 0.029, $n = 4$, $p < 0.05$), being significantly different from that in the amyloid-negative CN subjects. The increase rate of regional FMM SUVR in the frontal cortical region was also greater in focal positive MCI patients (0.093 ± 0.053, $n = 4$), but not significantly. There was no significant difference in annual rate of change in regional FMM SUVR between these cortical regions in the AD, typical and focal positive MCI, and amyloid-positive CN group.

When the individual annual rate of change in cortical FMM SUVR was correlated to the baseline FMM SUVR in all subjects, there was no significant correlation between them with simple model ($R^2 = 0.002$, $n = 41$, $p = 0.73$) and inversed U-shape model ($R^2 = 0.07$, $n = 41$, $p = 0.23$). In contrast, among amyloid-positive patients, the individual annual rate of increase in cortical FMM SUVR had significantly inverse correlation with the baseline FMM SUVR ($r = -0.44$, $n = 26$, $p < 0.05$).

Comparison Between FMM SUVR and PIB SUVR

The mean cortical FMM and PIB SUVRs at baseline, and the annual rate of change in cortical FMM and PIB SUVRs in the same AD, MCI, and CN subjects are shown in **Table 3**. The baseline value and the annual increase rate of cortical FMM SUVR in each group were not different from those of cortical PIB SUVR. The individual cortical FMM SUVR was significantly correlated with cortical PIB SUVR at baseline ($r = 0.96$, $n = 41$, $p < 0.001$) and at follow-up ($r = 0.95$, $n = 41$, $p < 0.001$; **Figure 4**). Furthermore, an individual annual rate in change of cortical FMM SUVR was significantly correlated with that in cortical PIB SUVR ($r = 0.69$, $n = 41$, $p < 0.01$; **Figure 5**).

Aβ Deposition, Cognition, Age, and APOE Genotype

Of the 26 amyloid-positive patients, the mean cortical FMM SUVR at baseline in the 14 APOEε4 carriers (1.76 ± 0.33, $n = 14$, $p = 0.77$) did not differ significantly from that in the 12 non-carriers (1.73 ± 0.22, $n = 12$). The annual rate of increase in FMM SUVR in the APOEε4 carriers (0.043 ± 0.028, $n = 14$) was greater than that in non-carriers (0.026 ± 0.029, $n = 12$), but the difference was not significant. There was no significant relationship between cortical FMM SUVR at baseline and MMSE score in individual amyloid-positive subjects ($r = -0.29$, $n = 26$, $p = 0.14$). Furthermore, the annual rate of changes in cortical FMM SUVR was not significantly correlated to that of the MMSE score in individual amyloid-positive subjects ($r = 0.30$, $n = 26$, $p = 0.12$) or that of the CDR SB score ($r = -0.27$, $n = 26$, $p = 0.18$). The baseline age was not significantly correlated to the cortical FMM SUVR at baseline ($r = 0.14$, $n = 26$, $p = 0.48$) or the annual rate of increase in cortical FMM SUVR ($r = -0.14$, $n = 26$, $p = 0.49$) in individual amyloid-positive subjects.

DISCUSSION

We demonstrated that the cortical FMM SUVR in AD, amyloid-positive MCI, and CN subjects increased over follow-up. The annual rate of increase in cortical FMM SUVR was significantly greater in amyloid-positive MCI and CN subjects while it was relatively small in AD patients, and it was the greatest in focal positive MCI patients. A previous [11C]-PIB PET study revealed that MCI patients with high PIB retention had faster increase rates of Aβ deposition, similarly to HC subjects with high PIB retention, but AD patients had a slower rate (Jack et al., 2013). Our previous study demonstrated that the patients with MCI due to AD had greater rates of increase in Aβ deposition during the process of progression to AD, followed by smaller rates of increase at the stage of AD dementia (Hatashita and Wakebe, 2017). These findings indicate that the increase of Aβ deposition does not occur at a constant rate across the clinical stages of the AD spectrum. Aβ deposition could increase faster in MCI patients than in AD patients, and if MCI patients have focal amyloid-positive scans, the Aβ deposition would increase further faster.

TABLE 2 | Annual rate of change in regional [18F]-flutemetamol (FMM) standardized uptake value ratio (SUVR) in four different cortical regions of AD, MCI and CN subjects.

	LTC	FC	Pre	PC
AD	0.022 ± 0.031	0.034 ± 0.046	0.015 ± 0.038	0.031 ± 0.059
MCI typ	0.036 ± 0.025	0.048 ± 0.034	0.037 ± 0.046	0.049 ± 0.020
MCI foc	0.077 ± 0.031	0.093 ± 0.053	0.097 ± 0.029*	0.053 ± 0.025
MCI−	0.009 ± 0.030	0.033 ± 0.030	0.013 ± 0.051	0.037 ± 0.029
CN+	0.054 ± 0.036	0.041 ± 0.032	0.048 ± 0.038	0.046 ± 0.054
CN−	−0.013 ± 0.028	0.022 ± 0.030	−0.001 ± 0.041	−0.019 ± 0.031

*typ, typical amyloid-positive; foc, focal amyloid-positive; +, amyloid-positive; −, amyloid-negative; LTC, lateral temporal cortex; FC, frontal cortex; Pre, precuneus; PC, parietal cortex; Data are presented as means ± SD. *Statistically significant difference from CN- by Bonferroni test ($p < 0.05$).*

TABLE 3 | Mean cortical FMM and Pittsburgh Compound-B (PIB) SUVRs at baseline and annual rate of change in cortical FMM and PIB SUVRs in AD, MCI and CN subjects.

	n	[18F]-FMM SUVR		[11C]-PIB SUVR	
		Baseline	Δchange/year	Baseline	Δchange/year
AD	11	1.87 ± 0.28*	0.020 ± 0.018	1.88 ± 0.36*	0.027 ± 0.024
MCI typ	7	1.86 ± 0.14*	0.033 ± 0.024*	1.91 ± 0.10*	0.033 ± 0.035*
MCI foc	4	1.32 ± 0.02*	0.076 ± 0.034*	1.45 ± 0.06*	0.053 ± 0.036*
MCI−	6	1.25 ± 0.06	0.014 ± 0.030	1.18 ± 0.06	0.008 ± 0.013
CN+	4	1.64 ± 0.08*	0.039 ± 0.023*	1.55 ± 0.15*	0.047 ± 0.018*
CN−	9	1.19 ± 0.09	0.007 ± 0.016	1.14 ± 0.05	0.005 ± 0.010

*Δchange/year, annual rate of change; typ, typical amyloid-positive; foc, focal amyloid-positive; +, amyloid-positive; −, amyloid-negative; n, number of subjects; Data are presented as means ± SD. *Statistically significant difference from CN- by Student's t-test ($p < 0.05$).*

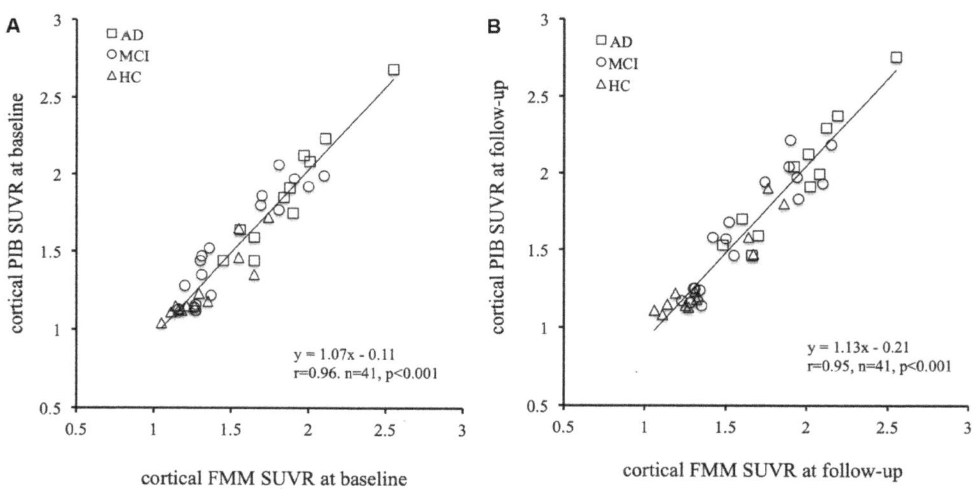

FIGURE 4 | Relationship of cortical FMM SUVR and cortical Pittsburgh Compound-B (PIB) SUVR in individual AD (squares), MCI (circles), and CN subjects (triangles) at baseline **(A)** and follow-up **(B)**. The FMM SUVR is significantly correlated to PIB SUVR at baseline ($r = 0.96$, $n = 41$, $p < 0.001$) and follow-up ($r = 0.95$, $n = 41$, $p < 0.001$).

In the present study, the annual rate of increase in regional FMM SUVR differed between the cortical regions in the amyloid-positive groups. The increase rate of regional FMM SUVR was the greatest in the precuneus in focal positive MCI patients, followed by the frontal cortical region. Previous [11C]-PIB PET studies have reported that the parietal and frontal cortices and the posterior cingulate showed the most prominent increase in [11C]-PIB uptake in MCI patients (Villemagne et al., 2011; Kemppainen et al., 2014). These findings indicate that Aβ deposition increases faster in precuneus/posterior cingulate in amyloid-positive MCI patients. On the other hand, the AD pathophysiological process has been demonstrated to be temporoparietal and/or precuneus hypometabolism. In the patients with MCI due to AD, we have reported that a regional hypometabolism in the temporal, parietal, and/or precuneus cortices detected by [18F]-fluorodeoxyglucose (FDG) PET is associated to the progression to AD (Hatashita and Yamasaki, 2013). Therefore, we suggest that the faster increase of Aβ deposition, particularly in precuneus, could cause primarily downstream neurodegeneration in the predementia stage.

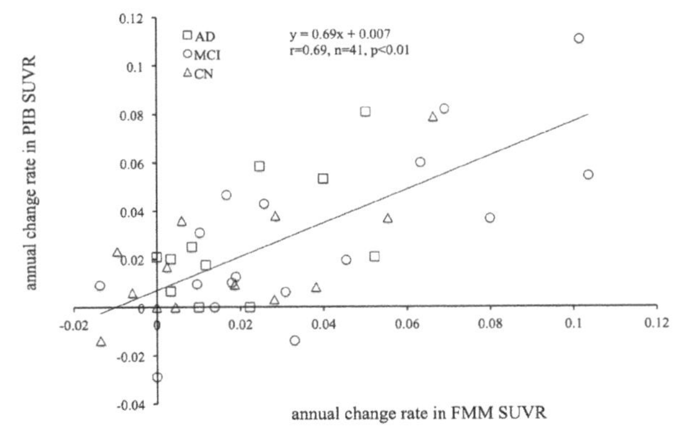

FIGURE 5 | Relationship between annual rate of changes in cortical FMM SUVR and PIB SUVR in AD (squares), MCI (circles), and CN subjects (triangles). Annual rate of change in FMM SUVR is significantly correlated to that in PIB SUVR ($r = 0.69$, $n = 41$, $p < 0.01$).

The annual rate of change in Aβ deposition has been described as providing the estimation for the duration of clinical progression of disease according to individual current Aβ deposition. The time span of disease progression has been estimated at 19.2 years for an individual to go from a PIB SUVR threshold of 1.5 in HC to a PIB SUVR of 2.33 in AD, equivalent to a 0.043 SUVR increase per year (Villemagne et al., 2013). The present study has demonstrated that the estimated time for disease progression to MCI was 6.15 years in amyloid-positive CN subjects to move from the mean cortical FMM SUVR of 1.62 in CN subjects to FMM SUVR of 1.86 in MCI patients based on a mean 0.039 FMM SUVR increase per year. In contrast, we have recently reported that 63% of 16 HC subjects with preclinical AD progressed to MCI within 7 years based on each clinical core criteria of the NIA-AA diagnostic guidelines (Hatashita and Wakebe, 2019). The time of clinical progression that is estimated by the amount and increased rate of Aβ deposition might actually be smaller than what occurs. The time of clinical progression in the preclinical stage of the AD spectrum would vary with APOE genotype, age, education, cognitive reserve and combined brain pathologies, in addition to increase of Aβ deposition.

On the other hand, in the typical positive MCI patients who had almost the same high level of FMM SUVR of 1.86 at baseline as AD, the present study found that the estimation of time for progression to AD dementia was 0.30 years, based on the annual rate of increase in FMM SUVR of 0.033. However, none of these MCI patients actually progressed to AD within 2 years. This implies that the typical positive MCI patients do not progress to AD quickly, even if Aβ deposition reaches the same level as AD. Furthermore, the present study showed that the increased rate of FMM SUVR was not correlated to the decline of MMSE or CDR SB scores in amyloid-positive subjects. In the predementia stage of AD, the increase rate of Aβ deposition does not appear to cause progressive cognitive deterioration directly but rather to trigger downstream AD neuropathological change.

The comparison of the [18F]-FMM PET and [11C]-PIB PET imaging has been studied along the continuum from normal cognitive status to the dementia of AD (Mountz et al., 2015; Lowe et al., 2017). We had already reported that the quantitative measurement of [18F]-FMM PET images, in addition to visual assessment, was consistent with that of [11C]-PIB PET (Hatashita et al., 2014). In this longitudinal study of [18F]-FMM PET and [11C]-PIB PET, we have demonstrated that the individual cortical FMM SUVR was significantly correlated with PIB SUVR at follow-up, in addition to at baseline, in the same AD, MCI, and CN subjects. In addition, the annual rate of change in cortical FMM SUVR was significantly related to that in cortical PIB SUVR. These findings imply that [18F]-FMM PET imaging successfully evaluates the longitudinal assessment of Aβ deposition across the AD spectrum, similarly to a standard approach of [11C]-PIB PET. Therefore, [18F]-FMM PET imaging can reliably detect longitudinal Aβ deposition in the brain and provide a potential prognostic timeframe based on the amount and increased rate of Aβ deposition. Furthermore, it is likely to play a critical role in the development of anti-amyloid therapies by establishing critical periods suitable for intervention along the disease pathway.

Certain limitations of our study should be noted. We conducted a successful longitudinal assessment of Aβ deposition across the AD spectrum during a follow-up period. The quantification was performed by regional FMM and PIB SUVRs normalized to a reference region of cerebellar gray matter. The number of participants included in the assessment was also relatively small, especially for the amyloid-positive CN subjects and focal positive MCI patients.

In conclusion, the [18F]-FMM PET imaging can clarify the longitudinal assessment of Aβ deposition and the increase rate of Aβ deposition across the AD spectrum, similarly to [11C]-PIB PET. The increase of Aβ deposition is faster in the predementia stage of AD and slower in the dementia stage. The amount and increased rate of Aβ deposition could not directly affect a potential prognostic timeframe across AD spectrum.

AUTHOR CONTRIBUTIONS

YK and DW provided substantial contribution to the acquisition of data. SH and AI provided the analysis of data. YK, AI, DW and SH reviewed the article.

REFERENCES

Albert, M. S., DeKosky, S. T., Dickson, D., Dubois, B., Feldman, H. H., Fox, N. C., et al. (2011). The diagnosis of mild cognitive impairment due to Alzheimer's disease: recommendation from the National Institute on Aging-Alzheimer's Association workgroups on diagnostic guidelines for Alzheimer's disease. *Alzheimers Dement.* 7, 270–279. doi: 10.1016/j.jalz.2011.03.008

Folstein, M. F., Folstein, S. E., and McHugh, P. R. (1975). "Mini-mental state" A practical method for grading the cognitive state of patients for the clinician. *J. Psychiatr. Res.* 12, 189–198. doi: 10.1016/0022-3956(75) 90026-6

Hatashita, S., and Wakebe, D. (2017). Amyloid-β deposition and long-term progression in mild cognitive impairment due to Alzheimer's disease defined with amyloid PET imaging. *J. Alzheimers Dis.* 57, 765–773. doi: 10.3233/JAD-161074

Hatashita, S., and Wakebe, D. (2019). Amyloid β deposition and glucose metabolism on the long-term progression of preclinical Alzheimer's disease. *Future Sci. OA* 5:FSO356. doi: 10.4155/fsoa-2018-0069

Hatashita, S., and Yamasaki, H. (2010). Clinically different stages of Alzheimer's disease associated by amyloid deposition with [^{11}C]-PIB PET imaging. *J. Alzheimers Dis.* 21, 995–1003. doi: 10.3233/JAD-2010-100222

Hatashita, S., and Yamasaki, H. (2013). Diagnosed mild cognitive impairment due to Alzheimer's disease with PET biomarkers of β amyloid and neuronal dysfunction. *PLoS One* 14:e66877. doi: 10.1371/journal.pone.0066877

Hatashita, S., Yamasaki, H., Suzuki, Y., Tanaka, K., Wakebe, D., and Hayakawa, H. (2014). [^{18}F] Flutemetamol amyloid-β PET imaging compared with [^{11}C] PIB across the spectrum of Alzheimer's disease. *Eur. J. Nucl. Med. Mol. Imaging* 41, 290–300. doi: 10.1007/s00259-013-2564-y

Ikonomovic, M. D., Klunk, W. E., Abrahamson, E. E., Mathis, C. A., Price, J. C., Tsopelas, N. D., et al. (2008). Post-mortem histopathology underlying β-amyloid PET imaging following flutemetamol F 18 injection. *Acta Neuropathol. Commun.* 4, 130–153. doi: 10.1186/s40478-016-0399-z

Jack, C. R. Jr., Albert, M., Knopman, D. S., McKhann, G. M., Sperling, R. A., Carillo, M., et al. (2011). Introduction to the recommendations from the National Institute on Aging-Alzheimer's Association Workgroups on diagnostic guidelines for Alzheimer's disease. *Alzheimers Dement.* 7, 257–262. doi: 10.1016/j.jalz.2011.03.004

Jack, C. R. Jr., Wiste, H. J., Lesnick, T. G., Weigand, S. D., Knopman, D. S., Vemuri, P., et al. (2013). Brain β-amyloid load approaches a plateau. *Neurology* 80, 890–896. doi: 10.1212/wnl.0b013e3182840bbe

Kemppainen, N. M., Scheinin, N. M., Koivunen, J., Johannson, J., Toivonene, J. T., Någren, K., et al. (2014). Five-year follow-up of [^{11}C]-PIB uptake in Alzheimer' disease and MCI. *Eur. J. Nucl. Med. Mol. Imaging* 41, 283–289. doi: 10.1007/s00259-013-2562-0

Klunk, W. E., Engler, H., Nordberg, A., Wang, Y., Blomqvist, G., Holt, D. P., et al. (2004). Imaging brain amyloid in Alzheimer' disease with Pittsburgh Compound-B. *Ann. Neurol.* 55, 306–319. doi: 10.1002/ana.20009

Lowe, V. J., Lundt, E., Knopman, D., Senjem, M. L., Gunter, J. L., Schwarz, C. G., et al. (2017). Comparison of [^{18}F] flutemetamol and [^{11}C] Pittsburgh Compound-B in cognitively normal young, cognitively normal elderly, and Alzheimer's disease dementia individuals. *Neuroimage Clin.* 16, 295–302. doi: 10.1016/j.nicl.2017.08.011

McKham, G. M., Knopman, D. S., Chertkow, H., Hyman, B. T., Jack, C. R. Jr., Kawas, C. H., et al. (2011). The diagnosis of dementia due to Alzheimer's disease: recommendation from the National Institute on Aging-Alzheimer's Association workgroups on diagnostic guidelines for Alzheimer's Association. *Alzheimers Dement.* 7, 263–269. doi: 10.1016/j.jalz.2011.03.005

Morris, E., Chalkidou, A., Hammers, A., Peacock, J., Summers, J., and Keevil, S. (2016). Diagnostic accuracy of [^{18}F] amyloid PET tracers for the diagnosis of Alzheimer's disease: a systematic review and meta-analysis. *Eur. J. Nucl. Med. Mol. Imaging* 43, 374–385. doi: 10.1007/s00259-015-3228-x

Morris, J. C. (1998). The clinical dementia rating (CDR): current version and scoring rules. *Neurology* 43, 2412–2414. doi: 10.1212/wnl.43.11.2412-a

Mountz, L. M., Laymon, C. M., Cohen, A. D., Zhang, Z., Price, J. C., Boudhar, S., et al. (2015). Comparison of qualitative and quantitative imaging characteristics of [^{11}C]-PIB and [^{18}F]-flutemetamol in normal control and Alzheimer's disease. *Neuroimage Clin.* 14, 592–598. doi: 10.1016/j.nicl.2015.10.007

Villemagne, V. L., Bumham, S., Bourgeat, P., Brown, B., Ellis, K. A., Salvada, O., et al. (2013). Amyloid β deposition, neurodegeneration, and cognitive decline in sporadic Alzheimer's disease: a prospective cohort study. *Lancet Neurol.* 12, 357–367. doi: 10.1016/S1474-4422(13)70044-9

Villemagne, V. L., Pike, K. E., Chételat, G., Ellis, K. A., Mulligan, R. S., Bourgeat, P., et al. (2011). Longitudinal assessment of Aβ and cognition in aging and Alzheimer disease. *Ann Neurol.* 69, 181–192. doi: 10.1002/ana.22248

Wechsler, D. (1987). *Wechsler Memory Scale-Revised.* New York, NY: Psychological Corporation.

21

Cofilin 2 in Serum as a Novel Biomarker for Alzheimer's Disease in Han Chinese

Yingni Sun[1†], Lisheng Liang[2†], Meili Dong[3], Cong Li[4], Zhenzhen Liu[5] and Hongwei Gao[1*]*

[1] School of Life Sciences, Ludong University, Yantai, China, [2] Department of Pain, Qingdao University Medical College Affiliated Yantai Yuhuangding Hospital, Yantai, China, [3] Central Sterile Supply Department, Qingdao University Medical College Affiliated Yantai Yuhuangding Hospital, Yantai, China, [4] Chemical and Materials Engineering, University of Kentucky, Lexington, KY, United States, [5] Chemical Engineering and Materials Science, College of Chemistry, Shandong Normal University, Jinan, China

***Correspondence:**
Yingni Sun
17805459157@163.com
Hongwei Gao
gaohongw369@ms.xjb.ac.cn

† These authors have contributed equally to this work

The identification of biomarkers of Alzheimer's disease (AD) is an important and urgent area of study, not only to aid in the early diagnosis of AD, but also to evaluate potentially new anti-AD drugs. The aim of this study was to explore cofilin 2 in serum as a novel biomarker for AD. The upregulation was observed in AD patients and different AD animal models compared to the controls, as well as in AD cell models. Memantine and donepezil can attenuate the upregulation of cofilin 2 expression in APP/PS1 mice. The serum levels of cofilin 2 in AD or mild cognitive impairment (MCI) patients were significantly higher compared to controls (AD: 167.9 ± 35.3 pg/mL; MCI: 115.9 ± 15.4 pg/mL; Control: 90.5 ± 27.1 pg/mL; $p < 0.01$). A significant correlation between cofilin 2 levels and cognitive decline was observed ($r = -0.792$; $p < 0.001$). The receiver operating characteristic curve (ROC) analysis showed the area under the curve (AUC) of cofilin 2 was 0.957, and the diagnostic accuracy was 80%, with 93% sensitivity and 87% specificity. The optimal cut-off value was 130.4 pg/ml. Our results indicate the possibility of serum cofilin 2 as a novel and non-invasive biomarker for AD. In addition, the expression of cofilin 2 was found to be significantly increased in AD compared to vascular dementia (VaD), and only an increased trend but not significant was detected in VaD compared to the controls. ROC analysis between AD and VaD showed that the AUC was 0.824, which could indicate a role of cofilin 2 as a biomarker in the differential diagnosis between AD and VaD.

Keywords: Alzheimer's disease, cofilin 2, biomarker, diagnosis, serum

INTRODUCTION

Alzheimer's disease (AD) is the most common fatal neurodegenerative disease of the elderly worldwide (Jagust, 2018). The identification of early biomarkers of AD will allow earlier diagnosis and thus earlier intervention (Wood, 2016; Hampel et al., 2018). New therapeutic strategies in AD are likely to have the best efficacy if they can be implemented early in the disease course (Lansbury, 2004; Livingston et al., 2017).

The pathology of AD is characterized by the progressive loss of basal forebrain cholinergic neurons and by two hallmark features: extracellular senile plaques and intracellular neurofibrillary tangles (NFTs) (Sery et al., 2013). In addition, AD brains show clear signs of oxidative stress along with neuroinflammatory response (Verri et al., 2012). Cytoskeletal abnormalities and synaptic loss are common pathologies in both sporadic and familial AD (Lane et al., 2018). Mild cognitive impairment (MCI) is not a pathological entity but defines a level of decline in cognitive function not interfering with daily activities (Petersen and Negash, 2008; Sanford, 2017).

The diagnosis of AD remain problematic at present (Scheltens et al., 2016; Hampel et al., 2018; Molinuevo et al., 2018). Reduced levels of Aβ, increased total tau (T-tau) or phosphorylated tau (P-tau) in cerebrospinal fluid (CSF) are currently the most promising biomarkers that might predict disease progression (Blennow et al., 2010; Humpel, 2011; Olsson et al., 2016; Polanco et al., 2018). Yet, their changes are not entirely specific to AD (Lleo et al., 2015), and moreover, it is challenging for the combination of Aβ, T-tau or P-tau in CSF to distinguish early AD to controls (Wood, 2016). Some disruption of the blood–brain barrier has been suggested to happen in AD patients, which enables some proteins in CSF to enter into the peripheral blood (Sweeney et al., 2018). Thus, blood biomarkers could reflect the alterations in brains. Not surprisingly, the blood biomarkers were focused on Aβ, T-tau and P-tau, but it turned out to be disappointing (O'Bryant et al., 2015; Hampel et al., 2018). In recent years, many candidate proteins in blood have been found using the proteomic approach (Lista et al., 2013; Robinson et al., 2017; Hondius et al., 2018), but the following validation research was often ignored, or the results were unsatisfactory. Evidences suggest that miRNAs have great potential for use as a biomarker in AD and other neurodegenerative disorders (Bekris and Leverenz, 2015; Pan et al., 2016). However, challenges still exist due to the lack of extensive validation and follow-up in larger cohorts of patients, and miRNAs are not yet a viable diagnostic or therapeutic tool for AD (Martinez and Peplow, 2019).

Cofilin as the major ADF/cofilin isoform in mammalian neurons influences the dynamics of actin assembly by severing or stabilizing actin filaments (Shaw and Bamburg, 2017). Cofilin is crucial for normal structure, dynamics, and function of the cytoskeleton, thus abnormalities in this protein can cause significant cytoskeletal disruption (Maloney and Bamburg, 2007; Bernstein and Bamburg, 2010; Bravo-Cordero et al., 2013). Because cofilin plays the central role in the regulation of actin filaments dynamics, it is involved in the development of neurodegenerative diseases, cancer and cardiomyopathies (Wang et al., 2007; Bamburg et al., 2010; Bravo-Cordero et al., 2013; Schonhofen et al., 2014; Chang et al., 2015; Subramanian et al., 2015; Bamburg and Bernstein, 2016). Three isoforms are known: cofilin 1, destrin and cofilin 2 (Bamburg and Wiggan, 2002; Shishkin et al., 2016). Cofilin 1 was mainly presented in non-muscle cells and in embryonic muscle cells (Shishkin et al., 2016). Destrin was expressed primarily in epithelial and endothelial cells. Cofilin 2 has two isoforms, CFL2a and CFL2b (Ostrowska and Moraczewska, 2017). The former is expressed in a wide variety of tissues, whereas the latter is expressed predominantly in skeletal and cardiac muscle (Shishkin et al., 2016). The protein cofilin 2 is composed of 5 α helices, 5 β sheets, and 1 C-terminal β short chain, with a molecular weight of 18 kDa (Ostrowska and Moraczewska, 2017). Studies of cofilin pathology have helped explain the development of sporadic (late onset) AD and have furthered our understanding of familial AD (Maloney and Bamburg, 2007; Zempel et al., 2017; Borovac et al., 2018; Rush et al., 2018). However, little was known whether cofilin can act as a biomarker of AD. In addition, most of above studies involved in AD either did not differentiate cofilin 1 from cofilin 2 (Whiteman et al., 2009; Rahman et al., 2014; Woo et al., 2015a; Deng et al., 2016; Shaw and Bamburg, 2017), or have only focused on cofilin 1 (Barone et al., 2014; Rush et al., 2018), but only few has concerned about cofilin 2 in AD.

Our previous proteomics study showed that the protein level of cofilin 2 was elevated greatly in the hippocampus of APP/PS1 transgenic mice compared with wild type (WT) mice, as well as in small amounts of AD serum samples (Sun et al., 2015). In the present study, we validated this result in a larger population, and moreover, we analyzed the expression of cofilin 2 in different AD animal and cell models. The protein expression and phosphorylation of cofilin 2 in the hippocampus tissues from AD patients and controls were also evaluated. To test whether cofilin 2 could be proposed as a non-invasive biomarker of AD, we compared the serum levels of cofilin 2 in AD, MCI patients and controls by enzyme-linked immunosorbent assay (ELISA), and the diagnostic accuracy as a biomarker was evaluated through the receiver operator characteristic curve (ROC) analysis. The correlation analysis between cofilin 2 levels and cognitive decline was also performed to determine whether higher cofilin 2 expression was associated with more severe disease or not. Additionally, to test whether cofilin 2 could distinguish AD from another common dementia-vascular dementia (VaD), we measured cofilin 2 serum levels in VaD, compared the expressions between AD and VaD, and also performed the relevant ROC analysis.

MATERIALS AND METHODS

Control and AD Brains

Frozen hippocampal samples of 10 AD patients and 10 age-matched controls were obtained from the Brain Bank of Chinese Academy of Medical Sciences and Peking Union Medical College, which collects brains from donors through a whole-body donation program. All procedures were approved by the Institutional Review Board (IRB). All AD patients displayed progressive intellectual decline and met NINCDS-ADRDA Workgroup criteria for the clinical diagnosis (McKhann et al., 1984). All controls had test scores in the normal range. The written informed consents for using the donated body tissue were given all donors for medical search. After death, the bodies were transferred rapidly to a designated autopsy facility. The average postmortem intervals (PMIs) were less than 3 h. Brains were bisected along the sagittal plane. One half was fixed in 10% phosphate-buffered formaldehyde, the other was cut into coronal slices (1 cm), and stored in −80°C until ready to use. These fixed hemi-brain blocks were sampled systematically, paraffin-embedded, and processed for standard immunohistologic and histologic stains as recommended (Montine et al., 2012).

Hematoxylin-eosin and modified-Bielschowsky staining, Aβ antibody (10D5), and α-synuclein immunohistochemistry were used for diagnosis on multiple neocortical, hippocampal, cerebellum and entorhinal sections.

Human Serum Sample Collection and Preparation

A total of 181 AD subjects, 58 MCI subjects and 181 non-demented healthy controls matched for age and gender were recruited in Yuhuangding Hospital for this study. Detailed demographic information of the subjects enrolled in the study is presented in **Table 1**.

All the subjects underwent a standard set of evaluations including past medical history review, laboratory tests, neurologic examinations and brief neuropsychological assessments (Fernandez Montenegro and Argyriou, 2017; Vallejo et al., 2017). Cases had a clinical diagnosis of probable AD according to DSW-IV, ICD-10 and NINCDS-ADRDA criteria. The cognitive status and severity of dementia were assessed by the Mini-Mental State Exam (MMSE) and the Clinical Dementia Rating (CDR) testing. Controls had no signs suggesting cognitive decline, and had a MMSE score between 28 and 30 and a CDR score of zero. Controls were excluded if they presented or had a history of depression or psychosis, substance abuse, or use of medications that could impair cognitive function. All controls were followed clinically for 2 years in order to rule out the development of cognitive decline. AD patients were followed-up and their cognitive status was reassessed 6 months after enrollment. MCI subjects were otherwise healthy, without significant medical, neurological, or psychiatric disease and met the following Petersen's criteria: (i) memory complaints by participant or family; (ii) objective signs of decline in any cognitive domain; (iii) normal activities of daily living; and (iv) the clinical features do not satisfy the DSM-IV/ICD-10 criteria (Petersen et al., 1999). In this study, no subject, originating from Northern Han Chinese populations, was presented with major and known co-morbidities, including hypertension, cardiopathy, diabetes or renal dysfunction.

This study also included 32 patients with VaD whose diagnoses were confirmed using NINDS-AIREN criteria (Roman et al., 1993). They are matched with the control group in age of onset, gender, body mass index (BMI) and educational level. Written informed consents were acquired from all subjects. The protocol of the study was approved by the Institute Ethical Committee of the Affiliated Yuhuangding Hospital of Qingdao University.

TABLE 1 | Demographics characteristics of the study samples.

	Control (n = 181)	MCI (n = 58)	AD (n = 181)	ANOVA p-value
Age, years	73.5 ± 5.1	72.7 ± 5.9	74.2 ± 6.3	N.S.
Male patients	80 (44.2%)	27 (46.6%)	85 (47.0%)	N.S.
BMI	27.2 ± 4.6	26.0 ± (3.8	26.8 ± 4.5	N.S.
MMSE, points	28.8 ± 0.7	26.0 ± 2.9	16.8 ± 4.6	< 0.001
Education, years	9.4 ± 3.1	8.8 ± 2.8	9.6 ± 3.2	N.S.

Data presented as mean ± SD where appropriate. Post hoc Tukey test: MMSE: AD vs. Control, $p < 0.001$; AD vs. MCI, $p < 0.001$; MCI vs. Control, $p < 0.001$. N.S. not significant different. MCI, mild cognitive impairment; AD, Alzheimer's disease; BMI, body mass index; MMSE, mini-mental status examination.

Blood samples (5 ml) were drawn in the morning hours under standardized conditions after an overnight fasting period. Blood was collected in evacuated collection tubes without anticoagulant and allowed to clot for 2 h on ice prior to centrifugation at 4,000 *g* for 8 min at 4°C. Serum was aliquotted (50 μl/tube) and stored in Eppendorf tubes at −80°C until utilized.

AD Animal Models

Groups of APP/PS1 double transgenic mice and age-matched WT mice (n = 8–10 per group) were purchased from the Jackson Laboratory Company [strain name B6C3-Tg (APPswe, PSEN1dE9) 85Dbo/J; stock number 004499]. Memantine and Donepezil were purchased from Sigma-Aldrich. They were dissolved respectively in distilled water. APP/PS1 transgenic mice were randomly divided into three groups of 8–10 mice each: untreated APP/PS1 Tg model, Memantine (Tg + 30 mg/kg Memantine) and Donepezil (Tg + 30 mg/kg Donepezil) groups. WT and untreated Tg model groups received distilled water alone. The administration by oral gavage was started at 12 months old and lasted for 12 weeks.

Aβ oligomers were prepared according to the protocols published by our group (Li et al., 2014). Synthetic $A\beta_{25-35}$ was purchased from Sigma. The concentration of $A\beta_{25-35}$ depends on the volume of the rat CSF. Male Wistar rats (3 months old, 220–250 g) were obtained from the Experimental Animal Center of Ludong University. 1 nM $A\beta_{25-35}$ was injected into the lateral cerebral ventricle of these rats.

All the mice and rats were kept in a temperature-controlled room at 25°C under a 12-h light/dark cycle and provided water and a commercial pelleted feed *ad libitum*. All the experiments were approved in according to the institutional guidelines of the Experimental Animal Center of Ludong University.

Cell Culture

SK-N-SH/SK-N-SH APP_{695} human neuroblastoma cells were cultured using Dulbecco's modified Eagle's medium (DMEM) culture in supplement with 10% fetal bovine serum, 100 U/ml penicillin and 100 μg/ml streptomycin, and maintained in a humidified atmosphere containing 5% CO_2 at 37°C. In addition, the SK-N-SH APP_{695} cells were supplemented with G418 (200 μg/ml). Cells were grown until nearly confluent, and then were collected.

The primary rat hippocampal neurons were separated from the brains of embryonic 18–19 (E18-19) Sprague-Dawley. Rat fetuses were dissociated for 20 min both enzymatically (0.25% trypsin-EDTA) and mechanically before filtering through a 100 μm cell strainer. The cell suspension was diluted in high glucose DMEM, 5% horse serum, 10% FBS, and 2 mM L-glutamine, and then plated into 6-well plates coated with poly-D-lysine (20 μg/ml) with the cell density of 1×10^5 cells/ml. Cells were maintained in a humidified atmosphere containing 5% CO_2 at 37°C. To inhibit the growth of glial cells, the medium was replaced by serum-free neurobasal medium containing supplement B27 and L-glutamine (0.5 mM) after almost 20 h. The half of the culture medium was changed every 3 days. Cells were incubated with 10, 30, and 100 μM $A\beta_{25-35}$ for 48 h separately, which was dissolved in distilled water for 7 days at 37°C before use. Cell culture reagents were obtained from Invitrogen, whereas all other reagents were purchased from Sigma.

Western Blot Analysis

Standard western blot analysis was carried out. All these mice and rats were sacrificed by CO_2 inhalation after behavioral testing was completed. The brains were removed and hippocampus was dissected on ice, and then were homogenized thoroughly in a RIPA lysis buffer [150 mM NaCl, 50 mM Tris (pH 7.4), 1% NP40, 0.5% sodium deoxycholate and 0.1% SDS]. The blood samples from mice and rats were collected into the evacuated collection tubes without anticoagulant, and treated in a similar manner with the human serum samples. Tissue sections from frozen hippocampus regions of AD patients and controls were dissected and resuspended in the above lysis buffer. These hippocampal samples were ultrasonicated for 1 min in cycles of 3 s on and 3 s off using a Fisher 550 Sonic Dismembrator. Then the samples were centrifuged at 20,000 *g* at 4°C for 60 min to remove the debris. The supernatants were collected and stored at –80°C before use.

All the cells were collected, and then total protein was extracted in the following lysis buffer containing 150 mM NaCl, 10 mM Tris, 10% glycerol, 1% NP40, 10 mM NaF, 1 mM Na_3VO_4, 1 mM EGTA and complete protease inhibitor. Then, the homogenate was centrifuged at 16,000 *g* at 4°C for 20 min. The protein solutions were collected and stored at –80°C before use. Protein concentration was measured with a BCA kit.

All the samples were subjected to electrophoresis, transferred onto PVDF membranes and incubated with the primary antibodies: rabbit anti-cofilin 2 (1:500, Cell Signaling Technology), rabbit anti-cofilin 2 (phospho S3) (1:1000, Abcam), mouse anti-β-actin (1:10000, Sigma) and mouse anti-IgG (1:10000, Abcam). Specifically, equal amounts of protein (40 μg) were run on 10% polyacrylamide gel, transferred on to PVDF membrance, blocked with 5% fat-free milk in Tris-Buffered Saline with Tween-20 (TBST) for 1 h, and subsequently incubated with primary antibody overnight. After washing with TBST for 5 times, the membranes were incubated with horseradish peroxidase (HRP)-coupled secondary antibody (1:10000, Cell Signaling Technology) at room temperature for 1 h with gentle agitation. Finally, membranes were revealed with the ECL Plus kit and High Performance Chemiluminescence Films (GE Healthcare, United States). Digital images of western blots were obtained with the LAS4000 FujiFilm imaging system (FujiFilm, Japan). The densitometric analysis was made by Quantity-One software (Bio-Rad, United States). The values were normalized to β-actin intensity levels.

Cofilin 2 ELISA

Serum cofilin 2 levels were detected using a commercially available human cofilin 2 quantitative sandwich enzyme immunoassay (Uscnk, Wuhan, China) according to the manufacturer's instructions. This kit was based on sandwich enzyme-linked immune-sorbent assay technology. Anti-cofilin 2 antibody was pre-coated onto 96-well plates. One hundred microliter of the standards and test samples were pipetted into the wells and were incubated for 2 h at 37°C subsequently. Any cofilin 2 present was bound by the immobilized antibody. The liquid of each well was removed without washing. After that, 100 μl of biotin-conjugated antibody specific for cofilin 2 was added to each well and incubated for 1 h at 37°C. During the incubation, biotin-antibody may appear cloudy. Then, they were warmed up to room temperature and mixed gently until solution appears uniform. Each well was aspirated and washed with wash buffer (200 μl) for three times. After the washing, the avidin conjugated HRP (100 μl) was added to each well and incubated for 1 h at 37°C. The aspiration/wash process was repeated for five times to remove any unbound avidin-enzyme reagent. TMB substrate (90 μl) was added to each well and incubated for 15–30 min at 37°C. After that, the stop solution (50 μl) was added to each well, and the optical density within 5 min was determined using a MQX200 microplate reader (Bio-Tek, United States) set to 450 nm. The serum level of cofilin 2 in the samples was interpolated from kit-specific standard curves generated using GraphPad Prism software.

Intra-assay Precision (Precision within an assay): CV% < 8%. Inter-assay Precision (Precision between assays): CV% < 10%. Three samples of known concentration were tested twenty times on one plate to assess. The detection range of the ELISA kit is 15.6–1000 pg/ml. The minimum detectable dose of human cofilin 2 is less than 3.9 pg/ml. The sensitivity of this assay, or Lower Limit of Detection (LLD) was defined as the lowest protein concentration that could be differentiated from zero. It was determined the mean OD value of 20 replicates of the zero standard added by their three standard deviations. This assay has high sensitivity and excellent specificity for detection of human cofilin 2. No significant cross-reactivity or interference between human cofilin 2 and analogs was observed.

Statistical Analysis

The data was analyzed using SPSS 13.0 software. Comparison between the groups was made using Student's *t*-test and one-way ANOVA. Correlations between cofilin 2 level and MMSE scores were performed with the Spearman correlation coefficient. Sensitivity and specificity of the measured variable for AD diagnosis were determined by ROC analysis. The best cut-off value was selected as those which minimize the sensitivity-specificity difference and maximize discriminating power of the tests. Statistical significance was set at $p < 0.05$.

RESULTS

Increased Cofilin 2 Expressions in Different AD Animal and Cell Models

Western blot analysis was performed to validate changes in protein expressions for cofilin 2 in different AD animal and cell models. As shown in **Figure 1A**, cofilin 2 was significantly increased in the hippocampus of APP/PS1 mice compared with

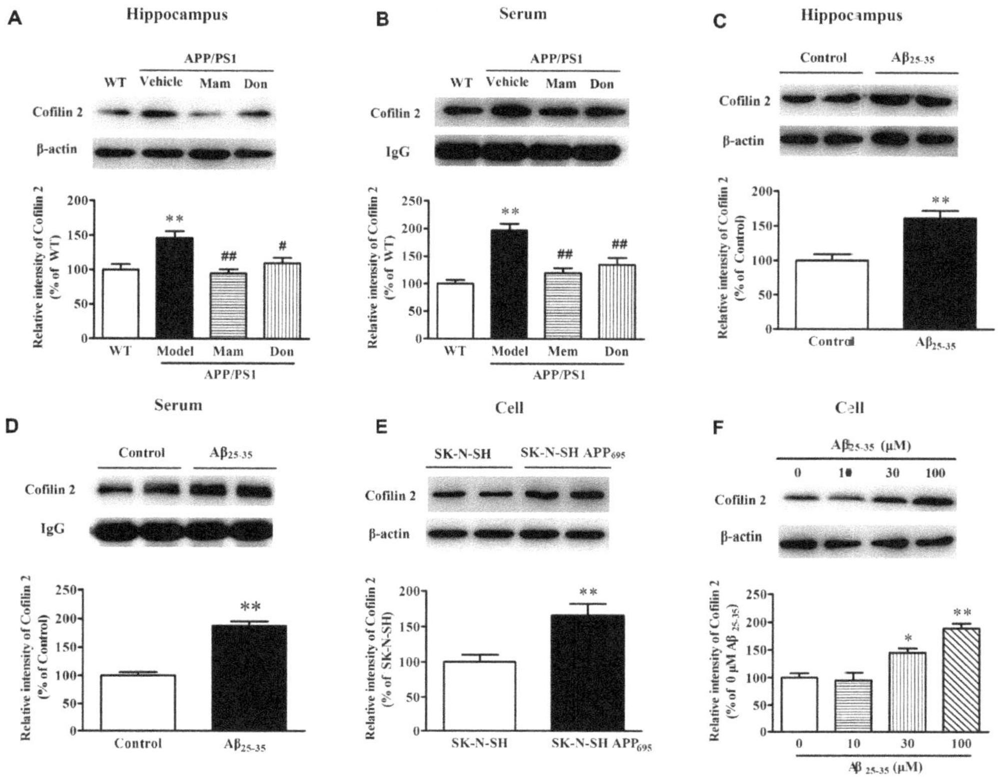

FIGURE 1 | Western blot analysis of cofilin 2 in different animal and cell models. **(A)** Cofilin 2 expression in the hippocampal brain homogenates of 12-month old APP/PS1 and WT mice and the effect of Memantine and Donepezil on cofilin 2. **(B)** Cofilin 2 levels in serum samples from 12-month old APP/PS1 and WT mice and the effect of Memantine and Donepezil on cofilin 2. **(C)** Cofilin 2 expression in the hippocampus of $A\beta_{25-35}$ intracerebroventricular-injected rats. **(D)** Cofilin 2 levels in serum samples from $A\beta_{25-35}$ intracerebroventricular-injected rats. **(E)** Cofilin 2 expression in the SK-N-SH APP_{695} cells. **(F)** Cofilin 2 expression in the primary-cultured hippocampal neurons from rats incubated with $A\beta_{25-35}$. Quantified results were normalized to β-actin/IgG expression. For all the results above, a representative experiment of three performed is shown. Values were expressed as percentages compared to the WT group (set to 100%), and represented as group mean ± SEM. n = 8–10 per group. $^{*}p < 0.05$, $^{**}p < 0.01$ vs. control group; $^{\#}p < 0.05$, $^{\#\#}p < 0.01$ vs. untreated APP/PS1 mice.

WT mice, consistent with our previous report (Sun et al., 2015). Similarly, a significant upregulation of cofilin 2 was observed in serum samples from APP/PS1 mice (**Figure 1B**). In order to observe the effects of positive anti-AD drugs on cofilin 2 expressions, APP/PS1 mice were orally administrated Memantine and Donepezil, respectively. After the long-term treatment, the expression of cofilin 2 was measured by western blot. Quantitative analysis exhibited that the increases of cofilin 2 in the hippocampus and serum samples were significantly attenuated with the treatment of Memantine or Donepezil (**Figures 1A,B**). In addition, we assessed the expression of cofilin 2 in $A\beta_{25-35}$ intracerebroventricular-injected rat AD model, and found that cofilin 2 was obviously increased by 61% in the hippocampus and by 88% in serum compared to the control rats (**Figures 1C,D**).

At the meantime, cofilin 2 expression was also detected in AD cell models. As shown in **Figures 1E,F**, cofilin 2 was increased significantly by 1.7-fold in SK-N-SH APP_{695} cells, and by 1.5/1.9-fold in 30/100 μM $A\beta_{25-35}$-treated primary-cultured hippocampal neurons from rats compared to control group. All these indicated that cofilin 2 was likely to be closely linked with AD pathology.

Increased Cofilin 2 in the Hippocampus Tissues of AD Patients

In different AD animal and cell models, cofilin 2 was validated to be increased significantly. To determine whether cofilin 2 was also upregulated in brain tissues of AD patients, we detected the expression of cofilin 2 in the hippocampal sections from AD patients and controls after death (**Figure 2A**). Meanwhile, the phosphorylation of cofilin 2 was also assessed (**Figure 2A**). The activity of cofilin 2 is regulated by reversible phosphorylation on ser3, rendering it inactive. Western blot analysis showed a statistically significant increase in protein expressions by 99% (**Figure 2B**), and by 29% in phosphorylation levels of cofilin 2 in AD samples (**Figure 2C**).

Serum Cofilin 2 Levels Detected by ELISA in AD, MCI and Controls

Results were validated subsequently by ELISA in a large population. All samples were comparable in terms of age, education and gender distribution. As expected, AD patients had a lower MMSE score than the healthy controls (mean MMSE score: 28.8 ± 0.7 versus 16.8 = 4.6) (**Table 1**).

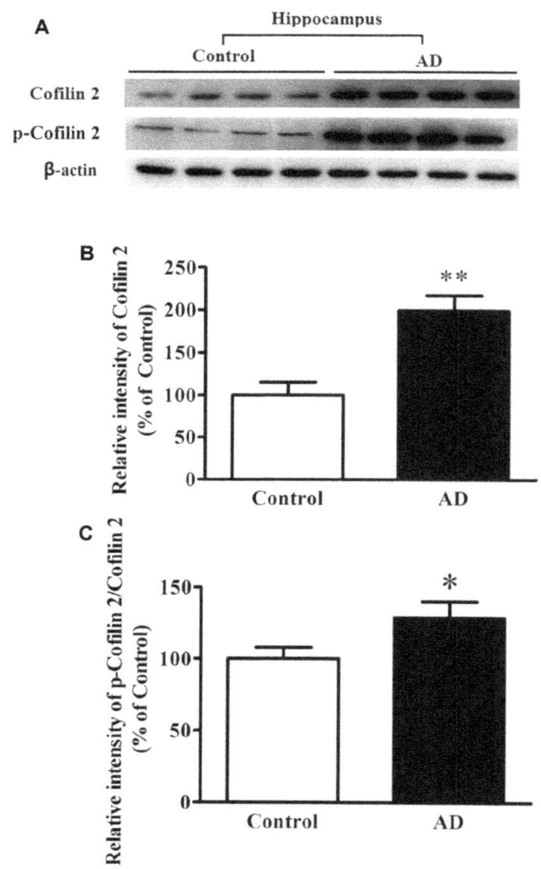

FIGURE 2 | Western blot analysis of cofilin 2 and phospho-cofilin 2 in the hippocampus tissues from AD patients and controls. **(A)** Representative western blot bands. **(B)** Quantitative analysis of cofilin 2 expression. **(C)** Quantitative analysis of cofilin 2 phosphorylation. Quantified results were normalized to β-actin expression. Values were expressed as percentages compared to the controls (set to 100%), and represented as mean ± SEM. $n = 10$ per group. $^*p < 0.05$, $^{**}p < 0.01$ vs. the control group, Student's *t*-test.

The ELISA results showed that AD patients presented higher serum levels of cofilin 2 in comparison to the controls, and cofilin 2 in MCI group was significantly higher than the control group and significantly lower than the AD group (AD: 167.9 ± 35.3 pg/ml, MCI: 115.9 ± 15.4 pg/ml, Control: 90.5 ± 27.1 pg/ml, $p < 0.01$). The 95% confidence intervals (CIs) were 162.7–173.1 pg/ml in AD, 111.9–119.9 pg/ml in MCI and 86.5–94.5 pg/ml in Control. The results showed no overlap of 95% CIs among AD, MCI and Control groups for cofilin 2, indicating the changes were statistically significant. Corresponding results are shown in **Table 2** and **Figure 3A**.

Correlation Analysis Between Cofilin 2 Serum Level and Cognitive Decline in AD Patients

The MMSE score is an important measure of the cognitive level of AD patients. The correlation between cofilin 2 serum levels and MMSE scores of patients is shown in **Figure 3B**. The results showed a significant negative correlation between cofilin 2 serum level and the cognition (evaluated by MMSE scores) within the AD group ($r = -0.792$, $p < 0.001$).

ROC Curve Analysis

To evaluate the diagnostic value of serum cofilin 2 as a potential biomarker of AD, ROC curve analysis of the ELISA results from AD and control groups was performed. As shown in **Figure 3C**, the area under the curve (AUC) was 0.957. The optimal cut-off value of 130.4 pg/ml was selected with sensitivity, specificity and diagnostic accuracy for serum cofilin 2 of 93, 87, and 80%, respectively, which could differentiate AD patients from controls.

Increased Serum Cofilin 2 Levels in AD Compared to VaD

There are many types of dementia that can be difficult to differentiate based on clinical features alone, despite vastly different underlying pathology. AD is characterized by the accumulation of Aβ peptides and hyperphosphorylated Tau (Hoppe et al., 2015; Bourdenx et al., 2017), whereas VaD is caused by the occurrence of many minor ischemic strokes over time (Ray et al., 2013). Other types of dementia include Lewy body dementia (LBD), frontotemporal dementia (FTD), multiple system atrophy dementia (MSA-D) and Parkinson's disease dementia (PDD), which also each have their own unique pathology. AD and VaD are the most common types (Posada-Duque et al., 2014). However, it can be challenging to differentiate them based on the clinical features alone.

Therefore, we detected cofilin 2 levels in VaD serum. Western blot analysis showed that cofilin 2 was obviously enhanced in serum of AD patients but only had an increased trend but not significantly in VaD patients compared to the control group (**Figures 4A,B**). ELISA analysis showed the similar results to the western blot, and the serum level of cofilin 2 in VaD was detected to be 107.1 ± 57.1 pg/mL (**Figure 4C**). It was also shown that cofilin 2 was significantly increased in AD compared to VaD in **Figure 4C**. ROC curve analysis of the levels of cofilin 2 between AD and VaD showed that AUC was 0.824 (**Figure 4D**), suggesting that cofilin 2 might act as a marker that could distinguish AD from VaD.

DISCUSSION

This study explored the potential of cofilin 2 as a candidate biomarker for AD. Our results indicated that cofilin 2 expression

TABLE 2 | Protein levels of cofilin 2 in serum of AD patients, MCI and controls.

	Control	MCI	AD
Protein Level (pg/ml)	90.5 ± 27.1	115.9 ± 15.4**	167.9 ± 35.3** ##
The 95% CIs	86.5–94.5	111.9–119.9	162.7–173.1

**p-value < 0.01 vs. Control, $^{\#\#}$p-value < 0.01 vs. MCI. One way ANOVA followed by Tukey–Kramer test. Data are means ± SD. n = 181 for Control and AD, and 58 for MCI. CIs, confidence intervals.

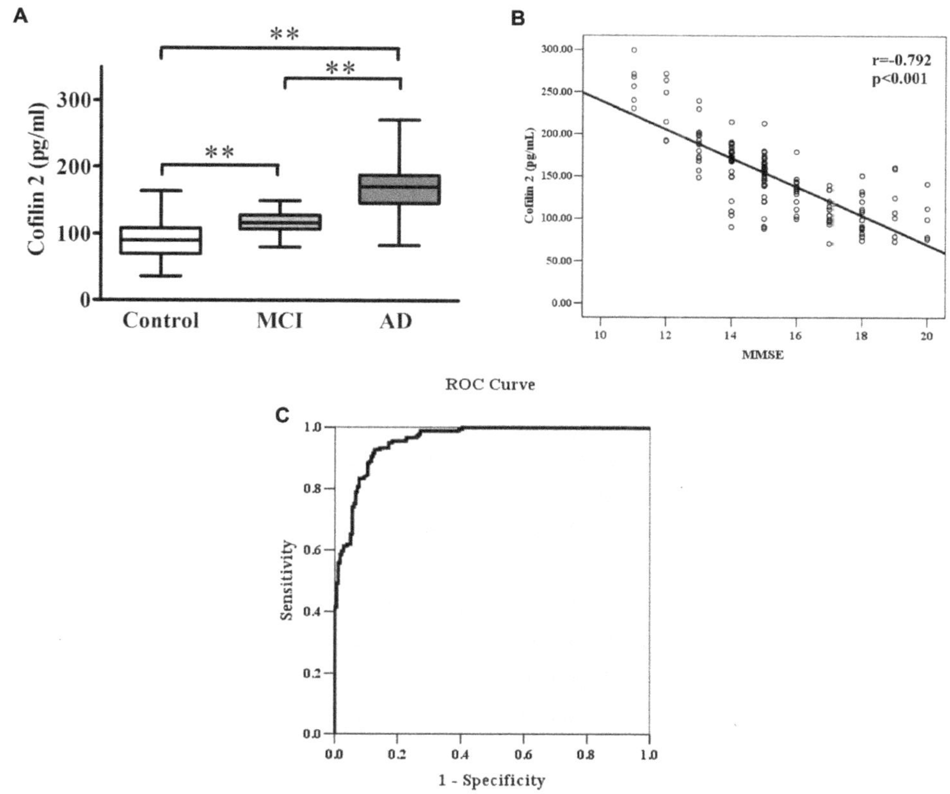

FIGURE 3 | (A) Cofilin 2 levels in serum are presented as box plots for AD (n = 181), MCI (n = 58) and healthy controls (n = 181). The lower and upper sides of the boxes indicate the 25th and 75th percentiles, and the horizontal lines indicate the means. Shown are also the lower and upper whiskers that indicate the minimum and maximum values, respectively. **p < 0.01 from one way ANOVA with Tukey–Kramer method as a *post hoc* test. **(B)** Correlation analysis between cofilin 2 serum levels and MMSE scores in AD patients. Correlation was assessed using the Spearman correlation coefficient. The concentration of serum cofilin 2 is plotted against MMSE scores for each patient. A significant negative correlation between serum cofilin 2 level and MMSE score (r = −0.792, p < 0.001) was observed. Correlation lines are also shown. **(C)** ROC curve analysis for serum cofilin 2 concentration and the prediction of the presence of AD. The AUC was 0.957. The optimal cut-off value (130.4 pg/ml) was selected. The diagnostic accuracy for cofilin-2 protein levels was 80% with the sensitivity and specificity 93 and 87%, respectively.

was significantly higher in different AD animal and cell models, as well as in AD patients. Memantine as *N*-methyl-D-aspartate (NMDA) receptor antagonist and Donepezil as acetylcholinesterase inhibitors, are currently effective drugs for AD (Standridge, 2004; Chen et al., 2017; Graham et al., 2017). In this study, the upregulated cofilin 2 was significantly attenuated after the treatment with Memantine and Donepezil in APP/PS1 mice, indicating that cofilin 2 might remain closely tied to the pathology of AD.

Many previous studies have demonstrated that cofilin may contribute to AD pathogenesis (Bamburg et al., 2010; Bamburg and Bernstein, 2016; Shaw and Bamburg, 2017; Rush et al., 2018). Cofilin and actin can form rod-like structures within neurites of AD brain (Minamide et al., 2000), and their dysfunction may mediate the loss of synapses, and production of the hallmark pathological features of AD: excess Aβ and NFTs (Maloney and Bamburg, 2007; Bamburg and Bernstein, 2016). Cofilin-actin rod formation represents a possible molecular mechanism for the chronic neuroinflammatory hypothesis of AD (Walsh et al., 2014). In all these cases, cofilin disrupts the normal balance of actin dynamics, thus exacerbating the oxidative cascade of neurodegeneration by accelerating mitochondrial decline and ATP depletion (Bernstein et al., 2006; Klamt et al., 2009; Kotiadis et al., 2012). The results presented here positively supports that cofilin might bridge and unite all the hypotheses of AD pathology.

Numerous studies have implicated the dysregulation of cofilin in AD (Bamburg and Bernstein, 2016; Shaw and Bamburg, 2017). It was reported that cofilin protein level was significantly increased in APP transgenic mouse brains and neurons (Yao et al., 2010). A recent study using cofilin immunofluorescence to compare the brains of human AD subjects with those of age-matched controls found that rod-like and aggregate cofilin pathology was four-fold greater in number and larger in area in the brains of AD subjects (Rahman et al., 2014). Studies of Aβ-overproducing mice have shown that decreasing cofilin dephosphorylation or decreasing total levels of cofilin expression are both effective in reducing the cognitive deficits (Woo et al., 2015a,b). However, to the best of our knowledge, there are few relevant studies of cofilin in blood of AD patients.

We confirmed that serum cofilin 2 levels were significantly higher in AD or MCI patients compared to controls. In

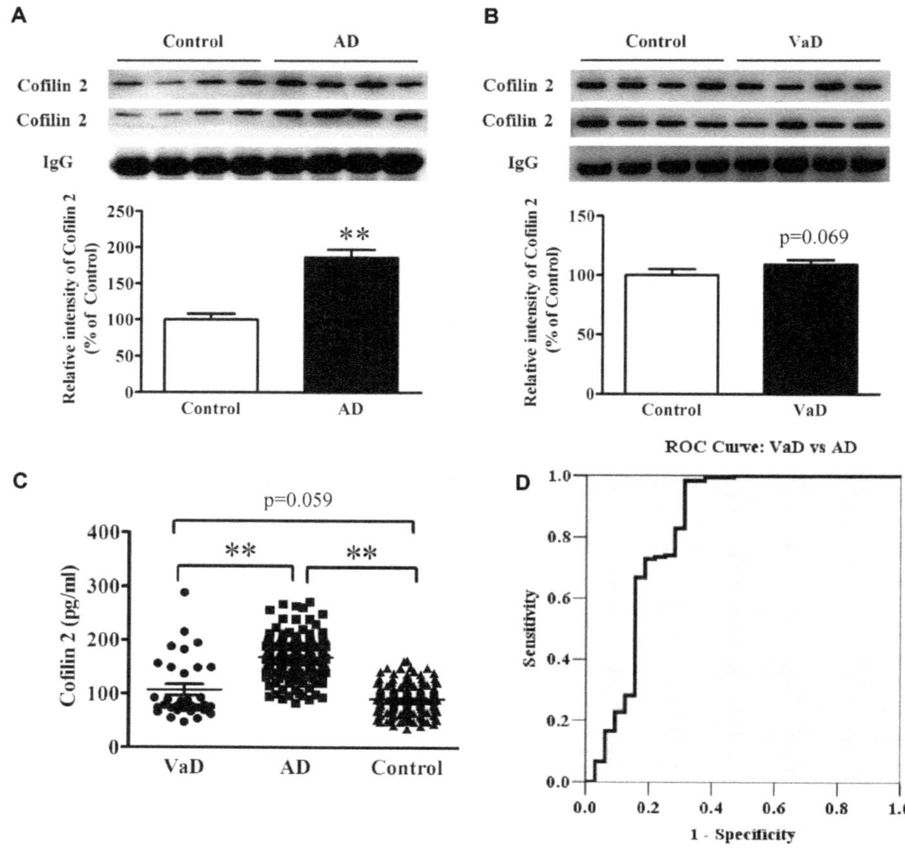

FIGURE 4 | Upregulation of serum cofilin 2 in AD samples **(A)**, and increased trends without significant difference in VaD samples compared to the controls **(B)**. The individual sera samples corresponding to AD/VaD and controls were analyzed by western blots for cofilin 2 protein expression. Equal volume of each sample was loaded and IgG was used as a loading control. Values were expressed as percentages compared to control group (set to 100%), and represented as group mean ± SEM. n = 32 per group. **p < 0.01 versus the control group, Student's t-test. **(C)** Scatter plots of cofilin 2 levels in serum of VaD (n = 32), AD (n = 181) and Controls (n = 181) measured by ELISA. Protein expression of cofilin 2 was significantly increased in AD compared to VaD. Data represent means ± SEM. **p < 0.01. **(D)** ROC curve analysis for serum cofilin 2 between VaD and AD. The AUC was 0.824.

addition, we observed a strong negative correlation between serum cofilin 2 levels and MMSE scores in AD patients, which suggested that higher cofilin 2 levels were associated with more severe disease. Through ROC curve analysis, we revealed that the sensitivity and specificity were 93 and 87% for serum cofilin 2 greater than 130.4 pg/ml, and its diagnostic accuracy was 80% in identifying AD patients. In addition, we found a significant increase of serum cofilin 2 in AD, and an increased trend but not significant in VaD compared to the controls. Cofilin 2 was previously reported to be significantly increased in protein expressions and phosphorylation levels, which was participated in the pathogenesis of idiopathic dilated cardiomyopathy with amyloid-like aggregates (Subramanian et al., 2015). Thus, it might be an overall marker for these degenerative diseases.

As we have ever known, there are 3 isoforms: cofilin-1, cofilin-2 and destrin, in which cofilin-1 and cofilin-2 have overlapping functions. Interestingly, we found in this study that cofilin 1 was undetectable in serum from both AD patients and controls by western blot. This is the first time to demonstrate the difference of expression of cofilin 1 from cofilin 2 in serum. As for why there is this discrepancy, and the exact roles in AD for cofilin 1 and cofilin 2, respectively, it remains to study further. Though we can't identify the exact role of cofilin 2 in AD, however, we detected the increased levels of cofilin 2 in human serum during the process. Furthermore, cofilin 2 performed well as a diagnostic and non-invasive biomarker with high sensitivity and specificity. So, it is still meaningful to develop cofilin 2 as a diagnostic biomarker of AD.

In summary, cofilin 2 expression was demonstrated to be significantly increased in AD patients and different AD models (animal and cell) in our present study. The good correlation between MMSE scores and cofilin 2 levels suggests that cofilin 2 might be used to diagnose disease severity. ROC analysis showed that cofilin 2 had high diagnostic values as a reliable biomarker to distinguish patients with AD from healthy subjects. Accordingly, our results highlight potential serum biomarkers of AD, which may facilitate AD diagnosis and assist in the evaluation of anti-AD drugs in both animal models and patients. Further investigation is needed to explore the value of cofilin 2 as a predictor of AD in a larger and independent population of AD and MCI patients.

AUTHOR CONTRIBUTIONS

HG and YS conceived and designed the studies. MD enrolled all the subjects and collected the serum samples. YS, LL, and ZL performed the research. CL modified the figures. YS and LL analyzed the data and wrote the manuscript.

FUNDING

This study was supported by the high-end talent team construction foundation (Grant No. 108-10000318), by the Startup Funds of Ludong University for New Faculty with PHD (No. 32830301), and by Natural Science Foundation of Shandong Province (Grant No. ZR201808030032).

ACKNOWLEDGMENTS

We thank all the subjects of our study who kindly agreed to participate. We also would like to thank Dr. Rachel Corbin, resident physician at Ventura County Medical Center for her assistance with English Language editing of the manuscript.

REFERENCES

Bamburg, J. R., and Bernstein, B. W. (2016). Actin dynamics and cofilin-actin rods in alzheimer disease. *Cytoskeleton (Hoboken)* 73, 477–497. doi: 10.1002/cm.21282

Bamburg, J. R., Bernstein, B. W., Davis, R. C., Flynn, K. C., Goldsbury, C., Jensen, J. R., et al. (2010). ADF/Cofilin-actin rods in neurodegenerative diseases. *Curr. Alzheimer Res.* 7, 241–250. doi: 10.2174/156720510791050902

Bamburg, J. R., and Wiggan, O. P. (2002). ADF/cofilin and actin dynamics in disease. *Trends Cell Biol.* 12, 598–605. doi: 10.1016/s0962-8924(02)02404-2

Barone, E., Mosser, S., and Fraering, P. C. (2014).). Inactivation of brain cofilin-1 by age, Alzheimer's disease and gamma-secretase. *Biochim. Biophys. Acta* 1842(12 Pt A), 2500–2509. doi: 10.1016/j.bbadis.2014.10.004

Bekris, L. M., and Leverenz, J. B. (2015). The biomarker and therapeutic potential of miRNA in Alzheimer's disease. *Neurodegener. Dis. Manag.* 5, 61–74. doi: 10.2217/nmt.14.52

Bernstein, B. W., and Bamburg, J. R. (2010). ADF/cofilin: a functional node in cell biology. *Trends Cell Biol.* 20, 187–195. doi: 10.1016/j.tcb.2010.01.001

Bernstein, B. W., Chen, H., Boyle, J. A., and Bamburg, J. R. (2006). Formation of actin-ADF/cofilin rods transiently retards decline of mitochondrial potential and ATP in stressed neurons. *Am. J. Physiol. Cell Physiol.* 291, C828–C839.

Blennow, K., Hampel, H., Weiner, M., and Zetterberg, H. (2010). Cerebrospinal fluid and plasma biomarkers in Alzheimer disease. *Nat. Rev. Neurol.* 6, 131–144. doi: 10.1038/nrneurol.2010.4

Borovac, J., Bosch, M., and Okamoto, K. (2018). Regulation of actin dynamics during structural plasticity of dendritic spines: signaling messengers and actin-binding proteins. *Mol. Cell Neurosci.* 91, 122–130. doi: 10.1016/j.mcn.2018.07.001

Bourdenx, M., Koulakiotis, N. S., Sanoudou, D., Bezard, E., Dehay, B., and Tsarbopoulos, A. (2017). Protein aggregation and neurodegeneration in prototypical neurodegenerative diseases: examples of amyloidopathies, tauopathies and synucleinopathies. *Prog. Neurobiol.* 155, 171–193. doi: 10.1016/j.pneurobio.2015.07.003

Bravo-Cordero, J. J., Magalhaes, M. A., Eddy, R. J., Hodgson, L., and Condeelis, J. (2013). Functions of cofilin in cell locomotion and invasion. *Nat. Rev. Mol. Cell Biol.* 14, 405–415. doi: 10.1038/nrm3609

Chang, C. Y., Leu, J. D., and Lee, Y. J. (2015). The actin depolymerizing factor (ADF)/cofilin signaling pathway and DNA damage responses in cancer. *Int. J. Mol. Sci.* 16, 4095–4120. doi: 10.3390/ijms16024095

Chen, R., Chan, P. T., Chu, H., Lin, Y. C., Chang, P. C., Chen, C. Y., et al. (2017). Treatment effects between monotherapy of donepezil versus combination with memantine for Alzheimer disease: a meta-analysis. *PLoS One* 12:e0183586. doi: 10.1371/journal.pone.0183586

Deng, Y., Wei, J., Cheng, J., Zhong, P., Xiong, Z., Liu, A., et al. (2016). Partial amelioration of synaptic and cognitive deficits by inhibiting cofilin dephosphorylation in an animal model of Alzheimer's Disease. *J. Alzheimers Dis.* 53, 1419–1432. doi: 10.3233/JAD-160167

Fernandez Montenegro, J. M., and Argyriou, V. (2017). Cognitive evaluation for the diagnosis of alzheimer's disease based on turing test and virtual environments. *Physiol. Behav.* 173, 42–51. doi: 10.1016/j.physbeh.2017.01.034

Graham, W. V., Bonito-Oliva, A., and Sakmar, T. P. (2017). Update on Alzheimer's Disease therapy and prevention strategies. *Annu. Rev. Med.* 68, 413–430. doi: 10.1146/annurev-med-042915-103753

Hampel, H., O'Bryant, S. E., Molinuevo, J. L., Zetterberg, H., Masters, C. L., Lista, S., et al. (2018). Blood-based biomarkers for Alzheimer disease: mapping the road to the clinic. *Nat. Rev. Neurol.* 14, 639–652. doi: 10.1038/s41582-018-0079-7

Hondius, D. C., Eigenhuis, K. N., Morrema, T. H. J., van der Schors, R. C., van Nierop, P., Bugiani, M., et al. (2018). Proteomics analysis identifies new markers associated with capillary cerebral amyloid angiopathy in Alzheimer's disease. *Acta Neuropathol. Commun.* 6:46. doi: 10.1186/s40478-018-0540-2

Hoppe, J. B., Salbego, C. G., and Cimarosti, H. (2015). Sumoylation: novel neuroprotective approach for Alzheimer's Disease? *Aging Dis.* 6, 322–330. doi: 10.14336/AD.2014.1205

Humpel, C. (2011). Identifying and validating biomarkers for Alzheimer's disease. *Trends Biotechnol.* 29, 26–32. doi: 10.1016/j.tibtech.2010.09.007

Jagust, W. (2018). Imaging the evolution and pathophysiology of Alzheimer disease. *Nat. Rev. Neurosci.* 19, 687–700. doi: 10.1038/s41583-018-0067-63

Klamt, F., Zdanov, S., Levine, R. L., Pariser, A., Zhang, Y., Zhang, B., et al. (2009). Oxidant-induced apoptosis is mediated by oxidation of the actin-regulatory protein cofilin. *Nat. Cell Biol.* 11, 1241–1246. doi: 10.1038/ncb1968

Kotiadis, V. N., Leadsham, J. E., Bastow, E. L., Gheeraert, A., Whybrew, J. M., Bard, M., et al. (2012). Identification of new surfaces of cofilin that link mitochondrial function to the control of multi-drug resistance. *J. Cell Sci.* 125(Pt 9), 2288–2299. doi: 10.1242/jcs.099390

Lane, C. A., Hardy, J., and Schott, J. M. (2018). Alzheimer's disease. *Eur. J. Neurol.* 25, 59–70. doi: 10.1111/ene.13439

Lansbury, P. T. Jr. (2004). Back to the future: the 'old-fashioned' way to new medications for neurodegeneration. *Nat. Med.* 10(Suppl.), S51–S57. doi: 10.1038/nrn1435

Li, P. P., Wang, W. P., Liu, Z. H., Xu, S. F., Lu, W. W., Wang, L., et al. (2014). Potassium 2-(1-hydroxypentyl)-benzoate promotes long-term potentiation in Abeta1-42-injected rats and APP/PS1 transgenic mice. *Acta Pharmacol. Sin.* 35, 869–878. doi: 10.1038/aps.2014.29

Lista, S., Faltraco, F., Prvulovic, D., and Hampel, H. (2013). Blood and plasma-based proteomic biomarker research in Alzheimer's disease. *Prog. Neurobiol.* 10, 1–17. doi: 10.1016/j.pneurobio.2012.06.007

Livingston, G., Sommerlad, A., Orgeta, V., Costafreda, S. G., Huntley, J., Ames, D., et al. (2017). Dementia prevention, intervention, and care. *Lancet* 390, 2673–2734.

Lleo, A., Cavedo, E., Parnetti, L., Vanderstichele, H., Herukka, S. K., Andreasen, N., et al. (2015). Cerebrospinal fluid biomarkers in trials for Alzheimer and Parkinson diseases. *Nat. Rev. Neurol.* 11, 41–55. doi: 10.1038/nrneurol.2014.232

Maloney, M. T., and Bamburg, J. R. (2007). Cofilin-mediated neurodegeneration in Alzheimer's disease and other amyloidopathies. *Mol. Neurobiol.* 35, 21–44.

Martinez, B., and Peplow, P. V. (2019). MicroRNAs as diagnostic and therapeutic tools for Alzheimer's disease: advances and limitations. *Neural Regen. Res.* 14, 242–255. doi: 10.4103/1673-5374.244784

McKhann, G., Drachman, D., Folstein, M., Katzman, R., Price, D., and Stadlan, E. M. (1984). Clinical diagnosis of Alzheimer's disease: report of the NINCDS-ADRDA work group under the auspices of department of health and human services task force on Alzheimer's Disease. *Neurology* 34, 939–944.

Minamide, L. S., Striegl, A. M., Boyle, J. A., Meberg, P. J., and Bamburg, J. R. (2000). Neurodegenerative stimuli induce persistent ADF/cofilin-actin rods that disrupt distal neurite function. *Nat. Cell Biol.* 2, 628–636. doi: 10.1038/35023579

Molinuevo, J. L., Ayton, S., Batrla, R., Bednar, M. M., Bittner, T., Cummings, J., et al. (2018). Current state of Alzheimer's fluid biomarkers. *Acta Neuropathol.* 136, 821–853. doi: 10.1007/s00401-018-1932-x

Montine, T. J., Phelps, C. H., Beach, T. G., Bigio, E. H., Cairns, N. J., Dickson, D. W., et al. (2012). National institute on aging-Alzheimer's association guidelines for the neuropathologic assessment of Alzheimer's disease: a practical approach. *Acta Neuropathol.* 123, 1–11. doi: 10.1007/s00401-011-0910-3

O'Bryant, S. E., Gupta, V., Henriksen, K., Edwards, M., Jeromin, A., Lista, S., et al. (2015). Guidelines for the standardization of preanalytic variables for blood-based biomarker studies in Alzheimer's disease research. *Alzheimers Dement* 11, 549–560. doi: 10.1016/j.jalz.2014.08.099

Olsson, B., Lautner, R., Andreasson, U., Ohrfelt, A., Portelius, E., Bjerke, M., et al. (2016). CSF and blood biomarkers for the diagnosis of Alzheimer's disease: a systematic review and meta-analysis. *Lancet Neurol.* 15, 673–684. doi: 10.1016/S1474-4422(16)00070-3

Ostrowska, Z., and Moraczewska, J. (2017). Cofilin - a protein controlling dynamics of actin filaments. *Postepy Hig. Med. Dosw.* 71, 339–351.

Pan, Y., Liu, R., Terpstra, E., Wang, Y., Qiao, F., Wang, J., et al. (2016). Dysregulation and diagnostic potential of microRNA in Alzheimer's disease. *J. Alzheimers Dis.* 49, 1–12. doi: 10.3233/JAD-150451

Petersen, R. C., and Negash, S. (2008). Mild cognitive impairment: an overview. *CNS Spectr.* 13, 45–53. doi: 10.1017/s1092852900016151

Petersen, R. C., Smith, G. E., Waring, S. C., Ivnik, R. J., Tangalos, E. G., and Kokmen, E. (1999). Mild cognitive impairment: clinical characterization and outcome. *Arch. Neurol.* 56, 303–308.

Polanco, J. C., Li, C., Bodea, L. G., Martinez-Marmol, R., Meunier, F. A., and Gotz, J. (2018). Amyloid-beta and tau complexity - towards improved biomarkers and targeted therapies. *Nat. Rev. Neurol.* 14, 22–39. doi: 10.1038/nrneurol.2017.162

Posada-Duque, R. A., Barreto, G. E., and Cardona-Gomez, G. P. (2014). Protection after stroke: cellular effectors of neurovascular unit integrity. *Front. Cell Neurosci.* 8:231. doi: 10.3389/fncel.2014.00231

Rahman, T., Davies, D. S., Tannenberg, R. K., Fok, S., Shepherd, C., Dodd, P. R., et al. (2014). Cofilin rods and aggregates concur with tau pathology and the development of Alzheimer's disease. *J. Alzheimers Dis.* 42, 1443–1460. doi: 10.3233/JAD-140393

Ray, L., Khemka, V. K., Behera, P., Bandyopadhyay, K., Pal, S., Pal, K., et al. (2013). Serum homocysteine, dehydroepiandrosterone sulphate and lipoprotein (a) in alzheimer's disease and vascular dementia. *Aging Dis.* 4, 57–64.

Robinson, R. A., Amin, B., and Guest, P. C. (2017). Multiplexing biomarker methods, proteomics and considerations for Alzheimer's Disease. *Adv. Exp. Med. Biol.* 974, 21–48. doi: 10.1007/978-3-319-52479-5_2

Roman, G. C., Tatemichi, T. K., Erkinjuntti, T., Cummings, J. L., Masdeu, J. C., Garcia, J. H., et al. (1993). Vascular dementia: diagnostic criteria for research studies. Report of the NINDS-AIREN international workshop. *Neurology* 43, 250–260.

Rush, T., Martinez-Hernandez, J., Dollmeyer, M., Frandemiche, M. L., Borel, E., Boisseau, S., et al. (2018). Synaptotoxicity in Alzheimer's Disease involved a dysregulation of actin cytoskeleton dynamics through cofilin 1 phosphorylation. *J. Neurosci.* 38, 10349–10361. doi: 10.1523/JNEUROSCI.1409-18.2018

Sanford, A. M. (2017). Mild cognitive impairment. *Clin. Geriatr. Med.* 33, 325–337. doi: 10.1016/j.cger.2017.02.005

Scheltens, P., Blennow, K., Breteler, M. M., de Strooper, B., Frisoni, G. B., Salloway, S., et al. (2016). Alzheimer's disease. *Lancet* 388, 505–517. doi: 10.1016/S0140-6736(15)01124-1

Schonhofen, P., de Medeiros, L. M., Chatain, C. P., Bristot, I. J., and Klamt, F. (2014). Cofilin/actin rod formation by dysregulation of cofilin-1 activity as a central initial step in neurodegeneration. *Mini. Rev. Med. Chem.* 14, 393–400. doi: 10.2174/1389557514666140506161458

Sery, O., Povova, J., Misek, I., Pesak, L., and Janout, V. (2013). Molecular mechanisms of neuropathological changes in Alzheimer's disease: a review. *Folia Neuropathol.* 51, 1–9. doi: 10.5114/fn.2013.34190

Shaw, A. E., and Bamburg, J. R. (2017). Peptide regulation of cofilin activity in the CNS: a novel therapeutic approach for treatment of multiple neurological disorders. *Pharmacol. Ther.* 175, 17–27. doi: 10.1016/j.pharmthera.2017.02.031

Shishkin, S., Eremina, L., Pashintseva, N., Kovalev, L., and Kovaleva, M. (2016). Cofilin-1 and other ADF/cofilin superfamily members in human malignant cells. *Int. J. Mol. Sci.* 18:10. doi: 10.3390/ijms18010010

Standridge, J. B. (2004). Pharmacotherapeutic approaches to the treatment of Alzheimer's disease. *Clin. Ther.* 26, 615–630. doi: 10.1016/s0149-2918(04)90064-1

Subramanian, K., Gianni, D., Balla, C., Assenza, G. E., Joshi, M., Semigran, M. J., et al. (2015). Cofilin-2 phosphorylation and sequestration in myocardial aggregates: novel pathogenetic mechanisms for idiopathic dilated cardiomyopathy. *J. Am. Coll. Cardiol.* 65, 1199–1214. doi: 10.1016/j.jacc.2015.01.031

Sun, Y., Rong, X., Lu, W., Peng, Y., Li, J., Xu, S., et al. (2015). Translational study of Alzheimer's disease (AD) biomarkers from brain tissues in AbetaPP/PS1 mice and serum of AD patients. *J. Alzheimers Dis.* 45, 269–282. doi: 10.3233/JAD-142805

Sweeney, M. D., Sagare, A. P., and Zlokovic, B. V. (2018). Blood-brain barrier breakdown in Alzheimer disease and other neurodegenerative disorders. *Nat. Rev. Neurol.* 14, 133–150. doi: 10.1038/nrneurol.2017.188

Vallejo, V., Wyss, P., Rampa, L., Mitache, A. V., Muri, R. M., Mosimann, U. P., et al. (2017). Evaluation of a novel serious game based assessment tool for patients with Alzheimer's disease. *PLoS One* 12:e0175999. doi: 10.1371/journal.pone.0175999

Verri, M., Pastoris, O., Dossena, M., Aquilani, R., Guerriero, F., Cuzzoni, G., et al. (2012). Mitochondrial alterations, oxidative stress and neuroinflammation in Alzheimer's disease. *Int. J. Immunopathol. Pharmacol.* 25, 345–353. doi: 10.1177/039463201202500204

Walsh, K. P., Minamide, L. S., Kane, S. J., Shaw, A. E., Brown, D. R., Pulford, B., et al. (2014). Amyloid-beta and proinflammatory cytokines utilize a prion protein-dependent pathway to activate NADPH oxidase and induce cofilin-actin rods in hippocampal neurons. *PLoS One* 9:e95995. doi: 10.1371/journal.pone.0095995

Wang, W., Eddy, R., and Condeelis, J. (2007). The cofilin pathway in breast cancer invasion and metastasis. *Nat. Rev. Cancer* 7, 429–440. doi: 10.1038/nrc2148

Whiteman, I. T., Gervasio, O. L., Cullen, K. M., Guillemin, G. J., Jeong, E. V., Witting, P. K., et al. (2009). Activated actin-depolymerizing factor/cofilin sequesters phosphorylated microtubule-associated protein during the assembly of alzheimer-like neuritic cytoskeletal striations. *J. Neurosci.* 29, 12994–13005. doi: 10.1523/JNEUROSCI.3531-09.2009

Woo, J. A., Boggess, T., Uhlar, C., Wang, X., Khan, H., Cappos, G., et al. (2015a). RanBP9 at the intersection between cofilin and Abeta pathologies: rescue of neurodegenerative changes by RanBP9 reduction. *Cell Death Dis.* 6:1676. doi: 10.1038/cddis.2015.37

Woo, J. A., Zhao, X., Khan, H., Penn, C., Wang, X., Joly-Amado, A., et al. (2015b). Slingshot-cofilin activation mediates mitochondrial and synaptic dysfunction via abeta ligation to beta1-integrin conformers. *Cell Death Differ.* 22, 1069–1070. doi: 10.1038/cdd.2015.41

Wood, H. (2016). Alzheimer disease: biomarkers of AD risk - the end of the road for plasma amyloid-beta? *Nat. Rev. Neurol.* 12:613. doi: 10.1038/nrneurol.2016.160

Yao, J., Hennessey, T., Flynt, A., Lai, E., Beal, M. F., and Lin, M. T. (2010). MicroRNA-related cofilin abnormality in Alzheimer's disease. *PLoS One* 5:e15546. doi: 10.1371/journal.pone.0015546

Zempel, H., Dennissen, F. J. A., Kumar, Y., Luedtke, J., Biernat, J., Mandelkow, E. M., et al. (2017). Axodendritic sorting and pathological missorting of tau are isoform-specific and determined by axon initial segment architecture. *J. Biol. Chem.* 292, 12192–12207. doi: 10.1074/jbc.M117.784702

22

Methodological Issues in the Clinical Validation of Biomarkers for Alzheimer's Disease: The Paradigmatic Example of CSF

Marco Canevelli[1,2]*, *Ilaria Bacigalupo*[2], *Giuseppe Gervasi*[2], *Eleonora Lacorte*[2], *Marco Massari*[3], *Flavia Mayer*[2], *Nicola Vanacore*[2] and *Matteo Cesari*[4,5]

[1]Department of Human Neuroscience, Sapienza University, Rome, Italy, [2]National Center for Disease Prevention and Health Promotion, National Institute of Health, Rome, Italy, [3]National Center for Drug Research and Evaluation, National Institute of Health, Rome, Italy, [4]Fondazione IRCCS Ca' Granda Ospedale Maggiore Policlinico, Milan, Italy, [5]Geriatric Unit, Department of Clinical Sciences and Community Health, University of Milan, Milan, Italy

***Correspondence:**
Marco Canevelli
marco.canevelli@gmail.com

The use of biomarkers is profoundly transforming medical research and practice. Their adoption has triggered major advancements in the field of Alzheimer's disease (AD) over the past years. For instance, the analysis of the cerebrospinal fluid (CSF) and neuroimaging changes indicative of neuronal loss and amyloid deposition has led to the understanding that AD is characterized by a long preclinical phase. It is also supporting the transition towards a biology-grounded framework and definition of the disease. Nevertheless, though sufficient evidence exists about the *analytical validity* (i.e., accuracy, reliability, and reproducibility) of the candidate AD biomarkers, their *clinical validity* (i.e., how well the test measures the clinical features, and the disease or treatment outcomes) and *clinical utility* (i.e., if and how the test improves the patient's outcomes, confirms/changes the diagnosis, identifies at-risk individuals, influences therapeutic choices) have not been fully proven. In the present review, some of the methodological issues and challenges that should be addressed in order to better appreciate the potential benefits and limitations of AD biomarkers are discussed. The ultimate goal is to stimulate a constructive discussion aimed at filling the existing gaps and more precisely defining the directions of future research. Specifically, four main aspects of the clinical validation process are addressed and applied to the most relevant CSF biomarkers: (1) the definition of reference values; (2) the identification of reference standards for the disease of interest (i.e., AD); (3) the inclusion within the diagnostic process; and (4) the statistical process supporting the whole framework.

Keywords: biomarkers, Alzheimer's disease, validation, diagnostic research, epidemiology, mild cognitive impairment

INTRODUCTION

A biomarker is defined as a characteristic that is objectively measured and evaluated as an indicator of normal biological processes, pathogenic processes, or pharmacological responses to a therapeutic intervention (Biomarkers Definitions Working Group, 2001). The use of biomarkers is profoundly transforming medical research and practice (the so called "biomarker revolution";

Schisterman and Albert, 2012). In fact, they may: (1) support the identification of pathophysiological processes causing or contributing to diseases; (2) define and predict the individual's health trajectories and clinical outcomes; and (3) help in selecting interventions and monitoring the response to treatments. Thus, they play a relevant role within the promise of precision medicine approaches where medical choices are driven by individually targeted genetic and biological profiles (Jameson and Longo, 2015).

Biomarkers are particularly relevant in the study of pathological conditions affecting the central nervous system (CNS), considering that brain tissue is not readily accessible for diagnostic or research purposes. Specifically, their adoption has triggered major advancements in the field of Alzheimer's disease (AD) over the past years. For instance, the analysis of the cerebrospinal fluid (CSF) and neuroimaging abnormalities indicative of neuronal loss and protein deposition has led to the understanding that AD is characterized by a long preclinical phase (Jack et al., 2013). This finding has been responsible for opening new perspectives in researching novel preventive/therapeutic strategies. It has also supported the transition towards a biology-grounded framework and definition of the disease (Jack et al., 2018). Furthermore, the use of these markers, when adopted as surrogate measures of AD in animal models, has contributed in accelerating the development of possible disease-modifying treatments (Cummings et al., 2018).

To date, although increasingly adopted in specialized clinical settings (Frisoni et al., 2017), the use of biomarkers to detect AD is still recommended only for research purposes and in selected atypical cases (McKhann et al., 2011; Dubois et al., 2014; Jack et al., 2018). Their adoption in the routine clinical practice remains controversial as confirmed by different systematic reviews and meta-analyses reaching heterogeneous results on the topic (Noel-Storr et al., 2013; Olsson et al., 2016; Ritchie et al., 2017). In particular, though sufficient (albeit inconclusive) evidence exists about the *analytical validity* (i.e., is the test accurate, reliable, and reproducible?) of the proposed AD biomarkers (Hansson et al., 2018; Lewczuk et al., 2018), their *clinical validity* (i.e., how well the test measures the clinical features, and the disease or treatment outcomes) and *clinical utility* (i.e., if and how the test improves the patient's outcomes, confirms/defines the diagnosis, identifies at-risk individuals, influences therapeutic choices) have not yet been fully proven (Frisoni et al., 2017; Kraus, 2018).

In the present article, we discuss some of the methodological issues and challenges that should be addressed in order to better assess the potential benefits and limitations of AD biomarkers. Without the intent of underestimating what has been done over the years in the field, the ultimate goal of the present article is to stimulate a constructive discussion aimed at filling the existing gaps and more precisely defining the directions of future research. The work is structured around four main aspects to be considered when adopting a biomarker in clinical practice: (1) the definition of reference values; (2) the identification of reference standards specific for the disease of interest (i.e., AD); (3) the proper inclusion and contextualization within the diagnostic process; and (4) the statistical process supporting the whole framework. In particular, these points will be addressed with regard to the most relevant CSF biomarkers.

DEFINITION OF REFERENCE VALUES

The validation of a candidate biomarker should follow two preliminary steps: (1) the assessment of its distribution in healthy people; and (2) the definition of the index test reference values (e.g., those included between the 2.5th and 97.5th percentile of the distribution, or within the interval of the mean ±1.96 standard deviations in case of symmetric distribution). The impact of common sociodemographic characteristics (e.g., age, sex, race/ethnicity) on the identified normal and abnormal values should also be considered (Sackett and Haynes, 2002; Haynes and You, 2009; Colli et al., 2014). It should be underlined, within this framework, how challenging (or even arbitrary) the selection of the reference group (i.e., healthy controls) to be used to define the 95% range of reference values might be.

To assess the methodology of the studies providing reference intervals for possible CSF biomarkers [i.e., amyloid peptides Aβ1–42 (Aβ42), total tau (T-tau), and 181-phospo-tau (P-tau)] in AD, we retrieved all available literature published up to May 2019. To this purpose, we performed a structured search on PubMed using the following search terms: (Aβ* OR A-β* OR A-beta* OR abeta* OR AB-42 OR *tau) AND (CSF OR liquor OR cerebrospinal OR cerebro-spinal) AND [(population* OR reference* OR normative*) AND (value* OR limit*)] AND (healthy OR normal OR normality OR average OR "general population"). The search strategy led to the identification of 155 abstracts. The full-texts of six selected studies were retrieved and assessed for inclusion based on the following predefined inclusion/exclusion criteria: being published in English; having sample size >50 subjects; defining as explicit aim the identification of reference intervals or limits for the considered biomarkers. Only two studies were included based on their pertinence with and relevance to the topic of interest (Sjögren et al., 2001; Burkhard et al., 2004). As reported in **Table 1**, the two included studies showed a high heterogeneity in how both methods and results were reported, thus limiting their hypothetical summarization. Both studies investigated the CSF dosage of Aβ42 and T-tau in hospital-based samples of subjects with a wide spectrum of age (i.e., ranging from less than 30 years to even more than 90 years). The studies adopted the 10th fractile (or percentile) to calculate the reference limit for Aβ42 and the 90th fractile (or percentile) to define the reference limit for T-tau. Important differences were observed for what concerns the age distribution and sex composition of the enrolled study samples. Although the inconsistencies in the reporting of results (e.g., different stratification for age groups) preclude the possibility of a direct comparison of the findings, a relevant discrepancy in the identified reference limits was evident in the two studies (e.g., for Aβ42: 150 ng/L vs. 500 ng/L, respectively). Finally, none of them assessed the role of individual characteristics (e.g., race and genetics) that could potentially affect results and conclusions.

TABLE 1 | Studies reporting reference limits for CSF Aβ42 and T-tau in healthy people.

Author	Setting	Sample size	Age	Sex	Diagnostic criteria for healthy individuals	Statistics	Reference limits
Sjögren et al. (2001)	Norwegian University Norwegian Hospital	231 (total) 175 (age >50 years)	61.3 ± 18 (mean age ± SD) 21–93 (range)	177 F 54 M	No symptoms or signs of psychiatric or neurological disorders: • People aged ≥60 years: MMSE score = 28–30 • People aged <60 years: no criteria listed	• >0.10 fractile (i.e., 10th percentile) for Aβ42 • <0.9 fractile (i.e., 90th percentile) for tau	**Aβ42** 500 ng/L (not age dependent) **T-tau** • 300 ng/L (for age range 21–50) • 450 ng/L (for age range 51–70) • 500 ng/L (for age range ≥71)
Burkhard et al. (2004)	University Hospital of Geneve	105 (total) 82 (age >50 years)	69, 56–78 (median, interquartile range) 29–96 (range)	61 F 44 M	• Historical referral of absence of any CNS or PNS condition, or psychiatric condition, or chronic systemic illness possibly modifying the CSF proteins • Face-to-face questionnaire covering the most common neurological symptoms • Intake of medication potentially interfering with brain functions • Neuropathological findings confirming the absence of any dementia (for 10 autopsy proven cases)	• >10th percentile for Aβ42 • <90th percentile for tau	**Aβ42** 150 ng/L, 90% Confidence Interval 90–172 ng/L (for age >49 years) **T-tau** 385 ng/L, 90% Confidence Interval 332–451 ng/L (for age >49 years)

DEFINING DIAGNOSTIC REFERENCE STANDARDS FOR AD

The clinical validation of AD biomarkers is complicated by the lack of a unique diagnostic reference (Noel-Storr et al., 2013). Furthermore, the biological and clinical approaches to the diagnosis of AD have some relevant limitations. Neuropathology has traditionally been considered as the gold standard for the evaluation and judgment of clinical manifestations (McKhann et al., 1984). Nevertheless, its large-scale implementation is hampered by the difficulty of obtaining samples. However, the neuropathological characteristics of AD have a weak correlation with its phenotypic and clinical expression. In fact, it is well established that many individuals showing a high burden of AD pathology do not exhibit any clinical signs of the disease, whereas others with a limited amount of neuropathological changes had developed overt AD in life (Wallace et al., 2019). Beyond the absence of clear evidence supporting their causal role, some of the biological processes resulting in the AD neuropathological hallmarks (e.g., amyloid deposition) may have different pathogenic implications (Espay et al., 2019). They may, in fact, alternatively contribute to and accelerate neurodegeneration, represent epiphenomena, or even constitute compensatory mechanisms to molecular/cellular stress (Espay et al., 2019). Moreover, different latent factors, such as the individual's frailty status, may moderate the relationship between AD pathology and dementia (Wallace et al., 2019). Finally, most of dementia cases (including AD dementia) are underlined by a mixed neuropathology (Boyle et al., 2018).

On the other hand, the adoption of clinical standards can be itself prevented by several obstacles. Logically, the cross-sectional validation of biomarkers against clinical criteria cannot result in an optimal diagnostic accuracy (Noel-Storr et al., 2013). Therefore, their use as prognostic markers, using longitudinal reference standards such as the conversion from MCI to AD dementia, are being increasingly considered for this purpose (Ritchie et al., 2014). However, the marked heterogeneity of these clinical outcomes may strongly confound their performance. For instance, the phenomenon of MCI conversion may occur in extremely variable times and ways, and be potentially affected by several additional, interacting factors (Grande et al., 2014). Moreover, it has been observed that a sizeable proportion of subjects with MCI shows a normalization of neuropsychological tests over time (Canevelli et al., 2016). Some subjects may follow even more complex clinical trajectories, by, for example, first reverting to normal cognition and subsequently progressing to dementia (Roberts et al., 2014). Theoretically, such a potential for multiple evolutions of MCI, shared by most of the risk conditions (Canevelli et al., 2017), implies the need to overcome the adoption of "classic" dichotomous outcomes (i.e., normal vs. pathological) preferring endpoints including at least 3 levels (i.e., improvement vs. stability vs. worsening). In other words, biomarkers could potentially support the identification not only of those subjects progressing to dementia, but also of those

TABLE 2 | The diagnostic research questions.

Phase I: Do the test results in patients with the target disorder differ from those in normal people? This preliminary phase is important to provide novel insights on the pathophysiological mechanisms of the disease. It can be addressed by conducting cross-sectional studies confronting a convenience group of subjects known to have the disease and a group of people definitely known to not have it.
Phase II: Are patients with certain test results more likely to have the target disorder than patients with other test results? The answer to this question can be derived by classic 2 × 2 contingency tables (or Error Matrices). The accuracy of the test (in terms of its results or cut-points) at distinguishing patients with the disease from normal controls is expressed by means of sensitivity, specificity, positive and negative predictive values and likelihood ratios
Phase III: Does the test result distinguish patients with and without the target disorder among patients in whom it is clinically reasonable to suspect that the disease is present? Differently from the previous phase, the accuracy of the test is here explored in a "real world" scenario of routine clinical practice, that is among subjects whose clinical status is not already established (e.g., subjects referred from their general practitioners to specialist services for a clinical suspicion). Participants should, blindly, be assessed with both the test and what is considered as the diagnostic reference standard (ideally a gold standard).
Phase IV: Do patients who undergo this diagnostic test have better health outcomes than similar patients who are not tested? This question strongly deals with the clinical utility of the test and concerns the health outcomes following the diagnostic/therapeutic choices resulting from the test findings. Ideally, such information could be obtained by the follow-up of subjects randomized to perform the test or not to perform it.
Phase V: Does the use of the diagnostic test lead to better health outcomes at acceptable costs? This question refers to the cost-effectiveness (the so-called "value-for-money") of the index test and can be answered by randomized controlled trials.

Adapted from Haynes and You (2009) and Sackett and Haynes (2002).

individuals showing an "inverse" trajectory towards normality. In this framework, the possibility of combining different biomarkers (or sets of biomarkers) should be considered with the objective of detecting the risk of decline as well as the possibility of restoration of a normal status.

THE ARCHITECTURE OF THE DIAGNOSTIC PROCESS

The actual validity and utility of a diagnostic test (e.g., a biomarker) can be summarized in a multistep process that should answer some crucial diagnostic questions, included in five iterative phases (**Table 2**; Sackett and Haynes, 2002; Haynes and You, 2009).

In the AD literature, a relevant number of Phase I and Phase II studies has indicated that the CSF levels of biomarkers reflecting amyloid deposition (i.e., Aβ42) and neurodegeneration (i.e., T-tau and P-tau) are significantly different between subjects diagnosed with AD and to normal controls. In this context, a recent meta-analysis of 231 studies enrolling a total of 15,699 patients with AD and 13,018 controls reported an estimate of the following AD-to-control ratios: Aβ42 (average ratio 0.56, 95% CI 0.55–0.58, $p < 0.0001$), T-tau (2.54, 2.44–2.64, $p < 0.0001$), and P-tau (1.88, 1.79–1.97, $p < 0.0001$; Olsson et al., 2016). These biomarkers could also help in distinguishing those subjects with mild cognitive impairment (MCI) that will convert to dementia from non-converting subjects (Ritchie et al., 2017). Specifically, according to a recent Cochrane systematic review (Ritchie et al., 2017), the observed accuracy ranges of CSF biomarkers in predicting the conversion from MCI to AD dementia are:

- T-tau: sensitivity: 51%–90%; specificity: 48%–88%;
- P-tau: sensitivity: 40%–100%; specificity: 22%–86%;
- P-tau/Aβ42 ratio: sensitivity: 80%–96%; specificity: 33%–95%.

Such wide variability can be attributed to relevant discrepancies in the adopted reference standards, in the source of recruitment and sampling of participants, and in the index test methodology across the retained studies. It is to be noted that most of these results were obtained in research settings, evaluating highly selected patients in whom the presence of the target disease had already been ascertained under ideal/almost utopic circumstances (e.g., by expert clinicians with the best available equipment, adopting the same reference standard for those with and without AD). These samples are unlikely to represent the overall population of patients with AD under multiple socio-demographic and clinical aspects. Therefore, it seems reasonable to expect these same biomarkers to yield different results when transferred from the research to the clinical setting (Dyer et al., 2016; Frisoni et al., 2017). To date, only few studies have provided realistic information on the validity of AD biomarkers in the "real world" (thus answering pragmatic Phase III questions). As expected, a lower accuracy in the discrimination of patients with and without AD was observed in these works (Mattsson et al., 2009; Tariciotti et al., 2018). Moreover, to our knowledge, no Phase IV and V evidence are available in this field of AD research. In other words, no study has yet robustly explored how the use of biomarkers can actually affect health outcomes (e.g., mortality, disability, response to treatment; Frisoni et al., 2017) nor their cost-effectiveness.

STATISTICAL APPROACHES ACROSS THE DIAGNOSTIC RESEARCH PROCESS

According to the previously discussed phases, different statistical approaches are required in each sequential step (Moons et al., 2012a,b; Collins et al., 2015). Phase I is exploratory by nature and is typically based on null hypothesis significance testing focused on isolating variables deemed individually relevant according to the *P*-value. The statistical methods for investigating Phase II and III questions belong to the field of prediction models (both diagnostic and prognostic) that typically focus on identifying sets of variables that can accurately predict the outcomes of interest. Considering the wide range of options and the differing

TABLE 3 | Definition and interpretation of the Likelihood Ratio (LR).

LR values	Change from pre-test to post-test probability	Results
>10 or <0.1	Large	Conclusive
5–10 or 0.1–0.2	Moderate	Moderately important
2–5 or 0.2–0.5	Small	Sometimes important
1–2 or 0.5–1	Small/minimum	Rarely important
1	None	Not important/useless

Adapted from Jaeschke et al. (1994).

perspectives of researchers, clinicians and public health decision makers, it is crucial to be aware about the trade-off between *model transparency* (allowing for easy interpretability and transparent scientific understanding) and *model complexity* (maximizing the predictive power through very sophisticated predictions that may often appear as an Opaque Black Box; Bzdok and Ioannidis, 2019). To this purpose, simple univariable classifications where Error Matrices (i.e., 2 × 2 contingency tables that report the number of *false positives*, *false negatives*, *true positives*, and *true negatives*) are derived by predefined cut-off values of single biomarkers as well as long-trusted multivariable statistical methods (e.g., Logistic and Cox Regression models) still remain the most suitable tools in the box. Regarding the Error Matrix and its derived measures (Akobeng, 2007), the Positive Predictive Value (PPV) and the Likelihood Ratio (LR) should always be preferred in prediction studies. In fact, Sensitivity and Specificity are indicative of the accuracy of a test (i.e., the biomarker), thus they are mostly useful for comparing the performance of different ones (with the possibility of combining two single tests in "OR"/"AND" modality to enhance the overall sensitivity/specificity; Sackett et al., 1985). The PPV and LR are, instead, informative about the single, specific individual. The PPV measures the individual probability to develop (or to have) the disease if the test is positive. The LR expresses the probability that the test is positive (or negative) in people with the disease compared to the probability that it is positive (or negative) in healthy people. It thus allows to simply update the pre-test probability of having the disease (based on the individual's characteristics and clinical history) to the post-test probability (given the test results) according to its direction and magnitude (**Table 3**; Jaeschke et al., 1994; Kent and Hancock, 2016). Candidate CSF biomarkers for AD have so far shown small to minimum LR values (i.e., LR+ 2.72, LR− 0.32 at the median specificity of 72% for T-tau; LR+ 1.55, LR− 0.39 at the median specificity of 47.5% for P-tau; Ritchie et al., 2017).

The predictive performance of a model is usually measured using discrimination measures (such as c-index that is equal to the area under the Receiver Operating Curve) and calibration plots. These measures can be inflated in the data sample from which they are derived when compared to new but comparable data samples (overfitting). K-fold cross-validation and bootstrap are the preferred internal validation techniques to evaluate a potential overfitting. However, external validation is still necessary to guarantee the generalizability of the model in the real word setting (Phase III). Finally, the appropriate reporting, communication and use of the resulting model are crucial. Therefore, the output of the predictive model (in terms of coefficient estimates, standard error and confidence intervals) can be combined to graphic tools, such as nomograms, thus easily allowing to obtain the final outcome probability for a new patient based on his/her profile of predictive variables. This graphical approach, although not widely used in the field of AD (Jang et al., 2017), may have important practical implications in the clinical and regulatory setting (e.g., patient's counseling, risk stratification, elaboration of guidelines, drug reimbursement). Phase IV studies, while sharing inferential testing tools that are similar to those used in Phase I, are usually framed within an evidence-based decision-making context where the statistical methods are derived from the domain of well-controlled experimental study design (typically a randomized clinical trial). Phase V studies, instead, focus on the evaluation of the most effective or cost-effective diagnostic strategies through specific cost-effectiveness analysis.

CONCLUSION

Overall, various methodological issues remain to be addressed in order to perform an adequate and complete clinical validation of candidate CSF biomarkers for AD. First, studies reporting the distribution of biomarkers in normal/healthy subjects and their variability according to major sociodemographic and clinical attributes are still lacking. In this regard, significant sex and race disparities for Aβ42 and tau levels have recently been reported both in healthy subjects and in patients with AD (Koran et al., 2017; Morris et al., 2019). Second, there is no conclusive agreement on the most appropriate reference standard for AD (e.g., clinical vs. biological) to be adopted to test the performance of new biomarkers. Third, no biomarker has yet consistently gone through all the phases that compose the architecture of diagnostic research. In particular, their actual impact on "hard" health outcomes and their cost-effectiveness has to be clarified. Similar conclusions have been reached by Mattsson et al. (2017) who have adopted an alternative model for developing the framework concerning AD biomarkers. Their approach, borrowed from oncology and structured around the natural history of the disease, should be regarded as complimentary to that adopted in the present work, essentially based on the methodological validation of biomarkers from the lens of clinical epidemiology. It is also crucial that, in each phase, the scientific contributions meet the highest quality standards. To this end, the widespread application of the checklist on reporting standards in dementia and cognitive impairment (STARDdem; Noel-Storr et al., 2014) can be a useful tool to improve consistency and transparency, and the application of the QUADAS 2 checklist (Whiting et al., 2011) can allow the identification of potential methodological biases, thus enabling a more effective assessment of candidate diagnostic tests. Moreover, multivariate statistical methodologies, possibly resulting in clinically-oriented tools such as nomograms, should be increasingly used to capture the complexity of the disease, both from a pathophysiological and phenotypic perspective, and to understand the actual clinical relevance of potential new biomarkers. It should be emphasized how these considerations, here paradigmatically referred to CSF, can be extended to all the candidate biomarkers for

AD, regardless of their origin and nature (e.g., plasma, serum, urine, neuroimaging).

In conclusion, despite the enormous progress made in the field, there is still insufficient evidence to promote the use of candidate CSF biomarkers for AD in the routine clinical practice, As already pointed out by previous works on this topic, leaving the discussed methodological issues unaddressed raises the risk to provide clinicians with tools and tests whose answers are difficult to interpret and translate into concrete decisions. This might ultimately result in potential harm to patients, families, and healthcare systems.

AUTHOR CONTRIBUTIONS

MCa: study conception and writing of the manuscript. IB, GG, EL, MM and FM: literature search and drafting of the manuscript. NV and MCe: study conception and revision of the manuscript for important intellectual content.

REFERENCES

Akobeng, A. K. (2007). Understanding diagnostic tests 1: sensitivity, specificity and predictive values. *Acta Paediatr.* 96, 338–341. doi: 10.1111/j.1651-2227.2006.00180.x

Biomarkers Definitions Working Group. (2001). Biomarkers and surrogate endpoints: preferred definitions and conceptual framework. *Clin. Pharmacol. Ther.* 69, 89–95. doi: 10.1067/mcp.2001.113989

Boyle, P. A., Yu, L., Wilson, R. S., Leurgans, S. E., Schneider, J. A., and Bennett, D. A. (2018). Person-specific contribution of neuropathologies to cognitive loss in old age. *Ann. Neurol.* 83, 74–83. doi: 10.1002/ana.25123

Burkhard, P. R., Fournier, R., Mermillod, B., Krause, K.-H., Bouras, C., and Irminger, I. (2004). Cerebrospinal fluid tau and Aβ42 concentrations in healthy subjects: delineation of reference intervals and their limitations. *Clin. Chem. Lab. Med.* 42, 396–407. doi: 10.1515/cclm.2004.071

Bzdok, D., and Ioannidis, J. P. A. (2019). Exploration, inference, and prediction in neuroscience and biomedicine. *Trends Neurosci.* 42, 251–262. doi: 10.1016/j.tins.2019.02.001

Canevelli, M., Bruno, G., Remiddi, F., Vico, C., Lacorte, E., Vanacore, N., et al. (2017). Spontaneous reversion of clinical conditions measuring the risk profile of the individual: from frailty to mild cognitive impairment. *Front. Med. Lausanne.* 4:184. doi: 10.3389/fmed.2017.00184

Canevelli, M., Grande, G., Lacorte, E., Quarchioni, E., Cesari, M., Mariani, C., et al. (2016). Spontaneous reversion of mild cognitive impairment to normal cognition: a systematic review of literature and meta-analysis. *J. Am. Med. Dir. Assoc.* 17, 943–948. doi: 10.1016/j.jamda.2016.06.020

Colli, A., Fraquelli, M., Casazza, G., Conte, D., Nikolova, D., Duca, P., et al. (2014). The architecture of diagnostic research: from bench to bedside—research guidelines using liver stiffness as an example. *Hepatology* 60, 408–418. doi: 10.1002/hep.26948

Collins, G. S., Reitsma, J. B., Altman, D. G., and Moons, K. G. M. (2015). Transparent reporting of a multivariable prediction model for individual prognosis or diagnosis (TRIPOD): the TRIPOD statement. *Ann. Intern. Med.* 162, 55–63. doi: 10.7326/l15-0078-4

Cummings, J., Lee, G., Ritter, A., and Zhong, K. (2018). Alzheimer's disease drug development pipeline: 2018. *Alzheimers Dement.* 4, 195–214. doi: 10.1016/j.trci.2018.03.009

Dubois, B., Feldman, H. H., Jacova, C., Hampel, H., Molinuevo, J. L., Blennow, K., et al. (2014). Advancing research diagnostic criteria for Alzheimer's disease: the IWG-2 criteria. *Lancet Neurol.* 13, 614–629. doi: 10.1016/S1474-4422(14)70090-0

Dyer, S. M., Flicker, L., Laver, K., Whitehead, C., and Cumming, R. (2016). The clinical value of fluid biomarkers for dementia diagnosis. *Lancet Neurol.* 15:1204. doi: 10.1016/S1474-4422(16)30238-1

Espay, A. J., Vizcarra, J. A., Marsili, L., Lang, A. E., Simon, D. K., Merola, A., et al. (2019). Revisiting protein aggregation as pathogenic in sporadic Parkinson and Alzheimer diseases. *Neurology* 92, 329–337. doi: 10.1212/WNL.0000000000006926

Frisoni, G. B., Boccardi, M., Barkhof, F., Blennow, K., Cappa, S., Chiotis, K., et al. (2017). Strategic roadmap for an early diagnosis of Alzheimer's disease based on biomarkers. *Lancet Neurol.* 16, 661–676. doi: 10.1016/S1474-4422(17)30159-X

Grande, G., Vanacore, N., Maggiore, L., Cucumo, V., Ghiretti, R., Galimberti, D., et al. (2014). Physical activity reduces the risk of dementia in mild cognitive impairment subjects: a cohort study. *J. Alzheimers Dis.* 39, 833–839. doi: 10.3233/jad-131808

Hansson, O., Mikulskis, A., Fagan, A. M., Teunissen, C., Zetterberg, H., Vanderstichele, H., et al. (2018). The impact of preanalytical variables on measuring cerebrospinal fluid biomarkers for Alzheimer's disease diagnosis: a review. *Alzheimers Dement.* 14, 1313–1333. doi: 10.1016/j.jalz.2018.05.008

Haynes, R. B., and You, J. J. (2009). "The architecture of diagnostic research," in *The Evidence Base of Clinical Diagnosis: Theory and Methods of Diagnostic Research, 2nd Edn*, eds J. A. Knottnerus and F. Buntinx (Blackwell Publishing Ltd), 20–41.

Jack, C. R. Jr., Bennett, D. A., Blennow, K., Carrillo, M. C., Dunn, B., Haeberlein, S. B., et al. (2018). NIA-AA research framework: toward a biological definition of Alzheimer's disease. *Alzheimers Dement.* 14, 535–562. doi: 10.1016/j.jalz.2018.02.018

Jack, C. R. Jr., Knopman, D. S., Jagust, W. J., Petersen, R. C., Weiner, M. W., Aisen, P. S., et al. (2013). Tracking pathophysiological processes in Alzheimer's disease: an updated hypothetical model of dynamic biomarkers. *Lancet Neurol.* 12, 207–216. doi: 10.1016/S1474-4422(12)70291-0

Jaeschke, R., Guyatt, G. H., and Sackett, D. L. (1994). Users' guides to the medical literature. III. How to use an article about a diagnostic test. B. What are the results and will they help me in caring for my patients? The Evidence-Based Medicine Working Group. *JAMA* 271, 703–707. doi: 10.1001/jama.271.9.703

Jameson, J. L., and Longo, D. L. (2015). Precision medicine—personalized, problematic, and promising. *N. Engl. J. Med.* 372, 2229–2234. doi: 10.1056/NEJMsb1503104

Jang, H., Ye, B. S., Woo, S., Kim, S. W., Chin, J., Choi, S. H., et al. (2017). Prediction model of conversion to dementia risk in subjects with amnestic mild cognitive impairment: a longitudinal, multi-center clinic-based study. *J. Alzheimers Dis.* 60, 1579–1587. doi: 10.3233/JAD-170507

Kent, P., and Hancock, M. J. (2016). Interpretation of dichotomous outcomes: sensitivity, specificity, likelihood ratios, and pre-test and post-test probability. *J. Physiother.* 62, 231–233. doi: 10.1016/j.jphys.2016.08.008

Koran, M. E. I., Wagener, M., and Hohman, T. J. (2017). Sex differences in the association between AD biomarkers and cognitive decline. *Brain Imaging Behav.* 11, 205–213. doi: 10.1007/s11682-016-9523-8

Kraus, V. B. (2018). Biomarkers as drug development tools: discovery, validation, qualification and use. *Nat. Rev. Rheumatol.* 14, 354–362. doi: 10.1038/s41584-018-0005-9

Lewczuk, P., Gaignaux, A., Kofanova, O., Ermann, N., Betsou, F., Brandner, S., et al. (2018). Interlaboratory proficiency processing scheme in CSF aliquoting: implementation and assessment based on biomarkers of Alzheimer's disease. *Alzheimers Res. Ther.* 10:87. doi: 10.1186/s13195-018-0418-3

Mattsson, N., Lönneborg, A., Boccardi, M., Blennow, K., Hansson, O., and Geneva Task Force for the Roadmap of Alzheimer's Biomarkers. (2017). Clinical validity of cerebrospinal fluid Aβ42, tau, and phospho-tau as biomarkers for Alzheimer's disease in the context of a structured 5-phase development framework. *Neurobiol. Aging* 52, 196–213. doi: 10.1016/j.neurobiolaging.2016.02.034

Mattsson, N., Zetterberg, H., Hansson, O., Andreasen, N., Parnetti, L., Jonsson, M., et al. (2009). CSF biomarkers and incipient Alzheimer disease in patients with mild cognitive impairment. *JAMA* 302, 385–393. doi: 10.1001/jama.2009.1064

McKhann, G. M., Drachman, D., Folstein, M., Katzman, R., Price, D., and Stadlan, E. M. (1984). Clinical diagnosis of Alzheimer's disease: report of the NINCDS-ADRDA work group under the auspices of department of health and human services task force on Alzheimer's disease. *Neurology* 34, 939–944. doi: 10.1212/wnl.34.7.939

McKhann, G. M., Knopman, D. S., Chertkow, H., Hyman, B. T., Jack, C. R., Kawas, C. H., et al. (2011). The diagnosis of dementia due to Alzheimer's disease: recommendations from the National Institute on Aging-Alzheimer's Association workgroups on diagnostic guidelines for Alzheimer's disease. *Alzheimers Dement.* 7, 263–269. doi: 10.1016/j.jalz.2011.03.005

Moons, K. G. M., Kengne, A. P., Grobbee, D. E., Royston, P., Vergouwe, Y., Altman, D. G., et al. (2012a). Risk prediction models: II. External validation, model, updating and impact assessment. *Heart* 98, 691–698. doi: 10.1136/heartjnl-2011-301247

Moons, K. G. M., Kengne, A. P., Woodward, M., Royston, P., Vergouwe, Y., Altman, D. G., et al. (2012b). Risk prediction models: I. Development, internal validation and assessing the incremental value of a new (bio)marker. *Heart* 98, 683–690. doi: 10.1136/heartjnl-2011-301246

Morris, J. C., Schindler, S. E., McCue, L. M., Moulder, K. L., Benzinger, T. L. S., Cruchaga, C., et al. (2019). Assessment of racial disparities in biomarkers for Alzheimer disease. *JAMA Neurol.* 76, 264–273. doi: 10.1001/jamaneurol. 2018.4249

Noel-Storr, A. H., Flicker, L., Ritchie, C. W., Nguyen, G. H., Gupta, T., Wood, P., et al. (2013). Systematic review of the body of evidence for the use of biomarkers in the diagnosis of dementia. *Alzheimers Dement.* 9, e96–e105. doi: 10.1016/j. jalz.2012.01.014

Noel-Storr, A. H., McCleery, J. M., Richard, E., Ritchie, C. W., Flicker, L., Cullum, S. J., et al. (2014). Reporting standards for studies of diagnostic test accuracy in dementia. *Neurology* 83, 364–373. doi: 10.1212/WNL. 0000000000000621

Olsson, B., Lautner, R., Andreasson, U., Öhrfelt, A., Portelius, E., Bjerke, M., et al. (2016). CSF and blood biomarkers for the diagnosis of Alzheimer's disease: a systematic review and meta-analysis. *Lancet Neurol.* 15, 673–684. doi: 10.1016/S1474-4422(16)00070-3

Ritchie, C., Smailagic, N., Noel-Storr, A. H., Takwoingi, Y., Flicker, L., Mason, S. E., et al. (2014). Plasma and cerebrospinal fluid amyloid-β for the diagnosis of Alzheimer's disease dementia and other dementias in people with mild cognitive impairment (MCI). *Cochrane Database Syst. Rev.* 6:CD008782. doi: 10.1002/14651858.CD008782.pub4

Ritchie, C., Smailagic, N., Noel-Storr, A. H., Ukoumunne, O., Ladds, E. C., and Martin, S. (2017). CSF tau and the CSF tau/Aβ ratio for the diagnosis of Alzheimer's disease dementia and other dementias in people with mild cognitive impairment (MCI). *Cochrane Database Syst. Rev.* 3:CD010803. doi: 10.1002/14651858.CD010803.pub2

Roberts, R. O., Knopman, D. S., Mielke, M. M., Cha, R. H., Pankratz, V. S., Christianson, T. J. H., et al. (2014). Higher risk of progression to dementia in mild cognitive impairment cases who revert to normal. *Neurology* 82, 317–325. doi: 10.1212/wnl.0000000000000055

Sackett, D. L., and Haynes, R. B. (2002). The architecture of diagnostic research. *BMJ* 324, 539–541. doi: 10.1136/bmj.324.7336.539

Sackett, D. L., Haynes, R. B., and Tugwell, P. (1985). *Clinical Epidemiology: A Basic Science for Clinical Medicine.* Boston: Little, Brown & Company.

Schisterman, E. F., and Albert, P. S. (2012). The biomarker revolution. *Stat. Med.* 31, 2513–2515. doi: 10.1002/sim.5499

Sjögren, M., Vanderstichele, H., Agren, H., Zachrisson, O., Edsbagge, M., Wikkelsø, C., et al. (2001). Tau and Aβ42 in cerebrospinal fluid from healthy adults 21–93 years of age: establishment of reference values. *Clin. Chem.* 47, 1776–1781.

Tariciotti, L., Casadei, M., Honig, L. S., Teich, A. F., McKhann Ii, G. M., Tosto, G., et al. (2018). Clinical experience with cerebrospinal fluid Aβ42, total and phosphorylated tau in the evaluation of 1,016 individuals for suspected dementia. *J. Alzheimers Dis.* 65, 1417–1425. doi: 10.3233/JAD-180548

Wallace, L. M. K., Theou, O., Godin, J., Andrew, M. K., Bennett, D. A., and Rockwood, K. (2019). Investigation of frailty as a moderator of the relationship between neuropathology and dementia in Alzheimer's disease: a cross-sectional analysis of data from the Rush Memory and Aging Project. *Lancet Neurol.* 18, 177–184. doi: 10.1016/s1474-4422(18) 30371-5

Whiting, P. F., Rutjes, A. W. S., Westwood, M. E., Mallett, S., Deeks, J. J., Reitsma, J. B., et al. (2011). QUADAS-2: a revised tool for the quality assessment of diagnostic accuracy studies. *Ann. Intern. Med.* 155, 529–536. doi: 10.7326/0003-4819-155-8-201110180-00009

23

Correlation Between Diabetic Cognitive Impairment and Diabetic Retinopathy in Patients with T2DM by ^{1}H-MRS

*Xuefang Lu†, Wei Gong†, Zhi Wen, Lanhua Hu, Zhoufeng Peng and Yunfei Zha**

Department of Radiology, Renmin Hospital, Wuhan, China

***Correspondence:**
Yunfei Zha
mona_666666@163.com

†These authors have contributed equally to this work and share first authorship

Objective: To explore the correlation between diabetic cognitive impairment (DCI) and diabetic retinopathy (DR) through examining the cognitive function and the metabolism of the cerebrum in Type 2 diabetes mellitus (T2DM) by ^{1}H-MRS.

Methods: Fifty-three patients with T2DM were enrolled for this study. According to the fundus examination, the patients were divided into the DR group ($n = 26$) and the T2DM without DR group (T2DM group, $n = 27$). Thirty healthy adults were selected as a control group (HC group, $n = 30$). Cognitive function was measured by Montreal Cognitive Assessment (MoCA). The peak areas of N-acetylaspartate (NAA), Cho-line (Cho), Creatine (Cr), and Myo-inositol (ml) as well as their ratios were detected by proton magnetic resonance spectroscopy (^{1}H-MRS). The difference analysis between the three groups was performed by one-way ANOVA. When $p < 0.05$, LSD-t was applied. A partial correlation analysis (with age as a covariate) was used to analyze the correlation between metabolites in the DR group and MoCA scores. Among all T2DM patients, Chi-square test age, gender, education level, BMI, SBP, DBP, FPG, HbA1c, TC, TG, HDL-C, LDL-C, DR, and DCI correlation were measured. Differences were statistically significant while $P < 0.05$.

Results: 1. The scores of MoCA in the DR group or in the T2DM group were significantly less than those in the HC group ($F = 3.54$, $P < 0.05$), and the scores of MoCA in the DR group were significantly less than those in the other groups ($F = 3.61$, $P < 0.05$). 2. There were significant differences for NAA in the bilateral hippocampus in DR patients, T2DM patients, and healthy controls ($P < 0.05$). 3. The NAA/Cr was significantly positively correlated with the score of MoCA in DR patients' left hippocampus ($r = 0.781$, $P < 0.01$). 4. Chi-square analysis found that there was a correlation between DR and DCI ($x^2 = 4.6$, df $= 1$, $p = 0.032$, plt: 0.05). There was no correlation between other influencing factors and DCI ($P > 0.05$).

Conclusion: DCI is closely correlated with the DR in patients with T2DM. Hippocampal brain metabolism may have some changes in two sides of NAA in patients with DR, ^{1}H-MRS may provide effective imaging strategies and methods for the early diagnosis of brain damage and quantitative assessment cognitive function in T2DM.

Keywords: T2DM, diabetic brain damage, diabetic retinopathy, hippocampus, ^{1}H-MRS, MoCA

Type 2 diabetes mellitus (T2DM) is a comprehensive metabolic disease caused by insufficient insulin secretion or insulin resistance and is associated with a variety of systemic complications (1). The incidence of T2DM in China has reached 9.7% (2). T2DM has similar pathological changes with Alzheimer's disease (AD), namely axonal degeneration, neuronal loss, and extensive fibrosis of the meninges, while the hippocampus undergoes one of the early changes in T2DM brain structure (3), with varying degrees of cognitive impairment. The Montreal Cognitive Assessment Scale (MoCA) is able to assess cognitive impairment, including naming abilities, visual space, and executive ability. Studies have shown that diabetic patients with diabetic cognitive impairment (DCI) have a higher risk of cardiovascular accidents and death than diabetic patients without cognitive impairment (4). Studies (5) found that diabetic retinopathy (DR) may be closely related to DCI and provide indirect evidence of cognitive dysfunction in diabetes, but its clinical symptoms are diverse and unstable, and there is still a lack of prevention. The gold standard for prevention is often easily underestimated or ignored. ^{1}H-MRS (proton magnetic resonance spectroscopy) is a powerful tool for early detection and quantitative assessment of brain microstructural and functional changes in T2DM patients and brings the unique advantages of virtual biopsy. The correlation between cognitive impairment and DR is explored through examining the cognitive function and the metabolism of the cerebrum in T2DM by ^{1}H-MRS and MoCA.

OBJECTS AND METHODS

Objects

This study was approved by the patients and the ethics committee. Subjects were recruited from January 2016 to December 2018 in our hospital, according to the T2DM diagnostic criteria promulgated by the American Diabetes Association (ADA) in 2010. To avoid as much as possible the course of diabetes, the drugs taken, the way of treatment and the complications of diabetes and other neurological diseases. The course of diabetes was more than 15 years but <30 years. The patients were not using insulin and had standardized oral medication. There were differences in diabetic retinopathy, and none had any other diabetic complications or microangiopathies. Fundus examination was used to diagnose the presence or absence of DR lesions, microaneurysms, and/or small hemorrhage as it is the earliest and most accurate characteristics of DR lesions, and 53 patients with T2DM were enrolled for this study. According to the fundus examination, the patients were divided into the DR group ($n = 26$) and the T2DM without DR group (T2DM group, $n = 27$). HC (healthy control group) group inclusion criteria were as follows: no abnormal glucose metabolism, and other conditions were matched with DR and T2DM. Thirty healthy adults were selected as the control group (HC group, $n = 30$).

Exclusion criteria were organized into three groups: (1) patients who could not complete the MoCA test; (2) patients with a history of mental and neurological diseases; (3) those with organic diseases of the nervous system; (4) patients who were dependent on smoking, alcoholism and psychotropic substances; (5) impaired glucose tolerance or fasting glucose, and ketoacidosis; and (6) patients with contraindications with MRI. There were differences in diabetic retinopathy, they all had no other diabetic complications, and there were no significant differences in gender, age, education, height, and weight ($P > 0.05$); there were statistical differences among three groups of GLU and HbA1c ($P < 0.05$) (**Table 1**).

Cognitive function was measured by MoCA. The peak areas of N-acetylaspartate (NAA), Cho-line (Cho), Creatine (Cr), and Myo-inositol (mI), and their ratios, were detected by ^{1}H-MRS.

TABLE 1 | Comparison of the general conditions of the three groups of subjects.

Project	DR group	T2DM group	HC group	t	P
Gender (M/F)	26 (14/12)	27 (10/17)	30 (17/13)	5.163	0.076
Age (y)	61.19 ± 8.41	61.04 ± 7.54	59.81 ± 3.68	0.249	0.780
Education (y)	9.50 ± 1.90	10.54 ± 3.40	11.12 ± 2.70	1.587	0.212
BMI (kg/m^2)	23.94 ± 2.52	23.69 ± 3.04	23.37 ± 3.64	0.169	0.845
SBP/mmHg	160.24 ± 9.43	160.01 ± 7.74	150.18 ± 9.81	8.291	0.801
DBP/mmHg	96.19 ± 8.54	96.22 ± 8.75	90.01 ± 9.85	7.342	0.786
FPG (mmol/L)	9.23 ± 0.46	7.18 ± 0.82	5.13 ± 0.37	11.203	0.000*
HbA1c (%)	8.98 ± 2.24	7.98 ± 0.89	5.31 ± 0.40	3.670	0.000*
TC (mmol/L)	6.32 ± 1.07	5.37 ± 1.16	4.31 ± 1.12	1.037	0.000*
TG (mmol/L)	1.98 ± 0.97	1.92 ± 1.09	1.07 ± 0.79	0.901	0.000*
HDL-C (mmol/L)	0.89 ± 0.13	1.02 ± 0.46	1.38 ± 0.72	0.870	0.000*
LDL-C (mmol/L)	3.81 ± 0.71	3.76 ± 0.57	3.51 ± 0.45	1.015	0.000*

**There were statistical differences among three groups in FPG, HbA1c, TC, TG, HDL-C, and LDL-C ($P < 0.05$).*
There were no significant differences among three groups in gender, age, education, BMI, SBP, and DBP ($P > 0.05$).

Methods

Cognitive Function Test and Fundus Examination

The MoCA assessment was performed by a neurology professional and an ophthalmologist performed the fundus examination. This study used an internationally recognized version developed in November 2004. The scale was developed by Nasreddine et al. (6) with reference to the Mini-mental State Examination and based on clinical experience. It is an assessment tool for rapid screening of cognitive dysfunction. It includes 11 inspection projects in 8 cognitive areas, including concentration, executive function, memory, language, visual structural skills, abstract thinking, calculation, and positioning. It possesses high sensitivity, covers important cognitive areas, has a short test time and is suitable for clinical settings.

$$n = \frac{2\bar{p}\bar{q}(Z_\alpha + Z_\beta)^2}{(p1 - p2)^2}$$

Abbreviations: T2DM, Type 2 diabetes mellitus; DCI, diabetic cognitive impairment; DR, diabetic retinopathy; ^{1}H-MRS, proton magnetic resonance spectroscopy; HC group, healthy control group; MoCA, Montreal Cognitive Assessment; NAA, Nacetylaspartate; Cr, Creatine; Cho, Cho-line; mI, myo-inositol; ANOVA, Analysis of Variance.

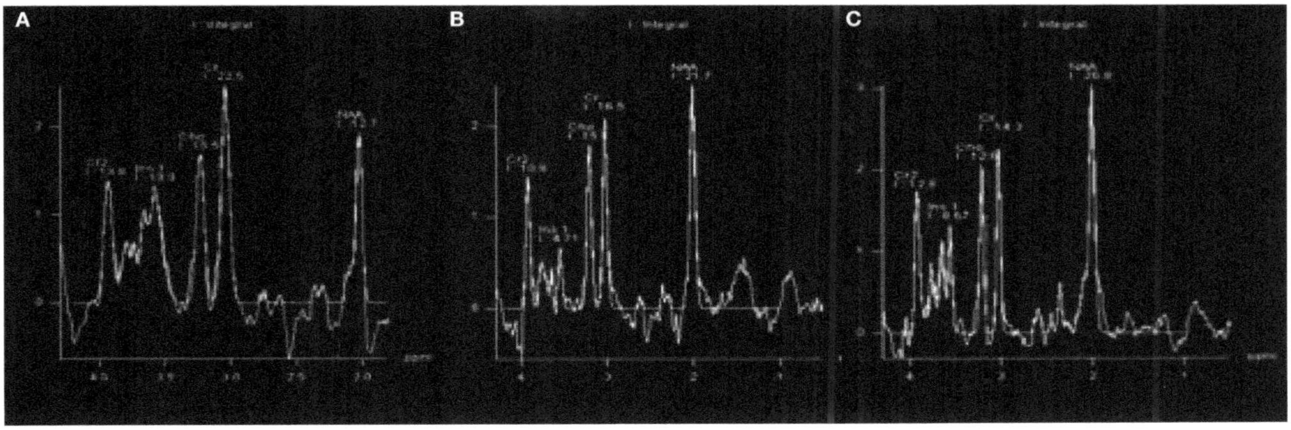

FIGURE 1 | There were statistically significant differences in NAA on bilateral hippocampus. **(A)** DR group, **(B)** T2DM group, **(C)** HC group.

Here, n indicates the number of samples, and the table shows that Z_{α}, $Z_{\beta}$is 1.96 and 1.28, respectively. p_1 and p_2 represent the prevalence of the intervention group and the control group, with $\bar{p}$ representing the average of p_1 and p_2, and $\bar{q}$ representing the average of $(1-p_1)$ and $(1-p_2)$.

The incidence of T2DM in China is as high as 9.7% (2). According to the above formula, we get n is equal to 6.38, and the total number of diabetic patients enrolled is 53, so the sample size is reasonable and the result is credible.

Equipment and Methods

This study used a GE (Discovery 750w) 3.0T superconducting magnetic resonance imaging scanner and matching head coil (8 channels), and quality testing was employed before each scan to ensure the stability of the machine signal. All objects underwent a T2WI scan in advance, and two professional imaging physicians evaluated the images to rule out brain lesions. A high-resolution 3D-T1 multi-planar image was obtained by 3D-T1 MPRAGE for subsequent scan positioning. The following conditions were present: hippocampus ^{1}H-MRS, STEAM (Stimulated Echo Acquisition Method) mode, point probe Probe-SV35 sequence scan (7), TR 1700 ms, TE 30 ms, FA 90°, ST 15 mm, FOV 16 cm × 16 cm, MS 320 × 320, VS 10 mm × 10 mm × 15 mm. The scan time is usually 6 min 53 s. Coastal horse long axis, according to the axial ROI, supplemented by sagittal, oblique coronal plane, try to avoid air cavity, skull, cerebrospinal fluid, and fat. The bilateral ROI was the same and the whole hippocampus was included as much as possible. The scan was manually corrected and the value was read at the workstation.

GE (Discovery 750w) 3.0T workstation spectroscopy software was used for phase and baseline calibration of the measured line, signal averaging, metabolite identification and spectral line fitting, automatic reading of the bilateral hippocampus, the area under the peak curve of NAA, Cho, Cr, and mI and to calculate the ratio of NAA/Cr, Cho/Cr, and mI/Cr.

Statistical Method

All data were tested and conformed to a normal distribution by SPSS21.0 software package. The statistical analysis of the analytes obtained by ^{1}H-MRS was performed. The data are represented as the mean ± standard deviation. The difference analysis between the three groups was performed by one-way ANOVA. When $p < 0.05$, LSD-t was applied. A partial correlation analysis (with age as a covariate) was used to analyze the correlation between metabolites in the DR group and MoCA scores. Among all T2DM patients, Chi-square test was used on age, gender, education level, BMI, SBP, DBP, FPG, HbA1c, TC, TG, HDL-C, LDL-C, DR, and DCI correlation. Differences were statistically significant while $P < 0.05$.

RESULTS

MoCA

One-way ANOVA statistical analysis showed that the MoCA scores in the DR group were significantly less than those in the other groups ($P < 0.05$), and the MoCA scores in the T2DM group were significantly less than those in the HC group ($P < 0.05$).

Comparison of Bilateral Hippocampal ^{1}H-MRS Detection Values Between DR Group, T2DM Group, and HC Group

There were statistically significant differences in NAA on the bilateral hippocampus between the DR group, the T2DM group and the HC group ($F_{\text{left}} = 10.052, p < 0.05; F_{\text{right}} = 10.316, p < 0.05$). Further examination with LSD-t showed that the DR group was significantly lower than the T2DM and HC groups ($p < 0.05$) (**Figures 1, 2, Tables 2, 3**); the differences of the other indicators were not statistically significant ($P > 0.05$).

Correlation Between ^{1}H-MRS and MoCA Scores in DR Group

The NAA/Cr is significantly positively correlated with the MoCA score in DR patients on the left hippocampus ($r = 0.774$, $P < 0.01$). There were no correlations among the other detection values of the two hippocampus detection values and the MoCA scores ($P > 0.05$) (**Table 4**).

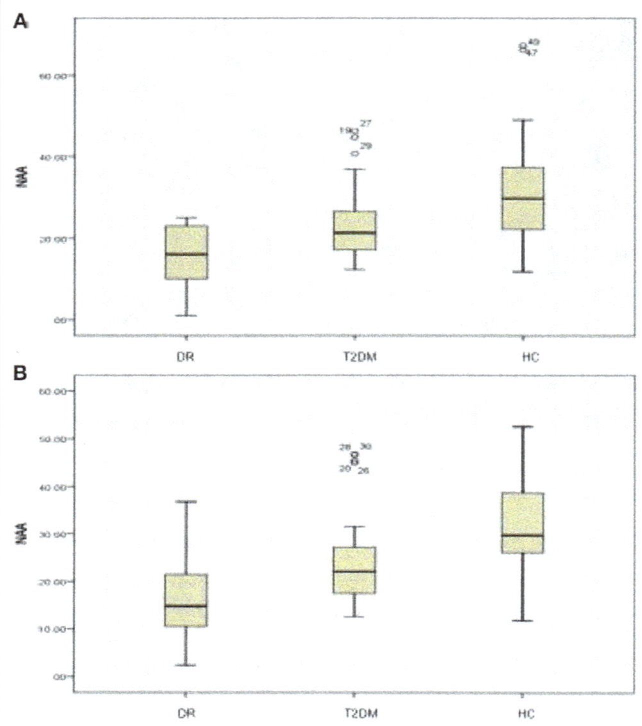

FIGURE 2 | There were statistically significant differences in NAA on the bilateral hippocampus among the DR group, the T2DM group and the HC group. **(A)** Left hippocampal, **(B)** right hippocampal.

TABLE 2 | Multiple comparisons of left hippocampal NAA.

Group		Mean	SD	*p*	95% confidence interval	
					Lower limit	Upper limit
DR	T2DM	-8.12260*	3.56952	0.026*	−15.2494	−0.9958
	HC	-15.29449*	3.54425	0.000*	−22.3708	−8.2182
T2DM	DR	8.12260*	3.56952	0.026*	0.9958	15.2494
	HC	-7.17189*	3.08675	0.023*	−13.3348	−1.0090
HC	DR	15.29449*	3.54425	0.000*	8.2182	22.3708
	T2DM	7.17189*	3.08675	0.023*	1.0090	13.3348

**The left hippocampal NAA were compared between any two groups, $p < 0.05$, the difference was statistically significant. T2DM, Type 2 diabetes mellitus; DR, diabetic retinopathy; NAA, Nacetylaspartate.*

Among all T2DM patients, Chi-square tested age, gender, education level, BMI, SBP, DBP, FPG, HbA1c, TC, TG, HDL-C, LDL-C, DR, and DCI for correlation. Chi-square analysis found that there was a correlation between DR and DCI ($x^2 = 4.6$, df $=$ 1, $p = 0.032$, plt: 0.05). There was no correlation between other influencing factors and DCI ($P > 0.05$).

DISCUSSION

With changes in modern lifestyles, the incidence of T2DM is increasing year by year (8). The incidence of cognitive dysfunction caused by T2DM is 10.8–17.5% (9), and its occurrence is related to hippocampus and amygdala atrophy (10). In addition, T2DM not only causes metabolic disorders but also involves multiple systems. DR is one of the more common lesions, and studies have shown that diabetic retinopathy is closely related to DCI (11). The occurrence of these two diseases is parallel (12, 13): (1) mass accumulation of glycosylation end products; (2) the protein kinase C (PKC) pathway is activated at high glucose; (3) oxidative stress: there is an excessive amount of reactive oxygen species, resulting in vascular cell damage, diabetic brain damage, or DR; and (4) DR is also a neurovascular disease, which, like diabetic brain injury, can be specifically reflected by the neuronal marker NAA in the ^{1}H-MRS.

TABLE 3 | Multiple comparisons of right hippocampal NAA.

Group		Mean	SD	*p*	95% confidence interval	
					Lower limit	Upper limit
DR	T2DM	−7.24610*	3.06174	0.021*	−13.3557	−1.1365
	HC	−13.85166*	3.06174	0.000*	−19.9613	−7.7421
T2DM	DR	7.24610*	3.06174	0.021*	1.1365	13.3557
	HC	−6.60556*	2.69142	0.017*	−11.9762	−1.2349
HC	DR	13.85166*	3.06174	0.000*	7.7421	19.9613
	T2DM	6.60556*	2.69142	0.017*	1.2349	11.9762

**The right hippocampal NAA was compared between any two groups, $p < 0.05$, the difference was statistically significant. T2DM, Type 2 diabetes mellitus; DR, diabetic retinopathy; NAA, Nacetylaspartate.*

TABLE 4 | Correlation between the detection values of bilateral hippocampus and MoCA score in DR group.

Project	NAA	Cr	Cho	ml	NAA/Cr	Cho/Cr	ml/Cr
r_{left}	0.312	−0.523	−0.411	−0.046	0.684	0.441	0.292
p_{left}	>0.05	>0.05	>0.05	>0.05	<0.01**	>0.05	>0.05
r_{right}	−0.271	−0.299	−0.121	0.312	0.041	0.402	0.476
p_{right}	>0.05	>0.05	>0.05	>0.05	>0.05	>0.05	>0.05

***The ratio of NAA/Cr in the left hippocampal of DR patients was positively correlated with MoCA score, $p < 0.01$, and the difference was statistically significant. NAA, Nacetylaspartate; Cr, Creatine; Cho, Cho-line; ml, myo-inositol.*

The literature reports that there is early brain tissue damage in patients with diabetic retinopathy, and ^{1}H-MRS can detect this change early (12, 13). In recent years, ^{1}H-MRS has been reported in the diagnosis of cognitive impairment-related diseases, but there are few reports on the relationship between DCI caused by T2DM and DR. Based on the above problems, the research team—based on the previous animal experiments—explored the correlation between DCI and DR through examining the cognitive function and the metabolism of the cerebrum in T2DM by ^{1}H-MRS.

Studies have shown that individual factors such as education level and age group have different degrees of impact on MoCA scores (14). In this study, because the subjects were matched as much as possible in addition to the diabetes itself, the credibility of DCI judgment was higher, and these objects mainly showed memory loss, which is similar to previous reports (15). This indicates that T2DM is a risk factor for developing mild cognitive impairment. The MoCA scores were significantly different between the DR group and the HC group, the T2DM group and the HC group, and the DR group and the T2DM group, which may suggest differences in cognitive function among the three groups, which in turn may prompt diagnosis and early warning. Early clinical support in terms of dysfunction should be provided.

T2DM can play a significant role in the occurrence and/or development of AD either directly or as a cofactor (16). Clinical manifestations such as white matter lesions, cognitive dysfunction, etc., represent the various types of diabetic brain injury (17). Studies have shown that T2DM can cause cognitive decline through changes in hippocampal formation, neurophysiological activity and neurotransmitters (18), and hippocampal formation is one of the first brain structures to be altered (19). Its possible pathological mechanisms are similar to AD at the molecular level, including insulin resistance, metabolic mechanism damage, beta-amyloid (Aβ) formation, oxidative stress, and the presence of advanced glycation end products (AGEs), neuronal apoptosis. van Eldren et al. (19) and most scholars believe that the most important pathological feature of AD is the activation of astrocytes induced by Aβ deposition, which triggers the associated inflammatory response and oxidative stress (17). Although the damage of these nervous systems can be manifested by a variety of examination methods, MRS is uniquely and non-invasively embodied by its unique imaging method, that is, the specific and sensitive expression of the neuronal marker NAA (13). The results of this study showed that the NAA value of the bilateral hippocampal DR group was lower than that of the T2DM group and the HC group, and the NAA value of the bilateral hippocampal T2DM group was lower than that of the HC group ($P < 0.05$). Similar to the results of some studies (20, 21), the above changes suggest that DM can cause neurological damage. Studies have confirmed that NAA reduction is associated with neuronal or axonal loss (22) and is independently associated with the development of T2DM (23). Increased anaerobic glycolysis in the brain is accompanied by elevated blood sugar. When the accumulation of lactic acid increases, acidosis can occur, which in turn destroys the blood-brain barrier. The damage of nerve cells and glial cells is also aggravated by brain edema caused by the process (24). In addition, mitochondrial damage and cell death, DNA fragment breaks and increased cerebral ischemic damage are also caused by persistently elevated hyperglycemia, the mechanism of which is associated with excessive Ca^{2+} channel opening (21). Since Cr is a marker of creatine phosphate, it plays a buffer role in energy metabolism, and its changes in the body are relatively stable. Therefore, the main influences of NAA and NAA/Cr are NAA, and NAA is less sensitive and direct, but it may be weaker than NAA/Cr. There were no statistical differences in the rest of the indicators in this study, similar to previous studies (25).

The results of this study indicate that NAA/Cr, which represents neurons in DR patients, is significantly associated with MoCA scores that reflect cognitive function. Some studies found that there is consistency between the change of MoCA score and ^{1}H-MRS, which is partially consistent with the results we obtained (26, 27). It was shown that in the DR patient group, there was synaptic functional remodeling in the hippocampus, which was confirmed in an animal model (28). T2DM spatial learning memory defects (29) are also related. In this study, it was found that anaerobic glycolysis caused by hyperglycemia and excessive opening of Ca^{2+} channels may damage the blood-brain barrier and cause damage to nerve cells and glial cells (30). This damaging change may be specific to NAA or NAA/Cr. In addition, there is insulin receptor resistance in the left hippocampus (31), and the hippocampus is the pancreatic exocrine structure of human insulin, which can produce a small amount of insulin. As an important neuro-influence factor, insulin maintains nerve function, and nerve cell structure. It has an important role in integrity and post-injury regeneration, which means that the damage and degeneration of the left hippocampal neurons in this study are particularly significant (20). There were no statistical differences in the rest of the indicators in this study, similar to previous studies (30). In summary, NAA/Cr can be considered as a biochemical indicator for evaluating cognitive function.

This study shows that DR was the main risk factor for DCI, similar to the results of the study (31). Some Chinese scholars believe that cognitive dysfunction in patients with type 2 diabetes is associated with diabetic microvascular complications (32). Studies have pointed out that in the early stage of diabetic retinopathy, the pathological changes of the nerve fiber layer precede the retinal microangiopathy (33). The mechanism is that the swelling of the nerve cells causes compression of the surrounding microvessels and stenosis (34). Diabetic microvascular disease caused by diabetes may also cause abnormalities in the metabolism of retinal neurons and glial cells, which may cause degeneration of retinal nerve tissue (35). The typical manifestation is a decrease in retinal ganglion cells and a thinning of the retinal nerve fiber layer (34), causing changes in vision. T2DM microangiopathy is very common in patients with diabetic cerebrovascular disease, mainly caused by changes in brain microvascular structure, which increases arteriovenous short circuiting, resulting in reduced transfer of essential nutrients to nerve tissue, insufficient nutrition, decreased perfusion pressure, and reduced cerebral blood (36, 37). It makes brain tissue more susceptible to hypoxic damage. DR with microvascular disease and brain with cognitive decline have many similarities in microvascular structures, such as capillary basement membrane thickening, lumen narrowing, and increased vascular permeability. Both DCI and DR belong to diabetic microangiopathy. Due to their common pathogenesis: AGEs, activation of polyol pathway, oxidative stress, PKC, inflammatory factors, hemodynamic changes, etc., the occurrence and development of both Parallelism, but due to the genetic susceptibility of the two, the difference in the involvement of cytokines, some differences in diagnosis, etc., the non-parallelism of the two, so the severity of DR and DCI have a certain correlation, but not completely related (36, 37).The 5-year incidence of DR is 8%, and the 10-year incidence is 43%; although, DCI is usually seen in diabetic patients for more than 10 years, the incidence of both increases with the duration of diabetes (36, 37). DR and DCI are not only diabetic microangiopathy but also neuropathy, which is sensitive to hypoxia, ischemia, and metabolic disorders.

Therefore, diabetic patients may suffer from both diseases after a period of illness. The difference is that the optic nerve, as part of the peripheral nervous system, is relatively more sensitive to hyperglycemia, leading to abnormal hemodynamics, impaired optic nerve nutrient metabolism, and possibly DR earlier than DCI. In addition to the similar pathological mechanisms of DR, DCI also has a large amount of amyloid deposits, which occurs slightly later than DR, but overall, the longer the duration of diabetes, the greater the likelihood of DR and DCI.

Limitation

DR and DCI with the regularity and correlation of T2DM specific disease course changes, we will improve the group expansion study in the next step.

CONCLUSION

Diabetic cognitive impairment is closely correlated with the DR in patients with T2DM. Hippocampal brain metabolism may have some changes in two sides of NAA in patients with DR, and ^{1}H-MRS may provide effective imaging strategies and methods for the early diagnosis of brain damage and quantitative assessment of cognitive function in T2DM.

AUTHOR CONTRIBUTIONS

All authors listed have made a substantial, direct and intellectual contribution to the work, and approved it for publication.

FUNDING

This work was supported by the National Natural Science Foundation of China 81871332.

REFERENCES

WHO. *About Diabetes [C]*. Beijing: World Health Organization (2018).

Liu ZQ, Liu AP, Wang PY. Epidemiological investigation of prevalence of diabetes in China. *Chin J Mult Organ Dis Eld.* (2015) 14:547–50. doi: 10.11915/j.issn.1671-5403.2015.07.125

Gold SM, Dziobek I, Sweat V, Tirsi A, Rogers K, Bruehl H, et al. Hippocampal damage and memory impairments as possible early brain complications of type 2 diabetes. *Diabetologia.* (2007) 50:711–9. doi: 10.1007/s00125-007-0602-7

Yang W, Lu J, Weng J, Jia W, Ji L, Xiao J, et al. Prevalence of diabetes among men and women in C hina. *N Engl J Med.* (2010) 362:1090–101. doi: 10.1056/NEJMoa0908292

Demir N, Akkoyunlu G, Yargicoglu P, Agar A, Tanriöver G, Demir R. Fiber structure of optic nerve in cadmium-exposed diabetic rats: an ultrastructural study. *Int J Neurosci.* (2003) 113:323–37. doi: 10.1080/002074503901 62128

Nasreddine ZS, Phillips NA, Bédirian V, Charbonneau S, Whitehead V, Collin I, et al. The Montreal Cognitive Assessment, MoCA: a brief screening tool for mild cognitive impairment. *J Am Geriatr Soc.* (2005) 53:695–9. doi: 10.1111/j.1532-5415.2005.53221.x

Barnhart CD, Yang D, Lein PJ. Using the Morris water maze to assess spatial learning and memory in weanling mice. *PLoS ONE.* (2015) 10:e0124521. doi: 10.1371/journal.pone.0124521

Nathan DM, DCCT/Edic Research Group. The diabetes control and complications trial/epidemi ology of diabetes interventions and complications study at 30 years: overview. *Diabetes Care.* (2014) 37:9–16. doi: 10.2337/dc13-2112

Tong J, Geng H, Zhang Z, Zhu X, Meng Q, Sun X, et al. Brain metabolite alterations demonstrated by proton magnetic resonance spectroscopy in diabetic patients with retinopathy. *Magn Reson Imaging.* (2014) 32:1037–42. doi: 10.1016/j.mri.2014.04.020

Zhang J, Liu Z, Li Z, Wang Y, Chen Y, Li X, et al. Disrupted white matter network and cognitive decline in type 2 diabetes patients. *J Alzheimers Dis.* (2016) 53:185–95. doi: 10.3233/JAD-160111

Ryan CM, Geckle MO, Orchard TJ. Cognitive efficiency declines over time in adults with Type 1 diabetes: effects of micro— and macrovascular complications. *Diabetologia.* (2003) 46:940–8. doi: 10.1007/s00125-003-1128-2

Zhang X, Saaddine JB, Chou CF, Cotch MF, Cheng YJ, Geiss LS, et al. Prevalence of diabetic retinopathy in the United States, 2005–2008. *JAMA.* (2010) 304:649–56. doi: 10.1001/jama. 2010.1111

TongJia, BanBo. *Evaluation of the Brain Damage in Patients with Diabetic Retinopathty Using Magnetic Resonance Spectroscopy and Diffusion Weighted Imaging.* Shandong: Shandong University (2014).

Datusalia AK, Sharma SS. NF-kappa B inhibition resolves cognitive deficits in experimental type 2 diabetes mellitus through CREB and Glutamate/GABA neurotransmitters pathway. *Curr Neurovasc Res.* (2016) 13:22–32. doi: 10.2174/1567202612666151030104810

Tang Y, Yu C, Wu J, Chen H, Zeng Y, Wang X, et al. Lychee seed extract protects against neuronal injury and improves cognitive function in rats with type II diabetes mellitus with cognitive impairment. *Int J Mol Med.* (2018) 41:251–63. doi: 10.3892/ijmm.2017.3245

Mushtaq G, Khan JA, Kamal MA. Biological mechanisms linking Alzheimer's disease and type-2 diabetes mellitus. *CNS Neurol Disord Drug Targets.* (2014) 13:1192–201. doi: 10.2174/18715273136661409171 14537

van Elderen SG, de Roos A, de Craen AJ, Westendorp RG, Blauw GJ, Jukema JW, et al. Progression of brain atrophy and cognitive decline in diabetes mellitus: a 3-year follow-up. *Neurology.* (2010) 75:997–1002. doi: 10.1212/WNL.0b013e3181f25f06

Kimura N. Diabetes mellitus induces Alzheimer's disease pathology: histopathological evidence from animal models. *Int J Mol Sci.* (2016) 17:503–11. doi: 10.3390/ijms17040503

van Elderen SG, Brandts A, Westenberg JJ, van der Grond J, Tamsma JT, van Buchem MA, et al. Aortic stiffness is associated with cardiac function and cerebral small vessel disease in patients with type 1 diabetes mellitus: assessment by magnetic resonance imaging. *Eur Radiol.* (2010) 20:1132–8. doi: 10.1007/s00330-009-1655-4

Ma XC, Wang GZ, Wang YC, Fang Q, Wang KL. Clinical analysis of hydrogen proton spectroscopy in hippocampus of type 2 diabetic patients. *Modern J Integr Tradit Chinese Western Med.* (2010) 32:45–8.

Brundel M, van den Berg E, Reijmer YD, de Bresser J, Kappelle LJ, Biessels GJ, et al. Cerebral ha-emodynamics, cognition and brain volumes in patients with type 2 diabetes. *J Diabetes Complications.* (2012) 26:205–9. doi: 10.1016/j.jdiacomp.2012.03.021

Sinha S, Ekka M, Sharma U, P R, Pandey RM, Jagannathan NR. Assessment of changes in brain metabolites in Indian patients with type-2 diabetes mellitus using proton magnetic resonance spectroscopy. *BMC Res Notes.* (2014) 41:1–7. doi: 10.1186/1756-0500-7-41

Choi MH, Kim HS, Gim SY, Kim WR, Mun KR, Tack GR, et al. Differences in cognitive ability and hippocampal volume between Alzheimer's disease, amnestic mild cognitive impairment, and healthy control groups, and their correlation. *Neurosci Lett.* (2016) 620:115–20. doi: 10.1016/j.neulet.2016.03.044

Biessels GJ, Strachan MW, Visseren FL, Kappelle LJ, Whitmer RA. Dementia and cognitive decline in type 2 diabetes and prediabetic stages: towards targeted interventions. *Lancet Diabetes Endocrinol.* (2014) 2:246–55. doi: 10.1016/S2213-8587(13)70088-3

Brundel M, Kappelle LJ, Biessels GJ. Brain imaging in type 2 diabetes. *Eur Neuropsychopharmacol.* (2014) 24:1967–81. doi: 10.1016/j.euroneuro.2014.01.023

Li W, Huang E. An update on type 2 diabetes mellitus as a risk factor for dementia. *J Alzheimers Dis.* (2016) 53:393–402. doi: 10.3233/JAD-160114

Li J, Deng J, Sheng W, Zuo Z. Metformin attenuates Alzheimer's disease like neuropathology in obese, leptin-resistant mice. *Pharmacol Biochem Behav.* (2012) 101:567–74. doi: 10.1016/j.pbb.2012.03.002

Zheng H, Zheng Y, Zhao L, Chen M, Bai G, Hu Y, et al. Cognitive decline in type 2 diabetic db/db mice may be associated with brain region- specific metabolic disorders. *Biochim Biophys Acta.* (2017) 1863:266–73. doi: 10.1016/j.bbadis.2016.11.003

Lin B, Koibuchi N, Hasegawa Y, Sueta D, Toyama K, Uekawa K, et al. Glycemic control with empagliflozin, a novel selective SGLT2 inhibitor, ameliorates cardiovascular injury and cognitive dysfunction in obese and type 2 diabetic mice. *Cardiovasc Diabetol.* (2014) 13:148. doi: 10.1186/s12933-014-0148-1

Chu X, Zhao Y, Liu F, Mi Y, Shen J, Wang X, et al. Rapidly raise blood sugar will aggravate brain damage after severe hypoglycemia in rats. *Cell Biochem Biophys.* (2014) 69:131–9. doi: 10.1007/s12013-013-9779-1

Wang WT, Lee P, Yeh HW, Smirnova IV, Choi IY. Effects of acute and chronic hyperglycemia on the neurochemical profiles in the rat brain with streptozotocin induced diabetes detected using *in vivo* ^{1} H MR spectroscopy at 9.4 T. *Neurochem.* (2012) 121:407–17. doi: 10.1111/j.1471-4159.2012. 07698.x

Zuo LJ, Xu JM, Ji JL, Jiang KD, Zhao JC, Yu YP. Cognitive function of type 2 diabetics with micro-angiopathy. *Chinese J Clin Psychol.* (2001) 9: 103–5.

Yau JW, Rogers SL, Kawasaki R, Lamoureux EL, Kowalski JW, Bek T, et al. Global prevalence and major risk factors of diabetic retinopathy. *Diabetes Care.* (2012) 1:45–8. doi: 10.2337/dc11- 1909

Li J, Zhang S, Zhang L, Wang R, Wang M. Effents of L-3-n-Butylphthalide on cognitive dysfunction and NR2B expression in hippocampus of streptozotocin (STZ) -induced diabetic rats. *Cell Biochem Biophys.* (2014) 71:315–22. doi: 10.1007/s12013-014-0200-5

Wang Y, Bai C, Guan H, Chen R, Wang X, Wang B, et al. Subchronic exposure to arsenic induces apoptosis in the hippocampus of the mouse brains through the Bc12/Bax pathway. *J Occup Health.* (2015) 57:212–21. doi: 10.1539/joh.14-0226-OA

Domínguez RO, Pagano MA, Marschoff ER, González SE, Repetto MG, Serra JA. Alzheimer disease and cognitive impairment associated with diabetes mellitus type 2: associations and a hypothesis. *Neurologia.* (2014) 29:567–72. doi: 10.1016/j.nrl.2013.05.006

Peng GP, Feng Z, He FP, Chen ZQ, Liu XY, Liu P, et al. Correlation of hippocampal volume and cognitive performances in patients with either mild cognitive impairment or Alzheimer's disease. *CNS Neurosci Ther.* (2015) 21:15–22. doi: 10.1111/cns.12317

Permissions

All chapters in this book were first published by Frontiers; hereby published with permission under the Creative Commons Attribution License or equivalent. Every chapter published in this book has been scrutinized by our experts. Their significance has been extensively debated. The topics covered herein carry significant findings which will fuel the growth of the discipline. They may even be implemented as practical applications or may be referred to as a beginning point for another development.

The contributors of this book come from diverse backgrounds, making this book a truly international effort. This book will bring forth new frontiers with its revolutionizing research information and detailed analysis of the nascent developments around the world.

We would like to thank all the contributing authors for lending their expertise to make the book truly unique. They have played a crucial role in the development of this book. Without their invaluable contributions this book wouldn't have been possible. They have made vital efforts to compile up to date information on the varied aspects of this subject to make this book a valuable addition to the collection of many professionals and students.

This book was conceptualized with the vision of imparting up-to-date information and advanced data in this field. To ensure the same, a matchless editorial board was set up. Every individual on the board went through rigorous rounds of assessment to prove their worth. After which they invested a large part of their time researching and compiling the most relevant data for our readers.

The editorial board has been involved in producing this book since its inception. They have spent rigorous hours researching and exploring the diverse topics which have resulted in the successful publishing of this book. They have passed on their knowledge of decades through this book. To expedite this challenging task, the publisher supported the team at every step. A small team of assistant editors was also appointed to further simplify the editing procedure and attain best results for the readers.

Apart from the editorial board, the designing team has also invested a significant amount of their time in understanding the subject and creating the most relevant covers. They scrutinized every image to scout for the most suitable representation of the subject and create an appropriate cover for the book.

The publishing team has been an ardent support to the editorial, designing and production team. Their endless efforts to recruit the best for this project, has resulted in the accomplishment of this book. They are a veteran in the field of academics and their pool of knowledge is as vast as their experience in printing. Their expertise and guidance has proved useful at every step. Their uncompromising quality standards have made this book an exceptional effort. Their encouragement from time to time has been an inspiration for everyone.

The publisher and the editorial board hope that this book will prove to be a valuable piece of knowledge for researchers, students, practitioners and scholars across the globe.

List of Contributors

Laura Pelizzari, Maria M. Laganà, Sonia Di Tella, Federica Rossetto and Francesca Baglio
IRCCS, Fondazione Don Carlo Gnocchi, Milan, Italy

Niels Bergsland
IRCCS, Fondazione Don Carlo Gnocchi, Milan, Italy
Department of Neurology, Buffalo Neuroimaging Analysis Center, Jacobs School of Medicine and Biomedical Sciences, University at Buffalo, State University of New York, Buffalo, NY, United States

Raffaello Nemni and Mario Clerici
IRCCS, Fondazione Don Carlo Gnocchi, Milan, Italy
Department of Pathophysiology and Transplantation, Università degli Studi di Milano, Milan, Italy

Sara Lorio
Developmental Neurosciences, UCL Great Ormond Street Institute of Child Health, University College London, London, United Kingdom
Roche Pharma and Early Development, Neuroscience, Ophthalmology and Rare Diseases, F. Hoffmann-La Roche Ltd., Basel, Switzerland
Laboratory for Research in Neuroimaging, Department of Clinical Neurosciences, Lausanne University Hospital, University of Lausanne, Lausanne, Switzerland

Fabio Sambataro
Roche Pharma and Early Development, Neuroscience, Ophthalmology and Rare Diseases, F. Hoffmann-La Roche Ltd., Basel, Switzerland
Department of Experimental and Clinical Medical Sciences, University of Udine, Udine, Italy

Alessandro Bertolino
Roche Pharma and Early Development, Neuroscience, Ophthalmology and Rare Diseases, F. Hoffmann-La Roche Ltd., Basel, Switzerland
Department of Basic Medical Science, Neuroscience and Sense Organs, University of Bari, Bari, Italy

Bogdan Draganski
Laboratory for Research in Neuroimaging, Department of Clinical Neurosciences, Lausanne University Hospital, University of Lausanne, Lausanne, Switzerland
Max Planck Institute for Human Cognitive and Brain Sciences, Leipzig, Germany

Seung Joo Kim
Department of Neurology, Gyeongsang National University School of Medicine and Gyeongsang National University Changwon Hospital, Changwon, South Korea

Juergen Dukart
Roche Pharma and Early Development, Neuroscience, Ophthalmology and Rare Diseases, F. Hoffmann-La Roche Ltd., Basel, Switzerland
Institute of Neuroscience and Medicine, Brain and Behaviour (INM-7), Research Centre Jülich, Jülich, Germany
Institute of Systems Neuroscience, Medical Faculty, Heinrich Heine University Düsseldorf, Düsseldorf, Germany

Jin San Lee
Department of Neurology, Samsung Medical Center, Sungkyunkwan University School of Medicine, Seoul, South Korea
Neuroscience Center, Samsung Medical Center, Seoul, South Korea
Department of Neurology, Kyung Hee University Hospital, Seoul, South Korea

Yu Hyun Park, Seongbeom Park, Yeongsim Choe, Bo Kyoung Cheon, Alice Hahn, Jun Pyo Kim, Young Hee Jung, Hee Jin Kim, Hyemin Jang and Duk L. Na
Department of Neurology, Samsung Medical Center, Sungkyunkwan University School of Medicine, Seoul, South Korea
Neuroscience Center, Samsung Medical Center, Seoul, South Korea

Uicheul Yoon
Department of Biomedical Engineering, Daegu Catholic University, Gyeongsan, South Korea

Soo Hyun Cho
Department of Neurology, Chonnam National University Medical School, Gwangju, South Korea

Key-Chung Park
Department of Neurology, Kyung Hee University Hospital, Seoul, South Korea

Sang Won Seo
Department of Neurology, Samsung Medical Center, Sungkyunkwan University School of Medicine, Seoul, South Korea
Neuroscience Center, Samsung Medical Center, Seoul, South Korea
Samsung Alzheimer Research Center, Center for Clinical Epidemiology, Samsung Medical Center, Seoul, South Korea
Department of Health Sciences and Technology, Clinical Research Design and Evaluation, SAIHST, Sungkyunkwan University, Seoul, South Korea

Zhanxiong Wu
School of Electronic Information, Hangzhou Dianzi University, Hangzhou, China
Department of Biomedical Engineering, University of Houston, Houston, TX, United States

Dong Xu
School of Electronic Information, Hangzhou Dianzi University, Hangzhou, China
Zhejiang Key Laboratory of Equipment Electronics, Hangzhou, China

Thomas Potter and Yingchun Zhang
Department of Biomedical Engineering, University of Houston, Houston, TX, United States

Sander C. J. Verfaillie and Tessa Timmers
Department of Neurology and Alzheimer Center, Amsterdam University Medical Center, Vrije Universiteit Amsterdam, Amsterdam, Netherlands
Department of Radiology and Nuclear Medicine, Amsterdam Neuroscience, Amsterdam University Medical Center, Vrije Universiteit Amsterdam, Amsterdam, Netherlands
Amsterdam Neuroscience, Amsterdam, Netherlands

Rosalinde E. R. Slot, Linda M. P. Wesselman, Niels D. Prins and Philip Scheltens
Department of Neurology and Alzheimer Center, Amsterdam University Medical Center, Vrije Universiteit Amsterdam, Amsterdam, Netherlands
Amsterdam Neuroscience, Amsterdam, Netherlands

Chris W. J. van der Weijden, Maqsood Yaqub, Adriaan A. Lammertsma and Bart N. M. van Berckel
Department of Radiology and Nuclear Medicine, Amsterdam Neuroscience, Amsterdam University Medical Center, Vrije Universiteit Amsterdam, Amsterdam, Netherlands
Amsterdam Neuroscience, Amsterdam, Netherlands

Sietske A. M. Sikkes and Wiesje M. van der Flier
Department of Neurology and Alzheimer Center, Amsterdam University Medical Center, Vrije Universiteit Amsterdam, Amsterdam, Netherlands
Amsterdam Neuroscience, Amsterdam, Netherlands
Department of Epidemiology and Biostatistics, Amsterdam Neuroscience, Amsterdam University Medical Center, Vrije Universiteit Amsterdam, Amsterdam, Netherlands

Bianca Weinstock-Guttman, Shumita Roy, Michael Jaworski III, Alissa Nizinski, Pavitra Srinivasan, Kinga Szigeti and Ralph H. B. Benedict
Department of Neurology, Jacobs School of Medicine and Biomedical Sciences, University at Buffalo - The State University of New York, Buffalo, NY, United States

Annemiek Dols
Department of Neurology and Alzheimer Center, Amsterdam University Medical Center, Vrije Universiteit Amsterdam, Amsterdam, Netherlands
Amsterdam Neuroscience, Amsterdam, Netherlands
Department of Old Age Psychiatry, Amsterdam Neuroscience, GGZ inGeest, Amsterdam University Medical Center, Vrije Universiteit Amsterdam, Amsterdam, Netherlands

Rik Ossenkoppele
Department of Neurology and Alzheimer Center, Amsterdam University Medical Center, Vrije Universiteit Amsterdam, Amsterdam, Netherlands
Amsterdam Neuroscience, Amsterdam, Netherlands
Clinical Memory Research Unit, Lund University, Malmö, Sweden

Dejan Jakimovski and Tom A. Fuchs
Department of Neurology, Jacobs School of Medicine and Biomedical Sciences, University at Buffalo - The State University of New York, Buffalo, NY, United States
Buffalo Neuroimaging Analysis Center, Department of Neurology, Jacobs School of Medicine and Biomedical Sciences, University at Buffalo - The State University of New York, Buffalo, NY, United States

Laura Hancock
Department of Neurology, University of Wisconsin School of Medicine and Public Health, Madison, WI, United States

Robert Zivadinov
Department of Neurology, Jacobs School of Medicine and Biomedical Sciences, University at Buffalo - The State University of New York, Buffalo, NY, United States
Buffalo Neuroimaging Analysis Center, Department of Neurology, Jacobs School of Medicine and Biomedical Sciences, University at Buffalo - The State University of New York, Buffalo, NY, United States
Clinical Translational Science Institute, Center for Biomedical Imaging, University at Buffalo - The State University of New York, Buffalo, NY, United States

Ryota Kobayashi, Hiroshi Hayashi and Koichi Otani
Department of Psychiatry, Yamagata University School of Medicine, Yamagata, Japan

Shinobu Kawakatsu
Department of Neuropsychiatry, Aizu Medical Center, Fukushima Medical University, Aizuwakamatsu, Japan

Nobuyuki Okamura
Department of Pharmacology, Faculty of Medicine, Tohoku Medical and Pharmaceutical University, Sendai, Japan

Masanori Yoshioka
Department of Radiology, Yamagata University Hospital, Yamagata, Japan

Xin Chen, Yingqian Zhu, Shasha Geng, Qingqing Li and Hua Jiang
Department of Geriatrics, Shanghai East Hospital, Tongji University School of Medicine, Shanghai, China

Pengyun Wang, Rui Li and Juan Li
CAS Key Laboratory of Mental Health, Center on Aging Psychology, Institute of Psychology, Chinese Academy of Sciences, Beijing, China

Bei Liu
Department of Human Resources, Institute of Disaster Prevention, Beijing, China

Cheng Wang
Department of Psychology, Zhejiang Normal University, Jinhua, China

Zirui Huang
Department of Anesthesiology and Center for Consciousness Science, University of Michigan, Ann Arbor, MI, United States

Rui Dai
State Key Laboratory of Brain and Cognitive Science, Institute of Biophysics, Chinese Academy of Sciences, Beijing, China

Bogeng Song
School of Psychology, Capital Normal University, Beijing, China

Xiao Yuan
School of Sociology, China University of Political Science and Law, Beijing, China

Jing Yu
Faculty of Psychology, Southwest University, Chongqing, China

Alessandra Bandera and Andrea Gori
Infectious Disease Unit, Department of Internal Medicine, Fondazione IRCCS Ca' Granda Ospedale Maggiore Policlinico, Milan, Italy
Department of Pathophysiology and Transplantation, University of Milano, Milan, Italy

Elio Angelo Scarpini
Department of Pathophysiology and Transplantation, Dino Ferrari Center, Faculty of Medicine and Surgery, University of Milan, Milan, Italy
Neurodegenerative Diseases Unit, Fondazione IRCCS Ca' Granda, Ospedale Maggiore Policlinico, Milan, Italy

Lucia Taramasso
Infectious Disease Unit, Department of Internal Medicine, Fondazione IRCCS Ca' Granda Ospedale Maggiore Policlinico, Milan, Italy
Infectious Diseases Clinic, Department of Health Sciences, School of Medical and Pharmaceutical Sciences, Policlinico Hospital San Martino, University of Genova (DISSAL), Genova, Italy

Giorgio Bozzi and Antonio Muscatello
Infectious Disease Unit, Department of Internal Medicine, Fondazione IRCCS Ca' Granda Ospedale Maggiore Policlinico, Milan, Italy

Jake A. Robinson and Tricia H. Burdo
Department of Neuroscience, Lewis Katz School of Medicine at Temple University, Philadelphia, PA, United States

Daiana R. Pur
School of Biomedical Engineering, Western University, London, ON, Canada

Roy A. Eagleson
School of Biomedical Engineering, Western University, London, ON, Canada
Department of Electrical and Computer Engineering, Western University, London, ON, Canada

Anik de Ribaupierre and Nathalie Mella
Department of Psychology, University of Geneva, Geneva, Switzerland

Sandrine de Ribaupierre
School of Biomedical Engineering, Western University, London, ON, Canada
Department of Clinical Neurological Sciences, Schulich School of Medicine, Western University, London, ON, Canada

Marianna D'Anca, Chiara Fenoglio and Maria Serpente
Department of Pathophysiology and Transplantation, Dino Ferrari Center, Faculty of Medicine and Surgery, University of Milan, Milan, Italy

Beatrice Arosio
Department of Clinical Sciences and Community Health, Faculty of Medicine and Surgery, University of Milan, Milan, Italy

Matteo Cesari
Department of Clinical Sciences and Community Health, Faculty of Medicine and Surgery, University of Milan, Milan, Italy
Geriatrics Unit, Fondazione IRCCS Ca' Granda, Ospedale Maggiore Policlinico, Milan, Italy

Daniela Galimberti
Neurodegenerative Diseases Unit, Fondazione IRCCS Ca' Granda, Ospedale Maggiore Policlinico, Milan, Italy
Department of Biomedical, Surgical and Dental Sciences, Dino Ferrari Center, Faculty of Medicine and Surgery, University of Milan, Milan, Italy

Anastasia Falconi, Martina Di Bartolomeo, Marcella Massimini and Enrico Dainese
Faculty of Bioscience, University of Teramo, Teramo, Italy

Alessandra Bonito-Oliva and Gilberto Fisone
Department of Neuroscience, Karolinska Institute, Stockholm, Sweden

Francesco Fattapposta and Nicoletta Locuratolo
Department of Human Neurosciences, Sapienza University, Rome, Italy

Esterina Pascale
Department of Medical-Surgical Sciences and Biotechnologies, Sapienza University, Rome, Italy

Claudio D'Addario
Faculty of Bioscience, University of Teramo, Teramo, Italy
Department of Clinical Neuroscience, Karolinska Institute, Stockholm, Sweden

Noa Zifman, Ofri Levy-Lamdan, Hilla Fogel and Iftach Dolev
QuantalX Neuroscience, Tel Aviv-Yafo, Israel

Gil Suzin
Sagol Center for Hyperbaric Medicine and Research, Assaf Harofeh Medical Center, Ramle, Israel

Shai Efrati
Sagol Center for Hyperbaric Medicine and Research, Assaf Harofeh Medical Center, Ramle, Israel
Sackler School of Medicine and Sagol School of Neuroscience, Tel-Aviv University, Tel Aviv-Yafo, Israel

David Tanne
Sackler School of Medicine and Sagol School of Neuroscience, Tel-Aviv University, Tel Aviv-Yafo, Israel
Stroke and Cognition Institute, Rambam Healthcare Campus, Haifa, Israel

Xingqi Wu and Zhi Geng
Department of Neurology, The First Affiliated Hospital of Anhui Medical University, Hefei, China
Anhui Province Key Laboratory of Cognition and Neuropsychiatric Disorders, Hefei, China

Shanshan Zhou, Tongjian Bai, Ling Wei and Yanghua Tian
Department of Neurology, The First Affiliated Hospital of Anhui Medical University, Hefei, China
Anhui Province Key Laboratory of Cognition and Neuropsychiatric Disorders, Hefei, China
Collaborative Innovation Center of Neuropsychiatric Disorders and Mental Health, Hefei, China

Gong-Jun Ji
Anhui Province Key Laboratory of Cognition and Neuropsychiatric Disorders, Hefei, China
Collaborative Innovation Center of Neuropsychiatric Disorders and Mental Health, Hefei, China
Department of Medical Psychology, The First Affiliated Hospital of Anhui Medical University, Hefei, China

Wanqiu Zhu and Yongqiang Yu
Department of Radiology, The First Affiliated Hospital of Anhui Medical University, Hefei, China

Kai Wang
Department of Neurology, The First Affiliated Hospital of Anhui Medical University, Hefei, China
Anhui Province Key Laboratory of Cognition and Neuropsychiatric Disorders, Hefei, China
Collaborative Innovation Center of Neuropsychiatric Disorders and Mental Health, Hefei, China
Department of Medical Psychology, The First Affiliated Hospital of Anhui Medical University, Hefei, China

Laura Tay
Department of General Medicine, Sengkang General Hospital, Singapore, Singapore

Bernard Leung
Department of Rheumatology, Allergy and Immunology, Tan Tock Seng Hospital, Singapore, Singapore
Health and Social Sciences, Singapore Institute of Technology, Singapore, Singapore

Audrey Yeo
Institute of Geriatrics and Active Ageing, Tan Tock Seng Hospital, Singapore, Singapore

Mark Chan and Wee Shiong Lim
Institute of Geriatrics and Active Ageing, Tan Tock Seng Hospital, Singapore, Singapore
Department of Geriatric Medicine, Tan Tock Seng Hospital, Singapore, Singapore

Runrun Wang, Peidong Chen, Guisen Lin, Zhuozhi Dai, Yuanfeng Chen, Lihua Lai, Xiaodan Zong, Yan Li, Yanyan Tang and Renhua Wu
Department of Medical Imaging, The Second Affiliated Hospital, Shantou University Medical College, Shantou, China

Zhiwei Shen
Department of Medical Imaging, The Second Affiliated Hospital, Shantou University Medical College, Shantou, China
Philips Healthcare, Shantou, China

Gang Xiao
Department of Mathematics and Statistics, Hanshan Normal University, Chaozhou, China

Bingna Zhang
Translational Medicine, The Second Affiliated Hospital, Shantou University Medical College, Shantou, China

Lih-Fen Lue
Civin Neuropathology Laboratory, Banner Sun Health Research Institute, Sun City, AZ, United States

Ming-Chyi Pai
Division of Behavioral Neurology, Department of Neurology, National Cheng Kung University Hospital, College of Medicine, National Cheng Kung University, Tainan, Taiwan

Ta-Fu Chen, Jian-Shing Jeng and Ming-Jang Chiu
Department of Neurology, National Taiwan University Hospital, College of Medicine, National Taiwan University, Taipei, Taiwan

Chaur-Jong Hu and Li-Kai Huang
Department of Neurology, Taipei Medical University, Taipei, Taiwan
Department of Neurology, Shuang Ho Hospital, Taipei Medical University, New Taipei City, Taiwan

Wei-Che Lin
Department of Neurology, Kaohsiung Chang Gung Memorial Hospital, Kaohsiung, Taiwan

Chau-Chung Wu
Department of Internal Medicine, National Taiwan University Hospital, College of Medicine, National Taiwan University, Taipei, Taiwan

Kaj Blennow
Clinical Neurochemistry Laboratory, Sahlgrenska University Hospital, Mölndal, Sweden
Department of Psychiatry and Neurochemistry, Institute of Neuroscience and Physiology, University of Gothenburg, Mölndal, Sweden

Marwan N. Sabbagh
Lou Ruvo Center for Brain Health, Cleveland Clinic Nevada, Las Vegas, NV, United States

Sui-Hing Yan
Department of Neurology, Renai Branch, Taipei City Hospital, Taipei, Taiwan

Pei-Ning Wang
Department of Neurology, National Yang-Ming University, Taipei, Taiwan
Department of Neurology, Taipei Veterans General Hospital, Taipei, Taiwan

Shieh-Yueh Yang
MagQu Company Limited, New Taipei City, Taiwan
MagQu LLC, Surprise, AZ, United States

Hiroyuki Hatsuta
Hatsuta Neurology Clinic, Osaka, Japan
Department of Neurology, Osaka City University Graduate School of Medicine, Osaka, Japan

Satoru Morimoto
Hatsuta Neurology Clinic, Osaka, Japan
Department of Physiology, School of Medicine, Keio University, Tokyo, Japan

Akitoshi Takeda and Yoshiaki Itoh
Department of Neurology, Osaka City University Graduate School of Medicine, Osaka, Japan

Jun Liu
Departemnt of Neurology, Sun Yat-Sen Memorial Hospital, Sun Yat-Sen University, Guangzhou, China

Haiqun Xie
Department of Neurology, Foshan Hospital of Sun Yat-Sen University, Foshan, China

Cindy K. Barha, Chun-Liang Hsu, Lisanne ten Brinke and Teresa Liu-Ambrose
Department of Physical Therapy, University of British Columbia, Vancouver, BC, Canada
Djavad Mowafaghian Centre for Brain Health, University of British Columbia, Vancouver, BC, Canada
Centre for Hip Health and Mobility, Vancouver Coastal Health Research Institute, Vancouver, BC, Canada

Shizuo Hatashita
Department of Neurology, Shonan-Atsugi Hospital, Atsugi, Japan

Daichi Wakebe
Department of Radiology, Shonan-Atsugi Hospital, Atsugi, Japan

Yuki Kikuchi and Atsushi Ichijo
Department of Radiopharmacology, Shonan-Atsugi Hospital, Atsugi, Japan

Lisheng Liang
Department of Pain, Qingdao University Medical College Affiliated Yantai Yuhuangding Hospital, Yantai, China

Yingni Sun and Hongwei Gao
School of Life Sciences, Ludong University, Yantai, China

Meili Dong
Central Sterile Supply Department, Qingdao University Medical College Affiliated Yantai Yuhuangding Hospital, Yantai, China

Cong Li
Chemical and Materials Engineering, University of Kentucky, Lexington, KY, United States

Zhenzhen Liu
Chemical Engineering and Materials Science, College of Chemistry, Shandong Normal University, Jinan, China

Marco Canevelli
Department of Human Neuroscience, Sapienza University, Rome, Italy
National Center for Disease Prevention and Health Promotion, National Institute of Health, Rome, Italy

Ilaria Bacigalupo, Giuseppe Gervasi, Eleonora Lacorte, Flavia Mayer and Nicola Vanacore
National Center for Disease Prevention and Health Promotion, National Institute of Health, Rome, Italy

Marco Massari
National Center for Drug Research and Evaluation, National Institute of Health, Rome, Italy,

Matteo Cesari
Fondazione IRCCS Ca' Granda Ospedale Maggiore Policlinico, Milan, Italy
Geriatric Unit, Department of Clinical Sciences and Community Health, University of Milan, Milan, Italy

Xuefang Lu, Wei Gong, Zhi Wen, Lanhua Hu, Zhoufeng Peng and Yunfei Zha
Department of Radiology, Renmin Hospital, Wuhan, China

Index